Key Clinical Topics in
Ophthalmology

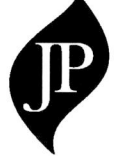

Ophthalmology

Key Clinical Topics in Ophthalmology

Parham Azarbod BSc (Hons) MBBS MRCS (Surgery) FRCOphth
Consultant Ophthalmic Surgeon,
Moorfields Eye Hospital, London, UK
Former Director of Training, Glaucoma Service,
Moorfields Eye Hospital

Professor Sir Peng Tee Khaw PhD FRCP FRCS FRCOphth FCOptom Hon DSc FSBiol FRCPath FMedSci FARVO
Consultant Ophthalmic Surgeon
Director, National Institute for Health Biomedical Research Centre, Moorfields Eye Hospital and UCL Institute of Ophthalmology, London, UK
Director of Research and Development
Programme Director Eyes and Vision UCL Partners
Former President of Association for Research in
Vision and Ophthalmology (ARVO)

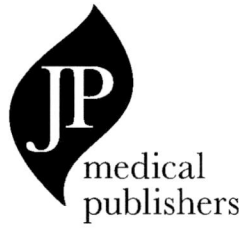

London • New Delhi

© 2021 Jaypee Brothers Medical Publishers

Published by Jaypee Brothers Medical Publishers,
4838/24 Ansari Road, New Delhi, India

Tel: +91 (011) 43574357   Fax: +91 (011)43574390

Email: info@jpmedpub.com, jaypee@jaypeebrothers.com
Web: www.jpmedpub.com, www.jaypeebrothers.com

JPM is the imprint of Jaypee Brothers Medical Publishers.

The rights of Parham Azarbod and Professor Sir Peng Tee Khaw to be identified as the editors of this work have been asserted by them in accordance with the Copyright, Designs and Patents Act 1988.

All rights reserved. No part of this publication may be reproduced, stored or transmitted in any form or by any means, electronic, mechanical, photocopying, recording or otherwise, except as permitted by the UK Copyright, Designs and Patents Act 1988, without the prior permission in writing of the publishers. Permissions may be sought directly from Jaypee Brothers Medical Publishers (P) Ltd. at the address printed above.

All brand names and product names used in this book are trade names, service marks, trademarks or registered trademarks of their respective owners. The publisher is not associated with any product or vendor mentioned in this book.

Medical knowledge and practice change constantly. This book is designed to provide accurate, overview information about the subject matter in question. However readers are advised to check the most current information available on procedures included and check information from the manufacturer of each product to be administered, to verify the recommended dose, formula, method and duration of administration, adverse effects and contraindications. It is the responsibility of the practitioner to take all appropriate safety precautions. Neither the publisher nor the editors assume any liability for any injury and/or damage to persons or property arising from or related to use of material in this book.

This book is sold on the understanding that the publisher is not engaged in providing professional medical services. If such advice or services are required, the services of a competent medical professional should be sought.

ISBN: 978-1-909836-76-1

British Library Cataloguing in Publication Data
A catalogue record for this book is available from the British Library

Library of Congress Cataloging in Publication Data
A catalog record for this book is available from the Library of Congress

Development Editor: Harsha Madan
Editorial Assistant: Keshav Kumar
Cover Design: Seema Dogra

Printed at: Sterling Graphics Pvt. Ltd.

Preface

The field of Ophthalmology is rapidly changing. Over the past few years, we have seen the introduction of novel minimally invasive surgical techniques particularly in the field of Glaucoma; new medical therapies such as vascular endothelial growth factor antagonists which have revolutionised the treatment of conditions such as age-related macular degeneration; and the use of new ocular imaging techniques such as ocular coherence tomography and OCT angiography which provide unparalleled, non-invasive detailed fundal images. This book was written for those wishing to embark on a career in this very exciting speciality or for those non-specialists who are seeking to expand their knowledge. In this ever changing field with the recent explosion of information, the task can seem a rather daunting challenge. With this in mind, we set out to bring together experts in the field and organise the information into concise chapters. This makes a quick overview of topics available to the interested reader, while the subject matters are covered in a comprehensive manner for those in ophthalmic training or ophthalmologists wishing to seek further knowledge on topics outside of their subspecialist area. Whilst we have made every effort to ensure the most accurate and up to date information is presented here, given the rapidly changing ophthalmic horizon, omissions, and errors are possible. We hope you enjoy ready the book as much as it was a pleasure for us to edit and complete this project.

Parham Azarbod
Professor Sir Peng Tee Khaw
July 2020

Acknowledgements

The editors would like to thank all the contributing authors for their hard work and expertise. This book would not have been possible without you.

Parham Azarbod
Professor Sir Peng Tee Khaw

Dedication

I would like to dedicate this book to my parents (Rafi and Katayoun) for their continual guidance on my journey in life: my wife (Shirin) and three boys (Arya, Nima, and Kasra) for their unconditional love and patience that bring joy to every moment. Their continual support is the backbone of my achievements.

Parham Azarbod

I would like to dedicate this book to my parents, wife, and children who have supported and made possible all that we have been able to achieve.

Professor Sir Peng Tee Khaw

Contents

Preface v
Acknowledgements vi
Contributors x

Topics		Page
1	Age-related macular degeneration	1
2	Angle closure glaucoma	6
3	Anisocoria	10
4	Anterior uveitis	14
5	Benign lid lesions	17
6	Biometry and lens implant power calculation	22
7	Birdshot chorioretinopathy	29
8	Blepharitis	32
9	Blepharoptosis	35
10	Carotid-cavernous fistula	39
11	Cataract – acquired	43
12	Cataract – complications of surgery	50
13	Cataracts – congenital	55
14	Central serous chorioretinopathy	59
15	Chalazion	63
16	Chemical injuries	67
17	Conjunctivitis	72
18	Contact lens-related problems of the eye	75
19	Corneal dystrophies	79
20	Corneal ectasia	84
21	Corneal grafts	90
22	Corneal topography	94
23	Cranial nerve palsy – abducens nerve palsy	98
24	Cranial nerve palsy – facial nerve palsy	101
25	Cranial nerve palsies – multiple cranial nerves palsies	104
26	Cranial nerve palsy – oculomotor (third) nerve palsy	109
27	Cranial nerve palsy – trochlear nerve palsy	113
28	Diabetic eye disease	116
29	Dry eye syndrome	122

30	Ectropion	125
31	Entropion	128
32	Epiphora	131
33	Episcleritis	134
34	Esotropia	137
35	Exotropia	142
36	Eyelid trauma	146
37	Femtosecond laser-assisted phacoemulsification	149
38	Full-thickness macular holes	152
39	Giant cell arteritis	156
40	Glaucoma – inflammatory	159
41	Glaucoma – medical management	162
42	Glaucoma – primary open angle	165
43	Glaucoma in children	169
44	Headache	172
45	Imaging in ophthalmology	176
46	Infectious keratitis	181
47	Intermediate uveitis	185
48	Intraocular lenses	188
49	Intravitreal injection therapies	193
50	Lacrimal infections	198
51	Lacrimal surgery	201
52	Leucocoria	205
53	Minimally invasive glaucoma surgery	208
54	Myasthenia gravis	212
55	Neovascular glaucoma	216
56	Normal tension glaucoma	219
57	Nystagmus	222
58	Ocular hypertension	226
59	Ophthalmia neonatorum	229
60	Optic disc imaging	232
61	Optic neuritis	236
62	Optic neuropathies	239
63	Orbital cellulitis	242
64	Papilloedema	245
65	Perimetry	248
66	Peripheral retinal degenerations	253

67	Pigmentary glaucoma	256
68	Posterior uveitis	259
69	Refractive surgery	263
70	Retinal arterial occlusion	267
71	Retinal detachment	270
72	Retinal dystrophies	272
73	Retinal imaging	277
74	Retinal lasers	282
75	Retinal vasculitis	286
76	Retinal vein occlusion	290
77	Retinoblastoma	294
78	Retinopathy of prematurity	298
79	Scleritis	302
80	Secondary open angle glaucoma	305
81	Sickle cell retinopathy	309
82	Strabismus surgery	312
83	Thyroid eye disease	316
84	Trauma – globe rupture	319
85	Tumours – eyelid	323
86	Tumours of the choroid	329
87	Tumours – conjunctival neoplasia	336
88	Tumours of the uvea	340
89	Tumours of the retina	345
90	Vitreoretinal surgery – retinal breaks and detachment and vitreomacular interface disorders	350
91	Vitreoretinal surgery – management of complications of cataract surgery, post-operative endophthalmitis and vitreoretinal biopsy	360
92	Vitreoretinal surgery – intraocular haemorrhage, complications of vitreoretinal surgery and modern developments	365
93	White dot syndromes	372
	Index	375

Contributors

Joseph Abbott FRCOphth
Topics 52, 59, 78
Consultant Ophthalmic Surgeon
Birmingham Women's & Children's Hospital, UK

Jonathan Aboshiha MA(Cantab) MRCS(Ed) FRCOphth CertLRS PgDipCRS PhD
Corneal fellow
Topics 19, 21
Consultant Ophthalmic Surgeon
Moorfields Eye Hospital, UK

Ahmed El Amir FRCOphth
Topic 71
Consultant Opthamic Surgeon
Royal Berkshire NHS Foundation Trust, UK

Owen Anderson BSc PhD MBChB MRCP FRCOphth
Topic 1
Consultant Ophthalmologist,
Royal Bournemouth Hospital, UK

Romesh I Angunawela BM MD FRCOphth FRCS(Ed) Cert LRS
Topics 37, 48
Consultant Ophthalmic Surgeon
Moorfields Eye Hospital, UK

Parham Azarbod BSC (Hons) MRCS (Surg) FRCOphth
Topics 2, 11, 12, 15, 41, 42, 53, 56, 58, 65, 80
Consultant Ophthalmic Surgeon
Moorfields Eye Hospital, UK

Philip Banerjee BMedSci BMBS FRCOphth PhD
Topic 66
Consultant Ophthalmic Surgeon,
Frimley Health NHS Foundation Trust, UK

Victoria Barnett BMBS BMedSci
Topic 69
Specialist Trainee in Ophthalmology
Western Eye Hospital, London, UK

Allon Barsam MA MB BS FRCOphth
Topics 22, 69
Consultant Ophthalmic Surgeon,
Luton and Dunstable NHS foundation Trust,
Ophthalmic Consultants of London, UK

Fion Bremner BSc MB BS PhD FRCOphth
Topics 23, 24, 26, 27
Consultant Neuro-ophthalmologist
Department of Neuro-ophthalmology
National Hospital for Neurology & Neurosurgery,
Queen Square, London, UK

John Brookes FRCOphth
Topic 43
Consultant Ophthalmic Surgeon
Moorfields Eye Hospital, Great Ormand Street Hospital for Children, UK

Roberto Fernández Buenaga MD
Topic 20
Consultant Ophthalmologist
Vissum Madrid, Spain

Pilar Casas-Llera MD PhD
Topic 65
Ophthalmologist
Vissum Corporacion Oftalmologica, Spain

Aman Chandra FRCOphth PhD MFSTEd FRCSEd
Topic 38
Consultant Ophthalmic Surgeon
Southend University Hospital, Southend, Essex, UK

Victor Chong MD FRCOphth
Topic 73
Consultant Ophthalmic Surgeon
Royal Free Hospital and Optegra Eye Hospital,
London, UK

Sophie Coutts BMedSci(Neuroscience) MBBS FRCOphth
Topic 22
Consultant Ophthalmic Surgeon
North East London NHS Treatment Centre, UK

Nicky Cronbach MBBS
Topic 5
Ophthalmology Specialist Registrar
Buckinghamshire Healthcare NHS Trust, UK

Maria-Laura Dari MD FEBO
Topics 16, 18
Ophthalmologist
Moorfields Eye Hospital, UK

Indran Davagnanam MB Bch BAO BMedSci FRCR
Topic 45
Consultant Neuroradiologist
The National Hospital for Neurology and Neurosurgery & Moorfields Eye Hospital
Honorary Senior Lecturer
UCL Institute of Neurology, UK

Ryan Davies FRCOphth
Topic 3
Consultant Ophthalmologist
Royal Gwent Hospital
Newport, UK

Navpreet Dhillon MBChB FRCOphth FEBO BMedSc
Topic 37
Cornea Consultant
Moorfields Eye Hospital and University Hospitals of Leicester
NHS Trust, London, UK

Jennifer Doyle MBBS
Topic 36
Ophthalmology Specialist Registrar
Buckinghamshire NHS Trust, UK

Mostafa Elgohary MB ChB MSc MD FRCSEd FRCSI FRCOphth
Topics 90, 91, 92
Consultant Ophthalmologist and Vitreoretinal Surgeon
Kingston Hospital NHS Foundation Trust, UK

Neil Finer MA MBBS FRCOphth
Topic 14
Locum Consultant Ophthalmologist
Royal London Hospital, Barts Health NHS Trust
London, UK

Konstantinos Fotis MD FEBO
Topic 38
Vitreoretinal Service
Southend University Hospital, Southend, Essex, UK

Seyed MS Ghazi-Nouri MD BSc (hons) MBBS FRCOphth
Topics 30, 31, 32
Consultant Ophthalmologist and Oculoplastic Surgeon
Mid and South Essex University NHS foundation Trust, UK

Sam Gurney BSc (Hons) MB ChB (Hons) FRCOphth
Topic 52
Senior Specialist Trainee in Ophthalmology
Birmingham Children's Hospital, UK

Lamis Al Harby MD
Topic 87
Ocular Oncology Service
Moorfields Eye Hospital and UCL Institute of Ophthalmology, London, UK

Nashila Hirji MBBS MRCP FRCOphth
Topic 72
Clinical Research Fellow
UCL Institute of Ophthalmology, University College London, London, UK

Henrietta Ho FRCOphth FAMS
Topics 41, 56
Ophthalmology Specialist Registrar
St Thomas' Hospital, London, UK

Jason Ho MBBS (Hons) BSc (Hons) FRCOphth
Topic 66
Consultant Ophthalmologist and Vitreoretinal Surgeon
Royal Berkshire NHS Foundation Trust and Honorary Consultant Vitreoretinal Surgeon, Imperial College Healthcare NHS Trust, UK

Richard Imonkhe BEng MSc MBBS FRCOphth ARSM
Topics 42, 58
Consultant Ophthalmic Surgeon
University Hospital Southampton, UK

Saurabh Jain FRCOphth FHEA
Topics 13, 77
Consultant Ophthalmologist and Clinical Director
Royal Free Hospital
Training Director for Ophthalmology
Health Education England, UK

Fiona Jazayeri FRCOphth
Topic 85
Consultant Ophthalmic Surgeon
Buckinghamshire Healthcare NHS Trust, UK

Hugh Jewsbury FRCOphth
Topics 3, 25, 54
Consultant Ophthalmologist
University Hospital of Wales, Cardiff, UK

Ashkan Khalili MD PhD FRCOphth
Topic 80
Fellow in Ophthalmology
Birmingham and Midlands Eye Centre, UK

Usman Khan BSc (Hons) MBBS FRCP PhD
Topics 10, 44
Consultant Neurologist
St George's Hospital NHS Foundation Trust, UK

Michelle lai BSc (Medicine) MBChB FRCOphth
Topics 23, 24, 26, 27
Neuro-ophthalmologist Fellow
Department of Neuro-ophthalmology, National Hospital for Neurology & Neurosurgery, Queen Square, London, UK

Andre Litwin FRCOphth
Topics 50, 51, 83
Consultant Ophthalmic Surgeon, Queen Victoria Hospital NHS Foundation Trust, UK

Bita Manzouri BSc MBBS MRCP FRCOphth PhD CertLRS
Topics 16, 18
Consultant Ophthalmic Surgeon & Lead for Primary Care Services
Queen's Hospital, BHR University Hospitals NHS Trust, UK
Honorary Clinical Senior Lecturer
Barts and The London School of Medicine, UK

Ali Mearza MBBS FRCOphth
Topics 29, 46
Consultant Ophthalmic Surgeon and Clinical Director, Imperial College Healthcare NHS Trust, Ophthalmic Consultants of London, UK

Hemal Mehta MBBS (London) MD (Cambridge), FRCOPHTH
Topic 49
Consultant Ophthalmologist
Royal Free London NHS Foundation Trust, UK
Macular Research Group, Save Sight Institute, Sydney University, Australia

Michel Michaelides MD(Res) FRCOphth
Topic 72
Consultant Ophthalmologist
Moorfields Eye Hospital,
UCL Institute of Ophthalmology
University College London, London, UK

Zahir Mirza MBChB BSc FRCOphth CertLRS
Topics 29, 46
Consultant Ophthalmic Surgeon
Barts Health NHS Trust, London, UK

Sonali Nagendran FRCOphth
Topic 9
Oculoplastics Fellow
Queen Victoria Hospital NHS Foundation Trust, UK

James E Neffendorf MA (Cantab) MBBS FRCOphth
Topic 71
Specialist Registrar and Vitreoretinal Research Fellow
King Edward VII Hospital, Windsor & King's College London, UK

Guy Negretti MB BChir MA FRCOphth
Topic 84
Fellow in Vitreoretinal Surgery
Moorfields Eye Hospital, London, UK

Hon Shing Ong FRCOphth
Topics 11, 12
Consultant Ophthalmic Surgeon
Singapore National Eye Centre, Singapore

Eoin O'Sullivan MD MRCP FRCOphth
Topic 39
Consultant Ophthalmologist
King's College Hospital
London, UK

Sally Painter MA MB BChir FRCOphth
Topics 57, 78
Ophthalmology Specialist Trainee
Birmingham Women's & Children's Hospitals, UK

Vasilios Papastefanou MD PhD ASIS FRPS MRCOphth
Topics 86, 88, 89
Consultant Ophthalmologist
Moorfields Eye Hospital & Barts Health NHS Trust, London, UK

Manoj V Parulekar MS FRCS FRCOphth
Topics 34, 35, 82
Consultant Ophthalmologist
Birmingham Womens and Children's Hospital NHS Trust
Oxford University Hospitals NHS Trust, UK

Darshak Kumar Patel MSc FRCOphth
Topic 15
Senior Ophthalmology Specialist Registrar,
Moorfields Eye Hospital, UK

Elizabeth Pearce MSc
Topic 73
Clinical Research Fellow
UCL Institute of Ophthalmology, London, UK

Marie Restori PhD
Topic 6
Consultant Physicist
Moorfields Eye Hospital, UK

Mandeep S Sagoo BSc MB PhD MRCOphth FRCS (Ed)
Topic 87
Professor of Ophthalmology and Ocular Oncology
NIHR Biomedical Research Centre for Ophthalmology at UCL Institute of Ophthalmology and Moorfields Eye Hospital;
Barts Health NHS Trust, London, UK

Amanjeet Sandhu FRCOpth
Topic 55
Consultant Ophthamic Surgeon
Moorfields Eye Hospital, UK

Richard Scawn FRCOphth
Topics 5, 36
Consultant Ophthalmologist and Oculoplastic Surgeon
Chelsea & Westminster NHS Trust,
The Royal Marsden NHS Trust, Buckinghamshire Healthcare NHS Trust, UK

Senthil Selvam PhD
Topic 49
Honoraryy Research Fellow
Moorfields Eye Hospital NHS Trust and UCL Institute of Ophthalmology, UK

Ameet Shah MD (Res) FRCOphth
Topic 40
Consultant Ophthalmologist
Royal Free Hospital, London, UK

Parth R Shah MB BS BSc(Med)Hons MMed(Ophth Sc) FRANZCO
Topics 34, 35, 82
Consultant Ophthalmologist
Sydney Children's & Prince of Wales Hospitals
Sydney NSW Australia

Pari Shams BSc MRCP FRCOphth
Topics 9, 63
Consultant Ophthalmic Surgeon
Moorfields Eye Hospital, London, UK

Marianne Shiew MBBS FRCSEd (Ophthalmol)
Topic 81
Consultant Ophthalmologist
Hinchingbrooke Hospital, UK

Vasuki Sivagnanavel FRCOphth MD BSc MBBS PG Cert Healthcare Management
Topics 70, 74, 76
Consultant Ophthalmologist,
Kingston Hospital NHS Foundation Trust, UK

Elisabeth de Smit MBBS BSc MSc PhD
Topic 39
Ophthalmology Specialist Registrar
Kingston Hospital NHS Foundation Trust, UK

Mala Subash BSc (Hons) BM FRCOphth
Topic 28
Consultant Ophthalmic Surgeon
Luton and Dunstable University Hospital NHS Foundation Trust, UK

Paul M Sullivan MD FRCOphth
Topic 84
Consultant Ophthalmic Surgeon
Director of Education
Moorfields Eye Hospital, London, UK

Rajan Tailor BSc MBBS MRCP FRCOphth
Topic 67
Consultant Ophthalmologist
Oxford University Hospitals, UK

Naomi Tan MBChB BSc(hons) FRCOphth
Topic 13
Subspecialty Fellow in Paediatric Ophthalmology and Strabismus
Moorfields Eye Hospital NHS Trust, UK

Andrew Tatham MBChB FRCOphth FRCS(Ed) FEBO
Topic 60
Consultant Ophthalmic Surgeon
Honorary Senior Clinical Lecturer
Princess Alexandra Eye Pavilion Edinburgh, UK

William Tucker BMBS BSc FRCOphth
Topics 4, 47, 68, 75,
Consultant Ophthalmologist and Moorfields South Director
Moorfields Eye Hospital NHS Foundation Trust, UK

Miodrag Vojcic MD FEBO
Topics 57, 61, 62, 64
Locum Consultant Ophthalmologist
Moorfields Eye Hospital, UK

Martin Watson MBChB FRCOphth PhD DIC CertLRS
Topics 19, 21
Consultant Ophthalmic Surgeon
Moorfields Eye Hospital, UK

Mark Westcott FRCOphth MD CCST
Topics 7, 33, 79, 93
Consultant Ophthalmic Surgeon
Moorfields Eye Hospital
Barts Health NHS Trust
Honorary Senior Lecturer at UCL Institute of Ophthalmology, London, UK

Gynn Williams FRCOphth
Topics 7, 33, 79, 93
Consultant Ophthalmolgist
Singleton Hospital, Swansea, UK

Damien Yeo FRCOphth
Topic 25
Consultant Ophthalmologist,
Alder Hey Children's Hospital, Liverpool, UK

Mohammed Ziaei MBChB (Hons) MD FRCOphth FRANZCO
Topics 8, 17
Consultant Ophthalmic Surgeon
Senior Lecturer – Faculty of Medical and Health Sciences
University of Auckland, New Zealand

Plate 1

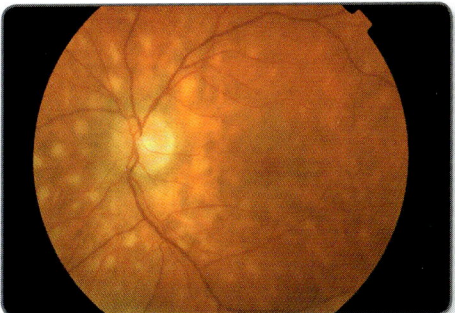

Figure 7.1 Fundal photo of birdshot.

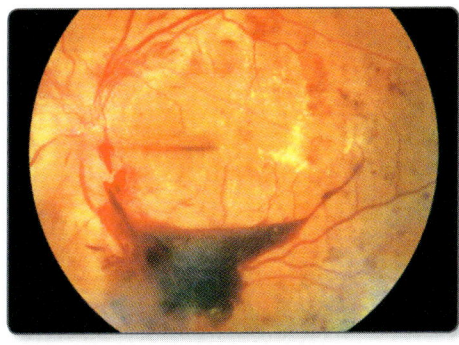

Figure 28.1 Fundus photo of severe diabetic retinopathy and neovascularisation.

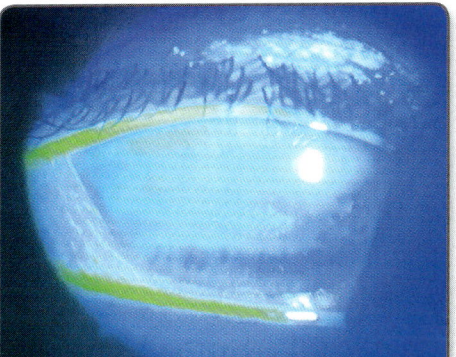

Figure 29.1 Punctate epithelial erosions on the cornea of a patient with dry eye.
Courtesy: M Bizrah Moorfields Eye Hospital.

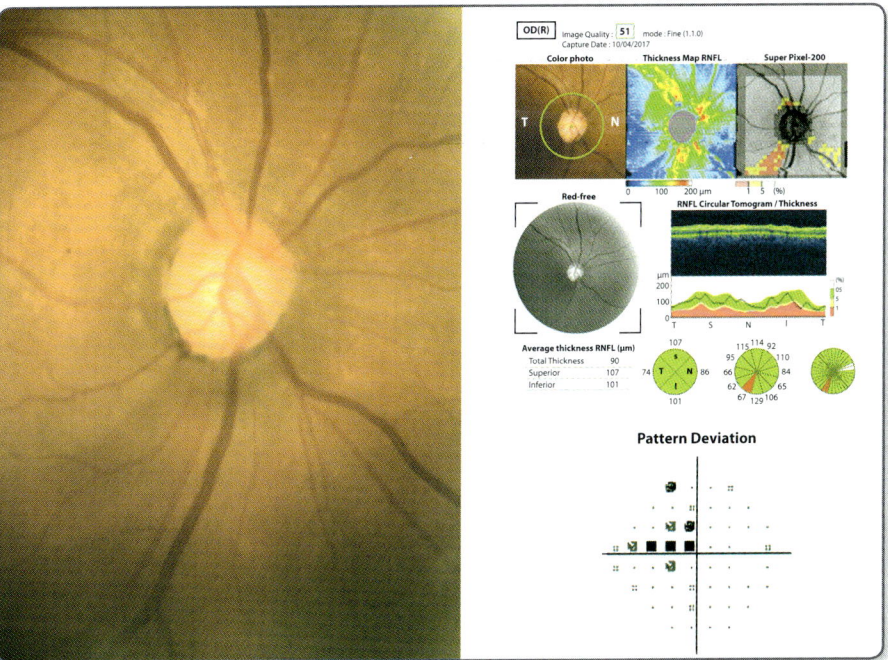

Figure 42.1 Typical findings in primary open angle glaucoma (POAG), showing optic disc photo (note the inferotemporal disc haemorrhage and neuroretinal rim thinning with an associated nerve fibre layer defect), optic disc optical coherence tomography (OCT) and corresponding visual field defect.

Plate 2

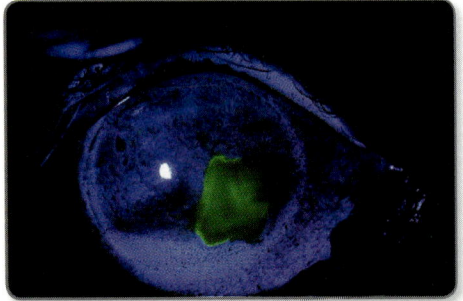

Figure 46.2 Epithelial defect, demonstrated by fluorescein staining, overlying an infiltrate caused by bacterial keratitis.
Courtesy: M Bizrah Moorfields Eye Hospital.

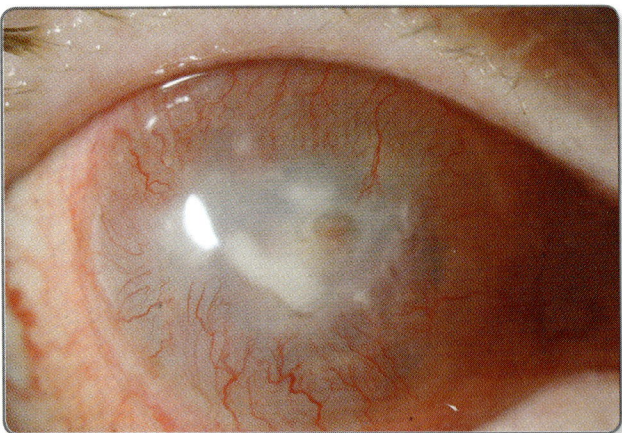

Figure 46.4 Fungal keratitis with satellite lesions.
Courtesy: M Bizrah Moorfields Eye Hospital.

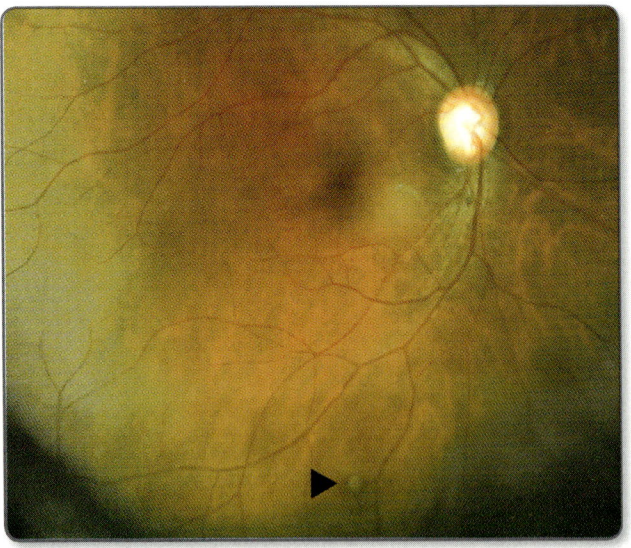

Figure 47.1 Wide field fundus photograph of a right eye showing (black arrowhead) a 'snowball' sitting just above the retina in the posterior vitreous.

Plate 3

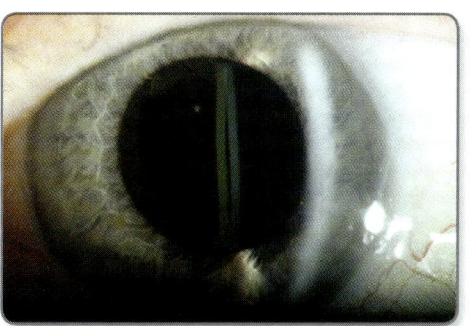

Figure 48.2 Anterior segment showing example of glistening.
Courtesy: Romesh Angunawela, Moorfields Eye Hospital, London.

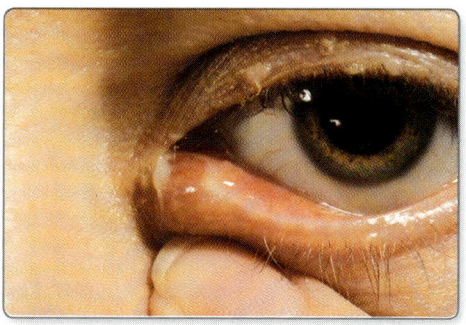

Figure 50.2 Photo of canaliculitis.

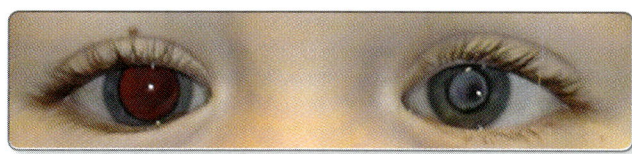

Figure 52.1 Leucocoria in the left eye due to lens capsule opacification following cataract surgery.

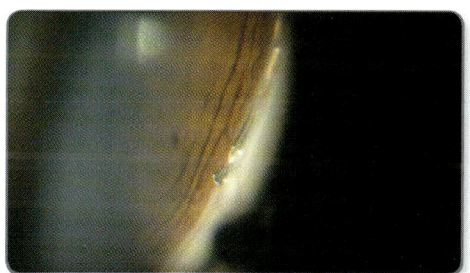

Figure 53.2 Gonioscopic view of Hydrus.
Courtesy: Mr Keith Barton, Moorfields eye Hospital.

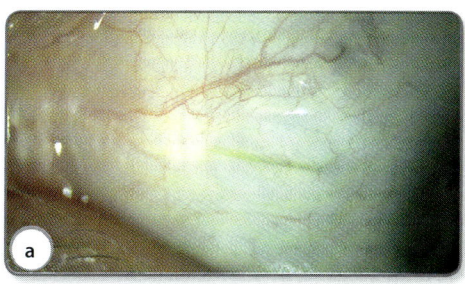
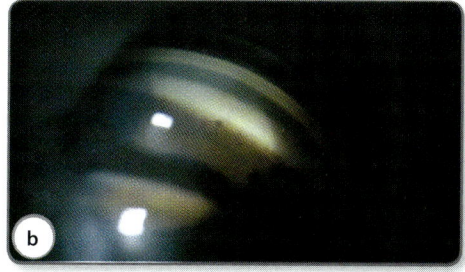

Figures 53.3a and b (a) Subconjunctival portion of XEN implant with a shallow diffuse bleb. (b) Gonioscopic view of the intraocular portion of the XEN implant.
Courtesy: Mr Keith Barton, Moorfields eye Hospital.

Plate 4

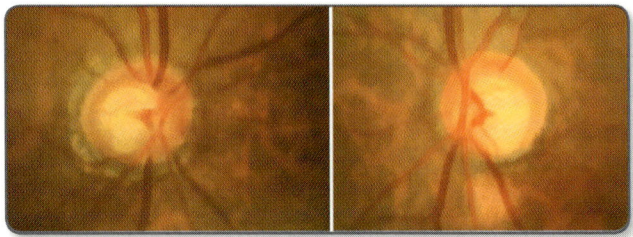

Figure 60.1 Optic disc photographs of patient with glaucoma in both eyes.

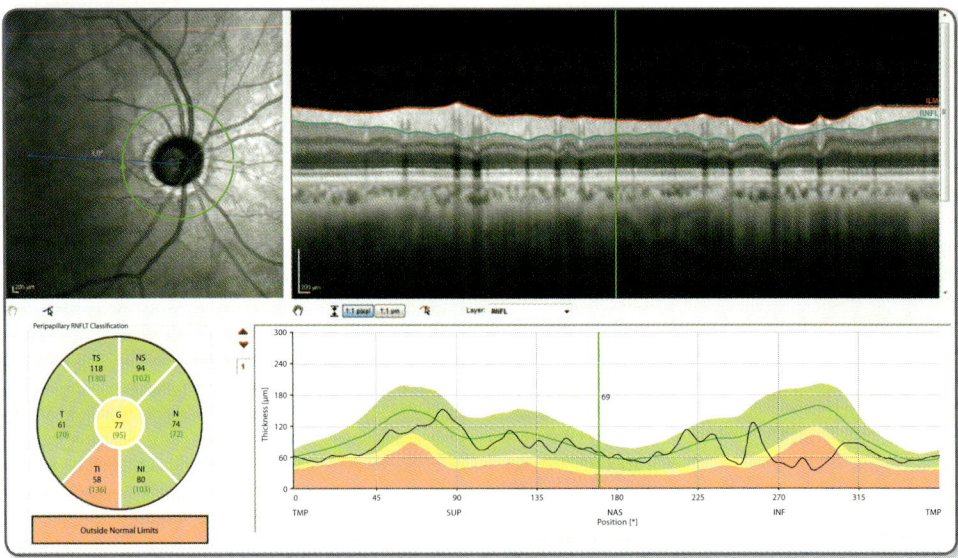

Figure 60.2 Optical coherence tomography (OCT) retinal nerve fibre layer (RNFL) scan for the right eye of the patient in Figure 1 showing segmentation of the RNFL and classification as outside normal limits.

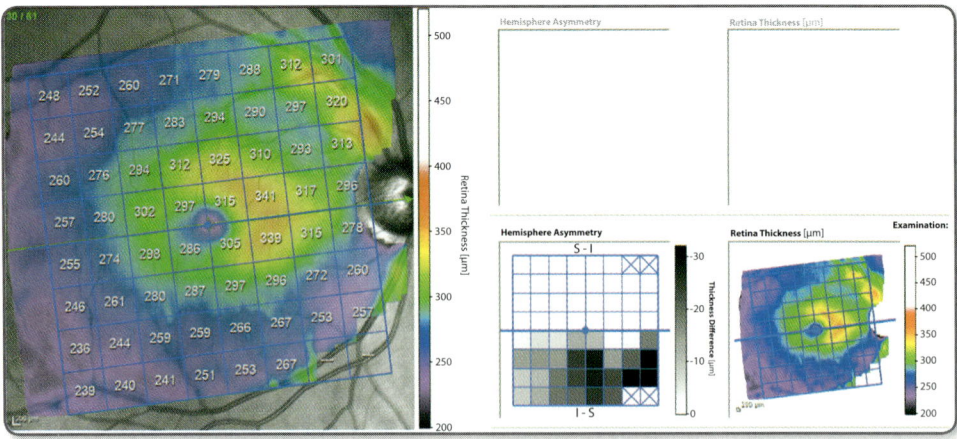

Figure 60.3 Macular retinal thickness analysis for the same patient.

Plate 5

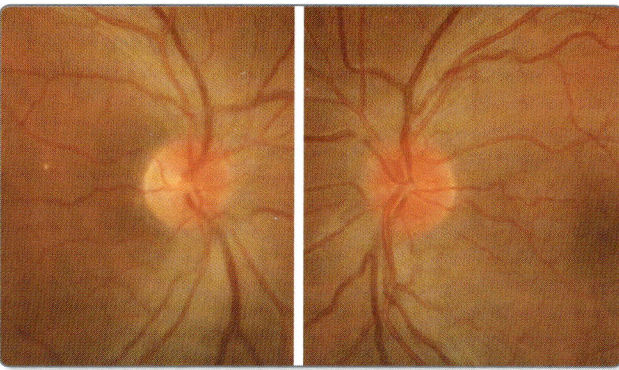

Figure 62.1 Leber's hereditary optic neuropathy. Description: patient presented with worsening vision in the left eye (6/24), and 6 week history of visual loss in the right eye (CF).

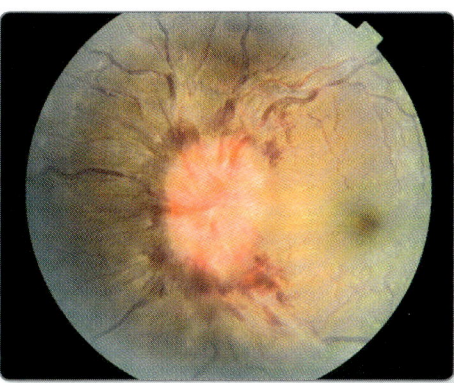

Figure 64.1 Acute papilloedema.

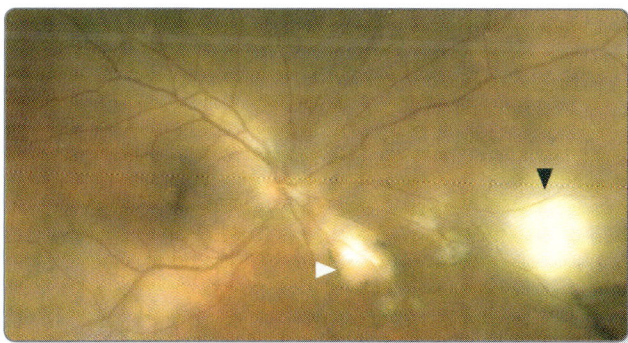

Figure 68.2 Wide field fundus colour photograph of a right eye showing (black arrowhead) an active focus of retinitis secondary to toxoplasmosis, note the fluffy poorly defined edges. In contrast older lesions are well defined with pigmented borders (white arrowhead). The view is hazy due to vitritis.

Plate 6

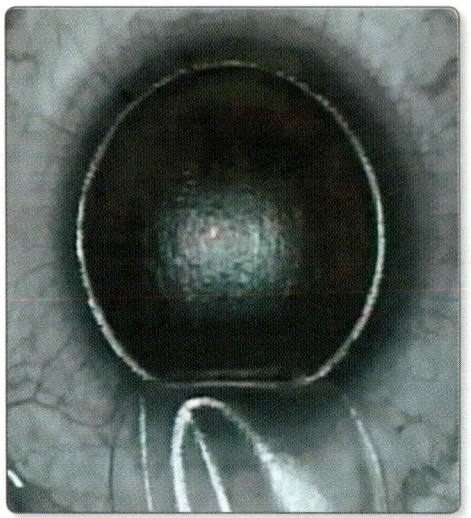

Figure 69.1 LASIK flap reflected back to expose the underlying stromal bed.

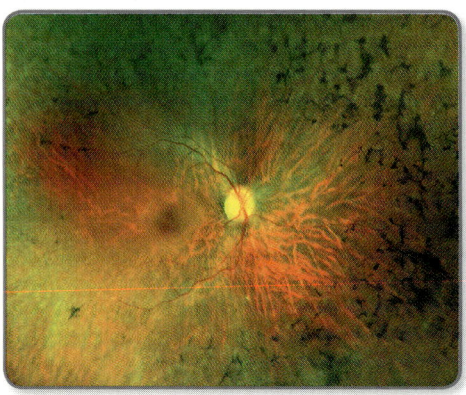

Figure 72.1 Fundus photograph showing the mid-peripheral 'bone-spicule' retinal pigmentation, optic disc pallor and arteriolar attenuation of retinitis pigmentosa.

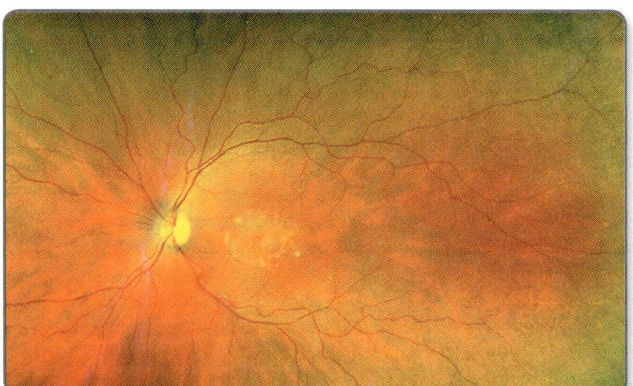

Figure 72.2 Fundus photograph of Stargardt disease showing areas of macular atrophy.

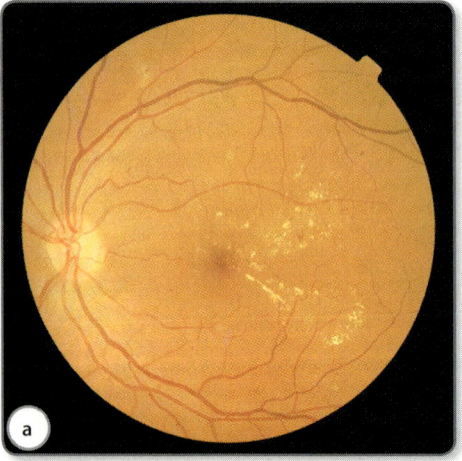

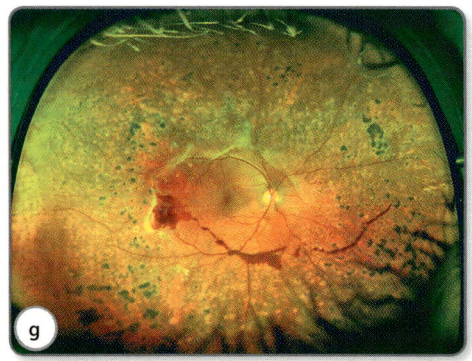

Figures 73.1 Fundus photos to show examples of different imaging modalities. (a) Fundus colour photography; (g) Ultra-widefield imaging.

Plate 7

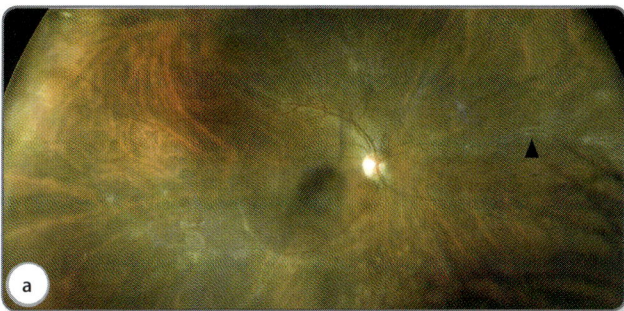

Figure 75.1a (a) Wide-field fundus colour photograph of a right eye showing (black arrowhead) cuffing of a retinal vein.

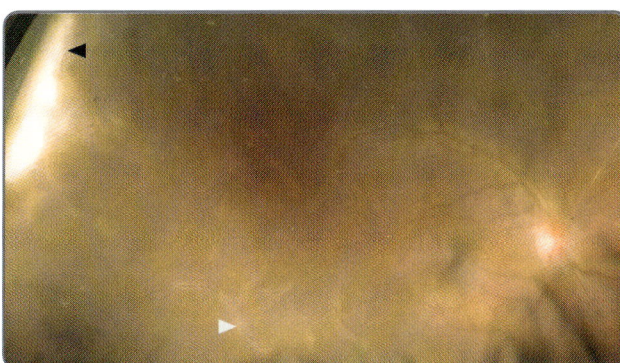

Figure 75.2 Wide-field fundus colour photograph of a right eye showing (black arrowhead) peripheral acute retinal necrosis with opaque whitening of the retina. There is additional vascular cuffing of arteries and veins leading towards the area (white arrowhead). The picture is hazy due to vitritis.

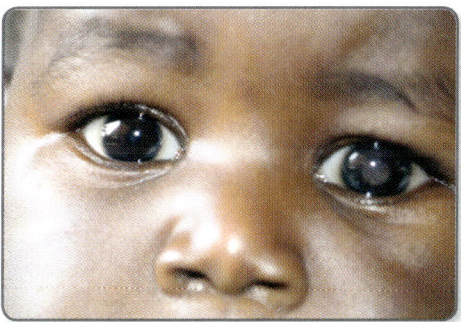

Figure 77.1 A child with leucocoria +/− squint.

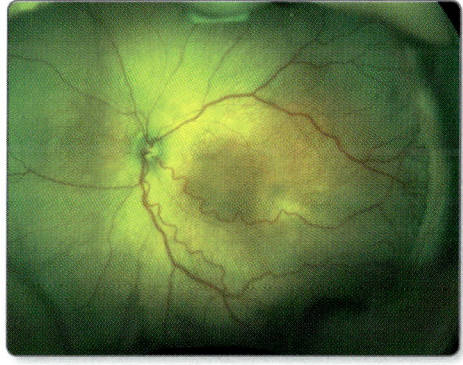

Figure 78.1 AP-ROP with extensive arteriolar and venular dilatation and tortuosity in zone I.

Figure 78.2 Temporal zone II, stage 3 ROP with plus disease in superotemporal and inferotemporal quadrants. This is type 1 ROP and should be treated as per ET-ROP criteria.

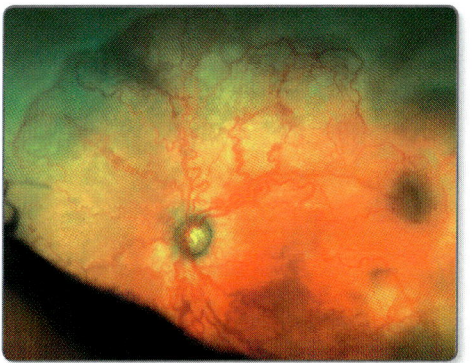

Plate 8

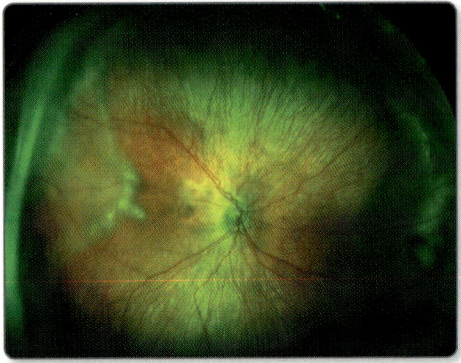

Figure 78.3 Temporal zone II, stage 4a ROP with a localised area of retina under traction extending towards the fovea.

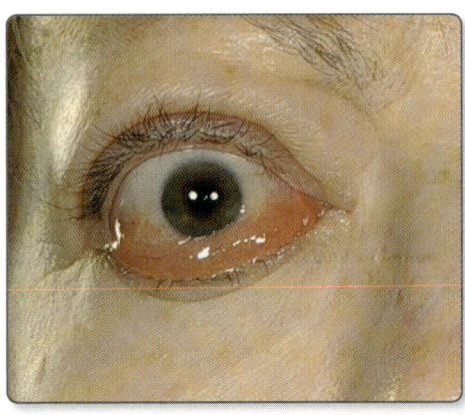

Figure 83.1 Patient demonstrating signs of thyroid eye disease.

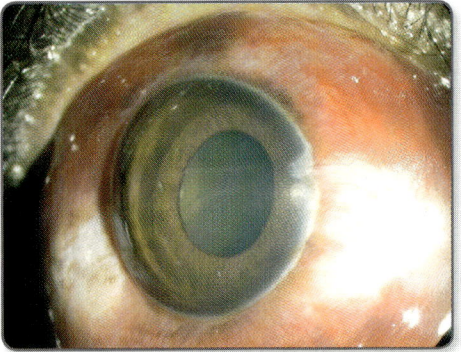

Figure 84.2 Haemorrhagic chemosis and deep anterior chamber following globe rupture.

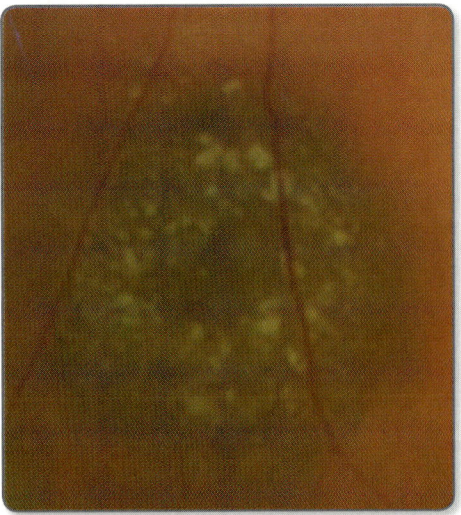

Figure 86.1 Choroidal naevus – note the presence of well defined drusen on the surface.

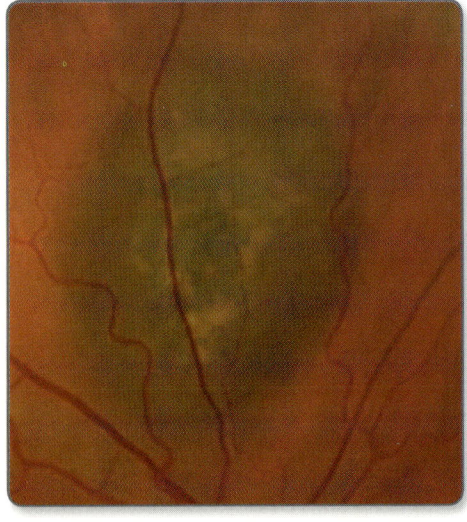

Figure 86.2 Small choroidal melanoma – note the presence of confluent lipofuscin on the surface.

Plate 9

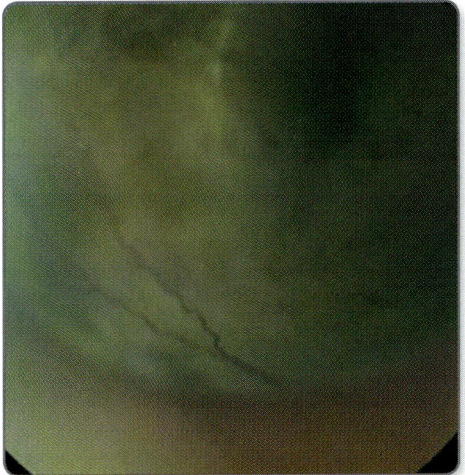

Figure 86.3 Large choroidal melanoma – protruding choroidal mass with associated detachment and disturbance of the overlying retina.

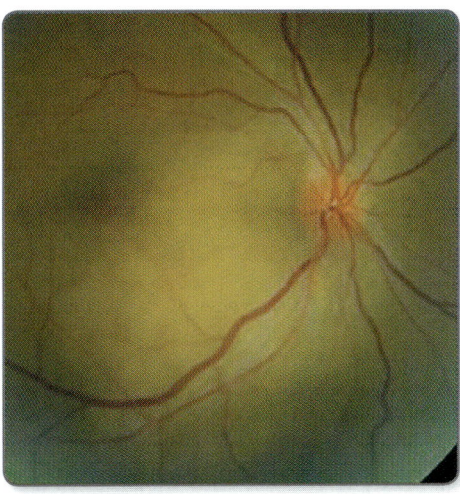

Figure 86.4 Choroidal metastasis – yellowish lesion with feathery margins.

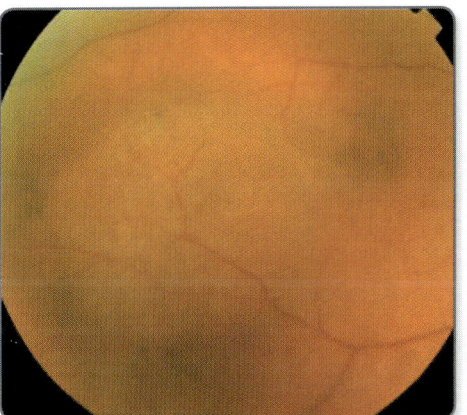

Figure 86.5 Circumscribed choroidal hemangioma – organe mass less distinct with superficial metaplastic features and associated fluid.

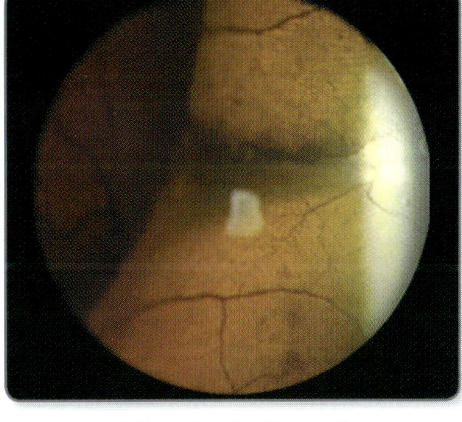

Figure 86.6 Diffuse choroidal hemangioma with extensive exudative detachment visible through the pupil.

Figure 86.7 Choroidal osteoma white yellow mass with circumferential peripapillary extension, decalcification and macular RPE changes.

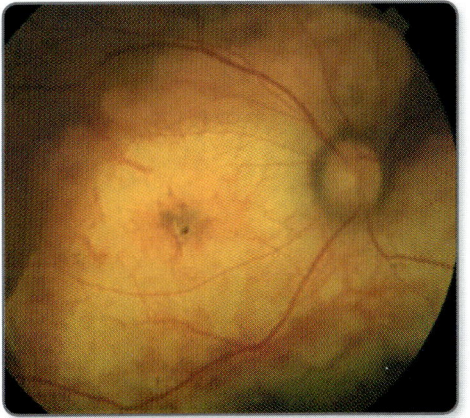

Plate 10

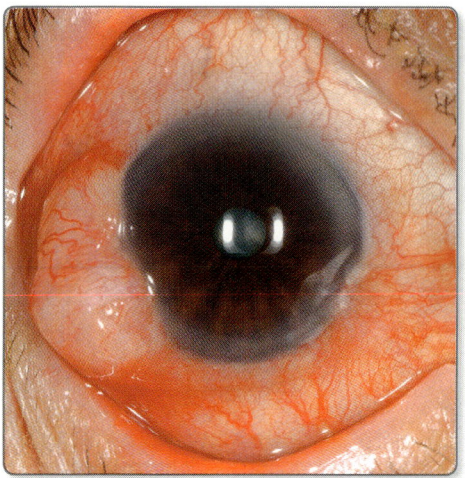

Figure 87.2 Conjunctival squamous carcinoma.

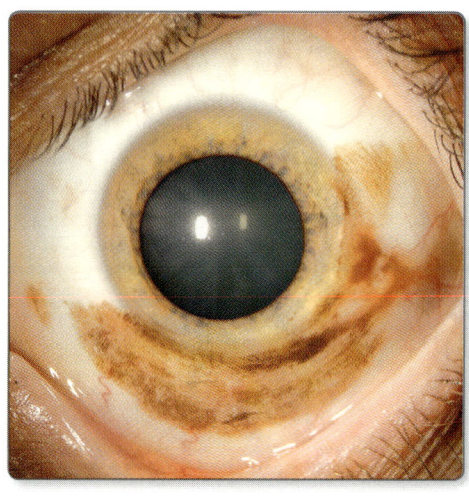

Figure 87.3 Primary acquired melanosis (PAM).

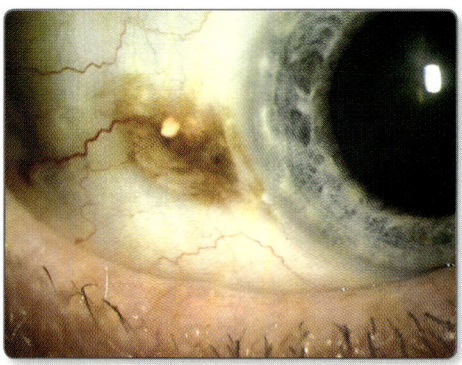

Figure 87.4 Conjunctival naevus.

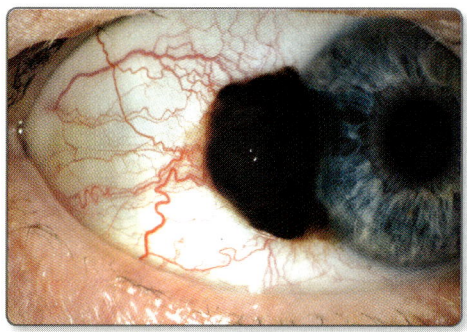

Figure 87.5 Conjunctival melanoma.

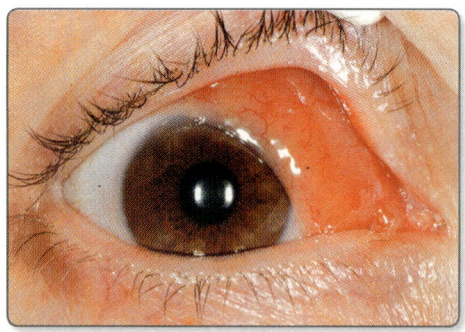

Figure 87.6 Conjunctival lymphoma.

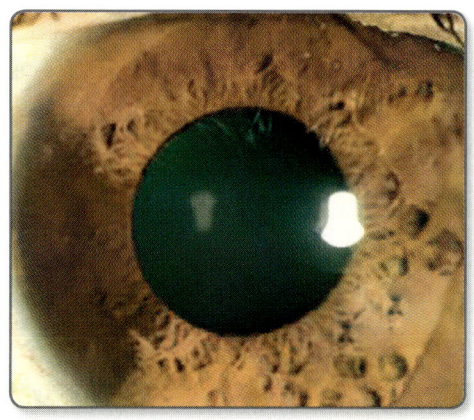

Figure 88.1 Melanocytic iris freckle – note there is no disturbance of the iris stroma.

Plate 11

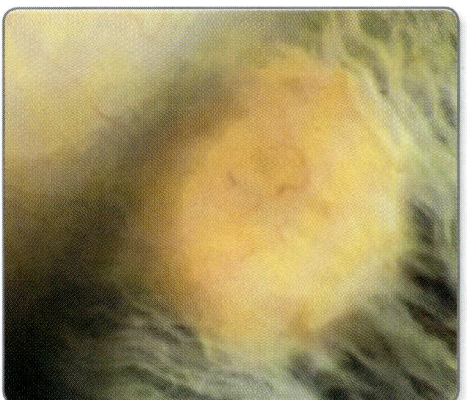

Figure 88.2 Amelanotic iris naevus – note the intrinsic vasculature being discernible.

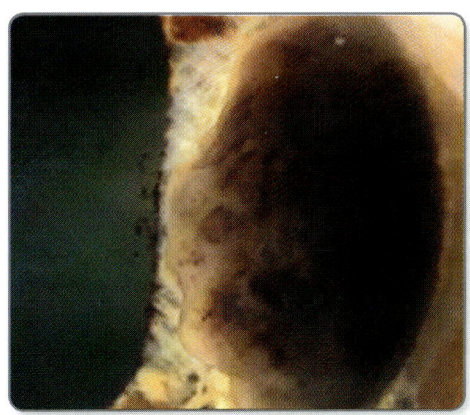

Figure 88.3 Iris melanoma – expansion of the tumour in the anterior chamber with displacement of the iris and shedding of pigment.

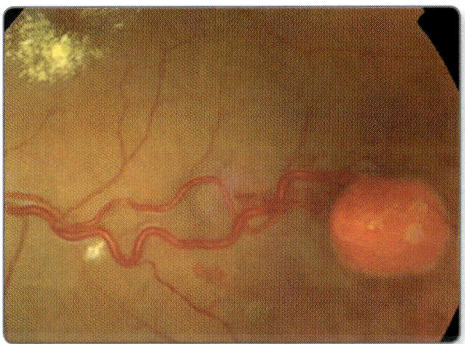

Figure 89.1 Peripheral capillary hemangioma – note the distended feeder vessels and the extent of edema to the macula creating a macular star.

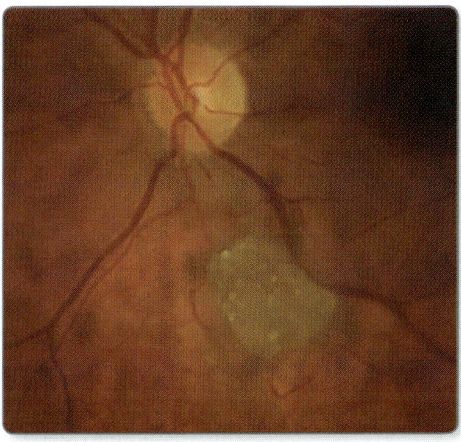

Figure 89.2 Calcified astrocytic hamartoma with discrete nodules on its surface.

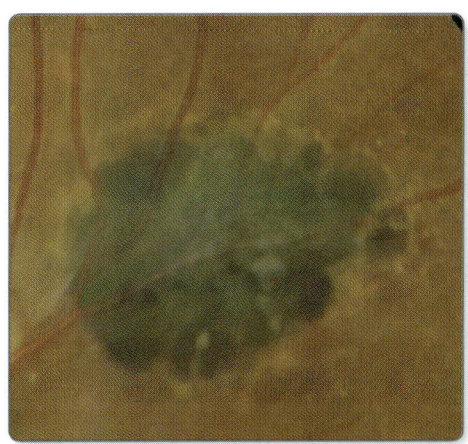

Figure 89.3 Solitary CHRPE with amelanotic lacunae on its surface.

Plate 12

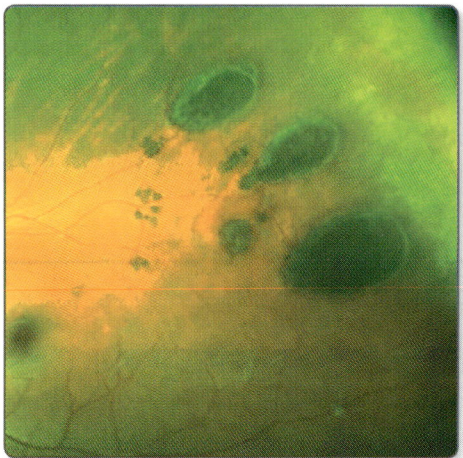

Figure 89.4 Multifocal CHRPE with avoid and spotted configuration.

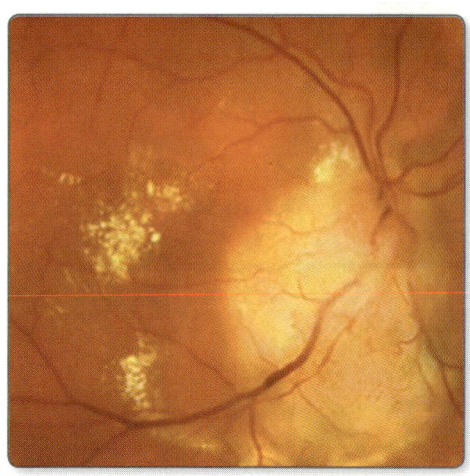

Figure 89.5 Combined hamartoma of the retina and the RPE with evidence of superficial gliosis and associated retinal traction and exudation.

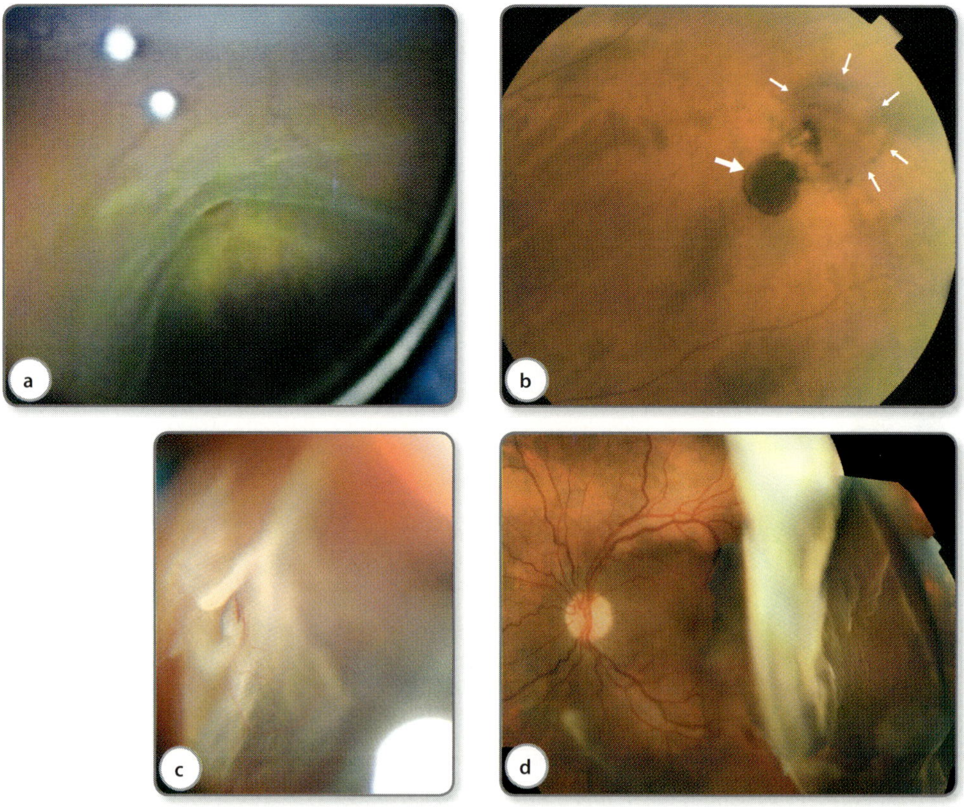

Figure 90.1 Retinal breaks. (a) An atrophic round hole; (b) An operculated tear (the edge–thin arrows and a pigmented operculum–thick arrow); (c) A 'horse-shoe' or U-shaped tear and retinal detachment; (d) A giant retinal tear (≥3 clock hours) with retinal detachment; and (e) Traumatic retinal dialysis. *Continues opposite...*

Plate 13

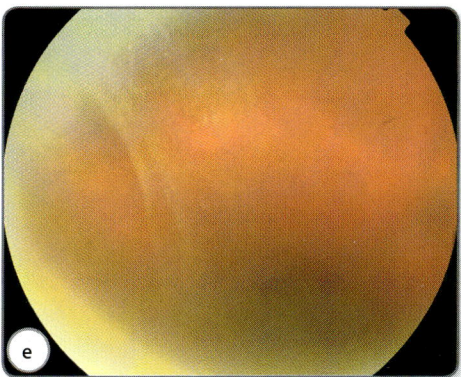

Figure 90.1 Continued..

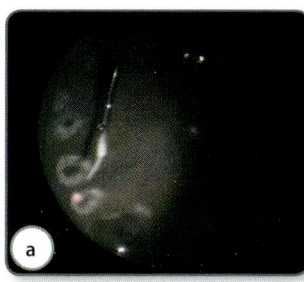

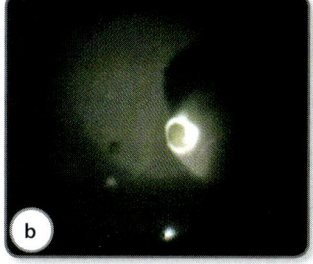

Figure 90.2 Treatment of retinal breaks. (a) Endolaser retinopexy to multiple retinal breaks (during pars plana vitrectomy); and (b) Cryotherapy.

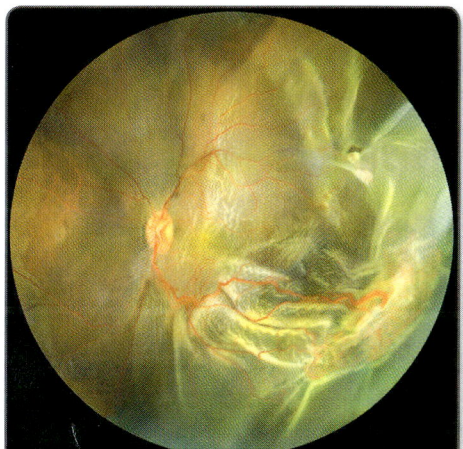

Figure 90.4 Combined tractional and rhegmatogenous retinal detachment in a patient with proliferative sickle cell retinopathy. Note the concave configuration of the area of tractional detachment. There is also a tear with surrounding rhegmatogenous RD that assumes a convex configuration.
Courtesy: Paul Sullivan, Moorfields Eye Hospital.

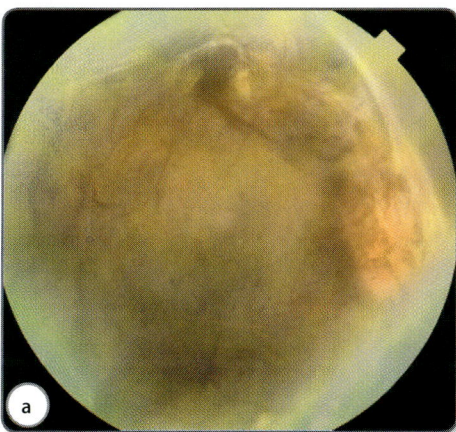

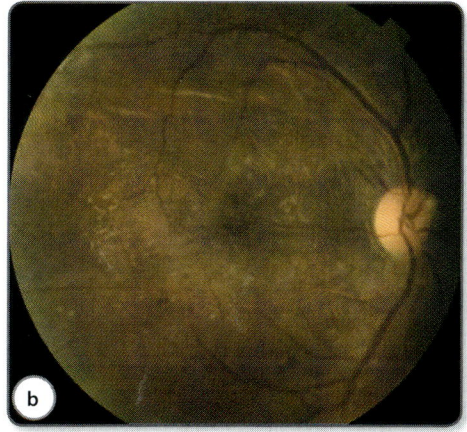

Figure 90.6 A case of proliferative diabetic retinopathy with fibrovascular membrane associated with macular traction along the arcades (a) before and (b) after surgery.

Plate 14

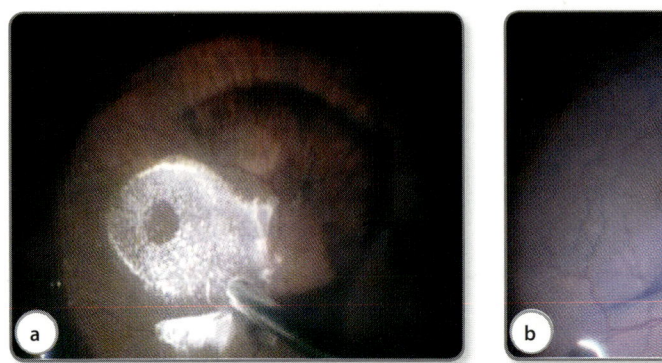

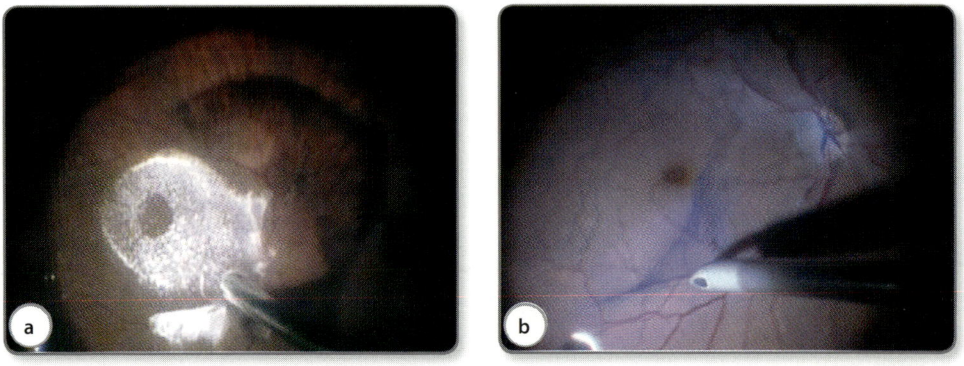

Figure 90.8 Treatment of vitreomacular interface disorders. (a) Posterior vitreous detachment inducement (triamcinolone is used to assist visualisation); (b) Internal limiting membrane peeling during vitrectomy for full-thickness macular hole (trypan blue dye is used to assist visualisation).

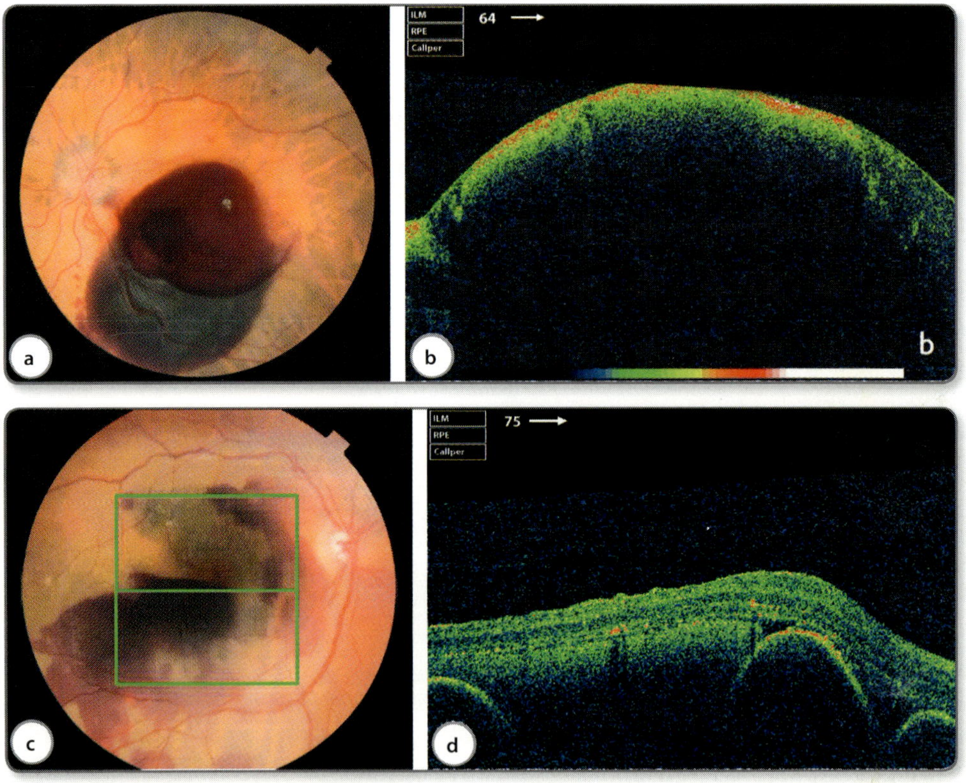

Figure 92.1 Bright sub-internal limiting membrane (ILM) and slightly darker sub-retinal haemorrhage (notice that it masks all the underlying structures) and dark sub-retinal pigment epithelium (RPE) haemorrhage (a and b). Both sub-retinal and sub-RPE haemorrhages have the retinal structures clearly visible over the area of the blood. The cause of submacular haemorrhage in the bottom frames (c and d) is due to choroidal polyps, which appear as saccular protrusions underneath the retina on the optical coherence tomography (OCT) scan.

Plate 15

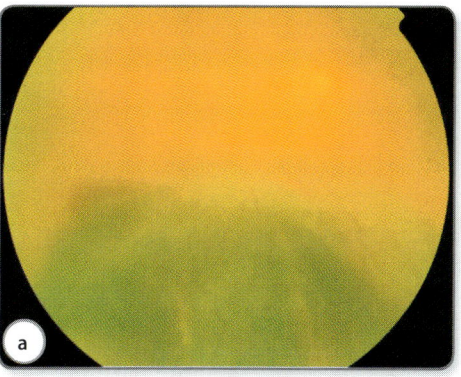 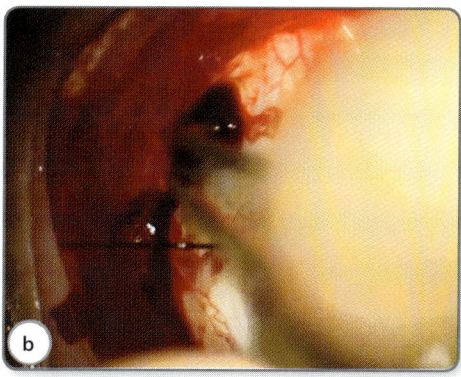

Figure 92.5 (a) Acute (intraoperative) suprachoroidal haemorrhage; (b) Drainage through a sclerotomy incision 2 weeks after the onset of the haemorrhage.

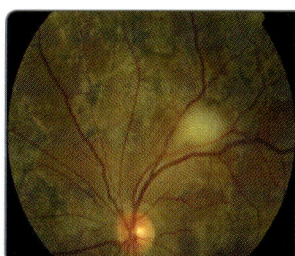 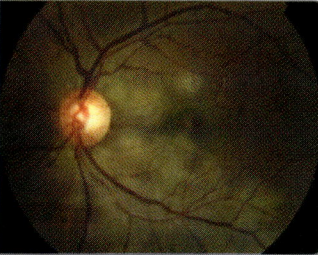

Figure 93.2 Acute posterior multifocal placoid pigment epitheliopathy (APMPPE).

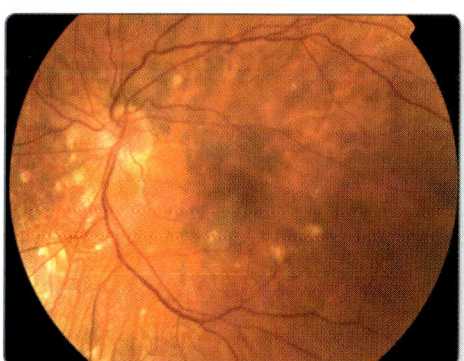

Figure 93.3 Punctate inner choroidopathy (PIC).

1 Age-related macular degeneration

Key points
- Age-related macular degeneration (AMD) can be broadly divided into two sub-groups: dry AMD and wet AMD
- There is currently no treatment for dry AMD, while anti-vascular endothelial growth factor (anti-VEGF) inhibitors are used to treat wet-AMD
- Rapid assessment of concerning visual symptoms, via optical coherence tomography (OCT) +/− angiography, is essential in early detection of wet AMD

Epidemiology

Age-related macular degeneration (AMD) is the leading cause of blindness in over 60 years old in the western world. Prevalence increases with increasing age. Most patients suffer mild visual symptoms. However, 10–15% of patients with AMD suffer from severe central visual loss.

Pathophysiology

Genetic and environmental factors combine to produce an environment of oxidative stress and inflammation at the retinal-choroidal interface. With age adaptive mechanisms begin to fail and the pathological state of AMD ensues. This begins with a build-up of waste material at the retinal-choroidal interface (drusen). Subsequently the following changes occur:
- *Dry AMD*: The retinal pigment epithelium (RPE) becomes dysfunctional and atrophic, leading to secondary photoreceptor atrophy
- *Wet AMD*: New vessels grow from the choriocapillaris [choroidal neovascularisation (CNV)], or occasionally from the retina [retinal angiomatous proliferation (RAP)]

Clinical features

Symptoms

Patients may complain of blurred central vision in one or both eyes, often associated with distortion (when straight lines appear crooked or bent). They find it more difficult to read in dim illumination, often requiring good lighting when reading. Sometimes words appear and disappear when reading, as the words move in and out of parafoveal scotomas caused by AMD. Some patients are not aware of visual loss, if the other eye is dominant.

Signs

The AMD can be divided into two categories, dry AMD and wet AMD.

Dry AMD
- Areas of altered RPE pigmentation in the macular region: hyper- and hypopigmentation
- Patches of RPE hypopigmentation, in the shape of islands [geographic atrophy (GA)]

Wet AMD
- Haemorrhage at the macular region (intraretinal, subretinal or sub-RPE)
- Macular oedema and/or submacular fluid
- Intraretinal exudates
- A grey-green lesion in the macular region CNV
- A subretinal fibrotic scar

The AMD normally occurs in the presence of drusen. However drusen alone, in the absence of symptoms or features described above, do not indicate AMD, just the potential to develop it.

Wet AMD usually occurs on a background of preceding dry AMD.

Investigations

Optical coherence tomography

The OCT scanning is essential in determining if AMD is wet or dry. It is also vital when following up patients treated for wet AMD, as it shows response to treatment.

Key OCT features of dry AMD
- Sub-RPE deposits (drusen – between the RPE layer and Bruch's membrane)
- Subretinal deposits (reticular pseudo-drusen – between the photoreceptor outer segments and the RPE)
- Thinning/loss of the RPE layer (GA) with associated thinning of the overlying photoreceptor layer (outer nuclear and ellipsoid layer) and a bright area of choroid below (due to more OCT light reaching the choroid allowing more to be reflected back)

Key OCT features of wet AMD (Figure 1.1)
- Retinal thickening
- Fluid cysts within the retinal layers (intraretinal fluid – IRF)
- Fluid between the retina and the RPE (subretinal fluid – SRF)
- Fusiform shaped lesion between the retina and the RPE, between the RPE and Bruch's membrane, or both (choroidal neovascularisation – CNV)
- Associated subretinal and intraretinal hyper-reflective material (blood, exudate)

Fundus fluorescein angiography

Fundus fluorescein angiography (FFA) is a useful test in confirming wet AMD, in the presence of suspicious features on OCT scanning. It is also used where there is a diagnostic uncertainty, based on the clinical and OCT findings. If there are no concerning features on OCT scanning, FFA should not be performed.

Key FFA features of wet AMD
- Area of hyperfluorescence, seen early (typically a lacy network at 30 seconds) that gets brighter and bigger later in the FFA. This is a CNV between the retina and the RPE (classic CNV, type-2 CNV) (**Figure 1.2**)
- Area of hyperfluorescence, seen later in the FFA (1–2 minutes), that gets brighter and bigger later on, associated with a fibrovascular pigment epithelial detachment (PED) or late leakage of unknown origin. This is a CNV hidden underneath the RPE (occult CNV, type-1 CNV) (**Figure 1.3**)

OCT angiography

The OCT angiography enables the visualisation of choroidal neovascularisation (CNV) without the injection of dye. It is often used instead of traditional FFA imaging and has the following advantages:
- Non-invasive (no dye required)
- Able to detect CNV complexes in patients where traditional FFA is often inconclusive (e.g. elderly patients with only SRF [wet AMD vs. central serous chorioretinopathy (CSCR)]

Fundus autofluorescence

Fundus autofluorescence (FAF) is a non-invasive technique for imaging natural retinal fluorophores (predominantly lipofuscin in the RPE). Healthy RPE fluoresces. Sick/absent RPE has altered/absent autofluorescence. FAF is particularly useful in monitoring progression of GA.

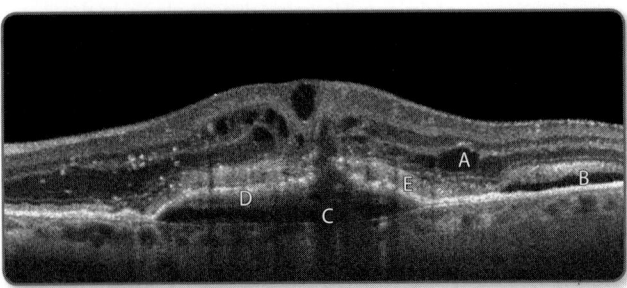

Figure 1.1 Macular OCT scan showing typical features of wet AMD. Intraretinal (A) and subretinal fluid (B). A pigment epithelial detachment (PED) (C) containing a fusiform lesion [D – choroidal neovascular membrane (CNV)]. Blood is seen as subretinal hyper-reflective material (E).

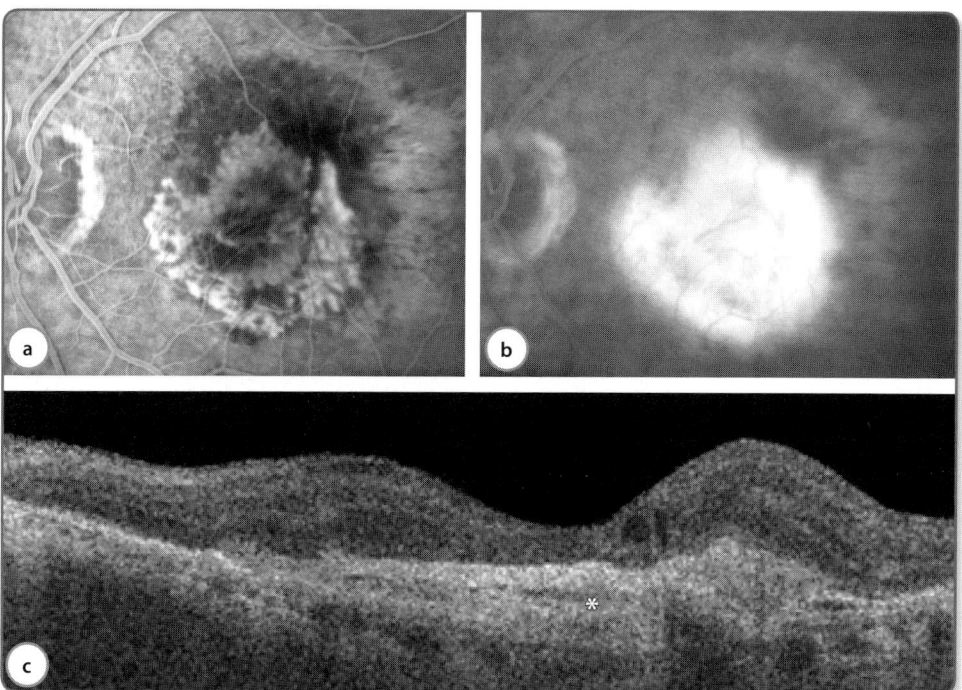

Figure 1.2 Fundus fluorescein angiogram (FFA) of a type-2 (classic) choroidal neovascular membrane (CNV). (a) Bright lesion seen at 15 seconds. Note: the lacy network and central feeder vessels. (b) At 3 minutes the lesion is brighter and bigger due to leak. (c) Corresponding OCT showing a choroidal neovascular membrane (CNV) between the retina and the RPE (*).

Key FAF features of dry AMD
- Areas of hypofluorescence, due to loss of lipofuscin laden RPE cells in GA
- Drusen have variable fluorescence

Indocyanine green angiography

Indocyanine green angiography (ICG) is used to visualise lesions under the RPE. Unlike fluorescein the excitation and emission wavelengths of ICG can penetrate the RPE. It is particularly useful in the detection of idiopathic polypoidal choroidal vasculopathy (IPCV) and retinal angiomatous proliferation (RAP) lesions.

Multimodal imaging

Multimodal imaging means imaging lesions in two or more different ways (e.g. OCT and FFA) and then reviewing the results together. It leads to both a better understanding of the pathology and also enables more accurate diagnosis.

Diagnosis

Dry AMD
Diagnosing dry AMD is based on the identification of typical RPE abnormalities in a patient over 50 years old. Drusen are invariably present to some degree. An OCT scan has ruled out wet AMD.

Wet AMD
Diagnosing wet AMD is based on typical OCT findings in the presence of macular drusen +/- blood/exudate. The diagnosis is confirmed with FFA or OCT angiography.

Treatment

Dry AMD
Currently there is no treatment for dry AMD. RPE atrophy, with associated photoreceptor atrophy, tends to slowly progress, leading to central and para-central visual loss. Current advice includes smoking cessation, a healthy

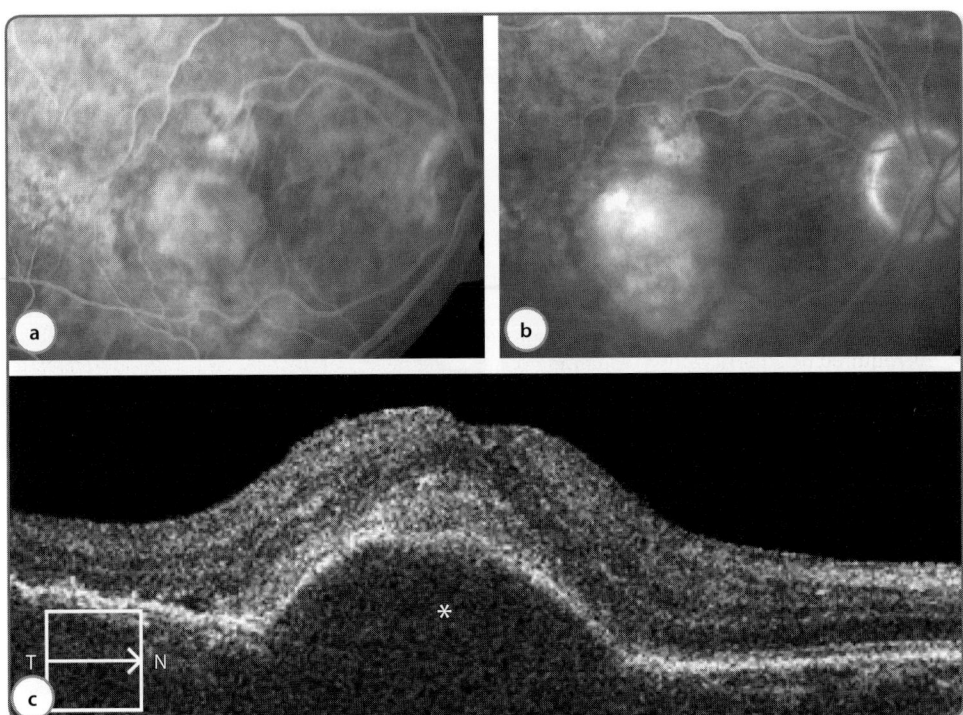

Figure 1.3 Fundus fluorescein angiogram (FFA) of a type-1 (occult) choroidal neovascular membrane (CNV). (A) Some hyperfluorescence seen at 1 minute. This is later and dimmer than in a type-2 (classic) CNV, due to the overlying retinal pigment epithelium (RPE) obscuring much of the underlying fluorescence. (B) At 4 minutes the lesion is brighter and bigger due to leak. (C) Corresponding OCT showing a fibrovascular pigment epithelial detachment (PED) (*).

Table 1.1 Summary of types of patients shown to benefit from vitamin supplementation (age-related eye disease study (AREDS) 1 & 2) and formula of AREDS-2 supplementation. Drusen can be sized by comparing their size with a retinal vein as it crosses the optic disc. This vein is approximately 125 µm in diameter	
Patient groups benefiting from AREDS formula	AREDS-2 formula

Extensive intermediate drusen (62.5–125 µm)
 ≥1 large drusen (>125 µm)
 Non-central geographic atrophy (GA)
 Fellow eye advanced AMD – Central GA
   Wet AMD
   Vision ≤6/12 due to AMD
	500 mg of vitamin C
	 400 IU of vitamin E
	 25 mg zinc as zinc oxide
	 2 mg copper as cupric oxide
	 10 mg lutein and 2 mg zeaxanthin

diet rich in colourful fruit and vegetables and consideration of vitamin supplementation (antioxidant vitamin formulation reduces progression by 25% – AREDS 1 and 2 trials) (Table 1.1).

Wet AMD

Wet AMD is treated with intravitreal injections. Three are in current use:

- Ranibizumab (Lucentis) is a monoclonal antibody fragment (FAb) against vascular endothelial growth factor (VEGF)
- Aflibercept (Eylea) is a recombinant human fusion protein against VEGF. It also binds to placental growth factor (PGF)
- Bevacizumab (Avastin) is a recombinant humanised monoclonal antibody against VEGF. Unlike ranibizumab and aflibercept

it is not licensed for use in the eye. It is licensed for the treatment of cancer. One vial of bevacizumab can be divided into many separate intravitreal injections. It is widely used worldwide and is considerably less expensive than ranibizumab or aflibercept

Patients are usually treated initially with three intravitreal injections, each 1 month apart. After that, treatment usually follows one of three pathways:
- As required treatment (PRN) – Patients are seen monthly and injected if there are signs of disease activity (OCT macular intra or subretinal fluid, new macular blood, five letter reduction in vision in the presence of macular fluid)
- Fixed dosing (maintenance) – This is traditionally every 4 weeks (ranibizumab) or every 8 weeks (aflibercept). Injections are given regardless of the clinical findings. This dosing regimen most closely mimics the clinical trials
- Treatment and extend (Rx & Extend) – Patients receive a clinical assessment and injection at every visit. However, the interval between visits increases if the condition is stable (vision stable/improving, no new macular blood, OCT dry). If there are signs of activity [new macular blood, OCT new macular fluid, increasing pigment epithelial detachment (PED)] then the interval between injections is reduced. Intervals tend to range between 8 and 16 weeks, occasionally being as short as every 4 weeks

Complications

Complications of the disease
- Central visual loss due to subfoveal GA (dry AMD) or subfoveal scar (wet AMD)
- Central visual loss due to large submacular haemorrhage (bleeding of neovascular tissue). A large macular haemorrhage can sometimes be moved away from the macular with recombinant tissue plasminogen activator (rTPA), intravitreal gas, and posturing

Complications of the treatment
Injection related complications
- Sore eye for 24 hours (corneal exposure, irritation from local anaesthetic and/or antiseptic)
- Subconjunctival haemorrhage
- Intravitreal haemorrhage (1:1000)
- Intravitreal infection (endophthalmitis – 1:1000)
- Mild increase in risk of myocardial infarction or cerebrovascular accidents as compared to controls

Further reading

National Institute for Health and Care Excellence (NICE) guidance for AMD – updated January 2018; https://www.nice.org.uk/guidance/ng82

Related topics of interest

- Retinal imaging (p. 277)
- Intravitreal injection therapies (p. 193)

2 Angle closure glaucoma

Key points
- Glaucoma is the leading cause of irreversible blindness worldwide
- Population surveys suggest that untreated angle-closure glaucoma blinds about half those affected
- Most angle closure cases are not symptomatic in the initial stages
- Acute angle closure is an ophthalmic emergency requiring immediate treatment

Epidemiology

Glaucoma is the world's commonest cause of irreversible blindness, currently affecting 60 million people with 8.4 million blind, and projected to rise to 80 million by 2020 with 11.2 million blind.

Recent evidence estimates primary angle closure glaucoma (PACG) prevalence in European derived populations as being 130,000 people in the UK, 1.60 million people in Europe, and 581,000 people in the USA. The prevalence of PACG in those 40 years or more is 0.4%. Three quarters of all cases occur in female subjects.

Risk factors for angle closure include increasing age, female gender, certain ethnic groups (e.g. Inuits and East Asians), shallow anterior chamber depth, shorter axial length, and more recently genetic factors have been identified.

Pathophysiology

There are four potential mechanisms that can lead to narrowing of the angle and angle closure:
- *Pupil-block:*
  - This is the most common mechanism by which angle closure occurs. In certain lighting condition, pupillary mydriasis results in contact between the iris and the lens at the pupillary margin, such that aqueous flow to the anterior chamber is block, whilst at the same time the increased pressure behind the iris causes further forward movement in peripheral and mid peripheral iris resulting in more iridotrabecular contact and outflow restriction
- *Peripheral iris crowding (e.g. plateau iris syndrome):*
  - In this condition, the short iris root is inserted anteriorly on the ciliary face, resulting in the anterior displacement of the peripheral iris into the angle
- *Lens-induced:*
  - This group of conditions is associated with mature cataracts, sudden swelling of the lens or anterior subluxation of lens secondary from trauma or other causes of disruption in normal zonular attachments
- *Retro-lenticular causes:*
  - The mechanism in this subgroup is often multifactorial. Some conditions associated with this mechanism include previous scleral buckling, posterior scleritis, aqueous misdirection following surgery, e.g. trabeculectomy, cataract surgery, uveal effusion, and intraocular tumours

Certain drugs and pharmacological agents and environmental factors have been linked to the development of angle closure in susceptible patients. These include, but are not limited to:
- Agents with sympathomimetic activity, e.g. β_2-agonists such as salbutamol; α-agonists such as phenylephrine, and nasal decongestants such as phenylpropanolamine and cocaine.
- Agents with anticholinergic activity, e.g. tricyclic antidepressants such as imipramine, clomipramine, trazadone; selective serotonin reuptake inhibitors (SSRIs) such as venlafaxine, paroxetine, citalopram, and muscarinic antagonists such as oxybutynin, atropine, botulinum toxin A, and tropicamide
- Other drug classes (idiosyncratic reactions): Antihistamines, e.g. promethazine; amphetamines, e.g.

ecstasy; sulpha-containing drugs, e.g. sulphamethoxazole, trimethoprim, acetazolamide; thiazide diuretic, e.g. hydrochlorothiazide; antiepileptic, e.g. topiramate; and antidepressant, e.g. escitalopram.

Clinical features

Most cases of narrow angles are asymptomatic. A recent survey examining the frequency of symptoms associated with primary angle closure in an East Asian population with high rates of disease found that symptoms of visual disturbance and ocular pain traditionally linked with angle closure were reported frequently by both normal and potentially affected people. Intermittent blurring of vision at night was the only common symptom of angle closure that was significantly more frequent in people with narrow angles and peripheral anterior synechiae. However, patients who are in acute angle closure often present with blurred vision, severe eye pain/headache, the appearance of rainbow coloured circles around light, nausea and vomiting, and potentially sudden loss of vision. The clinical features and classifications, differ depending on whether angle closure is primary or secondary.

Based on clinical features, primary angle closure is classified into three categories which also describe the evolution of the condition:

1. *Primary angle closure suspect:* This is where there is at least 180 degrees of appositional contact between the peripheral iris and posteior trabecular meshwork; Acute Angle closure is considered possible.
2. *Primary angle closure (PAC):* This stage describes an occludable drainage angle in the presence of features indicating that trabecular obstruction by the peripheral iris has occurred, these include peripheral anterior synechiae, elevated intraocular pressure, iris whorling (distortion of the radially orientated iris fibres), 'glaucomflecken' lens opacities, or excessive pigment deposition on the trabecular surface. However, the optic disc does not have glaucomatous damage at this stage.
3. *Primary angle closure glaucoma (PACG):* In this subgroup, there are features of PAC as described above, together with evidence of glaucomatous optic neuropathy.

Investigations

Van herick

This is a rapid, non-contact screening method aimed at identifying those at high risk of angle closure. A very fine bright beam of light to be shone on the temporal limbus giving an optical cross-section of the most peripheral part of the cornea where an estimate the depth of the limbal corneal depth as a percentage/fraction of peripheral corneal thickness is made.

Gonioscopy

This is currently the reference gold standard for assessment of the angle. The examination is performed in low ambient lighting ensuring that the slit lamp beam is kept away from the centre of the pupil. Both dynamic and static gonioscopy should be carried out and the findings are carefully recorded (see classification systems later).

Angle imaging

The two most widely used angle imaging devices are ultrasound biomicroscopy (UBM) and anterior segment OCT (AS-OCT), which provide a useful objective complementary record to clinical findings, particularly in cases where an atypical mechanism is suspected.

Central anterior chamber depth measurement

Measurement of central AC depth is useful when planning cataract surgery, particularly in risk stratification.

Diagnosis

Unlike an acute angle closure case where a sudden rise in intraocular pressure (IOP) results in severe acute symptoms of blurred vision, a red painful eye, corneal oedema, raised IOP, mid-dilated pupil, and potentially glaucomatous optic neuropathy, most patients with primary angle closure are asymptomatic. Diagnosis is based on the history and clinical examination with key components being assessment of anterior chamber angle using static and dynamic gonioscopy (in low ambient lighting), intraocular pressure, and fundoscopy.

There are several angle grading systems used to describe the angle including Scheie classification which was originally described in 1957, based on visible angle structures (**Table 2.1**), the Shaffer system which was originally described in 1960, based on angular width of the angle recess (**Table 2.2**), and the Spaeth grading, the most comprehensive, which was originally described in 1970, based on evaluating iris insertion, angular approach, peripheral iris configuration, and degree of trabecular meshwork pigmentation (**Table 2.3**).

Treatment

Acute angle closure glaucoma is an ophthalmic emergency requiring immediate treatment. Whilst the majority of cases are due to pupil block, it is important to fully assess the patient, given that in non-pupil-block cases, the immediate treatment will vary according to the underlying cause. The principles of management involve breaking the attack [systemic (e.g. acetazolamide) and topical (antihypertensives /pilocarpine) medication], iridoplasty or cyclodiode laser if required, and once this is achieved, the next step is prevention of further attacks (e.g. iridotomies/lens extraction), and detection and treatment optic disc and visual field damage (regular follow-up).

Medical treatment

Pilocarpine which causes pupil constriction and hence opening the angle by pulling the peripheral iris away from the angle is used in acute angle closure and as a pretreatment agent when performing an iridotomy. Topical and systemic antihypertensive can also play a role in the treatment of angle closure.

Laser iridotomy

This is the procedure where using laser, a full thickness hole in the peripheral iris is made. This is usually done using Nd:YAG laser (using single pulse, well targeted, low-energy

Table 2.1 Scheie classification of angle grading

Scheie classification	
Wide open	All structures visible
Grade I	Iris root not visible
Grade II	Angle apex not visible
Grade III	Posterior ½ trabecular meshwork obscured
Grade IV	No angle structures visible

Table 2.2 Shaffer system of angle grading

Shaffer system	
Grade 4	35° to 45° (wide open)
Grade 3	20° to 35° angle (wide open)
Grade 2	20° angle (narrow)
Grade 1	≤10° angle (extremely narrow)
Grade 0	0° angle (closed)

Table 2.3 Spaeth system of angle grading

Spaeth angle grading system					
Iris insertion	Angular approach	Curvature of peripheral iris		Pigmentation of trabecular meshwork	
A (Anterior to Schwalbe's Line) B (Between the Schwalbe's line and scleral spur) C (Scleral spur visible) D (Deep ciliary body visible) E (Extremely deep with > 1 mm of ciliary body visible)	0° to 40°	r (regular) s (steep) q (queer)	f (flat) b (bowed anteriorly) p (plateau iris) c (concave)	(0) no pigment (1+) minimal (2+) mild (3+) moderate (4+) intense	

shots). In patients where the iris is thick (e.g. Africans, Chinese), it is helpful to use Argon laser to pre-treat the area (two stage procedure) before using Nd:YAG to create a full thickness opening in the iris. In patients where a lot of laser energy use is anticipated, it may be better to perform a surgical iridectomy.

Iridoplasty

This procedure invloves applying argon laser burns to the peripheral iris causing it to contract away from the trabecular meshwork and, therefore, opening the angle. Whilst at one time, it was a treatment of choice in plateau iris patients where the angle remained occludable following iridotomy, it is generally not commonly performed for this indication. It is, however, more commonly used in cases of angle closure to break the attack.

Lens extraction

By deepening the anterior chamber angle, cataract extraction has a therapeutic effect on these cases. A recent randomised control trial (EAGLE study) comparing lens extraction versus peripheral iridotomy found that in selected cases particularly in those with angle-closure and intraocular pressure of > 30 or in those presenting with glaucomatous optic neuropathy, lens extraction had greater efficacy (better clinical and patient-reported outcomes) and was more cost effective as first line treatment.

Complications

Whilst primary angle closure glaucoma accounts for a smaller proportion (around a fourth) of all primary glaucoma cases compared with primary open angle glaucoma, it is generally more severe and the numbers of those blind from each of these conditions are almost equal. It is important that the condition is recognised and treated promptly (according to disease stage) if the blinding impact of angle closure is to be reduced.

Further reading

Azuara-Blanco A, Burr J, Ramsay C, et al. EAGLE study group. Effectiveness of early lens extraction for the treatment of primary angle-closure glaucoma (EAGLE): a randomised controlled trial. Lancet 2016; 388:1389–1397.

Foster PJ, Buhrmann R, Quigley HA, et al. The definition and classification of glaucoma in prevalence surveys. Br J Ophthalmol 2002; 86:238–242.

Tello C, Tran HV, Liebmann J, et al. Angle closure: classification, concepts, and the role of ultrasound biomicroscopy in diagnosis and treatment. Semin Ophthalmol 2002; 17:69–78.

Related topics of interest

- Glaucoma – inflammatory (p. 159)
- Glaucoma – medical management (p. 162)

3 Anisocoria

Key points

- Anisocoria can be a normal physiological finding in up to 20% of the population
- Slit lamp examination is necessary to exclude localised conditions of the anterior chamber and iris
- Reduced visual acuity, ptosis or diplopia are red flags when accompanying anisocoria
- Prompt diagnosis is essential as anisocoria can be indicative of serious, potentially life-threatening pathology

Epidemiology

Anisocoria is a term used to denote unequal sized pupils with a difference of > 0.4 mm. Anisocoria can be a normal physiological finding in up to 20% of the population. The size difference in physiological anisocoria is generally < 1 mm and the difference remains unchanged in light and dark conditions. Anisocoria that fluctuates with lighting conditions or is associated with ptosis can be indicative of life-threatening pathology including impending carotid dissection or expanding intracranial aneurysm. Knowledge and understanding of the autonomic supply to the iris is essential when assessing anisocoria and can allow localisation of a potential lesion based on history and clinical examination alone.

Pathophysiology

Anisocoria can arise from congenital and acquired causes (**Table 3.1**). Mechanisms include:

Local causes

- *Iris trauma*: Blunt trauma to the globe can result in rupture of the iris sphincter and traumatic mydriasis. This dilatation can often persist long term. Blunt trauma can also result in iridodialysis where a segment of the iris is detached from its root. In cases of globe rupture it is possible for uveal tissue to be expulsed with variable amount of iris loss. In such cases iris implants may be used which would also give the appearance of anisocoria
- *Iris inflammation*: Persistent or severe anterior uveitis can result in posterior synechiae formation and a miosed irregular pupil that dilates poorly. This can be segmental or 360° resulting in iris bombe. In cases of herpetic uveitis patients can develop iris atrophy, the

Table 3.1 Causes of anisocoria

Benign	Physiological
Congenital	Horner's syndrome
	Coloboma
	Ectopia lentis et pupillae
	Axenfeld-Rieger syndrome
	Persistent pupillary membrane
	Microcoria
	Congenital mydriasis
	Aniridia
Iatrogenic	Iris hooks
	Malyugin ring
	Phaco trauma
	Iris prolapse
	Urrets-Zavalia syndrome
Iris Pathology	Posterior synechiae
	Iris atrophy
	ICE syndrome
	Traumatic mydriasis
	AACG
	Rubeosis
	Tumour (Iris or ciliary body)
Pharmacological	Sympathomimetics
	Parasympathomimetics
Neurological	
Sympathetic	Horner's syndrome
	Benign episodic unilateral mydriasis
Parasympatheti	Third nerve palsy
	Adie's pupil

ICE, iridocorneal endothelial; AACG, acute angle closure glaucoma

appearance of which is often sectorial with iris transilluminations
- *Acute angle closure glaucoma (AACG)*: This can result in a fixed, mid-dilated pupil that is unresponsive. Raised pressure can quickly result in iris atrophy and the pupil may remain irregular in appearance. Rubeotic glaucoma can result in a similar appearance with a heavily vascularised iris
- *Iatrogenic*: The use of iris hooks during cataract surgery may result in an irregular pupillary appearance different to that of the fellow eye. Artisan intraocular lenses (IOL's) may also cause mechanical anisocoria. Urrets-Zavalia syndrome is a fixed dilated pupil following penetrating keratoplasty
- *Iris coloboma*: Inferior in location as a result of failed closure of the embryonic fissure
- *Iridocorneal endothelial (ICE) syndrome*: Three separate clinical sub-types arising from abnormal corneal endothelium which is migratory. This can result in varying degrees of unilateral iris atrophy, corectopia and pseudopolycoria. ICE can be differentiated from Axenfeld-Rieger syndrome with the latter being bilateral and hereditary

Neurological causes

- *Third cranial nerve palsy*: The third cranial nerve innervates the medial, inferior and superior recti, along with the inferior oblique and levator palpaebrae superioris. It also contributes para-sympathetic innervation to the constrictor pupillae. A third nerve palsy therefore classically results in a 'down and out eye', with a ptosis and dilated pupil. The anisocoria being more prominent in bright conditions. The term 'pupil involving' third nerve palsy is in reference to the fact that the pupillomotor fibres are most superficial in the nerve and therefore more prone to compression indicating a surgical cause, whereas a 'pupil sparing' third nerve palsy is more likely to be of microvascular origin. An important anatomical relationship is with that of the posterior communicating artery (PCA) to which it runs in close proximity. Berry aneurysms at the junction of the PCA and internal carotid artery are therefore an important cause of third nerve palsy. A painful pupil involving third nerve palsy is an aneurysm until proven otherwise
- *Aberrant regeneration and cranial nerve dysinnervation disorders*:
  - Adie's tonic pupil is thought to arise from aberrant regeneration of para-sympathetic fibres to the iris following a viral insult. The result is a dilated (tonic) pupil, which reacts poorly to light and exhibits classical vermiform movement as seen on slit lamp examination. Long standing Adie's can result in a miotic pupil
  - Following a third nerve palsy, synkinesis can occur which may result in miosis on adduction. The pupils may be equal in primary position but often react poorly to light (pseudo-Argyll Robertson)
- *Pharmacological*: It is important to take a full history for potential exposure to drug products. This could be accidental, e.g. nursing staff or caregivers administering treatment to a patient and accidentally cross contaminating. Illicit drug use also needs to be excluded
- *Benign episodic unilateral mydriasis (BEUM)*: This can be associated with migraine and thought to be a result of sympathetic overaction
- *Horner's syndrome*: Postganglionic sympathetic neurons innervate the dilator pupillae via the long cilary nerves. A lesion at any point along the sympathetic pathway, however, can result in Horner's syndrome. Characteristically there is a miosed pupil and slight ptosis. The anisocoria is most obvious in dim conditions. Knowledge of the anatomy is essential to aid focused history taking and guide examination. A painful Horner's syndrome is a carotid dissection until proven otherwise and requires prompt investigation and treatment. Congenital Horner's has the same features with the addition of iris heterochromia ipsilateral to the side of the lesion
- *Neurosyphilis*: Tertiary syphilis can cause an Argyll Robertson pupil. This is a miosed pupil that accommodates but doesn't

exhibit a light response. This is known as light-near dissociation of which there are a number of causes
- It is important to note that a Marcus Gunn pupil (relative afferent pupillary defect) should not result in anisocoria

Clinical features

A proportion of patients with anisocoria will be asymptomatic and detected incidentally. Vision can be normal, they may however complain of visual aberrations depending on the degree of dilation or constriction. The presence of reduced visual acuity in the setting of anisocoria should be a red flag.

It is important to determine whether the patient's symptoms and anisocoria are worse in dim conditions, bright conditions or remain constant. This information can help determine which is the abnormal pupil and narrow down the diagnosis (**Figure 3.1**).

A third cranial nerve palsy would typically present with sudden onset diplopia and drooping of the ipsilateral eyelid, with or without pain. The presence of pain in this scenario should raise suspicion of an intracranial aneurysm.

Horner's syndrome may be asymptomatic or may present with subtle drooping of the eyelid and anhidrosis on the ipsilateral side of the face. The presence of pain in this scenario could indicate carotid dissection.

Investigations

History taking

This is an essential component in the assessment of a patient with anisocoria. The history of presenting complaint should be detailed including duration of onset, when is it most prominent and any associated symptoms particularly headaches or any other focal neurology. Systemic review is also essential, e.g. respiratory symptoms in suspected Horner's syndrome. It can be useful to look at old photos at this stage for comparison.

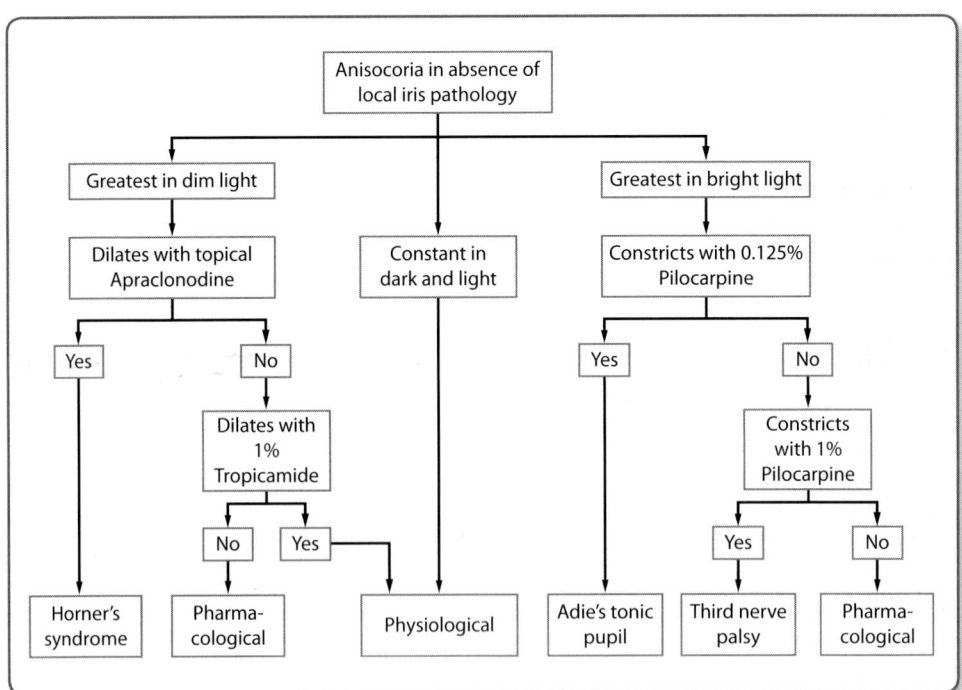

Figure 3.1 Flowchart demonstrating causes of anisocoria in the absence of localised iris pathology.

Slit lamp examination

This can be important for identifying clues as to the diagnosis. Including and not limited to, iris heterochromia, posterior synechiae, vermiform movements, iris atrophy and raised intraocular pressure.

Pharmacological tests

Dilated pupil

- Instill 0.125% pilocarpine. This can be reconstituted from 2% pilocarpine and normal saline. If the pupil constricts this is a hypersensitised Adie's pupil. If there is no response
- Instill 1% or 2% pilocarpine. If the pupil constricts this is a third nerve palsy. If there is no response
- This is a pharmacological dilation

Constricted pupil

- Iopidine 1% (apraclonidine) and cocaine 10% are useful for diagnosing a Horner's pupil. Iopidine is more readily available in most eye clinics. Dilation with Iopidine would suggest a Horner's pupil. Conversely, failure to dilate with cocaine would suggest a Horner's pupil
- Failure to dilate with 1% tropicamide is suggestive of a pharmacological constriction

Imaging

Neuroimaging plays an important role in the diagnosis and treatment of anisocoria.

If a painful Horner's syndrome or third nerve palsy is suspected then immediate discussion with a radiologist and medical/neurosurgical specialist should be sought to determine the most appropriate course of action. Usually a MRA or CTA head (+/- CT neck & thorax for Horner's syndrome) are required.

Treatment

The treatment for anisocoria is dependent on the aetiology. The primary role of the ophthalmologist is to diagnose and differentiate between local and systemic causes. Third nerve palsy and Horner's syndrome may need urgent referral to medical or neurosurgical colleagues for further investigation and emergency treatment.

Visual aberrations associated with anisocoria can be treated with medical therapy if necessary. Topical pilocarpine can be used for a troublesome dilated pupil. Sympathomimetics can be used for a constricted pupil. Brimonidine has been shown to be of use in treating anisocoria associated with Horner's syndrome.

Complications

Anisocoria and ptosis can often be subtle and easily missed. A low threshold of suspicion is necessary as this can be indicative of life-threatening pathology, most notably posterior communicating artery aneurysm or carotid artery dissection.

Further reading

Bruce BB, Biousse V, Newman NJ. Third nerve palsies. Semin Neurol 2007; 27:257–268.

Davagnanam I, Fraser CL, Miszkiel K, Daniel CS, Plant GT. Adult Horner's syndrome: a combined clinical, pharmacological, and imaging algorithm. Eye (Lond) 2013; 27:291–298.

Keane JR. Third nerve palsy: analysis of 1400 personally-examined inpatients. Can J Neurol Sci 2010; 37:662–670.

McDougal D, Gamlin P. Autonomic control of the eye. Compr Physiol 2015; 5:439–473.

Related topics of interest

- Cranial nerve palsies – multiple cranial nerves palsies (p. 104)

4 Anterior uveitis

Key points
- Occurs due to inflammation of the ciliary body and iris
- Characterised by recurrent attacks of pain, photophobia and a red eye
- Multiple different possible causes but 80% will remain idiopathic after investigation
- Must be differentiated from more serious infectious uveitis of the posterior segment with a dilated fundal examination

Epidemiology

Uveitis is an uncommon condition with an incidence of around 12 in 1000,000. Men and women are affected equally although the disease has been reported to be more severe in males. Uveitis can develop at any age but is most common in those aged over 20 years.

Risk factors

Most cases remain idiopathic with no cause found, however the human leucocyte antigen (HLA) B27 variant, which is present in up to 8% of the population, is found in up to 20–50% of uveitis cases so is a known genetic risk factor. The most common identifiable causation is an underlying disease which affects the immune system and predisposes to the dysregulation seen as part of the pathophysiology.

Pathophysiology

It is believed that an external antigen sets off the immune system which then reacts to the ocular tissues due to genetic and environmental risk factors which have sensitised it. While the initiating event is not fully understood we have evidence that the activated immune system, through T-lymphocytes and macrophages, leads to localised inflammation in the uveal tissue that breaks down the blood-ocular barrier. White blood cells and protein pass into the anterior chamber and lead to the clinical signs described below.

Although most remain idiopathic there are many cases where a source of antigen can be discovered, and these are divided into infectious and non-infectious causes.
- Non-infectious:
  - Seronegative spondyloarthropathies associated with HLA-B27 (ankylosing spondyloarthritis, psoriatic arthritis, reactive arthritis and inflammatory bowel disease associated)
  - Juvenile idiopathic arthritis (JIA)
  - Sarcoidosis
  - Behçet's disease
  - Localised ocular causes including trauma and hypermature cataracts
  - Specific syndromes – Fuchs' heterochromic cyclitis
- Infectious:
  - Bacterial – Syphilis, Lyme disease, tuberculosis
  - Viral – Herpesvirus family, Ebola virus
  - Fungal – Microsporidia

Clinical features

Symptoms

Inflammation in any organ is associated with pain and when the principle affected tissue is the muscles in ciliary body and iris, this produces aching pain on pupillary constriction and accommodation. This manifests as visual blurring, photophobia and pain on near focusing such as reading.

Examination

The affected eye will be red with a characteristic vasodilation around the limbus called ciliary flush. The characteristic signs of anterior uveitis are keratic precipitates (KP) and cells in the anterior chamber (AC) – the presence and amount of which are often used to grade severity and assess response to treatment. Keratic precipitates are deposits of inflammatory material and cells on the corneal endothelium. These can be small (dusting) or large and greasy (mutton-fat) KP. The same inflammatory material congregates and floats in the AC as cells and flare which is the proteinaceous element. These can be counted and graded using an angled 1 by 1 mm bright slit lamp beam (see **Tables 4.1** and **4.2**).

The pupil may be miosed due to a spasming painful pupillary constrictor muscle and may be adherent to the anterior lens capsule called posterior synechiae. If these posterior synechiae seal off the pupil in 360° then iris bombe may develop and cause angle closure and acute glaucoma. The iris may also show granulomatous nodules at the pupillary margin called Koeppe's nodules or present in the ciliary zone called Busacca's nodules. Intraocular pressure may be high due to bombe or inflammatory adhesions between the iris and trabecular meshwork, but conversely may be low due to reduced aqueous production. The fundus must be examined with a dilated examination to exclude posterior uveitis presenting with anterior signs.

Investigations

Given most cases are idiopathic, the majority of investigations performed for anterior uveitis will be normal or negative. They should therefore be targeted and restricted to cases which are recurrent, bilateral, granulomatous or have associated systemic signs or symptoms.

A good history is essential to tailor your investigations according to systemic symptoms, e.g. of rheumatic back pain for HLA-B27 or chronic cough for sarcoid. A history of tuberculosis (TB) exposure will lead you to TB testing and intravenous drug use to HIV testing.

Initial investigations

- Blood testing – full blood count (FBC), urea and electrolytes, treponemal (syphilis) serology
- Chest X-ray – sarcoid and tuberculosis
- Urinalysis – looking for blood and protein
- Optical coherence tomography (OCT) – may be normal or show cystoid macula oedema

Targeted investigations

Based on results of the initial investigations/suspicions:
- Tuberculosis testing – Mantoux skin testing or interferon-gamma (IFN-γ)release assay on blood
- Serology for HIV, Lyme disease
- HLA-B27 testing for seronegative spondyloarthropathies
- Further testing under medical physicians including sarcoid specific imaging, etc.

Diagnosis

Anterior uveitis has characteristic symptoms and signs which make diagnosis relatively easy. The skill comes in ensuring there is no other secondary cause or deeper inflammation and then deciding which cases to investigate to rule out causes as described above. Anterior uveitis can be classified in many different ways; non-granulomatous or granulomatous (mutton-fat KPs, iris nodules), acute or chronic (lasting > 3 months) and infectious or non-infectious based on the causes.

Differential diagnosis

- Conjunctivitis
- Keratitis
- Episcleritis
- Scleritis

Table 4.1 SUN classification for grading anterior chamber cells – count the cells	
0	–
1–5	+/–
6–15	+
16–25	++
26–50	+++
>50	++++

Table 4.2 SUN classification for grading anterior chamber flare – degree of blur when examining the iris	
None	–
Hardly any	+
Definite blur but still clear iris detail	++
Obvious blur and iris details hazy	+++
Fibrinous flare	++++

- Posterior, panuveitis or endophthalmitis (examine the whole eye and beware severe postoperative inflammation)
- Pigment dispersion syndrome (referred from optometry with iris transillumination, Krukenberg's spindle looking like KP)

Treatment
Treat the inflammation and pain
- Topical corticosteroids – start with intensive treatment and taper down over several weeks. Hourly dexamethasone 0.1% drops applied day and night should be reduced to 2 hourly then 6 times a day, 5 times a day etcetera. Steroid ointments can be used at night as an alternative but are not as effective as waking to put in the drop in the initial stage
- Cycloplegic agents – paralyse the spasming muscles relieving pain but blurring vision, e.g. cyclopentolate 1% given 3 times a day
- Very severe or resistant cases may require steroid injected either sub-conjunctivally or periocular

Prevent complications
- Cycloplegia also dilates the pupil and can prevent posterior synechiae formation
- Drops to lower intraocular pressure
- Taper the drops over time to prevent secondary iatrogenic complications of steroid use such as ocular hypertension or cataract formation

Complications
With the correct use of treatment these complications are less likely but include posterior synechiae and iris bombe, cataract, cystoid macula oedema and band keratopathy.

Glaucoma and uveitis are common partners due to multiple causes including iatrogenic steroid response, synechial angle closure, physical blockage of the trabecular meshwork with cells and iris bombe.

Prognosis for vision is good when chronic anterior uveitis doesn't develop but certain categories of disease such as JIA associated uveitis have a worse prognosis with a quarter developing severe visual loss.

Further reading
Williams GS, Westcott M (Eds). Practical Uveitis: Understanding the Grape. Taylor and Francis; 2017.

Related topics of interest
- Intermediate uveitis (p. 185)
- Posterior uveitis (p. 259)
- Retinal vasculitis (p. 286)

5 Benign lid lesions

Key points
- Benign lid lesions may arise from any cell type within the lid and may present in patients of all ages
- Histological analysis should be considered for lesions with atypical or concerning features such as lash loss, bleeding, and recurrence following prior excision
- Some benign tumours are associated with systemic conditions requiring further investigation

Introduction

Benign lid lesions may arise from any cell type within the eyelid and may be classified according to whether they are of epidermal, adnexal or stromal origin. This chapter will focus on the most common benign lid lesions arising from the epithelium, sebaceous glands, and vasculature of the lids.

Epidemiology

Benign lid lesions may present at any age and affect people of all ethnicities. The majority result from an isolated cause, but some may be associated with systemic or other localised disease. Vascular malformations causing benign lid lesions such as capillary haemangioma present within the first few years of life, whereas epithelial lesions such as seborrheic keratosis are often related to degenerative changes and ultraviolet (UV) exposure, and therefore occur later in life. Chalazia, which are of meibomian gland origin, may develop in patients with lid margin disease.

Pathophysiology

Seborrhoeic keratosis and keratoacanthoma are lesions of epithelial origin resulting from degenerative changes, often in the context of UV exposure. Squamous papillomata tend to be viral in origin and have been associated with human papillomavirus types 6 and 11, although other subtypes may also cause papilloma.

Chalazia result from a chronic granulomatous inflammatory reaction to retained material in a blocked meibomian gland. Secondary infection and acute inflammation may develop and, if untreated, may progress to cause preseptal cellulitis. The most common causative organism for this is *Staphylococcus aureus*.

The most common benign vascular lesion of the eyelid is capillary haemangioma, often called "strawberry naevus" when superficial. These develop within the first few months of life, may have an initial rapid growth in the first year followed by slower growth phase over 2–4 years with gradual involution thereafter.

Clinical features

Seborrhoeic keratoses are clearly demarcated, warty, flat lesions with variable pigmentation, and classically have a "stuck on" appearance (**Figure 5.1**). Patients will often have multiple seborrhoeic keratoses across the head, neck, and torso, but they may also present as a single lesion. The defining feature of keratoacanthoma is a central keratin horn or plaque. They are isolated lesions which grow rapidly in the initial stage. Squamous papilloma may be single or multiple lesions, which may be sessile or pedunculated (**Figure 5.2**). When a viral papilloma affects the lower lid margin, the corresponding area of the upper lid should be carefully examined to assess for a "kissing lesion".

Chalazia are well-defined, nontender, firm swellings along the lid margin, may be single or multiple, and affect any of the lids. They may be seen to be "pointing" to the lid margin and patients may report fluctuations in size with discharge from the lesion. When infected, they become tender, erythematous, and may enlarge in size. Examination of the lids and surrounding skin often reveals associated blepharitis or rosacea.

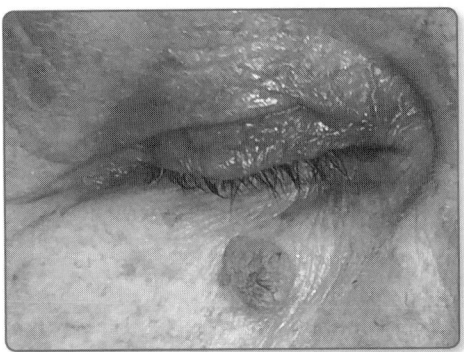

Figure 5.1 Seborrhoeic keratoses.

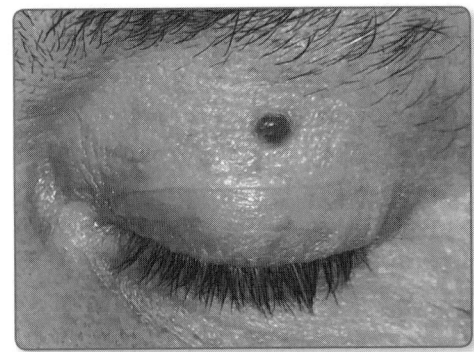

Figure 5.3 Superficial capillary haemangioma.

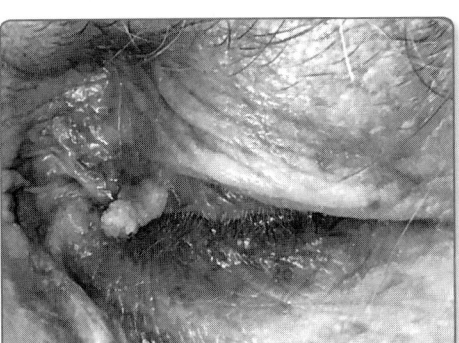

Figure 5.2 Squamous papilloma.

Superficial capillary haemangioma are well-demarcated, bright red lesions which blanch with pressure (**Figure 5.3**). They vary greatly in size and, if large, may cause ptosis or affect the visual axis such that there is a risk of amblyopia. Naevus flammeus (port-wine stain) are deeper red-purple lesions which do not blanch with pressure. They are large, unilateral, and may be associated with leptomeningeal angioma and glaucoma when part of Sturge–Weber syndrome. Varices or "venous lakes" are superficial venous dilations which display postural variation in size and enlarge on Valsalva manoeuvre.

Diagnosis

The diagnosis of benign lid lesions is primarily based on clinical history and examination. For confirmation of the diagnosis of epithelial and sebaceous gland lesions, histological testing is sometimes required. This is usually only necessary for lesions with atypical or concerning features, such as lash loss, ulceration, bleeding, or lesions which recur in the same location following excision or incision and curettage in the case of chalazia. It should be noted that a small proportion of lesions that are clinically considered benign, even in experienced hands, may be malignant. Therefore if any clinical doubt exists, diagnostic biopsy and histological analysis should be performed. Patients diagnosed with benign lesions should be advised to re-present if the lesion changes in character. If periocular lesions are excised, it is recommended all samples be sent for histological analysis.

Keratoacanthoma should be excised and sent for histological analysis as they are difficult to distinguish clinically from squamous cell carcinoma.

Investigations

Investigations are typically unnecessary for known benign lid lesions. Some lesions raise the suspicion of other associated or underlying conditions for which radiological or genetic testing may be required. If there is concern regarding the depth and flow of vascular lesions, then ultrasound with appropriate blood flow assessment may be useful. Computed tomography (CT) or magnetic resonance imaging (MRI)

Benign lid lesions

Table 5.1 Benign lid lesions. *Continues overleaf*

Lesion	Pathophysiology	Clinical features	Treatment
Acrochordon (squamous papilloma or fibroepithelial polyp)	Benign epithelial papilloma	Single or multiple, sessile or pedunculated soft lesions of variable size	Shave biopsy Excision
Chalazion	Chronic granulomatous inflammation of blocked meibomian or Zeis gland	Solid painless nodule within tarsal plate, may discharge spontaneously Usually associated with blepharitis or rosacea May become acutely inflamed	Hot compresses and lid hygiene Incision and curettage Intralesional triamcinolone Topical or oral antibiotics may be used
Epidermoid cyst	Inclusion cyst of epidermis within the dermis, usually following prior trauma but may be congenital	Smooth, firm, slow-growing lesion Does not transilluminate	Excision Marsupialisation
Apocrine hidrocystoma (cyst of Moll) or eccrine hidrocystoma	Retention cyst resulting from blockage of sweat gland duct May affect apocrine sweat glands of Moll or eccrine sweat glands	Smooth round pale non-tender cystic lesion on lid margin Does transilluminate	Excision Marsupialisation
Molluscum contagiosum	Epidermal infection with molluscum contagiosum virus	Multiple small pale nodules with umbilicated centres, more common in children and immunocompromised adults	Not usually required Excision or curettage Cryotherapy (depending on proximity to lid margin)
Pyogenic granuloma	Vascularised fibroblastic proliferation, usually following trauma	Rapidly enlarging painful vascular polypoid lesion	Excision
Syringoma	Benign adenoma of eccrine sweat gland	Multiple bilateral small hypopigmented lesions, usually on lower lids	Not usually required Excision Laser ablation
Xanthelasma	Collection of lipid-containing histiocytes within the dermis	Bilateral soft pale yellow plaques, associated with hyperlipidaemia in around 50% cases	Not usually required High recurrence rate Excision, laser or topical trichloroacetic acid
Capillary haemangioma (strawberry naevus)	Proliferation of capillaries within the dermis and subcutaneous tissues	Unilateral raised red lesion, blanches with pressure, usually on upper lid, presenting at or shortly after birth May be blue or purple if subcutaneous More common in girls than boys	Usually resolves spontaneously during childhood Treatment required if ocular or systemic complications Topical/oral beta-blockers Intralesional/systemic steroids Laser ablation Excision

Table 5.1 Continued...

Lesions	Pathophysiology	Clinical features	Treatment
Seborrheic keratosis	Basal cell papilloma	Slow-growing pigmented lesion with "stuck on" appearance and clearly defined margin, usually occur in sun-exposed areas in older patients	Not usually required Shave biopsy Cryotherapy, laser or chemical ablation (depending on proximity to lid margin)
Verruca vulgaris	Epidermal infection with human papilloma virus (usually HPV 6 or 11)	Small non-pigmented papilloma which may have elongated digitations on surface	Not usually required High recurrence rate Excision Cryotherapy (depending on proximity to lid margin)

with contrast may also be used. For facial naevus flammeus, contrast MRI with gadolinium is the first-line investigation for leptomeningeal angioma. Around half of all patients presenting with xanthelasma have hyperlipidaemia, so blood tests for this should be organised to ensure appropriate dietary and medication changes can be made to reduce the risk of other conditions associated with hyperlipidaemia.

Treatment

Treatment is only required when benign lid lesions are causing secondary problems such as mechanical changes in lid or punctal position, although other factors such as the psychological impact of lesions, particularly in children, should be taken into consideration. Removal of epithelial lesions is by shave, punch or excision biopsy. Management of chalazia is with warm compresses, massage, and lid hygiene measures. Topical antibiotics ± steroid ointments may be used, while oral tetracyclines are necessary in patients with rosacea. Incision and curettage should be reserved for chalazia that fail to respond or for those causing secondary problems.

Complications

Individuals who develop benign epithelial lesions related to UV exposure should have careful examination to ensure no other concerning lesions are present in the adnexal area. Referral to dermatology should be considered if suspicious lesions are present elsewhere on the skin.

Surgical excision or biopsy of small periocular lesions is usually uncomplicated in experienced hands; however, scarring and subsequent contracture of eyelid tissues is possible. Benign lid lesions may recur and patients should be counselled accordingly before excision.

Further reading

Hillson TR, Harvey JT, Hurwitz JJ, et al. Sensitivity and specificity of the diagnosis of periocular lesions by oculoplastic surgeons. Can J Ophthalmol 1998; 33:377–383.

Kanski J, Bowling B. Kanski's Clinical Ophthalmology, 8th edition. Amsterdam, Netherlands: Elsevier; 2016:1–62.

Lenci LT, Kirkpatrick CA, Clark TJ, et al. Benign Lesions of the External Periocular Tissues: A Tutorial, 2007. [online] Available from http://EyeRounds.org/tutorials/benign-lid-lesions/index.htm [Last accessed November, 2019].

Mohite AA, Johnson A, Rathore DS, et al. Accuracy of clinical diagnosis of benign eyelid lesions: is a dedicated nurse-led service safe and effective? Orbit 2016; 35:193–198.

Neff AG, Carter KD. Benign eyelid lesions. In: Yanoff M, Duker JS (Eds). Ophthalmology. 4th edition. Amsterdam, Netherlands: Elsevier; 2014;1295–1305.

The Royal College of Ophthalmologists. Periocular Basal Cell Carcinoma, 2011. [online] Available from https://www.rcophth.ac.uk/wp-content/uploads/2014/08/Focus-Winter-2011.pdf [Last accessed November, 2019].

Related topics of interest

- Chalazion (p. 63)
- Tumours – eyelid (p. 323)

6. Biometry and lens implant power calculation

Key points

- Accurate measurements are required to calculate the lens implant power to give a desired postoperative refraction
- Choice of an appropriate formula for this calculation is based on the measurements
- A sensible target is determined by patient choice, patient history and surgeon's viewpoint
- The lens model selected is based on the desired target, the availability of a model to achieve this and surgical experience with the chosen model

Introduction

Calculation of the lens implant power to replace the natural lens for any postoperative refraction requires a patient history/clinical examination and measurements including:

- Average anterior corneal curvature in two orthogonal meridians
- Ocular axial length
- Preoperative ACD (anterior corneal vertex to anterior crystalline lens surface)
- Central corneal thickness and posterior corneal curvature
- Lens thickness
- HWTW (horizontal white to white distance)
- Pupil diameter
- Refraction

Older formulae require only the first two measurements. Biometry should be repeated if a patient has undergone intervening surgery or has a condition affecting keratometry, axial length or anterior chamber depth measurements.

Corneal power

Corneal power is approximately twice that of the crystalline lens.

Tight fitting contact lenses affect corneal curvature so should be removed well in advance of biometry. Overall corneal power is usually calculated from the average anterior corneal curvature using a theoretical refractive index of 1.3375 (based on the fact that 7.5 mm curvature corresponds to 45Ds). Olsen, has suggested 1.332 is closer to true refractive index based on a lens model with 0.5 mm central corneal thickness and taking into account posterior corneal curvature.

Optical measurements

Optical interferometers are accurate and measure with ease, eyes with eccentric posterior staphyloma or with silicone oil in the vitreous. If fixation is not possible, then fellow fixation is used. In amblyopic eyes it helps to cover the fellow during measurements.

Dense opacities or excessive movements prevent measurements. A bi-lateral drop of corneal anaesthesia will reduce movement. A saline drop is useful if the tear film is poor. More viscous eye lubricants can affect curvature measurements.

In severe, ectasia or keratoconus, the corneal power is grossly overestimated by using the anterior corneal curvature measurement. An assumed corneal power (e.g. 44.4Ds) will leave the patient myopic for contact lens wear or if a corneal graft is intended. Successful grafts are usually steeper than average.

Images must be checked. **Figure 6.1a** shows an inaccurate axial length measurement taken with non-macular fixation and is 0.6mm too long. The correct measurement taken a few hours later is shown in **Figure 6.1b**. Optical axial length readings can appear artefactually short when pathology causes an abnormal reflex. An epi-retinal membrane (**Figure 6.2**) can cause a fluctuation in measurements of typically 0.2 mm.

If measurement of axial length is not possible using an optical system, the operator should use an ultrasonic technique.

Biometry and lens implant power calculation

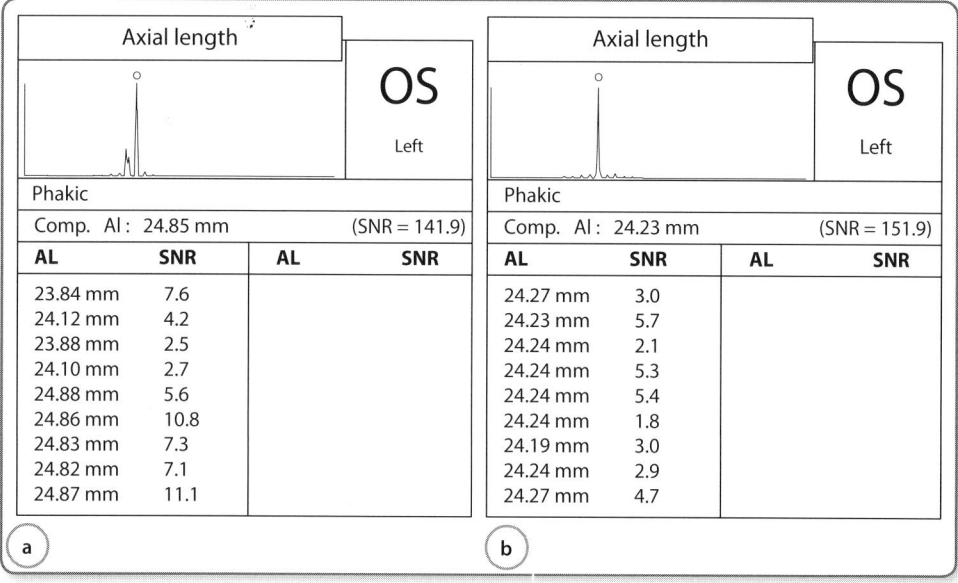

Figure 6.1 Incorrect (too long) optical measurement: Non-macular fixation – Note reflex anterior to tall spike and range of readings. Same eye as in (a) Correct measurement: Normal reflex – Macular fixation (patient asked to focus).

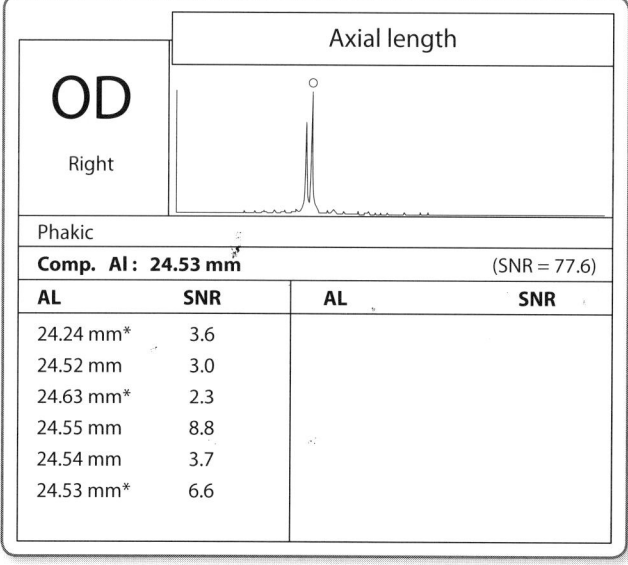

Figure 6.2 Optical measurements: Epi-retinal membrane gives rise to reflex 0.2 mm anterior to retina.

Ultrasound measurements

A-scan technique

Ultrasound A-scan is used to measure axial length in the presence of dense cataracts or, for patients who are unable to position their forehead against a support.

A small transducer, with a central embedded fixation light, emits pulses of ultrasound (typically 10 MHz). In the time

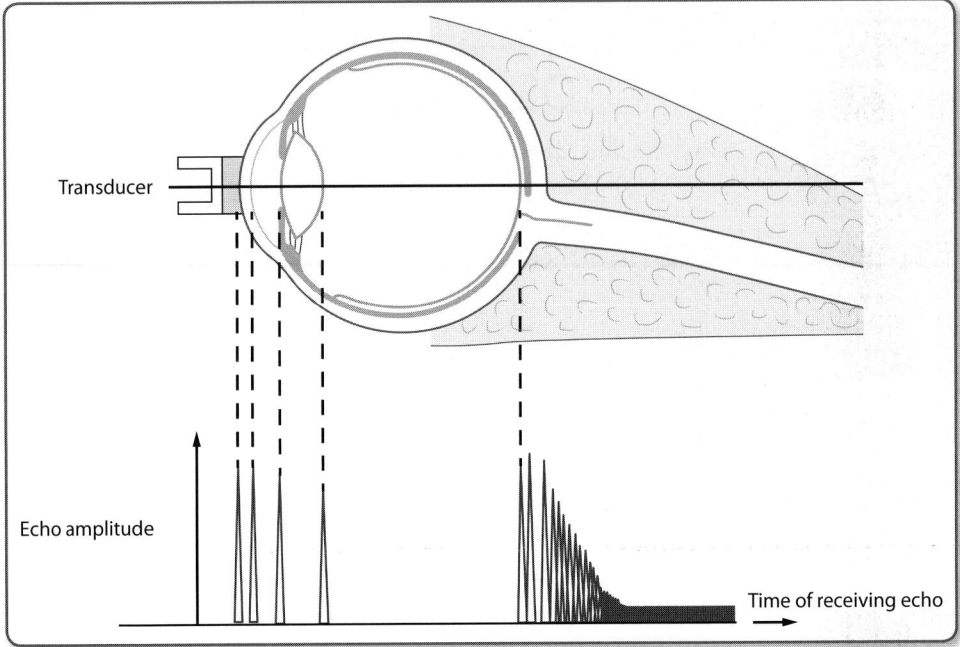

Figure 6.3 A-scan techniques.

interval between pulses, echoes received by the same transducer are converted to a display of data spikes (**Figure 6.3**). The spike height indicates the echo amplitude and their position along the X-axis the echo arrival time. Assumed velocities of ultrasound in tissue are used to convert the arrival times to distances. A-scans measure from the corneal vertex to the vitreoretinal interface.

There are two A-scan techniques, both require corneal anaesthesia:
1. Hand-held transducer: Must be coupled to the eye via a stand-off (saline or gel in a shell or bubble) to prevent indentation. Corneal reflexes help in alignment.
2. Mounted transducer (on a spring loaded assembly, e.g. tonometer head with pressure set to zero to prevent indentation): Direct contact, tear film providing couplant with saline drop if needed. Reflex of transducer light aids alignment.

Hand-held transducers should never be directly applied to the eye as indentation can be problematic (up to 0.3 mm seen by this author). Misalignment errors of the transducer with respect to the eye using either technique can be huge if the operator is careless. This author has seen a misalignment measurement 11 mm too long.

B-mode technique

B-scan measurement of axial length is used on infants or older patients who are unable to co-operate with other techniques. Central horizontal B-scans taken through a closed eyelid are shown in **Figure 6.4**. Adequate coupling gel and a light touch will prevent corneal flattening (**Figure 6.4a**). B-scans can be taken on the open eye through a liquid gel (**Figure 6.5**). B-mode measurements take approximately 1 second to obtain, inclusive of alignment time.

Calculation

Theoretical formulae are derived from Fyodorov's geometric optics formula published in 1967.

Recently authors have fine-tuned the expected lens position (ELP). Olsen's formula uses both the preoperative ACD and lens thickness to calculate ELP whereas Haigis uses a regression formula for different

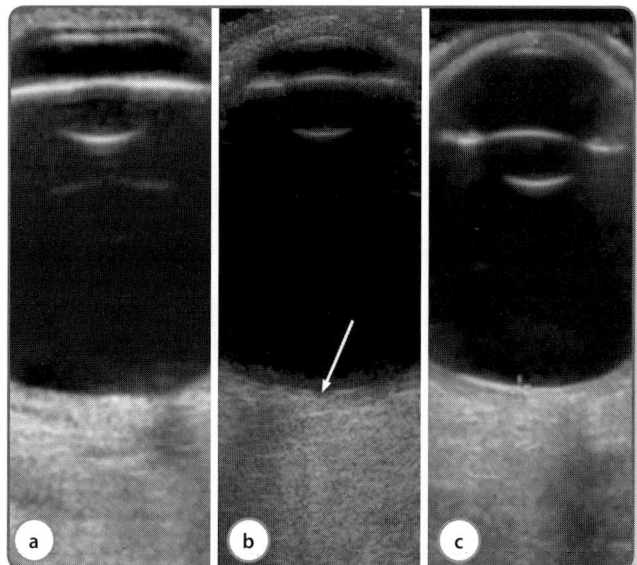

Figure 6.4 Central linear B-scans: Closed eyes (a) Intentional corneal flattening from applied pressure, (b) Foveal dip (arrow). (c) Megalocornea: High ratio of anterior chamber depth to axial length.

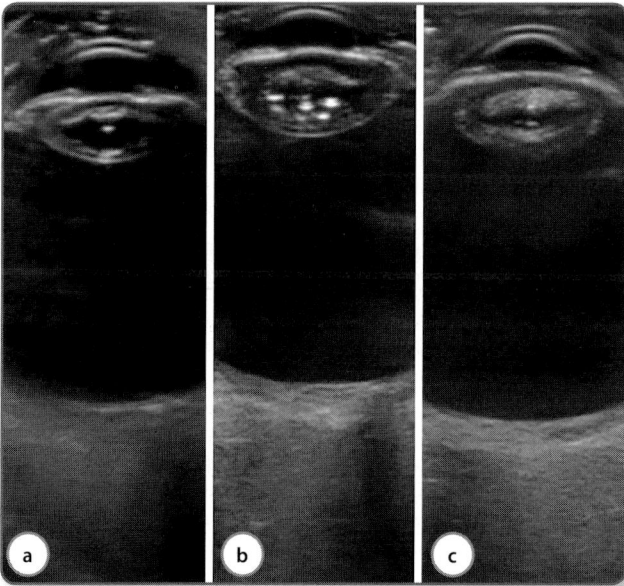

Figure 6.5 Central linear B-scans: Open eyes: anterior and posterior corneal interface echoes shown: (a) Dense cataract, (b) Dense intumescent cataract, micro-calcifications. (c) Very dense intumescent cataract.

implant models based on postoperative, world-wide data supplied from surgeons to the website ULIB. The ELP is based on the preoperative ACD, axial length and corneal power. The Holladay 2 formula also uses preoperative ACD, lens thickness preoperative refraction, HWTW, etc. to optimise ELP.

Barrett II universal formula has gained popularity and is available on-line. A choice of corneal refractive index is given of either 1.3375 or 1.332. Some A-constants for implants are listed and users are directed to the ULIB site for others.

Preussner has developed ray tracing software OKULIX which includes built-in manufacturer's data. Input of preoperative corneal topography data and AS OCT data are required (**Figure 6.6**). The software will highlight the suitability of a specific lens

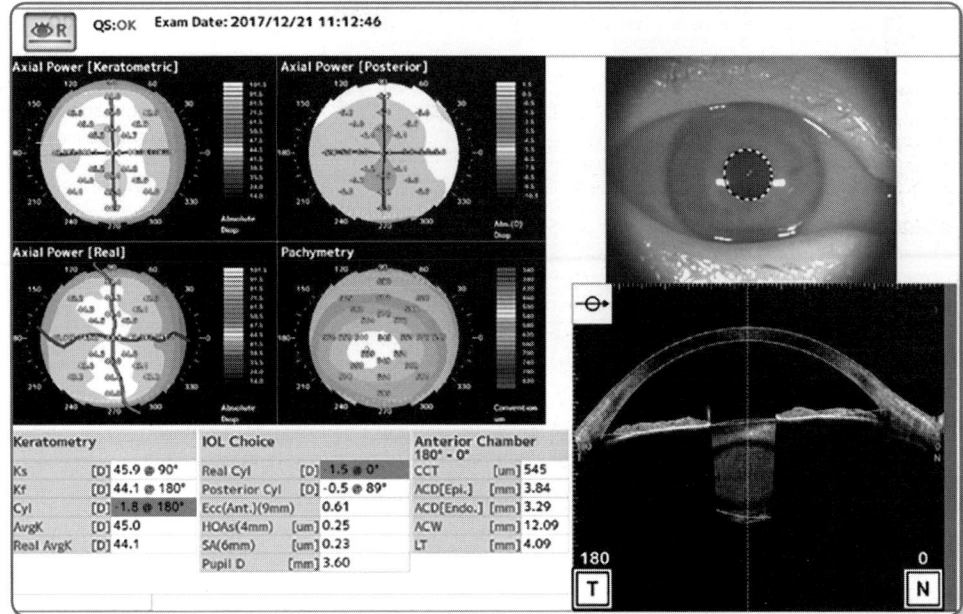

Figure 6.6 Topography and AS OCT (Casia Tomey).

implant based not only on the availability of strength of a particular lens implant model but the para axial and foveal focus dependant on pupil size and lens model (**Figure 6.7**) shows an OKULIX calculation on a long eye.

Although toric lens calculation is available on biometers, surgeons often use the on-line manufacturer's calculation facilities.

Different constants are needed in formulae for optical and ultrasound measurements.

Postrefractive corneal surgery

There are numerous techniques available on line to calculate the effective corneal power post corneal refractive surgery which can then be used in a chosen formula. Some require prerefractive surgery data and others require current keratometry or corneal topography readings. BESSt formula requires both pentacam readings and axial length. Formulae are also available on Optical Biometers. Many choose to average the results from as many techniques as possible and discard clear outliers. Others prefer to work with one or two formulae on their own database of surgical outcomes. Patients should be advised that refractive outcomes are less predictable than in eyes that have not undergone corneal refractive procedures and refractions may take longer to stabilise.

Postoperative refractive surprises

In unexpected postoperative outcomes, biometry should be repeated and compared to the preoperative biometry. The anterior cornea to anterior surface of lens implant should also be measured. If this is shallower or deeper than expected for the implant, B-mode ultrasound or AS OCT should be performed. Too shallow a postoperative distance may be due to several reasons including, capsular bag distention (**Figure 6.8**) or a bent haptic vaulting the implant anteriorly. Too deep a postoperative distance may indicate an incorrectly positioned implant. If all measurements appear consistent with preoperative measurements and postoperative lens position is within

Biometry and lens implant power calculation

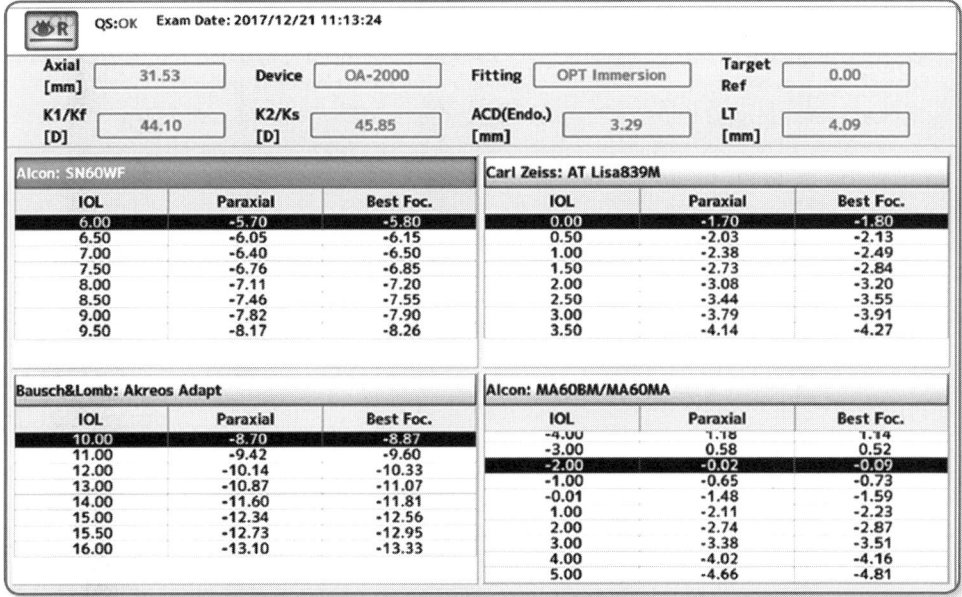

Figure 6.7 OKULIX ray tracing calculation. Axial length 31.5 mm – Four selected implants. Only MA60MA available in a negative power to target emmetropia. The para axial and foveal focus with each model is shown. SRKT and Haigis with optimised constants agree with this calculation.

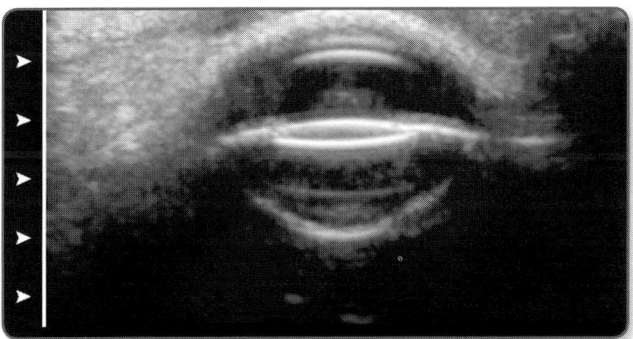

Figure 6.8 Zoomed B-scan showing pseudophakia with capsular bag distention.

the expected range, then a mislabelled lens implant should be considered. The thickness of the implant centrally should be measured using either an optical biometer or an AS OCT. The thickness of the implant can be compared to the same power implant model taken from a different batch using a preprepared calibration graph.

Further reading

Hoffer KJ, Savini G .Clinical results of the Hoffer h-5 formula in 2707 eyes: First 5th generation formula based on gender and race. Int Ophthalmol Clin 2017; 57:213–219.

Savini G, Negishi K, Hoffer KJ, Schiano Lomoriello D. Refractive outcomes of intraocular lens power calculation using different corneal power measurements with a new optical biometer. J Cataract Refract Surg 2018; 44:701–708.

Yang R, Yeh A, George MR, et al. Comparison of intraocular lens power calculation methods after myopic laser refractive surgery without previous refractive surgery data. J Cataract Refract Surg 2013; 39:1327–1335.

Related topics of interest

- Anisocoria (p. 10)
- Corneal ectasia (p. 84)
- Corneal topography (p. 94)
- Intraocular lenses (p. 188)

7 Birdshot chorioretinopathy

Key points

- Birdshot chorioretinopathy is a rare condition primarily affecting white Northern Europeans
- Clinical examination classically demonstrates creamy yellow oval lesions of a quarter of a disc diameter across that radiate out from the optic disc
- Human leucocyte antigen (HLA) A29 positivity is associated with a relative risk of birdshot of up to 224 in individuals with a suggestive clinical picture
- Systemic immunosuppression is almost always required, which is tapered according to serial electrophysiology and clinical examination

Epidemiology

Birdshot chorioretinopathy is a chronic, bilateral, and idiopathic posterior uveitis. Some textbooks include it within the description of 'white dot syndromes', but this is inappropriate and misleading. It is entirely separate and now stands alone as a well-described specific clinical entity. It is a rare disease, so its exact incidence is not known with great certainty, though it is estimated that there are approximately 1-6 cases per million population in Europe and North America. It is a condition of the white Northern Europeans with only very rare case reports published of other races being affected. There is a slight female preponderance.

Pathophysiology

The exact pathophysiology of birdshot chorioretinopathy is poorly understood, though is thought to be a combination of genetic susceptibility and exposure to an as yet unknown antigen that excites the immune system. More than 95% of birdshot sufferers are HLA-A29 positive, compared with around 7% of the Northern European population, with a relative risk ratio of 50–224 of being positive if the clinical picture was suggestive. In fact, from that perspective it is one of the most useful HLA tests available. The reason for the strong association is unknown, however.

Clinical features

The key here is the name itself. Birdshot is a type of lead shot used to shoot birds in flight and as such the lead separates out into a cone of smaller fragments in order to increase the chance of hitting a small moving target successfully. The alternative shot is buckshot, a small concentrated dose of lead that stays together and is best suited for larger stronger targets such as deer. The fundal lesions are yellowish ovals up to a quarter of a disc diameter in size with the long axis pointing toward the optic disc, exactly as if a hunter had taken aim at the disc with a shotgun full of birdshot; hence the name (**Figure 7.1**). They are predominantly posterior pole lesions, more frequent nasal to the optic disc, with the concentration diminishing rapidly as the distance from the optic disc increases. The lesions are usually non-pigmented and the creamy yellow colour may make distinction from the fundus itself difficult, especially in early disease. Although the disease is bilateral, it can present asymmetrically.

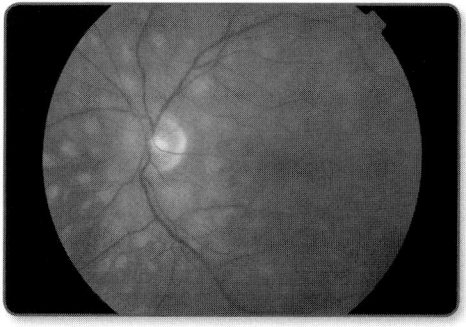

Figure 7.1 Fundal photo of birdshot. (*For colour version see plate 1*)

The typical presentation is with blurred vision, with floaters and photopsia, though nyctalopia can also be a feature. This is assessed by asking about visual difficulties in dark environments. Intriguingly patients commonly report 'vibrating vision', a wheel turning in their vision like a slow moving ceiling fan, or sometimes a shimmering effect such as the sun glinting off the surface of the sea in the distance. These features are highly suggestive of birdshot. There is usually only mild to moderate amounts of vitritis, but there is never anterior uveitis present. Lastly, as with most cases of uveitis, cystoid macular oedema (CMO) can develop, which can be detected either clinically or confirmed by optical coherence tomography (OCT) scanning. There are always signs of bilateral inflammation, but the degree of involvement can be asymmetrical between the two eyes.

Investigations

Investigations are primarily aimed at excluding other potential pathologies, the main differentials include sarcoidosis, TB, syphilis, and intraocular lymphoma, with sarcoidosis, the most likely condition to mimic birdshot. We recommend performing a full blood count, syphilis serology, and serum angiotensin-converting enzyme testing, along with a chest X-ray to exclude the main differential diagnoses, although detailed history taking is also essential in weighing up their relative likelihood. The investigation specific for this condition is HLA-A29. If the clinical picture is suggestiv, then this test is highly useful at confirming the diagnosis. Most clinicians would not make a diagnosis if HLA-A29 is negative, and in such cases the differential diagnoses should be explored again.

An electroretinogram (ERG) is useful in both diagnosing and monitoring patients with birdshot. Abnormal findings include a markedly reduced B-wave amplitude, reduction in 30 Hz flicker amplitude, and a delay in 30 Hz flicker – the latter being characteristic of this condition.

The fundus fluorescein angriogram (FFA) typically shows sub-clinical vasculitis and leakage at the disc, and if CMO is present,

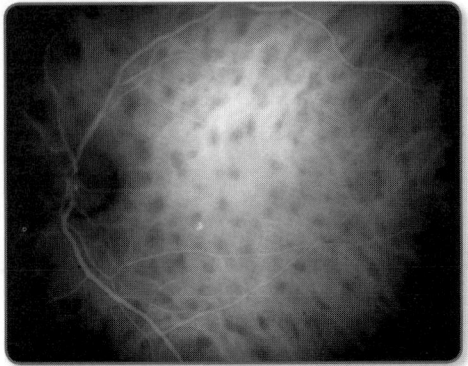

Figure 7.2 Indocyanine green of birdshot.

petalloid leakage around the fovea. The lesions themselves rarely show up well on FFA, though indocyanine green (ICG) angiography typically demonstrates them beautifully, with the lesions remaining hypofluorescent throughout the run (**Figure 7.2**). In fact, ICG commonly demonstrates many more lesions than seen on clinical examination. OCT scanning may show CMO.

Diagnosis

As with most entities in the field of inflammatory eye disease, the diagnosis is a clinical one supported by ancillary tests. If the above investigations have excluded other conditions and if the clinical picture is suggestive based on history and examination, HLA-A29 testing, ERG and/or angiography, then a diagnosis of birdshot chorioretinopathy can be made.

Treatment

Birdshot is a condition more akin to a slow burning fire than a full-out blaze. The clinical signs and symptoms can be subtle but treatment is needed in the form of immunosuppression in order to prevent lasting serious long-term damage. Oral steroids are commonly used to start with though the chronic nature of the condition means that a steroid-sparing agent is usually required. Should an acute flare up occur, it is possible to perform rescue therapy in the form of an intravitreal injection of steroid, commonly either an ozurdex implant or triamcinolone, though the latter is not licensed for intravitreal use. Orbital floor depot steroids have no role in the management of this disease and should be avoided.

As the clinical signs and symptoms can be subtle, the activity of the condition should be monitored via regularly ERG testing, automated visual fields, as well as wide-field angiography, so that new lesion development can be tracked. The ERG usually recovers after immunosuppression therapy is commenced and the tapering of medication is reliant on continued disease stability, monitored as mentioned above. If CMO is present, this can be monitored via serial OCT scanning after treatment initiation to ensure resolution. Ozurdex and triamcinolone have both got short durations of action so there is considerable interest in longer-lasting intravitreal implants such as iluvien. However the long-term efficacy of these implants, with or without systemic immunosuppression, remains to be determined.

Complications

Complications can broadly be divided into two categories: those arising as a result of active inflammation, or atrophic ones arising from the late consequences of that inflammation. The former includes CMO, vitritis, disc oedema, and rarely inflammatory choroidal neovascular membranes (CNV). The latter include photoreceptor loss, choroidal and retinal atrophy, and disc pallor. These are usually late consequences of the disease, and tend to occur if the disease presents late or is inadequately treated. For these reasons, the prognosis is highly variable.

Further reading

Abu-Yaghi NE, Hartono SP, Hodge DO, et al. White dot syndromes: a 20-year study of incidence, clinical features and outcomes. Ocul Immunol Inflamm 2011; 19:426.

Shah KH, Levinson RD, Yu F, et al. Birdshot chorioretinopathy. Surv Ophthalmol. 2005; 50:519–541.

Williams GS, Westcott M (Eds). Practical Uveitis: Understanding the Grape. Taylor and Francis; 2017.

Related topics of interest

- Posterior uveitis (p. 259)
- White dot syndromes (p. 372)

8 Blepharitis

Key points

- Blepharitis is a common ocular disorder that can lead to significantly altered quality of life
- Blepharitis can be anatomically subdivided into anterior and posterior forms but considerable overlap exists between the two categories
- Blepharitis is often difficult to manage satisfactorily but conventional treatment modalities include: lid hygiene, topical antibiotics/anti-inflammatories and systemic antibiotics

Epidemiology

Blepharitis is complex ocular disorder characterised by an imbalance in ocular flora, meibomian gland dysfunction and eyelid/ocular surface inflammation. Blepharitis is one of the most prevalent ocular disorders encountered by ophthalmologists. It affects patients of all ages and ethnicities with up to 37% of patients seen in ophthalmic clinics displaying signs of this condition.

Pathophysiology

Blepharitis is a descriptive term referring to a group of disorders resulting in chronic lid margin and adnexal inflammation. The pathophysiology of blepharitis is poorly understood with several reported pathogenic mechanisms:

- Chronic low-grade bacterial infection is likely present in a significant proportion of patients causing ocular surface inflammation as a result of direct tissue invasion or bacterial component related toxicity. Excess quantities of commensal bacteria or colonising species can disrupt the finely balanced ocular surface microenvironment. In recent years, Demodex infestation of the lash follicle and the resulting inflammatory response has been implicated in the pathogenesis of blepharitis, although the association has not been firmly established as the organism can also be found in asymptomatic patients
- Environmental factors such as exposure to pollutants, chemicals and low humidity environments
- Systemic diseases such as rosacea, seborrheic dermatitis and graft versus host disease have also been implicated in the disease process

Clinical features

There is no universally accepted classification system for the various forms of blepharitis, but the condition is typically categorised into anterior and posterior forms:

- *Anterior blepharitis*: Lid margin inflammation anterior to the grey line, predominately involving the base of lashes and their follicles. Anterior blepharitis may be further subcategorised into staphylococcal or seborrheic
- *Posterior blepharitis*: Lid margin inflammation posterior to the grey line with significant involvement of the meibomian glands
- Involvement is typically bilateral and symmetrical in both subtypes. The abnormal lid-margin secretions and dysfunctional pre-corneal tear film seen in blepharitis result in patients typically presenting with chronic symptoms such as ocular irritation, foreign body sensation, photophobia, eyelid discomfort, contact lens intolerance and decreased or fluctuating vision. The clinical features of the blepharitis categories often overlap, but certain signs are more commonly associated with particular subtypes. Typical features of blepharitis are summarised in **Table 8.1**

Investigations

Although blepharitis is a commonly seen clinical condition it still constitutes a diagnostic and therapeutic enigma. The diagnosis of blepharitis is typically clinical and rarely requires investigation. Culturing

Table 8.1 Summary of clinical features seen in patients with blepharitis

Presentation	Anterior blepharitis	Posterior blepharitis
Eyelid deposits	Collarettes (hard scales) in staphylocaccal blepharitis and scurf (greasy scales) in seborrheic blepharitis	Thick, foamy lipid secretions
Eyelid	Ulceration and tylosis (lid notching) can be seen in staphylococcal blepharitis	-
Eyelash misdirection	Frequent in staphylococcal blepharitis	Rare
Cyst	Hordeolum	Chalazion
Conjunctiva	Phlyctenules can be seen in staphylococcal blepharitis	Papillary reaction may be seen
Cornea	Inferior punctate epithelial erosions, marginal infiltrates, neovascularisation, pannus and phlyctenules can be seen in staphylococcal blepharitis	Inferior punctate epithelial erosions, marginal infiltrates, neovascularisation, pannus and phlyctenules can be seen
Tear film	Aqueous tear deficiency	Aqueous tear deficiency or tear foaming

the eyelid margins can be considered in cases of refractory or severe blepharitis but it should be noted that less than 50% of patients diagnosed with staphylococcal blepharitis will have positive cultures. In patients with chronic refractory blepharitis and cylindrical dandruff at the root of the lash, Demodex infestation should be suspected. In such patients lash sampling and microscopic examination provide a definitive diagnosis by identifying the mites along the lash. In recent years in-vivo confocal microscopy (IVCM) has also been utilised to diagnose.

Sebaceous gland carcinoma or nasolacrimal duct obstruction must also be considered in patients with chronic unilateral or highly asymmetrical lid margin inflammation refractory to conventional treatment and therefore, conjunctival/lid biopsy or nasolacrimal duct syringing/imaging should be considered in patients suspected of having a masquerading condition. Emerging investigations which may ultimately improve our understanding of the underlying disease process in blepharitis include lipid layer interferometry, tear osmolarity, meibometry (measurment of basal meibum levels at the eyelid margin) and meibography (direct visualisation of meibomian glands morphology in vivo).

Treatment

Blepharitis is a chronic condition and patients should be counselled at an early stage that a cure is unlikely and frequent exacerbations are possible. Therapy is directed at controlling symptoms, but it is currently not possible to permanently alter underlying factors such as gland dysfunction and skin flora imbalance. Current treatment is multifaceted and includes eyelid hygiene, topical/systemic antibiotics and topical anti-inflammatory agents (corticosteroids or cyclosporine).

Cleansing

The mainstay treatment for patients with blepharitis is regular lid hygiene and lid margin cleansing. The patient should be instructed to apply warm compressors to the eyelid to liquefy thickened meibomian secretions and soften crustations adherent to the eyelid margin. This should be followed by gentle cleansing of the lid margin to express the meibomian glands of their secretions. A diluted, non-irritating detergent, or a commercially available solution may facilitate cleansing. If Demodex infestation is suspected, the hygiene regimen should include a disinfectant scrub solution such as tea-tree oil. It is vital that patients continue the practice of good lid hygiene after disease control and symptom resolution has been achieved as maintenance therapy. It may also be helpful to advise patients with chronic disease to minimise the use of cosmetic products.

Antibiotics

Topical or systemic antibiotics can be used effectively in patients where a bacterial

aetiology is suspected or in patients with rosacea and posterior blepharitis. Macrolide antibiotics such as azithromycin are currently favoured as they:
- Reduce the production of bacterial lipases by *Staphylococcus epidermidis*, *Staphylococcus aureus* and *Propionibacterium acnes*
- Decrease the concentration of free fatty acids and their deleterious effects on the lipid layer of the tear film
- Have a long half-life and possess anti-inflammatory properties (antichemotactic effects on neutrophils and anticollagenase activity) in addition to their antibacterial properties

Anti-inflammatory

Severe cases of blepharitis with associated ocular inflammation may require the short-term use of topical anti-inflammatory medication to modulate the course of the disease process. To achieve this aim, non-potent corticosteroid drops should be used to minimise the risk of complications such as raised intraocular pressure. Corticosteroid therapy should, however, be avoided in patients requiring long term treatment and topical cyclosporine considered in such patients. The combination of a topical antibiotic and corticosteroid can be a useful treatment strategy in patients where lid/ocular surface bacterial infection and inflammation is thought to coexist. Antiseborrheic shampoos containing selenium sulphide or tar can be considered if seborrheic dermatitis is present.

Relapsing disease

Dietary supplementation with omega-3 fatty acids and novel interventional treatment modalities such as intraductal meibomian gland probing, thermal pulsation and intense pulsed light therapy should also be considered for patients with relapsing disease.

Complications

Chronic uncontrolled blepharitis can rarely lead to permanent alterations of the eyelid margin or vision threatening complications such as superficial keratopathy, corneal ulceration and neovascularisation.

Further reading

Duncan K, Jeng BH. Medical management of blepharitis. Curr Opin Ophthalmol 2015; 26:289–294.

Lindsley K, Matsumura S, Hatef E, Akpek EK. Interventions for chronic blepharitis. Cochrane Database Syst Rev 2012:CD005556.

Pflugfelder SC, Karpecki PM, Perez VL. Treatment of blepharitis: recent clinical trials. Ocul Surf 2014; 12:273–284.

Related topics of interest

- Chalazion (p. 63)
- Dry eye syndrome (p. 122)
- Infectious keratitis (p. 181)

9 Blepharoptosis

Key points

- Blepharoptosis is defined as an abnormally low-lying upper lid margin with the eye in primary gaze
- Blepharoptosis is a clinical sign and not a diagnosis. It may be the presenting sign of a serious or life-threatening systemic disorder
- Mild ptosis may cause cosmetic concerns but more severe forms may affect visual function
- Ptosis may be congenital or acquired. Causes include aponeurotic, neurogenic neuromuscular, myogenic, mechanical and traumatic
- A careful history and examination is needed to determine the aetiology and the most appropriate treatment

Epidemiology

Blepharoptosis is a common condition and over 5,000 ptosis repairs are performed annually in England. Ptosis has no race or gender predilection.

Pathophysiology

Anatomy of the eyelids

The upper eyelid normally lies 1.5 mm below the superior corneal limbus. The levator palpebrae superioris muscle and, to a lesser extent, Müller's muscle are responsible for raising the upper eyelid. The superior branch of the oculomotor nerve supplies the levator muscle. The smooth muscle fibres of Müller's muscle are innervated by sympathetic nervous system. Blepharoptosis can be classified as:

- Involutional or aponeurotic due to dehiscence of the levator aponeurosis or disinsertion from the tarsal plate
- Neurogenic or neuromuscular due to abnormal innervation of the levator or Müller's muscle
- Myogenic due to a myopathy affecting the levator muscle
- Mechanical due to the mechanical effects such a mass lesion within the upper eyelid
- Eyelid muscle trauma

Causes of a pseudoptosis should be excluded.

Involutional or aponeurotic ptosis

This is the most common type of acquired ptosis. The levator aponeurosis stretches and thins and, in some cases, detaches from the tarsal plate. It is associated with ageing but may occur earlier following long-term contact lens wear, intraocular surgery, severe periocular infection or inflammation or floppy eyelid syndrome.

Neurogenic ptosis and neuromuscular ptosis

Neurogenic ptosis arises from dysfunction of either the oculomotor nerve, which innervates the levator muscle, or the sympathetic fibres innervating Müller's muscle. A number of different insults including trauma, tumours, infection, inflammation and vasculopathy may affect these nerves at different points along their route and additional investigations are frequently required to determine the cause.

Neurogenic ptosis may be congenital or acquired. Congenital neurogenic ptosis includes congenital third nerve palsy, congenital Horner's syndrome and Marcus-Gunn jaw winking syndrome.

Causes of the acquired neurogenic ptosis include:

- Third nerve palsy
- Horner's syndrome
- Myasthenia gravis
- Synkinetic ptosis secondary to aberrant reinnervation of the oculomotor nerve
- Iatrogenic, e.g. complication of periocular Botulinum toxin injection Guillain–Barré syndrome
- Cerebral ptosis

Third nerve palsy is characterised by a variable degree of ptosis and weakness of the superior, inferior and medial rectus muscles, and the inferior oblique muscle. The pupillary fibres may be affected or spared depending on the underlying cause. Horner's syndrome is characterised by mild ptosis, miosis and anhydrosis and, in congenital forms, heterochromia.

Myasthenia gravis is a neuromuscular cause of ptosis that should be considered in any patient with an acquired ptosis and normal pupils. Ptosis may be unilateral, bilateral, asymmetric or alternating and may be associated symptoms of diplopia, orbicularis oculi weakness and a poor Bells phenomenon. Its hallmarks are variability and fatigability of eyelid ptosis with use.

Myopathic ptosis

This arises from abnormalities in the levator muscle, resulting in poor levator function. Myopathic ptosis may be congenital or acquired. Congenital myopathic ptosis is the most common type of congenital ptosis and is characterised by dysgenesis of the levator muscle, resulting in poor levator function and lid lag on downgaze. It can be separated into isolated ptosis (simple ptosis) and ptosis that occurs in association with other ocular or systemic abnormalities such as blepharophimosis-ptosis-epicanthus-inversus syndrome and congenital fibrosis of the extraocular muscles.

Causes of acquired myogenic ptosis include:
- Chronic progressive external ophthalmoplegia
- Oculopharyngeal dystrophy
- Myotonic dystrophy

A careful history and examination should be taken to elicit the symptoms and signs of other ocular and systemic features of these conditions.

Mechanical ptosis

Inflammation, infection or the presence of an orbital or lid mass (e.g. plexiform neurofibroma, capillary haemangioma, dermoid cyst) may cause mechanical ptosis.

Pseudoptosis

This is when the upper eyelid position is normal but appears ptotic due to:
- Dermatochalasis/brow ptosis
- Ipsilateral enophthalmos
- Contralateral eyelid retraction
- Hemifacial spasm
- Aberrant re-innervation of the facial nerve
- Post-enucleation socket syndrome
- Double elevator palsy
- Duane's retraction syndrome

Clinical features

History

A careful history will point to the possible aetiology and direct the examination and subsequent investigations. Old photographs may help determine if the ptosis has a congenital component.
- Acute, sub-acute onset or chronic ptosis; sudden onset following surgery or trauma or gradual onset, variability and fatigability
- Associated ocular symptoms including diplopia, head or neck pain or facial spasms
- Ocular history including contact lens wear, previous ocular surgery, trauma or botulinum toxin injections
- Past medical history and drug history with relevant systems enquiry if myogenic/neurogenic aetiology suspected

Examination

The face as a whole should be examined noting signs of facial weakness or asymmetry, frontalis overaction and brow ptosis.
Palpate the lids and orbital rim for masses and exophthalmometry if proptosis or enophthalmos is suspected. When examining the lids, note upper and lower lid position including the presence of lid laxity or swelling, skin lesions, dermatochalasis, and lash ptosis. Evert the eyelid to assess for conjunctival lesions, scarring and foreign bodies.
Measure and record the following:
- *Margin-reflex distance 1 (MRD1) with the frontalis muscle immobilised:* Vertical height from pupillary light reflex to upper lid margin in millimetres
- *Palpebral aperture with the frontalis muscle immobilised:* Vertical height from lower lid margin to upper lid margin in millimetres
- *Levator function:* Full excursion of upper lid margin from downgaze to upgaze with

the frontalis muscle immobilised (poor levator function < 4 mm, good levator function > 10 mm)
- A high or absent upper lid skin crease may indicate aponeurotic dehiscence
- Lid lag on downgaze may indicate levator muscle dysgenesis or previous surgery
- *Bell's phenomenon:* Patients have a higher risk of postoperative corneal exposure if absent
- Aberrant eyelid movements, e.g. jaw-winking, signs of facial dystonia or synkinesis
- Myasthenic signs, e.g. fatigability, variability, Cogan's twitch

The ocular examination should record the visual acuity, pupils, eye movements including cover test, an assessment of the ocular surface, and tear film. If a myogenic or neurogenic cause is suspected a full neurological, cranial nerve and orthoptic examination and dilated fundoscopy should be performed.

Investigations

The history and examination is sufficient to make the diagnosis in the majority of cases. A visual fields test, performed with and without lid taping, records the impact of ptosis on the visual field.

If systemic disease is suspected patients should be referred early to a relevant specialist. Patients with suspected myasthenia gravis should have blood tests to assess acetylcholine receptor antibody levels. Those with a suspected neurogenic cause, in particular third nerve palsy or Horner's syndrome, or inflammatory or infiltrative disease will require prompt neuroimaging.

Treatment

Children with congenital ptosis require a complete ophthalmic assessment. Signs of amblyopia, anisometropia, irregular astigmatism or an abnormal head posture induced by the ptotic eyelid would be indications for early surgical intervention.

Treatment for ptosis is primarily surgical but the exact timing and technique will depend on the underlying cause. Associated systemic disease should always be investigated and treated prior to considering ptosis surgery. Ptosis associated with myasthenia gravis may resolve with medical treatment alone. Many patients with neurogenic, traumatic or post-operative ptosis may recover spontaneously within the first 6 months.

The type of ptosis surgery depends on the severity of the ptosis and the levator function. Techniques will vary according to surgeon preference but as a guide the following is considered:
- *Poor levator function (< 4 mm):* Brow suspension/frontalis sling, where the eyelid is coupled to the frontalis muscle, using autogenous fascia lata or non-autogenous materials, e.g. supramid suture or silicone rods
- *Moderate levator function (4–10 mm):* Levator muscle resection
- *Good levator function (> 10 mm) with moderate-to-severe ptosis (> 2 mm):* Levator aponeurosis advancement
- *Good levator function (> 10 mm) with mild ptosis (< 2 mm):* Müllers muscle conjunctival resection

Preoperative and postoperative photographic documentation is recommended for all patients undergoing surgery.

Complications

All patients undergoing ptosis surgery should be counselled of the risk of asymmetry, abnormal lid contour, undercorrection or overcorrection. This may result in lagophthalmos, dry eye and exposure keratopathy and may require further surgical intervention. Patients also have a small risk of wound breakdown, infection and suture granulomas.

Further reading

Berry-Brincat A, Willshaw H. Paediatric blepharoptosis: a 10-year review. Eye (Lond) 2009; 23:1554–1559.

Collin JRO. A Manual of Systematic Eyelid Surgery. Oxford, England: Butterworth-Heinemann; 2006.

Crosby NJ, Shepherd D, Murray A. Mechanical testing of lid speculae and relationship to postoperative ptosis. Eye (Lond) 2013; 27:1098–1101.

Latting MW, Huggins AB, Marx DP, et al. Clinical Evaluation of Blepharoptosis: Distinguishing Age-Related Ptosis from Masquerade Conditions. Semin Plast Surg 2017; 31:5–16.

Leatherbarrow B. Oculoplastic Surgery, 2nd edition. New York: Informa Healthcare; 2010.

Satariano N, Brown MS, Zwiebel S, et al. Environmental factors that contribute to upper eyelid ptosis: a study of identical twins. Aesthet Surg J 2015; 35:235–241.

Related topics of interest

- Cranial nerve palsies – multiple cranial nerves palsies (p. 104)
- Optic disc imaging (p. 232)

10 Carotid-cavernous fistula

Key points

- Carotid-cavernous fistulas (CCFs) are rare, complex, acquired vascular lesions most commonly occurring after significant head injury
- High-flow fistulas present with dramatic eye signs and almost always require treatment
- Digital subtraction angiography is the gold-standard investigation
- If treatment is required, a multidisciplinary approach is important and usually the endovascular approach is preferred
- Regular ophthalmological monitoring of patients is essential to treat ocular complications

Epidemiology

The incidence of carotid cavernous fistulas (CCFs) follows that of the underlying aetiological mechanism and type of fistula (see **Table 10.1**). Post-traumatic, high-flow CCFs (Barrow Type A) have a 0.2% incidence in patients with head injury, rising to 4% in patients with basilar skull fracture. These account for about three-quarter of all types of CCF. In this group, young men are the demographic most affected. Low-flow or dural CCFs (Barrow Type B–D) are more common in older women and account for a quarter of cases.

Pathophysiology

Carotid cavernous fistulas are acquired abnormal communications between the carotid arteries and the cavernous sinus. The cavernous sinus is located adjacent to the sella turcica and is a lateral sellar trabeculated venous compartment within which runs the internal carotid artery and the oculomotor, trochlear, abducens nerve as well as the ophthalmic and maxillary branches of the trigeminal nerve. Several classifications systems exist, the Barrow classification being the most widely employed (see **Table 10.1** and **Figure 10.1**).

Trauma

Trauma, especially severe trauma, is the most important aetiological factor in Barrow Type A CCFs. These can develop immediately or after a latency of days to weeks. Penetrating injuries and iatrogenic CCFs, after carotid surgery, for example, are also reported as well as developing from the rupture of pre-existing cavernous carotid aneurysms. Idiopathic high-flow CCFs can also occur in the absence of trauma. They are also seen in genetic conditions associated with weakening of the vessel wall such as fibromuscular dysplasia, Ehlers–Danlos syndrome and pseudoxanthoma elasticum. It has been postulated that low-flow dural CCFs develop through venous thrombosis and increased venous pressure resulting in increased

Table 10.1 Barrow classification of carotid cavernous fistulas

Barrow classification	Anatomical classification	Haemodynamic classification	Aetiological classification	Anatomical vascular abnormality
Type A	Direct	High flow	Traumatic	Direct connection between intracavernous internal carotid artery and cavernous sinus
Type B	Indirect	Low flow	Spontaneous	Dural shunt between meningeal branches of the intracavernous internal carotid artery and cavernous sinus
Type C				Dural shunt between meningeal branches of external carotid artery and cavernous sinus
Type D				Dural shunt between both meningeal branches of intracavernous internal carotid artery (Type B) and meningeal branches of the external carotid artery (Type C) and cavernous sinus

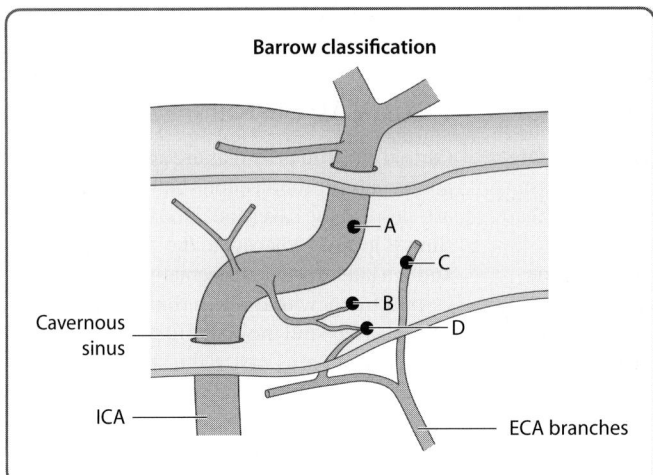

Figure 10.1 Anatomical vascular abnormalities in Barrow classification.

microscopic communications between dural arteries and venous sinuses. Hypertension has been proposed as a risk factor here.

Clinical features

High-flow CCFs

These present dramatically. Symptoms and signs are a result of high pressure in the orbital veins and compression of cranial nerves in the cavernous sinus giving rise to:
- Proptosis, chemosis and conjunctival injection
- Diplopia and ophthalmoplegia (abducens > oculomotor > trochlear)
- Bruit over globe
- Headache and orbital pain
- Blurred vision

Patients may also report loss of sensation in the distribution of the ophthalmic and maxillary branches of the trigeminal nerve. Fundoscopy may reveal changes consistent with venous stasis retinopathy (dilated retinal veins and intraretinal haemorrhages).

Low-flow CCFs

These present much more insidiously and there can be a significant latency between symptoms and diagnosis. Differing patterns of venous drainage can give rise to specific presentations:
- *Anterior draining* – most common, chemosis, conjunctival injection ('red-eye') with corkscrew vessels, proptosis, pain, abducens palsy
- *Posterior draining* – drainage into petrosal sinus gives rise to 'white-eyed' painful diplopia mostly involving single or multiple cranial nerves (oculomotor > abducens and trochlear)
- *Cortical vein draining* – high risk of venous infarction and intracranial haemorrhage resulting in focal neurological symptoms
- *Bilateral orbital venous drainage* – can present with bilateral or even contralateral symptoms and signs

Many patients with low-flow CCFs can demonstrate an ebb and flow of symptoms with changing presentations suggesting changes in drainage thought to be due to the formation and auto-lysis of venous thrombus.

Investigations

The gold-standard investigation for patients with a suspected CCF is digital subtraction angiography. Other non-invasive modalities do have clinical utility such as CT, CT angiography, MRI, MR angiography and orbital or transcranial Doppler ultrasound and are often carried out prior to angiography. These tests may identify the fistula, its cause (e.g. fractures) or its consequences (e.g. orbital proptosis) but MRI is also valuable in identifying other conditions mimicking CCF (see Diagnosis).

Digital subtraction angiography is necessary both to confirm the diagnosis as well as direct treatment. Certain patterns of venous drainage (e.g. cortical venous drainage) may suggest high risk of intracranial haemorrhage and prompt expedited treatment.

Diagnosis

Carotid cavernous fistulas present with painful ophthalmoplegia and the differential diagnosis is necessarily broad as any process that puts pressure on the cavernous sinus or the cranial nerves controlling eye movement may present in this fashion. Several differential diagnoses should be entertained:
- *Neoplastic* – Tumour (including lymphoma) or metastasis at cavernous sinus
- *Vascular* – Cavernous sinus thrombosis, intracavernous carotid artery aneurysm or dissection, posterior communicating artery aneurysm (painful occulomotor palsy)
- *Inflammatory* – Tolosa-Hunt syndrome, orbital psudotumour, sarcoidosis
- *Infective* – Abscess

Other diagnoses to consider are diabetic cranial nerve palsy, giant cell arteritis and orbital cellulitis.

Treatment

The management of patients with a confirmed CCF is complex and involves neuro-vascular multidisciplinary consultation (closure of the CCF) as well as ophthalmology input (monitoring and treatment of ophthalmological complications).

An understanding of the natural history of CCFs is important. Direct high-flow CCFs are unlikely to close spontaneously and present with significant symptoms and associated morbidity and therefore should be closed. Many dural CCFs, in contrast, will close spontaneously (20–60%) and could be managed conservatively unless there are concerning features on presentation and imaging (neurological symptoms, cortical venous drainage suggesting high bleeding risk, progressive visual loss). If managed conservatively, it is essential to ensure an adequate frequency of monitoring of ophthalmological status.

Approaches for intervention are endovascular, surgical, stereotactic radiosurgery and manual compression.
- *Endovascular approach*: This is the preferred approach for most CCFs and can achieve closure rates of 55–99% for high-flow CCFs with either transarterial or transvenous embolisation using coils, balloons, particulates and adhesives. Complication rates of 10–40% (carotid occlusion with cerebral infarction, cranial nerve damage) have been quoted. More favourable outcomes are seen with dural CCFs using these techniques (cure rate of 70–90%, complication rate 2–5%)
- *Neurosurgery*: This can be considered if the endovascular approach has failed or technically not possible. Several techniques can be employed including packing placement to occlude the fistula, suturing, clipping and sealing the fistula with glue. Ligation of the internal carotid may also be considered. Limited evidence suggests the surgical approach is inferior to the endovascular approach in terms of outcome and complication rates
- *Stereotactic radiosurgery*: This can be used as an adjunct to the endovascular approach or neurosurgery or if either of these techniques are not possible and can achieve long-term obliteration of the CCF in 75–100% of cases. However, the full therapeutic effect can take months and therefore is not feasible if immediate treatment is required. Long-term damage to cranial nerves and the cavernous internal carotid artery is possible
- *Manual vascular compression*: Intermittent manual compression of the ipsilateral carotid several times a day for several weeks is a technique that may result in dural CCF closure reported in case series

In conjunction with techniques employed to close CCFs, ophthalmological treatment of complications should be employed including lubrication of the eye to prevent exposure keratopathy and medical treatment of raised intraocular pressure. Eye patches, opaque contact lenses or eyeglasses and prisms can be employed to manage troublesome diplopia. Strabismus surgery may be warranted at a later time.

Complications

High-flow CCF patients are at risk of exposure keratopathy, corneal ulceration, secondary glaucoma and less commonly central retinal artery occlusion, subarachnoid haemorrhage and severe epistaxis.

A third of patients with anterior draining low-flow CCFs are at risk of visual loss due to:
- Orbital venous congestion and secondary glaucoma
- Venous stasis retinopathy
- Vitreous haemorrhage
- Proliferative retinopathy
- Ischaemic optic neuropathy
- Retinal detachment

Further reading

Barrow DL, Spector RH, Braun IF, et al. Classification and treatment of spontaneous carotid-cavernous sinus fistulas. J Neurosurg 1985; 62:248–256.

Ellis JA, Goldstein H, Connolly ES Jr, Meyers PM. Carotid-cavernous fistulas. Neurosurg Focus 2012; 32:E9.

Related topics of interest

- Cranial nerve palsies – multiple cranial nerves palsies (p. 104)
- Optic disc imaging (p. 232)

11 Cataract – acquired

Key points

- Cataract is the leading cause of blindness in the world
- The pathogenesis of cataract is multifactorial; in most patients, cataract is age-related
- Before performing cataract extraction surgery, the surgeon must establish that the benefits of surgery outweigh its risks
- A thorough clinical assessment must be performed to identify co-existing ocular morbidities that may affect the visual outcomes of surgery and factors that increase the risk of surgical complications
- Phacoemulsification surgery is the mainstay technique for cataract extraction in the developed world

Table 11.1 Risk factors for acquired cataracts

Individual factors:
- Increasing age
- Female sex
- Ethnicity (e.g. Asians have higher prevalence compared to Europeans; Caucasians have higher prevalence compared to Africans)
- Genetic factors (e.g. KCNAB1 up-regulation, CRYAA down-regulation)

Lifestyle factors:
- Smoking
- Ultraviolet light exposure
- Malnutrition

Drugs:
- Corticosteroids (topical or systemic)
- Phenothiazines
- Aspirin
- Amiodarone
- Miotic agents (e.g. pilocarpine)

Trauma:
- Blunt/penetrating injuries
- Chemical/thermal/electrical injuries
- Iatrogenic (e.g. vitrectomy, irradiation)

Secondary to systemic diseases:
- Diabetes mellitus
- Atopic dermatitis
- Metabolic abnormalities (e.g. hypocalcaemia, renal impairment)

Secondary to ocular disease:
- Myopia
- Uveitis
- Acute angle-closure glaucoma (glaukomflecken)
- Retinal dystrophies (e.g. retinitis pigmentosa)

Epidemiology

With significant refinements and advancements in surgical techniques, good visual outcomes are now achieved following modern cataract surgery. Indeed, cataract surgery has become one of the most commonly performed and cost-effective procedures in many countries.

Nevertheless, cataract remains the leading cause of blindness in the world. The World Health Organisation estimates that over 20 million individuals are blind as a result of cataract; the majority of these individuals living in developing countries. Indeed, cataract accounts for as high as 50% of blindness in developing countries compared to only 5% of blindness in developed countries. Such discrepancies exist as a result of a global inequality in health-care systems and limited access to cataract surgeries in developing countries. The result is a lower number of cataract surgeries performed per million per year [cataract surgical rate (CSR)] in these countries.

Several risk factors are associated with the development of cataracts. These are listed in **Table 11.1**.

Pathophysiology

Cataract formation is multifactorial. In most patients, the development of cataract is age-related. Large population-based studies have showed that the prevalence of cataract increases with age from approximately 4% at ages 50–60 years to over 90% at age 80 years and older.

The human crystalline lens can be conceptualised as consisting of a nucleus (central core), surrounded by a cortex and a capsule. The normal lens is transparent. Throughout life, lens epithelial cells migrate

Topic 11

to the lens equator to form lens fibres. As a continual process, these new cortical fibres are formed concentrically under the capsule, resulting in the older layers acquiring progressively deeper locations within the lens. The lens nucleus undergoes compression and hardening. The ageing lens thus increases in weight and thickness. Oxidative stress also causes changes in chemical compositions of the lens, proteolytic cleavage of lens proteins (crystallins), and a resultant formation of high-molecular weight protein aggregates. When these aggregates become sufficiently large, they alter the refractive index of the lens, causes scattering of light, and reduces the transparency of the lens. Changes in chemical composition with age also increase lens pigmentation (urochrome); the lens nucleus becomes increasingly yellow or brown.

Types of cataract

There are three main types of age-related cataracts (**Figure 11.1**). More than one type is found in most patients.

Nuclear cataracts (nuclear sclerosis)

An exaggeration of the normal ageing changes of the lens nucleus – protein modification and increased lenticular pigmentation (urochrome). In the early stages, nuclear sclerosis is characterised by a yellowish hue. With the progression of nuclear sclerosis, a myopic shift often results from an increase in the refractive index of the lens. In emmetropic or hypermetropic eyes, the myopic shift enables presbyopic individuals to read again without spectacles. This is sometimes known as 'second sight'.

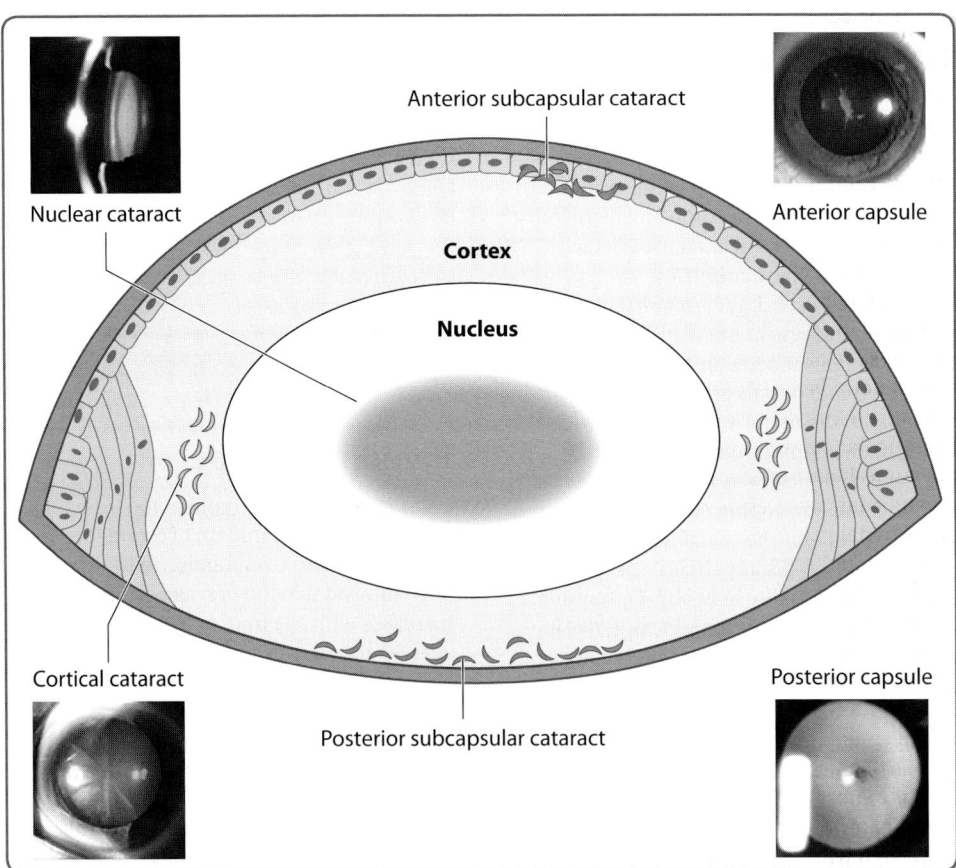

Figure 11.1 Schematic diagram of the human crystalline lens and main types of cataracts.

In advanced stages, the nucleus appears brown (brunescent cataract).

Cortical cataracts

Result from changes in the hydration of the lenticular cortex. They start as clefts and vacuoles between lens fibres. Progression results in typical radial wedge-shaped opacities extending from the cortex to the centre of the lens. Patients often report symptoms of glare due to the scattering of light. In advanced stages, cortical cataracts are associated with liquefaction of the cortical lens material and the lens appears white (intumescent cataract). A cataract is described as hypermature when liquefied cortical material leaks through the lens capsule, resulting in capsular shrinkage and wrinkling. A morgagnian cataract occurs when further liquefaction of the cortical lens allows the free movement of the nucleus within the capsular bag.

Subcapsular cataract

Posterior subcapsular cataracts are one of the main subsets of age-related cataracts. However, compared to nuclear or cortical cataracts, patients with posterior subcapsular cataracts present at younger ages. They are caused by a posterior migration of the lens epithelial cells from the lens equator to the axis on the inner surface of the posterior capsule. Such cataracts are also associated with the use of corticosteroids, trauma, inflammation, and exposure to ionising radiation. Posterior subcapsular cataracts appear as granular or plaque-like opacities of the posterior subcapsular cortex. Due to the proximity to the nodal point of the eye, even small posterior subcapsular cataracts can be highly symptomatic. Patients frequently report symptoms of glare and poor vision under conditions of miosis (e.g. bright light, accommodation). Near vision is often affected more than distance vision. Anterior subcapsular cataracts are less common. Causes of anterior subcapsular cataracts are similar to posterior subcapsular cataracts. Dense anterior subcapsular plaques are associated with atopic dermatitis.

Cataracts and diabetes mellitus

Cataract is a common cause of visual loss in patients with diabetes. There are two pathogenic mechanisms in diabetic cataracts. The first mechanism is the result of an osmotic effect of hyperglycaemia. High blood glucose levels are associated with high glucose levels in the aqueous humour. By diffusion, glucose from the aqueous humour enters the lens. Some of this intralenticular glucose is converted to sorbitol, by an enzyme, aldose reductase. As sorbitol cannot diffuse out of the intracellular compartment, it accumulates in lens cells cytoplasm. This creates an osmotic gradient and an influx of water into the lens fibres. This changes the refractive index of the lens and reduces its transparency. The second mechanism is the result of a direct damage from hyperglycaemia. Glucose can modify lens proteins via glycosylation, leading to protein aggregation and cataract formation.

As a consequence, patients with diabetes develop age-related lens changes earlier compared to the general population. 'Classical diabetic cataract' is less common. They are characterised by multiple snowflake subcapsular opacities seen initially in the superior anterior and posterior lens cortex. They typically occur in young patients with uncontrolled diabetes and can either resolve with improved glycaemic control or mature to intumescence rapidly.

Clinical features

Patients are often referred to the eye clinic by their primary care physicians or optometrists for the management of cataracts.

Common presentations include:
- *Deterioration in vision* – reduced visual acuity, contrast sensitivity, glare, monocular diplopia
- *Changes in refraction* – myopic shifts in nuclear cataracts, change in astigmatism
- *Difficulties in fundal view* – cataracts can obscure the view of the fundus, making clinical evaluation or photographic screening of posterior segment diseases (e.g. diabetes retinopathy) difficult

Less common presentations include:
- *Phacomorphic glaucoma* – Large cataractous lens causes anterior bowing of the iris and shallowing of the anterior chamber. The result is an acute or chronic secondary angle-closure glaucoma
- *Phacolytic glaucoma* – Leakage of soluble lens proteins through an intact anterior capsule of a hypermature cataract, obstructing the trabecular meshwork. The result is a secondary open-angle glaucoma
- *Phacoanaphylactic uveitis* – Inflammatory response to lens protein following traumatic capsular rupture or postoperative retention of lens material
- *Cosmetic* – Mature white cataract in a blind eye; patient requests for cataract extraction to restore a black pupil

Clinical evaluation of acquired cataract

A thorough clinical evaluation (history taking and ophthalmic examination) must be performed in all patients. This is important for all patients especially if cataract surgery is planned. In particular, the following should be established:
- Valid indications for surgery
- Co-existing ocular morbidities that may affect the visual outcomes of surgery and factors that may increase the risks of intraoperative and postoperative complications
- Patient's visual requirements
- Surgical planning including the type of anaesthesia, target refractive outcomes

Table 11.2 highlights the factors that may limit the visual outcome of surgery or increase the risk of surgical complications; for each factor, potential perioperative strategies to improve surgical outcomes are also listed.

Diagnosis

Cataract is a clinical diagnosis and the decision to proceed with cataract extraction surgery is based mostly on history and examination findings alone.

Table 11.2 Factors that may affect visual outcomes or increase the risk of operative complications. *Continues overleaf*

History	Factor(s)	Risk(s)	Action(s)
Past ophthalmic history	• Previous limited best corrected visual acuity (visual potential)	• Poor visual outcome	• Counsel patients – guarded prognosis
	• Ocular co-morbidities (e.g. amblyopia, strabismus, corneal pathologies, glaucoma, retinal pathologies, optic nerve disease, uveitis, trauma)	• Poor visual outcome	• Counsel patients – guarded prognosis
	• Previous corneal refractive surgery	• Refractive surprise	• Counsel patients – refractive surprise/need for further treatment
Past medical history	• Diabetes mellitus	• Infection/diabetic retinopathy • Cystoid macula oedema	• Optimise glycaemic control • Prophylactic non-steroidal anti-inflammatory drugs
	• Hypertension	• Suprachoroidal haemorrhage	• Optimise blood pressure control
	• Ability to lie flat and lie still (e.g. respiratory disease, neck or spine pathologies, tremor)	• Increased surgical difficulty	• Optimise positioning during surgery • Use of periocular local anaesthesia
	• Anaesthetic history (if general anaesthesia considered)	• Anaesthetic risk	• Preoperative anaesthetic review • Optimise general medical health

Cataract – acquired

Table 11.2 *Continued*

Drug history	• Anticoagulants or antiplatelets	• Risk of intraoperative haemorrhage	• Antiplatelets need not be stopped; check INR in patients taking warfarin (within therapeutic range)
	• α1-adrenergic receptor antagonists	• Intraoperative floppy iris syndrome/iris prolapse	• Intracameral sympathomimetics • Iris hooks
Ophthalmic examination			
	Factor(s)	Risk(s)	Action(s)
Globe	• Deep-set eyes	• Difficult surgical access	• Temporal position of surgeon
Lids / lacrimal/ conjunctiva	• Blepharitis +/– other ocular surface disease	• Endophthalmitis	• Treat blepharitis • Lid/conjunctival swab • Prophylactic antibiotics before surgery
	• Dacryocystitis/mucocele	• Endophthalmitis	• Postpone surgery • Treat infection before surgery
	• Conjunctivitis	• Endophthalmitis	• Postpone surgery • Treat infection before surgery
Cornea	• Guttata	• Corneal decompensation	• Counsel patient • Modify phaco technique (e.g. soft-shell, chop)
	• Corneal opacity/scar	• Poor visualisation	• Counsel patient • Capsular stains • Perform corneal surgery first
	• Corneal astigmatism	• Post-operative astigmatism	• Incision along steep axis (limited benefit) • Procedures to treat corneal astigmatism (e.g. limbal relaxing incisions, opposite clear corneal incisions) • Toric intraocular lenses
Anterior chamber	• Shallow	• Increased surgical difficulty • Corneal endothelial trauma	• Use of high viscosity cohesive viscoelastics
Intraocular pressure	• Uncontrolled high intraocular pressure	• Iris prolapse • Suprachoroidal haemorrhage	• Lower intraocular pressure before surgery
Pupil	• Relative afferent pupillary defect	• Poor visual outcome	• Counsel patients – guarded prognosis
	• Poor pupil dilatation	• Increased surgical difficulty	• Intra-cameral sympathomimetics • Pupil stretch • Iris hooks
	• Posterior synechiae	• Increased surgical difficulty	• Synechiolysis • Sphincterotomy • Pupil stretch • Iris hooks
Lens	• Very dense cataract	• Poor visualization of capsule • High levels of phacoemulsification power – affect corneal endothelium	• Capsular stains • Modify phaco techniques (e.g. chop) • Dispersive viscoelastics
	• Intumescent (white) cataract	• Poor visualization of capsule • Loss of capsulorrhexis	• Capsular stains • High viscosity viscoelastics • Decompress cataract before capsulorrhexis

Table 11.2 Continued

	• Instability / phacodenesis	• Zonular dehiscence • IOL decentration	• Anterior capsular hooks • Capsular tension ring • Iris- or scleral- fixated intraocular lens
Vitreous	• Posterior polar cataract	• Posterior capsular rupture	• Hydrodelineation (avoid hydrodissection)
	• Previous vitrectomy	• Unstable anterior chamber • Reverse pupil block	• Iris hooks • Low vacuum levels
	• Silicone oil in vitreous cavity	• Refractive surprise due to incorrect axial length measurement	• Use conversion factor for ultrasound biometry / appropriate settings for partial coherence interferometry
Fundus	• Optic nerve or retinal	• Poor visual outcome	• Counsel patients – guarded prognosis
Cover test	• Heterotropia	• Poor visual outcome (amblyopia) • Post-operative diplopia	• Counsel patients – guarded prognosis/risk of diplopia

Investigations

Investigations are not required to diagnose cataract.
- *Pre-operative refraction/focimetry* – Important for preoperative patient counselling and cataract surgical planning of postoperative target refraction
- *B-scan ultrasonography* – Useful to evaluate the posterior segment for co-existing pathologies (e.g. retinal detachments) in cases where a clear view of the fundus is not possible
- *Biometry* – (refer to chapter on Biometry)

Treatment

Conservative

Patients with early cataracts, good corrected visual acuities, and who are asymptomatic do not require surgery. In such cases, the risks of cataract surgery may outweigh its benefits. Thus, surgery should be deferred until the cataract progresses and causes worsening in visual quality, visual acuity, or clinical severity.

Surgical

In the developed world, phacoemulsification and intraocular lens implant is the mainstay technique for cataract extraction. Phacoemulsification surgery has superseded intracapsular cataract extraction (ICCE) and extracapsular cataract extraction (ECCE), achieving fast visual rehabilitation, good visual and refractive outcomes, and low rates of surgical complications. However, phacoemulsification is not feasible on a large scale in the developing world due to the high cost of surgery, the need for a steady source of electricity, and a lack of trained surgeons. Phacoemulsification is also not ideal for dense, hypermature cataracts, which are more common in the developing world; patients tend to wait longer for their surgeries in these countries. Manual small incision cataract surgery (SICS) has gained popularity in the developing world, where it has been shown to be more cost-effective. In experienced hands, manual SICS can achieve visual outcomes comparable to phacoemulsification surgery. Manual SICS is also suitable for dense, hypermature cataracts.

Complications

Refer to the chapter for 'complications of cataract surgery'.

Further reading

Liu YC, Wilkins M, Kim T, Malyugin B, Mehta JS.
  Cataracts. Lancet 2017; 390:600–612.

Related topics of interest

- Cataract – complications of surgery (p. 50)
- Cataract – congenital (p. 55)
- Biometry and lens implant power calculation (p. 22)
- Intraocular lens (p. 188)
- Femtosecond laser-assisted phacoemulsification (p. 149)

12 Cataract – complications of surgery

Key points

- Despite good visual and refractive outcomes with modern cataract surgery, sight-threatening complications do occur
- Complications can be divided into intraoperative, early postoperative, and late postoperative complications
- Many complications can potentially be prevented through the identification of risk factors and the modification of surgical technique
- Acute endophthalmitis is a sight-threatening ophthalmic emergency; patients require immediate intervention to avoid irreversible visual loss

Introduction

Modern cataract surgery is associated with rapid visual rehabilitation, good visual and refractive outcomes, and low rates of complications. However, complications of cataract surgeries do occur, some of which have the potential to cause loss of vision, or even the loss of eye. Many potential complications of cataract surgery can be prevented by:
- Thorough preoperative clinical assessment to identify factors that increase the risk of surgical complications (see Chapter 6)
- Detailed surgical planning and tailored perioperative measures to address such risk factors

A detailed description of the complications of cataract surgery is beyond the scope of this chapter but can be broadly classified into three categories: intraoperative, postoperative (early), and postoperative (late) complications.

Intraoperative complications

Complications can occur at any stage of cataract surgery.

1. **Anterior capsular complications**
   A tear in the anterior capsule (with potential posterior extension) can occur due to accidental trauma during surgery. In certain situations, there is an increased tendency for the capsulorrhexis to 'run out' or tear such as a high positive posterior pressure, young patients, poor red reflex (e.g. dense cataracts) or intumescent (white) cataracts.
   In anticipation, depending on the situation, measures such as use of appropriate anaesthesia, capsular stains (e.g. trypan blue), high viscosity viscoelastics (e.g. Helon GV or Helon 5), aspiration to decompress a white cataract can be used. The management of this complication depends on the stage of cataract surgery, extent of the tear and the experience of the operating surgeon.

2. **Posterior capsular complications**
   Rupture of the posterior capsule can occur at any stage of phacoemulsification surgery with increased risk of postoperative complications.
   The clinical signs of posterior capsular rupture among several include, sudden deepening from anterior chamber, vitreous seen in the anterior chamber and dropped nucleus.
   The management of posterior capsular rupture depends on the stage of the surgery at which it occurs, the size and extent of the rupture, the presence or absence of vitreous loss, and the amount and position of remnant lens matter, all of which will also determine the placement/type and the position of the intraocular lens (IOL), or requirement for referral to vitreoretinal surgeon and secondary surgery.

3. **Zonular dehiscence**
   Risk of intraoperative zonular dehiscence include, advanced age of patient, dense hypermature cataracts, pseudoexfoliation syndrome, Marfan's syndrome and trauma. In limited zonular dehiscence (< one quadrant), the capsular bag can be stabilised with anterior capsular hooks or capsular tension rings. In the presence

of vitreous loss, vitreous removal will be required. Depending on the extent of zonular dehiscence, the IOL can be implanted in the capsular bag or in the sulcus. In cases of extensive zonular dehiscence, the patient may be left aphakic. An anterior chamber IOL, iris-fixated IOL, or scleral-fixated IOL can be implanted at a later stage as a secondary procedure.

4. **Suprachoroidal haemorrhage**
This is a rare intraoperative sight-threatening complication. It is the result of a bleed into the suprachoroidal space usually from a long or short posterior ciliary artery. It may result in an extrusion of intraocular contents (expulsive haemorrhage) or apposition of retinal surfaces.

The risk factors of suprachoroidal haemorrhage can be patient factors such as age, hypertension and ocular factors such as high axial length or intraocular pressure (IOP).

There is a sudden increase in ocular pain with signs including a sudden increase in IOP (tense globe), iris prolapse, loss of vitreous, altered red reflex, extrusion of intraocular contents.

Once a suprachoroidal haemorrhage is recognised, the surgery should be immediately halted and all incisions sutured closed. Intravenous ocular antihypertensive medications (e.g. acetazolamide) can be administered. Patients should be started on intensive topical steroids. B-scan ultrasonography can be used to assess the severity of the bleed. In cases of small limited suprachoroidal haemorrhage, the bleed may be reabsorbed over days or weeks. In larger bleeds, a referral to a vitreoretinal surgeon is required to consider drainage sclerotomies to evacuate the clot with pars plana vitrectomy (PPV). Visual prognosis is often poor.

Early postoperative complications

1. **Corneal decompensation**
An optimal level of aqueous content of the cornea supports optimal interlamellar spacing of collagen fibrils and corneal transparency. Corneal hydration is regulated by the corneal endothelium. In cataract surgery, the corneal endothelium may be affected by direct mechanical trauma or by phacoemulsification energy, resulting in corneal oedema (decompensation). Risk factors including advancing age, endothelial diseases, dense cataracts, prolonged or complicated surgeries.

A Descemet's membrane (DM) detachment can be repaired by an intracameral air injection. In corneal oedema, IOPs and inflammation must also be controlled as these can affect endothelial cell function. Postoperative corneal decompensation generally resolves within 2–4 weeks. In situations where the cornea fails to clear with medical management, patients will need to be referred to corneal surgeons to consider endothelial keratoplasties.

2. **Wound leak +/- Iris prolapse**
In the presence of a wound leak, patients will have a shallow anterior chamber. There may be iridocorneal touch or iris prolapse. In wound leaks, the risk is postoperative endophthalmitis. Patients should be returned to the operating theatre for anterior chamber reformation and suturing of the incisions.

3. **Acute postoperative endophthalmitis**
This is a rare sight-threatening ophthalmic emergency requiring immediate intervention. Loss of vision is caused by rapid and irreversible photoreceptor damage from toxins produced by infecting pathogens and host inflammatory responses.

Since the introduction of phacoemulsification surgery and increasing awareness of risk factors the prevalence of acute endophthalmitis has fallen to under 0.1%.

In postoperative endophthalmitis, pathogens are inoculated into the eye during (or shortly after) surgery through the surgical incisions. The most common inciting micro-organisms causing endophthalmitis following cataract surgery are gram-positive bacteria, which are responsible of 90% of cases.

Patients typically present between 1-14 days following cataract surgery. Symptoms include increasing pain, redness, worsening vision, photophobia, and discharge. Clinical signs of endophthalmitis include lid swelling, chemosis and conjunctival injection, corneal oedema/infiltrate/keratic precipitates, anterior chamber activity (cells, flare)/fibrin/hypopyon, vitritis and loss of red reflex, blurred or absent view of posterior segment.

B-scan ultrasonography may be useful to assess the degree of vitritis and to rule out retinal pathologies. Aqueous humour and vitreous tap should be performed and samples obtained sent for microbiological investigations (gram stain, culture and sensitivities). Vitreous biopsies can also be taken using an automated vitreous cutter.

Management includes the immediate conjunctival swab, AC and vitreous tap and administration of intravitreal antibiotics such as vancomycin (gram-positive organisms) in combination with Amikacin/ceftazidime (gram-negative organisms) plus amphotericin voriconazole if fungal organisms are suspected. If the patient fails to respond after 24 hours of injection, consider repeating the aqueous and vitreous tap and intravitreal antibiotics. In addition fortified topical antibiotics, systemic broad-spectrum antibiotics, and steroids can be used and in selected cases, early vitrectomy is carried out.

The visual outcome following endophthalmitis depends on the duration of infection prior to treatment and the virulence of the organisms. Overall, 50-60% of patients do not recover vision better than 6/12. The sequelae of endophthalmitis include chornic uveitis, macular oedema, macular ischaemia, secondary glaucoma, retinal detachment, phthisis, or panophthalmitis.

Late postoperative complications

1. Chronic postoperative endophthalmitis

Endophthalmitis may rarely present weeks, months or even years after routine uncomplicated cataract surgery. It is thought to be caused by low virulence micro-organisms being sequestered within the capsular bag. It can thus occasionally occur following Nd:YAG posterior capsulotomy treatment, which releases trapped bacteria into the vitreous from the capsular bag. Causative organisms include *Propionibacterium acnes* (most common), *Staphylococcus epidermidis,* viridans-group streptococci, gram-negative rod bacteria, and fungi.

Patients often present with painless mild progressive visual loss and floaters. Clinical signs include a chronic low-grade anterior uveitis and vitritis. A capsular plaque in the peripheral capsular bag is characteristic of sequestered micro-organisms in the residual cortex. This can be visualised by performing a gonioscopy under mydriasis.

Growth of micro-organisms on cultures of the aqueous and vitreous can confirm the diagnosis. Anaerobic cultures should be requested to detect *Propionibacterium acnes.*

Low-grade inflammation often responds well to topical steroids but flares up when treatment is stopped. Eyes eventually become steroid resistant. As sequestered micro-organisms are isolated from host immune defences and antibiotics, antibiotic treatment alone is often not successful in the eradication of infection. Depending on the results of culture and sensitivities, appropriate intravitreal antimicrobials can be administered. In refractory cases, PPV with removal of the capsular bag and IOL implant may be required.

2. Cystoid macular oedema

In cystoid macular oedema (CMO), there is an accumulation of fluid in the outer plexiform and inner nuclear layers of the retina. It is seen best on OCT with a reported prevalence of up to 14% following cataract surgery depending on risk factors.

Treatment involves the control of inflammation using topical steroids and non-steroidal anti-inflammatory drugs (NSAIDs) such as ketorolac 0.5%/ nepafenac, bromfenac. Periocular or intravitreal/systemic steroids or oral carbonic anhydrase inhibitors (acetazolamide) may be considered. PPV may be useful for CMO refractory to medical therapy.

3. **Posterior capsule opacification**
Posterior capsule opacification (PCO) is the result of the proliferation of remnant lens epithelial cells onto the posterior capsule. This can result in a deterioration of vision, reduction in contrast sensitivity, symptoms of glare, or monocular diplopia.

It is the most common complication of cataract surgery with varying occurrence depending on risk factors. The prevalence has been reported to be about 12% at 1 year and as high as 28% in 5 years following surgery. Treatment is with Nd:YAG laser to create a posterior capsulotomy. The potential complications following laser posterior capsulotomy include transient rise in IOPs, IOL pitting or movement, uveitis, CMO and retinal tears/detachment.

4. **Anterior capsular contraction**
Several weeks or months following cataract surgery, the anterior capsule may opacify and the capsulorrhexis contract (anterior capsular phimosis). Significant contraction of the anterior capsule may affect the IOL position and prevent a complete view of the peripheral retina. An Nd:YAG laser anterior capsulotomy can be used to treat clinically significant anterior capsular phimosis.

5. **Intraocular lens malposition**
It may be caused by zonular instability or dialysis, inadequate capsular support (e.g. breach in anterior capsule, posterior capsular defect), poor intraoperative IOL positioning, or postoperative factors (e.g. trauma, capsular contraction). IOL may be tilted, subluxated, or completely dislocated into the anterior chamber or vitreous cavity.

Patients often present with reduced vision. When the edge of the IOL becomes displaced over patient's visual axis, symptoms of visual aberrations (glares and haloes) and monocular diplopia can result. Unstable IOL may cause ocular inflammation, raised IOP, corneal decompensation, CMO, and retinal detachment.

Mild malposition can be observed. Miotics may also be useful to reduce symptoms in these patients. Surgical intervention is required for significant malposition of IOL. Options include IOL repositioning, IOL exchange, or IOL removal.

6. **Retinal detachment**
Retinal detachment can occur anytime (months to years) following cataract surgery. The reported prevalence is between 1–2%. This requires immediate referral to a vitreoretinal surgeon.

Risk factors retinal detachment following cataract surgery include ocular factors, e.g. high myopia, intraoperative complications or laser posterior capsulotomy.

7. **Refractive surprise**
This is an unexpected failure to achieve the planned target refraction following cataract surgery with IOL implant. A systematic approach will help to identify the cause of the refractive error. This includes an in-depth case notes review, including the biometry and a thorough slit-lamp examination. A repeat of investigations (biometry, B-scan to confirm axial length, keratometry, corneal topography) may be useful (see Chapter on cataract surgery-biometry).

Management depends on the extent and cause of the refractive surprise. In patients with small refractive errors that are tolerable, no surgical intervention will be needed. Spectacle or contact lens correction may help in these patients. Intervention may be required for specific situations (e.g. Nd:Yag laser posterior capsulotomy for capsular bag distension syndrome or IOL repositioning for decentered IOL). For large refractive errors, surgical options include IOL exchange, secondary piggyback IOL, or laser refractive surgery.

Further reading

Endophthalmitis Vitrectomy Study Group. Results of the Endophthalmitis Vitrectomy Study. A randomized trial of immediate vitrectomy and of intravenous antibiotics for the treatment of postoperative bacterial endophthalmitis. Arch Ophthalmol 1995; 113:1479–1496.

Endophthalmitis Study Group, European Society of Cataract & Refractive Surgeons. Prophylaxis of postoperative endophthalmitis following cataract surgery: results of the ESCRS multicenter study and identification of risk factors. J Cataract Refract Surg 2007; 33:978–988.

Related topics of interest

- Cataract – acquired (p. 43)
- Cataract – congenital (p. 55)
- Biometry and lens implant power calculation (p. 22)
- Cataract - complications of surgery (p. 50)

13 Cataracts – congenital

Key points

- Congenital cataracts are a rare but important cause of severe visual impairment in children
- They may be a sign of systemic disease
- The timing of surgical management is very important
- Long term follow-up, occlusion, refraction and reassessment are key to successful management

Epidemiology

Congenital cataract is rare, but remains one of the most important causes of severe visual impairment in children. The incidence of congenital and infantile cataracts in the UK is approximately 2.5 per 10,000 by the age of 1 year, and 3.5 per 10,000 by age 15 years. Worldwide 200,000 children are thought to be blind from cataract and 20–40,000 children are born with congenital cataract each year.

Pathophysiology

Most unilateral cataracts and 50% of bilateral congenital cataract cases are idiopathic. Of the remaining 50%, the most common cause is autosomal dominant inheritance. Inheritance may also be X-linked or autosomal recessive. The systemic associations are summarised in **Table 13.1**.

Clinical features

Depending on the age at detection, clinical features may vary. Loss of red reflex and leucocoria are the most common features. Other features include strabismus, amblyopia and there may also be syndrome/aetiology specific signs (see **Tables 13.1** and **13.2**).

Table 13.1 Systemic associations		
Systemic association	System involved	Aetiology
Idiopathic		
Inherited		Autosomal dominant, X-linked, autosomal recessive
Chromosomal		Trisomy 13 (Patau), 18 (Edwards), 21 (Down's), deletions 5p, 18p, 18q
Metabolic		Diabetes
		Galactosaemia
		Hypoglycaemia
		Galactokinase deficiency
Syndromes	Ocular	Aniridia, anterior segment dysgenesis
	Renal	Lowe, Alport, Hallermann-Streiff-Francois
	Skeletal	Smith–Lemli-Opitz, Stickler
	CNS	Marinesco-Sjögren, Zellweger
	Musculoskeletal	Myotonic dystrophy
	Dermis	Cockayne, incontinentia pigmenti, ichthyosis
Infections	TORCH infections	(toxoplasma, other infections (syphilis, varicella zoster, parvovirus, B19), Rubella, cytomegalovirus and herpes infections)
Trauma		
Radiation		

Table 13.2 Cataract morphologies and possible aetiologies	
Cataract morphology	Possible aetiology
Sutural/nuclear cataract	Autosomal dominantly inherited
Pyramidal cataract	Aniridia
Anterior polar	Remnants of anterior pupillary membrane
Posterior polar	Remnants of hyaloid artery (Mittendorf's dot). Lenticonus/globus
Anterior subcapsular – sunflower cataract	Radiation, uveitis, trauma, atopy – Wilson's disease
Anterior lenticonus	Alport, Waardenburg, Fechtner syndromes
Posterior subcapsular	Steroid induced
Oil droplet	Galactosaemia
Cerulean blue dot cataract	Autosomal dominant, trisomy 21

Investigations

In the paediatric ophthalmology setting, diagnosis of congenital cataract should be accompanied by a full antenatal history including exposure to infections, radiation or toxins. A full family history, post-natal history and developmental history are also essential. Some developmental delay can be expected in children with visual impairment (bilateral cataracts), but hearing and speech development should be normal. A systemic cause is more likely in bilateral cataracts (though these too are commonly idiopathic). Referral to a paediatrician to assess for systemic associations or other congenital anomalies should be considered, especially when there are associated dysmorphic features or systemic findings.

Children should be screened for Rubella IgM titres where rubella vaccination is not commonly performed. If there is associated failure to thrive, metabolic and genetic testing for galactosaemia and urinary amino acids for Lowe's syndrome can be carried out. Next generation sequencing that detects mutations in genes coding for crystallins and connexions can help establish the aetiology of childhood onset cataracts.

Where there is no fundal view because of cataract, ocular ultrasound should be carried out to assess for posterior segment abnormality preoperatively.

Diagnosis

Congenital cataracts are usually detected on screening at birth or soon after by health professionals using the red reflex test. Childhood onset cataracts tend to develop later in life and may be associated with leucocoria, reduced vision or strabismus. Early detection of cataract in children is essential in instituting treatment measures.

Treatment

Optimal treatment of congenital cataract involves early diagnosis, timely removal of visually significant cataracts within the latent period for visual development (see below) and long-term compliance with occlusion therapy and optical correction.

A multidisciplinary approach involving the paediatric ophthalmology team, the GP and paediatricians is important. Parents and carers must be counselled to understand the diagnosis, realistic prognosis and the need for long-term rehabilitation beyond surgery. The diagnosis of congenital cataract can impact significantly on the child's immediate family.

Incomplete bilateral or unilateral cataracts can be treated non-surgically if felt to be visually insignificant. The density rather than the size correlates with visual prognosis in these cases. Patching of the other eye or chronic dilation of the pupil in the eye with incomplete cataract, along with appropriate refractive correction may be sufficient to maintain or even improve vision in the affected eye.

For visually significant cataracts in children, surgery remains the mainstay of treatment. The timing of surgery is critical; there is a latent period for visual development after birth before the densely amblyogenic effect of cataract begins. This period is shorter for unilateral cataracts (6 weeks) than for bilateral (10 weeks). The latent period for fixation stability is thought to be just 3 weeks from birth, when major form deprivation from cataract can result in nystagmus. The risk of developing postoperative aphakic glaucoma is higher in children operated within 1 month of birth. The balance of these factors means the optimal time for surgery is after 1 month postnatally, but within the latent period for visual development. Congenital nystagmus can convert to manifest latent nystagmus, which is more benign, after successful cataract surgery.

The treatment aim for unilateral cataract surgery is to give the child useful vision in the affected eye. About 60% of children who receive optimal intervention achieve better than 6/60 in the cataract eye. For children with bilateral cataract who undergo cataract surgery within 10 weeks of birth, the better seeing eye can attain 20/80 in 88% of cases. For surgery after 10 weeks, the visual prognosis is 20/100 or worse.

The surgery is performed through a clear corneal, limbal or scleral tunnel incision for the vitrector and the infusion. An anterior capsulorhexis can be carried out either through the vitrector or manually if intraocular lens (IOL) insertion is planned. The lens material can be aspirated through the vitrector and most surgeons will carry out a posterior capsulotomy and anterior virectomy to prevent posterior capsule opacification. If an IOL is implanted, the last step can be performed through the pars plicata following insertion of the IOL through an enlarged main wound. It is essential to suture all wounds in children due the lower scleral rigidity. Primary IOL implantation in eyes with a corneal diameter < 10 mm may result in pupil block and can require a primary peripheral iridectomy.

The decision to implant an IOL at the time of cataract surgery remains controversial. Its advantage is to reduce postoperative refractive error, anisometropia and aniseikonia. In children under 2 years of age at the time of surgery, primary IOL insertion is not associated with better visual outcomes or less secondary glaucoma when compared to aphakia primary IOL implantation is associated with more secondary procedures and consequently more general anaesthetics. Most commonly secondary procedures are for posterior capsule opacification, which occurs more in phakic than aphakic eyes. In some eyes it is not possible to implant a primary IOL – e.g. anterior segment dysgenesis, persistant hyperplastic primary vitreous (PHPV), glaucoma or microphthalmic eyes.

Biometry in young children is performed under general anaesthesia using A-scan ultrasound for axial length, and handheld keratometry for corneal curvature. IOL power calculation can be inaccurate in children < 36 months old and with axial lengths < 20 mm. The initial refractive target is hypermetropic overcorrection of +8.00 to +9.00DS for infants under 10 weeks at the time of surgery, to allow for later eye growth. Contact lens wear is then necessary until around 18 months of age – during which time most axial elongation occurs.

Where the patient is left aphakic, strong hypermetropic refractive correction is required in the form of aphakic glasses or contact lenses. The tolerability of aphakic glasses should be considered preoperatively as they are very heavy. Families' ability to comply with contact lens care must be assessed.

Children with unilateral cataract need long-term occlusion therapy, regular refraction and reassessment. Aggressive occlusion of 6–8 hours per day may be required to treat amblyopia.

Complications

Cataract surgery can be complicated by inflammation, which may be intense in young children, causing fibrin formation, seclusio pupillae and secondary angle closure. This can be treated with intensive topical steroids, peri-orbital depots or systemic steroids and can necessitate the use of intracameral tissue plasminogen activator or heparin, or surgical iridectomy.

Vitreous haemorrhage may occur in up to 10% of children with persistent foetal vasculature. The rate of retinal detachment following cataract surgery without IOL is 3.2%. PHPV may increase the risk of retinal detachment.

The rate of infectious endophthalmitis is < 1:1000 in children; *Staphylococcus* and *Streptococcus* being the most common causative organisms. Outcomes of paediatric endophthalmitis are poor (perception of light or less).

Glaucoma is a significant cause of postoperative morbidity. Glaucoma or ocular hypertension occurs in 20–59% of children who have undergone congenital cataract surgery. The onset of glaucoma peaks at 6 months postoperatively (angle closure glaucoma) and around 12 years (open angle glaucoma). Risk factors include cataract surgery within the first month of life and microphthalmia. Glaucoma necessitates treatment with medical therapy. Surgical management is required in 27% of eyes. Over half of these require more than one glaucoma procedure.

Cataract surgery causes loss of accommodation but some patients do show pseudoaccommodation, perhaps due to astigmatism, and have equal acuity for near and distance without presbyopic correction.

Further reading

Chan WH, Biswas S, Ashworth J, Lloyd IC. Congenital and infantile cataract: aetiology and management. Eur J Pediatr 2012; 171:625–630.

Jain S, Ashworth J, Biswas S, Lloyd IC. Duration of form deprivation and visual outcome in infants with bilateral congenital cataracts. J AAPOS 2010; 14:31–34.

Solebo AL, Cumberland PM, Rahi JS. 5-year outcomes after primary intraocular lens implantation in children aged 2 years or younger with congenital or infantile cataract: findings from the IoLunder2 prospective inception cohort study. Lancet Child Adolesc Health 2018; 2: 863–871.

Related topics of interest

- Cataract – acquired (p. 43)
- Glaucoma in children (p. 169)

14 Central serous chorioretinopathy

Key points

- Central serous chorioretinopathy (CSCR) is an uncommon but significant cause of visual impairment
- Acute CSCR usually resolves spontaneously, but recurrent or chronic disease can lead to varying degrees of visual loss
- Risk factors for CSCR (some modifiable) have been identified, but pathophysiological mechanisms are poorly understood
- Many different approaches to treatment have been proposed, and evidence is inconsistent

Epidemiology

Central serous chorioretinopathy is estimated to be the fourth commonest retinopathy after age-related macular degeneration (AMD), diabetic retinopathy, and branch retinal vein occlusion. It is most commonly seen in middle-aged men, with a male:female ratio of between 6:1 and 8:1. Incidence in men is 1:10,000 per year. Mean age of onset for acute CSCR is around 40–45 years in men, but may be older in women and in chronic presentations. Racial predilection is controversial, but it has been suggested that CSCR is less common yet more aggressive in African-Caribbean than in Hispanics, Asians or Caucasians.

Risk factors for CSCR include male sex, and (through a mechanism that remains poorly elucidated) both exogenous corticosteroid use and endogenous causes of hypercortisolism. Other known risk factors include type A personality and stress. Smoking, pregnancy, hypermetropia, and obstructive sleep apnoea have also been posited as independent risk factors.

Pathophysiology

The pathophysiology of CSCR is incompletely understood, but appears to be related to abnormal choroidal vascular hyperpermeability, perhaps secondary to choroidal ischaemia, inflammation, or vascular congestion. The resulting increase in subretinal pigment epithelium (RPE) hydrostatic pressure is believed to lead to a breakdown in the integrity and continuity of the RPE, allowing fluid ingress into the subretinal space. Impairment of the RPE's pump mechanism may inhibit spontaneous resolution. However, early fluid reabsorption is associated with reduced long-term photoreceptor damage and a lower risk of secondary choroidal neovascular membrane (CNV) formation.

Clinical features

Acute CSCR is typically unilateral at presentation. Patients may, in some cases, be asymptomatic, e.g. if the affected eye is amblyopic or the lesion is extrafoveal. Common symptoms include reduced visual acuity (VA) (usually between 6/9 and 6/18), metamorphopsia, micropsia, hyperopic shift, mild dyschromatopsia, and reduced contrast sensitivity.

Fundoscopy reveals a localised round or oval serous retinal detachment (SRD), which is typically central. Less commonly, multifocal SRDs may be seen. The SRD may be associated with pigment epithelial detachment (PED) and mild RPE changes.

In *chronic CSCR*, the SRD is typically shallower, but associated with more advanced RPE changes or atrophy ('diffuse retinal pigment epitheliopathy'). Other features may include retinal thinning, intraretinal cysts, and potentially irreversible reduction in VA. Large multifocal bullous SRDs or PEDs can occur, resulting in 'gravitational tracks' as fluid shifts to the inferior retina.

Investigations

Optical coherence tomography

This is the first-line, and often only, investigation required in suspected typical

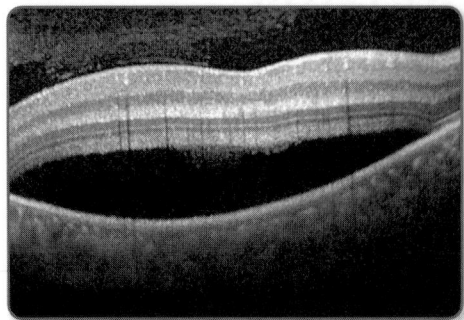

Figure 14.1 Spectral domain OCT of subfoveal fluid in acute right eye central serous chorioretinopathy.
Courtesy: Ms Angela Rees, Moorfields Eye Hospital; London, UK.

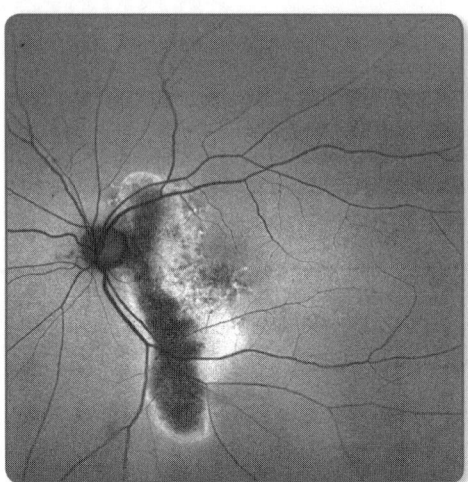

Figure 14.2 Fundus autofluorescence demonstrating hypoautofluorescent gravitational tracks with hyperautofluorescent borders in a patient with chronic left central serous chorioretinopathy.
Courtesy: Professor David Sarraf, Stein Eye Institute, UCLA, reproduced with kind permission of Biomed Central. Image first appeared in Yung M, Klufas MA, Sarraf D. Clinical Applications of Fundus Autofluorescence in Retinal Disease. Int J Retin Vitr 2016; 2:12.

acute CSCR, demonstrating subretinal fluid and possible mild RPE changes (**Figure 14.1**). Intraretinal cysts may be seen in chronic CSCR. In both acute and chronic CSCR, swept-source optical coherence tomography (OCT) may show a wider calibre of choroidal vessels, and choroidal thickening in one or both eyes.

Fundus autofluorescence

In acute CSCR, hyperautofluorescence is seen at the site of leakage, possibly reflecting increased RPE pump activity. In chronic CSCR, gravitational tracks are hypoautofluorescent with hyperautofluorescent borders (**Figure 14.2**).

Fundus fluorescein angiography

In typical acute CSCR, early phase fundus fluorescein angiography (FFA) shows a small spot of hyperfluorescence at the site of the focal RPE lesion. As fluorescein continues to leak into the subretinal space, it either rises superiorly in a 'smokestack' pattern or enlarges centrifugally in an 'inkblot' pattern (**Figure 14.3**) before filling the entire area of the SRD. A PED is present in about 5% of cases. In chronic CSCR with RPE changes, there may be diffuse or multifocal granular hyperfluorescence.

Indocyanine green angiography

Indocyanine green angiography (ICGA) can be helpful especially in older patients

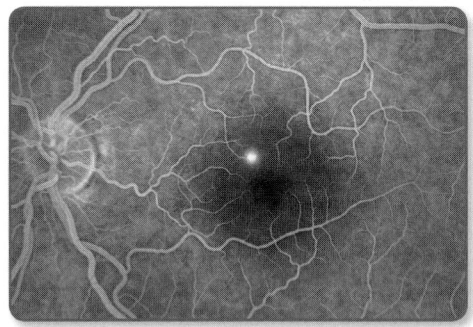

Figure 14.3: FFA shows left eye subretinal pooling of fluorescein in a characteristic expanding 'inkblot' pattern.
Courtesy: Professor Sobha Sivaprasad, Moorfields Eye Hospital; London, UK.

as it may help to differentiate CSCR from neovascular AMD. Early phase demonstrates dilatation of choroidal vessels and hypofluorescence, which is followed by mid-phase staining of the inner choroid. This washes out in the late phase, unlike the sustained hyperfluorescence of CNV.

Serum and urinary cortisol

Only indicated in cases where no risk factors are identified, where there is diagnostic uncertainty, or where there are clinical features of Cushing syndrome.

Diagnosis

The initial diagnosis of CSCR can usually be made on the basis of history, examination, and OCT. It is important to explore known and modifiable risk factors. Although patients may initially deny any use of exogenous steroids, careful questioning may reveal use of steroid inhalers or topical preparations, Chinese herbal medicines (which may be steroid-laced), or steroid preparations applied to a dependent family member (child or elderly parent) without protective gloves. Stress patterns and type A personality traits are important to elicit. Fundoscopy and OCT are usually sufficient to confirm the diagnosis, but further investigations (above) may be required. Recurrent CSCR may be defined as an active episode occurring at least 3 months after onset of a previous resolved episode, and chronic CSCR as an episode persisting for more than 4 months. These criteria vary. The differential diagnosis includes neovascular AMD, polypoidal choroidal vasculopathy, and Vogt-Koyanagi-Harada syndrome.

Treatment

In most cases, acute CSCR is observed during the first 3–4 months, during which spontaneous resolution is likely. It is helpful to counsel patients regarding stress reduction where possible, e.g. by modifying working patterns, or by interventions including exercise, yoga, or relaxation techniques. Where prescribed corticosteroid therapy is identified, patients should only consider tapering or ceasing treatment in consultation with their physician. Early medical intervention has not been shown to improve final VA, but may hasten resolution. It could therefore be considered for an 'only eye' (especially where contralateral visual loss is due to untreated CSCR), if CSCR is recurrent or atypical, or if quicker visual recovery is essential (professional drivers, pilots, etc.).

Numerous treatment modalities have been investigated for treatment of atypical, recurrent, and chronic CSCR, but until recently studies have mostly been limited by small numbers, lack of a control arm, short follow-up, or noncomparable treatment protocols. There is some evidence, albeit inconclusive, for each of the following as described here.

Laser photocoagulation

Its mechanism is unclear. It may hasten resolution of subretinal fluid, but at the risk of causing a permanent scotoma or CNV (10%).

FFA-guided micropulse diode laser

It localises effects of laser to the RPE. Promising results in some studies, and theoretically suitable for both subfoveal and extrafoveal lesions due to avoidance of damage to the neurosensory retina.

Half-dose or reduced-fluence verteporfin photodynamic therapy

It is thought to reduce choroidal hyperpermeability and leakage by narrowing and remodelling choroidal vessels. Poor evidence for improved final VA or for reduced recurrence risk when compared with observation, and may cause choroidal hypoperfusion or ischaemia.

Intravitreal anti-vascular endothelial growth factor injections

There is some evidence of anatomical improvement in chronic or recurrent CSCR, but inconclusive evidence for improved final VA.

Mineralocorticoid antagonists

Both eplerenone and spironolactone remain the focus of active research. Some studies have suggested efficacy in improving anatomical and visual outcomes, especially in chronic or recurrent CSCR.

Complications

Acute CSCR, resolving spontaneously within a few months, typically causes minimal if any, changes in measured VA, but may result in mild residual dyschromatopsia and reduced contrast sensitivity. Recurrence is estimated to occur in a third to a half of all the patients, and is associated with poorer anatomical and functional outcomes.

Longstanding SRDs may lead to irreversible photoreceptor damage and vision loss. Chronic CSCR is associated with a higher incidence of choroidal neovascularisation and RPE tears, with the risk of severe visual impairment.

Further reading

Daruich A, Matet A, Dirani A, et al. Oral Mineralocorticoid receptor antagonists: Real-life experience in clinical subtypes of nonresolving central serous chorioretinopathy with chronic epitheliopathy. Transl Vis Sci Technol 2016; 5:2.

Gupta B, Elagouz M, McHugh D, et al. Micropulse diode laser photocoagulation for central serous chorioretinopathy. Clin Exp Ophthalmol. 2009; 37:801–805.

Schwarz R, Habot-Wilner Z, Martinez MR, et al. Eplerenone for chronic central serous chorioretinopathy – a randomized controlled prospective study. Acta Ophthalmol 2017; 95:e610–e618.

Related topics of interest

- Retinal imaging (p. 277)
- Intravitreal injection therapies (p. 193)
- Retinal lasers (p. 282)

15 Chalazion

Key points

- Most will spontaneously regress without treatment
- Surgical options include intralesional steroid, incision, and curettage or a combination of both
- Sebaceous cell carcinoma may masquerade as recurrent chalazion

Epidemiology

Hordeola (chalazion and stye, internal vs. external respectively) are one of the most common eyelid lumps. The exact incidence and prevalence is unknown. They may present in any age group but are more common in adults, typically those over 30 years. There is no racial or gender predilection. They are associated with seborrheic dermatitis, blepharitis, acne rosacea, viral conjunctivitis (particularly in children), diabetes mellitus, pregnancy, and hyperlipidaemic states. Rarely, systemic infections such as tuberculosis or leishmaniasis may be responsible.

Pathophysiology

There are several sebaceous (meibomian and Zeis) and apocrine (Moll) glands that lie within the eye lids as shown in **Figure 15.1** which is a full-thickness sagittal section through the upper and lower lids. The glands of Zeis are sebaceous glands that secrete an oily substance into the lash follicle to lubricate them, whilst the oily secretion of the meibomian glands coats the ocular surface as part of the tear film. Meibomian gland ducts run vertically through the full length and width of the tarsal plate and are served by multiple acini that insert horizontally into the ducts. There are approximately 50 along the upper lid and 20 along the lower lid. Secretion is thought to be regulated by androgens and oestrogens which may explain changes in meibomian gland morphology during pregnancy and menopause. Gland expression is facilitated predominantly by gravity and is assisted by contraction of orbicularis oculi. Meibum, itself, is a lipid-rich substance secreted onto the lid margin and the ocular surface where it stabilises the tear film to impede evaporation.

Chalazia are chronic sterile lipogranulomatous inflammatory lesions of the lid. The source of inflammation is thought to be lipid breakdown products which occur because of meibomian gland obstruction. These products may leak into the tarsal plate stroma causing a granulomatous

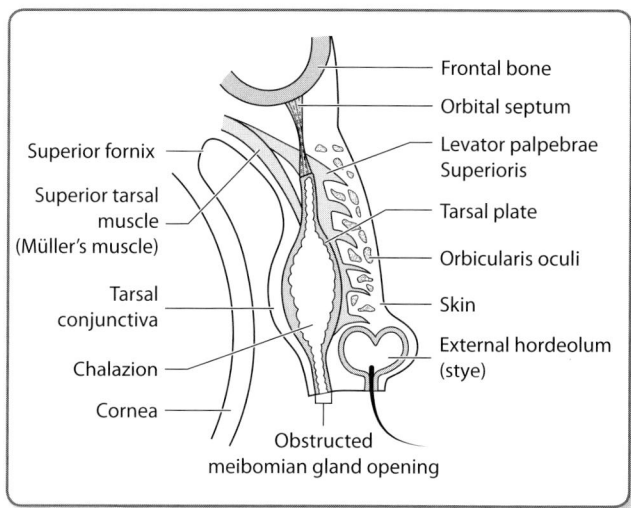

Figure 15.1 Sagittal section of the eyelid indicating the location of the internal and external hordeola.

reaction with multinucleated giant cells and prominent fat spaces on microscopy.

In the acute setting, blocked meibomian glands may give rise to an internal hordeolum (commonly referred to as a '*chalazion*'). Whereas an external hordeolum (commonly referred to as a '*stye*') results from blocked glands of Zeis or Moll. This results from staphylococcal infection of the gland leading to polymorphonuclear leucocyte infiltration and abscess formation.

Clinical features

Chalazia usually present as a painless, firm and non-tender nodule on the upper or, less commonly, lower lid (**Figure 15.2**). Patients normally describe a non-acute history with a lump that has been present and slowly enlarging over several weeks to months. Triggers for presentation include cosmetic concern or discomfort if the mass becomes acutely inflamed causing conjunctivitis or preseptal cellulitis.

Infected hordeola have a more acute presentation commensurate with the presence of an abscess including pain, erythema, tenderness, and focal swelling along the lid margin. Large collections of pus may point and spontaneously discharge to the skin (external hordeolum) or tarsal conjunctival surface (internal hordeolum). Hordeola are often associated with surrounding preseptal cellulitis and rarely may progress to frank orbital cellulitis, particularly in children. Hordeola may progress to chalazia once the initial infection has settled and chalazia themselves may undergo intermittent inflammation due to infection which can make it difficult to distinguish them. As both are generally benign conditions with similar conservative treatments, differentiating the two entities is not always clinically helpful.

Lid eversion may aid in identifying the lump if the diagnosis is not apparent on external examination. Chalazia may be visible under the tarsal conjunctiva as a firm yellow nodule and in chronic cases may be complicated by a pyogenic granuloma (**Figure 15.3**). Diseases affecting the lid margin may be present including rosacea, seborrheic dermatitis, and meibomian gland dysfunction.

Investigations

The diagnosis of chalazion and hordeolum is clinical and investigation by biopsy is rarely required unless recurrent. In cases of suspected orbital cellulitis, a CT scan or even an MRI is required.

Treatment

The majority of chalazia will resolve spontaneously over several weeks. Most of the remainder will resolve with conservative

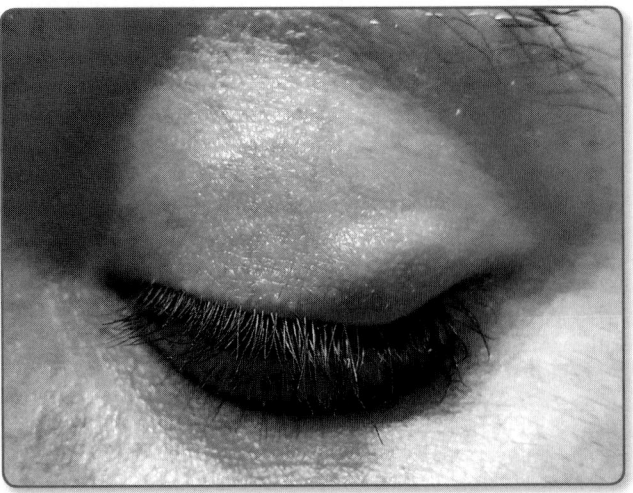

Figure 15.2 The typical appearance of an upper lid meibomian gland chalazion.

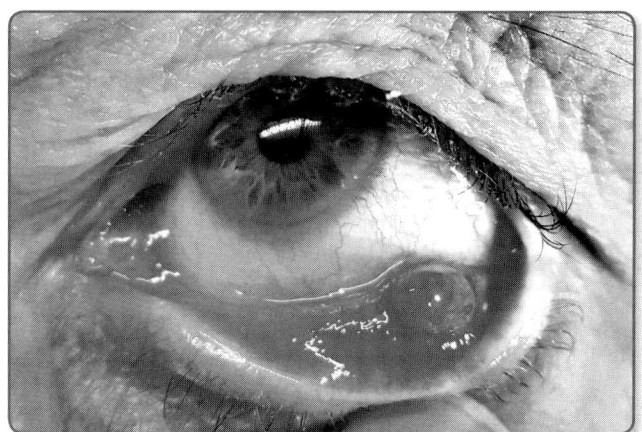

Figure 15.3 Pyogenic granuloma complicating a chronic chalazion.

treatment which should be initiated in a stepwise manner in primary care. This includes warm compression to soften inspissated secretions and massage of the lesion to aid expression of the obstructed gland. This should be repeated up to four times a day. Topical or oral antibiotics are generally not required unless there is evidence of infection.

Initial treatment for external hordeola is much the same consisting of warm compress. Topical antibiotics such as chloramphenicol may be used to shorten the duration of disease and treat any lid margin disease. The presence of preseptal cellulitis would require treatment with oral antibiotics.

For external hordeola, the lash at the centre of the affected follicle should be identified and removed to enhance drainage. Similarly, any obvious meibomian gland plug around which there is an internal hordeolum, can be removed with a cotton bud and topical anaesthetic. Following this, it is often possible to express the pus freely from the meibomian gland.

Surgical options for chalazia consist of an intralesional injection of steroid such as triamcinolone or incision and curettage. Intralesional steroids should be avoided in the presence of an abscess or suspected infection. There is no evidence that one method is superior to the other but steroid injections are generally employed for small, flat, multiple chalazia or those where surgery risks damage to the lacrimal puncta. The most common side effect is skin depigmentation around the injection site. Other potential adverse effects can include elevated intraocular pressure, cataract, fat atrophy and, rarely, globe perforation. Serious complications are probably less common with the transconjunctival route than with transcutaneous. Patients should be advised that recurrence is common, both at the same site and elsewhere along the lid margin.

Incision and curettage is generally the preferred method for larger chalazia and can be performed in the following fashion:

1. Mark the site of the chalazion with a surgical marker prior to the procedure as local anaesthetic can obscure its presence
2. Instill topical tetracaine and proxymetacaine into the inferior fornix.
3. Clean and drape the patient
4. Infiltrate local anaesthetic subcutaneously over the chalazion
5. Place the chalazion clamp over the chalazion and tighten.
6. Evert the lid to expose the tarsal conjunctiva overlying the chalazion. Depending on how posterior or anterior the chalazion sits within the lid, a yellow nodule may or may not be visible through the conjunctiva
7. Make a 3-mm vertical linear incision with a blade through the conjunctiva and tarsus, avoiding the lid margin
8. Use a curette to scrape out the contents of the chalazion, particularly the cyst wall to reduce recurrence. A sample may be

sent for histopathological or microbiology analysis if indicated (see complications section below)
9. Apply chloramphenicol ointment to the eye and remove the clamp
10. Bleeding may ensue following clamp removal, in which case apply firm pressure to the closed lids for a few minutes
11. Double pad the eye with a pressure bandage to achieve haemostasis

Surgical drainage is rarely required for external hordeola unless it is refractory to conservative measures. Drainage is best performed transconjunctivally unless the abscess is pointing onto the skin in which case a horizontal skin incision should be used, to minimise scarring.

Complications

The most common complication of hordeola is recurrence, the incidence of which is unrelated to the method of treatment.

Large chalazia can affect vision by inducing corneal astigmatism and a mechanical ptosis, both of which are potentially amblyogenic. Chronic chalazia that become recurrently inflamed may cause lid notching, lash loss, pyogenic granuloma formation, and scarring which may cause cosmetic deformity of the lid.

Recurrent chalazia in the same location or persistent thickening of the lid margin following treatment should raise suspicion of a masquerade syndrome, classically sebaceous cell or basal cell carcinoma. Biopsy guidelines vary based on location. The current Royal College of Ophthalmologists guidance on ophthalmic pathology recommends that a first occurrence of chalazion in any patient does not require samples to be sent for histopathological analysis. For patients under 40 years, the second recurrence (third occurrence) of a chalazion should prompt a biopsy. For patients over 40 years, the first recurrence (second occurrence) of a chalazion should prompt a biopsy.

Further reading

Aycinena AR, Achiron A, Paul M, et al. Incision and Curettage versus steroid injection for the treatment of chalazia: A Meta-analysis. Ophthalmic Plast Reconstr Surg 2016; 32:220–224.

Lindsley K, Nichols JJ, Dickersin K. Non-surgical interventions for acute internal hordeolum. The Cochrane Library. Cochrane Database Syst Rev 2017; 1:CD007742.

Özdal PÇ, Codere F, Callejo S, et al. Accuracy of the clinical diagnosis of chalazion. Eye 2004; 18:135.

Related topics of interest

- Blepharitis (p. 32)
- Benign lid lesions (p. 17)

16 Chemical injuries

Key points

- Chemical injuries to the eye represent one of the true ophthalmic emergencies, where time to treatment is critical
- Immediate and copious irrigation must precede clinical examination and history taking, as it will play an important role in the prognosis of the injury. The pH of both eyes should be checked. If the pH is not in the physiological range, the eye must be irrigated to bring the pH to an appropriate range (7–7.2)
- The causative agents of ocular chemical injuries are acids and alkalis. Alkalis tend to cause more severe damage compared with acid burns

Epidemiology

Chemical injuries to the eye constitute about a fifth of all ocular injuries with the majority occurring in the workplace as a result of industrial accidents; other causes are related to accidents at home or secondary to criminal assault. Acids, alkalis or neutral agents are the causative agents with alkalis causing more severe injuries due their ability to penetrate deeper into the eye. Where possible, safety glasses should be worn to prevent such injuries.

Pathophysiology

Acid burns are usually less severe than alkali burns as they cause damage by denaturing and precipitating proteins in the tissues. When a strong acid has a pH of less than 4, the acid dissociates into hydrogen ions in the cornea. The hydrogen molecules damage the ocular surface by altering the pH, while the anion causes protein denaturation, precipitation, and coagulation. The coagulated proteins act as a barrier to prevent further penetration of the acid and are responsible for the ground glass appearance of the corneal stroma following an acid injury; damage from acid burns is therefore more superficial. The one exception to this is hydrofluoric acid where the fluoride ion behaves like an alkaline substance because it has better penetrance through the stroma than most acids; it can therefore cause significant anterior segment destruction.

Alkali agents possess both hydrophilic and lipophilic properties giving them the ability to penetrate the corneal stroma and saponify the fatty acids of cell membranes, destroying proteoglycan ground substance and collagen bundles. Alkali substances dissociate into a hydroxyl ion and a cation on the ocular surface. The hydroxyl ion saponifies cell membrane fatty acids, while the cation interacts with stromal collagen and glycosaminoglycans; subsequent hydration of glycosaminoglycans results in stromal haze. This interaction facilitates deeper penetration into and through the cornea and into the anterior segment.

Both acid and alkali burns can cause conjunctival ischaemia which results in a reduced blood supply to the limbus. Limbal ischaemia can ultimately lead to stem cell deficiency and inhibition of normal corneal physiological resurfacing processes. This presents clinically as delayed epithelialisation, conjunctivalisation of the cornea, and neovascularisation or persistence of goblet cells in the corneal epithelium.

In case of deeper penetration into the stroma, the collagen fibrils are hydrated and become subsequently thicker and shorter. This can lead to an acute increase in the intraocular pressure (IOP) by reducing drainage of aqueous through distortion of the trabecular meshwork and by shrinkage of the eye contour caused by shrinkage and contraction of the corneal collagen fibrils.

Conjunctival burns, especially when extensive, may cause long-term problems such as symblepharon formation, scarring, cicatricial entropion, ectropion, and trichiasis.

Clinical features

The most common symptoms are severe pain (foreign body sensation), photophobia, epiphora, blepharospasm, red eyes, and reduced visual acuity.

Chemical injuries to the eye are one of the few true ocular emergencies. The initial mainstay of treatment is irrigation (see below) before any history is taken or clinical examination performed.

The physical examination should be used to assess the extent and depth of injury. A systematic examination of both eyes should be performed, specifically documenting the degree of corneal, conjunctival, and limbal involvement as these can be used to predict ultimate outcome. The examination should involve a check of the palpebral fissures and the fornices should be swept during the examination. Both the palpebral and bulbar conjunctiva, as well as the cornea, should be examined with white light and fluorescein under a cobalt blue light. The IOP should be documented. It is important to be able to distinguish an intact corneal epithelial surface from a corneal surface where the epithelium has been completely debrided; both will show similar fluorescein staining profiles but the luminosity of the corneal surface will be different.

The two major classification schemes for corneal burns are the Roper-Hall classification (**Table 16.1**) and the Dua classification (**Table 16.2**). The Roper-Hall classification is based on the degree of corneal involvement and limbal ischaemia. The Dua classification is based on an estimate of limbal involvement (in clock hours) and the percentage of conjunctival involvement.

Diagnosis

The severity of an ocular injury depends on four factors:
1. The toxicity of the chemical
2. The length of time the chemical was in contact with the eye
3. The depth of penetration, and
4. The area of involvement

A careful history, at an appropriate time, must be taken to note these factors. The patient should be asked when the injury occurred, whether they rinsed their eyes afterwards and for how long and with what

Table 16.1 Roper-Hall classification for ocular surface burns

Grade	Prognosis	Cornea	Conjunctiva/Limbus
I	Good	Corneal epithelial damage	No limbal ischaemia
II	Good	Corneal haze, iris details visible	< 1/3 limbal ischaemia
III	Guarded	Total epithelial loss, stromal haze, iris details obscured	1/3–1/2 limbal ischaemia
IV	Poor	Cornea opaque, iris and pupil obscured	> 1/2 limbal ischaemia

Table 16.2 Dua classification for ocular surface burns

Grade	Prognosis	Clinical findings	Conjunctival involvement	Analogue scale CH/percentage
I	Very good	0 clock hours of limbal involvement	0%	0/0%
II	Good	< 3 clock hours of limbal involvement	< 30%	0.1–3/1–29.9%
III	Good	Between 3 clock hours and 6 clock hours of limbal involvement	30–50%	3.1–6/31–50%
IV	Good to guarded	Between 6 clock hours and 9 clock hours of limbal involvement	50–75%	6.1–9/51–75%
V	Guarded to poor	Between 9 clock hours and 12 clock hours of limbal involvement	75–100%	9.1–11.9/75.1–99.9%
VI	Very poor	Total limbal involvement (12 clock hours)	Total conjunctival involvement (100%)	12/100%

Note: The analogue scale records the amount of limbal involvement in clock hours (CH) of affected limbus/percentage of conjunctival involvement. The conjunctival involvement should be calculated only for the bulbar conjunctiva, up to and including the conjunctival fornices.

liquid (e.g. tap water, boiled water or sterile water), the mechanism of injury (was the chemical under high pressure?), the nature of the chemical, and whether or not they were wearing eye protection.

Clinical course of chemical ocular injury

There are four phases of chemical injury, as devised by McCulley: immediate, acute, early reparative, and late reparative. These are further explained in **Table 16.3**.
- The immediate phase comprises the clinical findings on initial examination and gives an estimate of the severity and prognosis of the injury using one of the above-mentioned classification systems. The key elements for determining the extent of chemical ocular injury and prognosis are:
  - The total area of the corneal epithelial defect
  - The area of the conjunctival epithelial defect
  - The number of clock hours or degrees of limbal blanching
  - The area and density of corneal opacification
  - Evidence of increased IOP on presentation
  - Loss of lens clarity
- In the acute recovery phase, the key factor is re-epithelialisation which will protect the exposed stroma from the action of lytic enzymes. The IOP must be monitored and appropriately treated
- The early reparative phase is the healing period when the acute inflammatory response is replaced by chronic inflammation, stromal repair, and scarring
- The late reparative phase extends for 3 weeks following the chemical injury. This stage is characterised by completion of healing with good visual prognosis (Grade I and II) and complications in those with guarded visual prognosis (Grade III and IV)

Treatment

The first and most important step in management of an acute ocular chemical injury is copious irrigation, since the duration and area of exposure to the chemical agent will determine the extent and prognosis of the injury. First the pH of both eyes should be checked. If the pH is not in the physiological range, then the eye must be copiously irrigated to bring the pH to an appropriate range (7–7.2). Delivery of 1–2 litres of irrigating solution (normal saline, Ringer's lactate solution, and balanced salt solution) for at least 30 minutes is of great importance. However, immediate irrigation with even

Table 16.3 Stages of ocular recovery following chemical injury (McCulley)

Phase	Day	Recovery
Initial	0	Clinical findings relate to the severity of injury and can be graded according to the degree of limbal, corneal, and conjunctival involvement
Acute	0–7	Epithelial regrowth begins to occur if there is a sufficient amount of undamaged limbal stem cells. Treatment should be directed at encouraging growth while quelling inflammation.
Early repair	7–21	Corneal/conjunctival epithelium and keratocytes proliferate during this stage. Mild injuries show complete re-epithelialisation while more severe injuries can have persistent epithelial defects. Activity of collagenases peaks by day 14–21 while collagen synthesis continues. Treatment should attempt to maximise collagen synthesis while minimizing collagenase activity.
Late repair	After day 21	In mild injuries, where the limbal stem cell population is intact, repair is completed. In Grade II injuries, where there is focal stem cell loss, there may be a focal conjunctivalisation of the cornea. In more severe injuries, there is delayed re-epithelialisation of the cornea, ultimately leading to either repopulation by conjunctival epithelium or stromal ulceration and permanent scarring. In cases of severe limbal damage, despite optimal management, the eye often cannot be salvaged.

plain tap water is preferred over waiting for the ideal fluid. If the patient is unable to keep the eyelids open due to pain-induced blepharospasm or poor cooperation in the case of children, the use of a speculum can be considered. Instillation of topical anaesthetic drops prior to irrigation when available is very helpful. Irrigation should be continued until the achievement of a neutral tear pH measurement. After irrigation, it is imperative to wait at least for 5 minutes before checking the pH to ensure that the pH does not rise or fall secondary to retained particulate matter.

Only when the pH is within the normal range can a complete and thorough eye examination be performed. Care should be taken to examine the fornices and evert the upper lids for residual particles.

Grade I and II injuries usually respond very well to topical antibiotic treatment, steroid drops and cycloplegia for about a week. Treatment in more severe injuries aims to limit ocular damage and maximise visual potential.

Medical treatment

Medical treatment aims to promote ocular surface (epithelial) healing, to control inflammation and IOP, and to prevent infection.
- Steroids initially administered 2-hourly for the first 10–14 days followed by a tapering regime. Initial intensive steroid treatment reduces neutrophil infiltration and inflammatory response. Prolonged use of topical steroids causes reduction of collagen synthesis and inhibition of fibroblast migration which can lead to corneal ulceration. For this reason, they should be tailed off from day 14
- Topical ascorbic acid 10% 2-hourly and systemic vitamin C enhances corneal healing, acting as a cofactor in collagen synthesis
- Topical citric acid 10%, 2-hourly for 10 days, inhibits neutrophil activity and reduces inflammation, acting as a calcium chelator that decreases the intracellular calcium levels of neutrophils
- Doxycycline 100 mg bd initially, followed by od acts as a neutrophil and collagenase inhibitor, reducing corneal ulceration
- Cyclopentolate 1% tds is used as pain relief
- Topical antibiotics are used to prevent secondary bacterial infections
- Glaucoma medications are used to control high IOP, if present. Oral medication is preferable in the acute phase
- Ideally all topical preparations should be given preservative-free

Surgical treatment

Surgical intervention may be required if medical treatments alone do not result in epithelial healing within a few weeks.
- *Tenonplasty*: Advancement of Tenon's capsule to the limbus, aiming to re-establish limbal blood supply
- *Limbal cell transplantation*: Aims to restore the normal corneal epithelium. Should be delayed until optimal control of ocular surface inflammation has been achieved
- *Amniotic membrane transplant*: Provides a basement membrane for epithelialisation, reduces inflammation and corneal scarring
- *Corneal transplantation and gluing*: Should be considered in the presence of actual/imminent perforation. A penetrating or lamellar keratoplasty at a later stage can also be performed in the context of visual rehabilitation
- *Keratoprosthesis*: Used in more severe cases for visual rehabilitation, when conventional penetrating or lamellar keratoplasty survival has a poor prognosis

Complications

Severe chemical burns can have devastating and disfiguring consequences. Loss of vision, due to severe corneal damage or penetration of the chemical agent into the eye is the most serious complication; chronic dry eyes, corneal epithelial breakdown, corneal neovascularisation, loss of physiological corneal surface features, corneal thinning, and scarring are also common and depend on the severity of the injury. Problems related to high IOP or to the ocular adnexa (forniceal shortening, symblepharon formation, and cicatricial entropion or ectropion) could also coexist with other problems and render the management even more challenging.

Further reading

AAO. (2012). Treating Acute Chemical Injuries of the Cornea. [online] Available from https://www.aao.org/eyenet/article/treating-acute-chemical-injuries-of-cornea [Last accessed November, 2019].

Related topics of interest

- Corneal grafts (p. 90)
- Infectious keratitis (p. 181)

17 Conjunctivitis

Key points
- Infectious conjunctivitis can be classified into acute, hyperacute, and chronic
- Conjunctivitis is usually diagnosed based on clinical history and examination
- If the diagnosis is not obvious, laboratory studies can be a helpful way of determining the underlying aetiology
- Antibiotic therapy should be considered in the presence of severe purulent discharge, hyperacute disease, contact lens use, and in immunocompromised individuals

Epidemiology

The prevalence of conjunctivitis varies according to the underlying cause, which may be *infectious* [viral (including deno and herpetic)/bacterial (including *Staphylococcus*, *Streptococcus*, *Haemophilus*, chlamydial, and gonococcal)] or *non-infectious* (including allergic, drug/toxin induced/secondary to systemic disease). Acute infective conjunctivitis is seen in 2% of patients presenting to general practice, with viral disease accounting for up to 90% of all cases of acute conjunctivitis. Conjunctivitis imposes a significant socioeconomic burden as it affects millions of people annually with the cost of treatment estimated to be up to $857 million per year in the United States alone. As infectious conjunctivitis accounts for the majority of cases, discussions henceforth will be dedicated to this topic.

Pathophysiology

Conjunctivitis develops as a result of exposure to organisms, allergens, and toxins. The squamous epithelial layer of the conjunctiva provides a mechanical barrier against organism invasion. Once host defence mechanisms are overwhelmed, pathogenic organisms as well as commensal conjunctival species such as *Staphylococcus epidermidis*, *Staphylococcus aureus*, and *Corynebacterium* can cause infective conjunctivitis.

Infective conjunctivitis is highly contagious, and the risk of transmission has been estimated to be 10–50% in viral cases with the organism spreading through direct/indirect contact with contaminated individuals. Up to half of patients have positive cultures grown from their hands.

Clinical features

Conjunctivitis typically produces local symptoms such as discomfort, grittiness, and burning. Examination usually reveals conjunctival vessel dilatation, oedema, and discharge. Patients with severe disease should be examined for the following signs:

- *Pseudomembranes*: A loosely adherent mixture of exudate containing mucus, proteins, and inflammatory debris, which can be peeled away from the underlying conjunctival surface with little to no bleeding or damage to the underlying epithelium
- *True membranes*: A firmly adherent layer forming between necrotic conjunctival cells and overlying coagulum. Usually forms after intense inflammation and once peeled, the epithelium shreds, leaving behind a raw, bleeding surface
- *Subconjunctival haemorrhage*: Occasionally seen in pneumococcal or adenoviral conjunctivitis
- *Subepithelial corneal infiltrates*: Small, round, greyish lesions, usually seen bilaterally but frequently in an asymmetrical fashion. They are composed of antigen residues and lymphocyte accumulations adhered to stromal cells. They often lead to a reduction in visual acuity, halos, and photophobia. Whilst usually self-limiting, lesions can stay dormant for months or years
- *Lymphadenopathy*: More prevalent in viral cases and observed in up to 50% of patients

Table 17.1 summarises the key clinic features seen in conjunctivitis.

Table 17.1 Ocular signs in conjunctivitis

Sign	Bacterial	Viral
Injection	++	++
Haemorrhage	+	+
Chemosis	++	+
Exudate	Purulent/mucopurulent	Scant/watery
Pseudomembrane	+/−	+/−
Papillae	+/−	
Follicles	−	+
Perauricular lymphadenopathy	+	+

Table 17.2 Bacterial conjunctivitis pathogens

Hyperacute	Acute	Chronic*
Neisseria gonorrhoeae	S. aureus	S. aureus
N. meningitidis	S. pneumoniae	Moraxella lacunata
	H. influenzae	Klebsiella pneumoniae
	Moraxella catarrhalis	Serratia marcescens
	S. pyogenes	Escherichia coli

*Chronic bacterial conjunctivitis is used to describe any conjunctivitis lasting more than 4 weeks.

Viral

Viruses are responsible for the majority of cases of acute conjunctivitis with up to 90% of viral conjunctivitis resulting from adenoviral infection. Adenoviruses produce two distinct clinical entities:

1. *Pharyngoconjunctival fever*: It is characterised by bilateral conjunctivitis accompanied by an acute onset of fever, pharyngitis, and peri-auricular lymphadenopathy.
2. *Epidemic keratoconjunctivitis (EKC)*: Severe watery discharge, conjunctival injection, chemosis, and ipsilateral lymphadenopathy. EKC can lead to membranous or pseudomembranous conjunctivitis.

Bacterial

Patients with bacterial conjunctivitis typically present with purulent or mucopurulent discharge and conjunctival chemosis. Bilateral sticky eyelids, no history of conjunctivitis in the immediate family or friends, and a lack of itch are positive predictors for the presence of bacterial rather than viral disease. **Table 17.2** summarises the pathogens commonly leading to bacterial conjunctivitis.

Chlamydia

Chlamydia trachomatis is an obligate intracellular bacterium responsible for trachoma, inclusion conjunctivitis, and lymphogranuloma venereum. Trachoma is caused by subtypes A, B, Ba, and C, adult inclusion conjunctivitis by serotypes D-K, and lymphogranuloma venereum by L1, L2, and L3. A simplified World Health Organization (WHO) system widely used in endemic areas is presented in **Table 17.3**.

Table 17.3 The WHO trachoma grading system

Trachomatous inflammation – follicular (TF)	Five or more follicles at least 0.5 mm in diameter on the central area of the upper tarsal conjunctiva
Trachomatous inflammation – intense (TI)	Pronounced inflammatory thickening of the upper tarsal conjunctiva obscuring 50% or more of the normal deep tarsal vessels
Trachomatous scarring (TS)	Presence of visible scars on the tarsal conjunctiva
Trachomatous trichiasis (TT)	At least one lash touching the eyeball
Corneal opacity (CO)	Corneal opacity. Any corneal opacity blurring the pupil margin

Investigations

The diagnosis of conjunctivitis is typically clinical. Obtaining conjunctival cultures is generally reserved for recurrent or recalcitrant conjunctivitis, hyperacute cases or cases of suspected infectious neonatal conjunctivitis. To achieve the highest bacterial yield, antibiotic therapy should be initiated after obtaining conjunctival cultures or a short drug washout period.

Viral conjunctivitis is commonly misdiagnosed as bacterial conjunctivitis and in recent years rapid in-office antigen tests have become available, allowing for easy and highly specific tests for adenoviral disease, preventing unnecessary antibiotic use. A number of tests are available to detect chlamydial disease such as Giemsa staining, direct immunofluorescent staining or enzyme-linked immunosorbent assay.

Treatment

Because of the high rates of transmission, handwashing, strict instrument disinfection, and isolation of the infected patients from the rest of the clinic, are mandatory. Incubation and communicability are estimated to be 5–12 days and 10–14 days (prolonged with topical steroid use) respectively.

Viral

No effective treatment currently exists for viral conjunctivitis. Patients should be treated symptomatically with artificial tears or cold compresses. Topical antibiotics should be avoided as they do not reduce the duration of symptoms, do not protect against secondary infections, and may increase the risk of transmission to the other eye from contaminated bottles. Topical corticosteroids are often prescribed in severe cases or in the presence of visually significant subepithelial infiltrates, to reduce symptoms related to inflammation. However, their use may increase the duration of disease by promoting the replication of the virus. Some physicians favour the use of Povidone Iodine drops with or without concurrent steroid drops in cases of adenoviral conjunctivitis to reduce the duration of symptoms.

Bacterial

More than half of acute bacterial conjunctivitis episodes are self-limiting. Whilst topical broad-spectrum antibiotics reduce the duration of the disease and decrease transmissibility, they do not alter long-term outcomes nor reduce the risk of serious complications. Antibiotic therapy should, however, be considered in patients with severe purulent discharge, contact lens users, and in immunocompromised individuals.

Chlamydia

Patients suspected of having chlamydial inclusion conjunctivitis should be treated with systemic antibiotics such as oral azithromycin or doxycycline and their sexual partners traced for further investigation. Such patients also be screened for a co-infection with gonorrhoea and, if positive, treated with an intravenous or intramuscular cephalosporins. Management of trachoma in endemic areas consists of a multifaceted approach to prevent blindness. The WHO recommends the **SAFE** strategy to treat different stages of trachoma:

S: Surgery for trichiasis or entropion to reduce or prevent corneal blindness
A: Antibiotics for active disease (topical tetracycline or oral azithromycin)
F: Facial cleanliness
E: Environmental improvements

Complications

Late complications such as scarring of the eyelid, conjunctiva, and cornea may lead to loss of vision in chronic disease. Hyperacute conjunctivitis carries a high risk for corneal involvement and subsequent corneal perforation and should therefore be investigated in a timely fashion and treated aggressively.

Further reading

Azari AA, Barney NP. Conjunctivitis: a systematic review of diagnosis and treatment. JAMA 2013; 310:1721–1729.

Sheikh A, Hurwitz B, van Schayck CP, et al. Antibiotics versus placebo for acute bacterial conjunctivitis. Cochrane Database Syst Rev 2012:CD001211.

Related topics of interest

- Blepharitis (p. 32)
- Infectious keratitis (p. 181)

18 Contact lens-related problems of the eye

Key points

- Contact lenses (CLs) are widely used for therapeutic, optical, and cosmetic purposes
- Complications related to CL wear can occur with all lens types and vary from mild to severe
- The type of CL worn, the care taken of the lenses, and the patient's education play an important role in the risk of problems associated with CL wear

Epidemiology

Contact lenses are widely used for optical, cosmetic, and therapeutic purposes with an estimated 140 million individual users worldwide. Amongst wearers, about 6% will experience some CL-related problems although most of these are minor. However, an average of 3–5 per 10,000 CL wearers will face more serious sight-threatening complications such as microbial keratitis. The modality of use and previous underlying ocular conditions play an important role in the aetiology of CL-related problems.

Pathophysiology

Corneal infections are rare in the normal healthy eye. When they do occur, they are a result of an alteration in the defence mechanisms of the cornea allowing bacteria to invade in the presence of an epithelial defect. In CL-related infections, these microbes may come from the lid margins, the fingers upon lens insertion (or removal), the lens itself, the care solutions, or the storage case.

There are two main types of CLs: rigid gas permeable (RGP) CLs that allow oxygen penetration, and soft hydrogel CLs which have lower oxygen permeability. Hypoxia induced by CL wear is one of the main factors compromising the natural defences of the cornea. Hypoxia may increase bacterial binding, compromise corneal integrity, and impair wound healing.

Contact lens wear, especially extended and overnight wear, has been shown to cause changes in both the corneal and tear film physiology. An intact corneal epithelium together with the tear film allows for a high resistance against microbial invasion. Tears contain surfactants and antimicrobial proteins which prevent microbial adhesion to the corneal epithelium and initiate a defence response against virulent micro-organisms. A CL has the capacity to alter tear biochemistry at the corneal surface if it sits too close to the cornea (excludes tears), or if it shuts down exchange of tears (tear mixing) between the pre- and post-lens tear compartments during blinking. This lack of tear exchange may also reduce the ability to remove microbes from under the lens.

The physiological changes affecting the corneal epithelium, which are likely to affect the mechanisms of resistance to infection, include the inhibition of normal corneal epithelial shedding, corneal epithelial thinning, increased binding of bacteria to normal corneal cells, increased internalisation of bacteria through the expression of membrane lipid rafts on corneal epithelial cells, and the disruption to the normal lid/cornea/tear resurfacing mechanism.

The adhesion of bacteria to CLs is considered a major risk factor for serious corneal problems (particularly *Staphylococcus epidermidis* and *Pseudomonas aeruginosa*). CLs are a suitable surface for bacterial adhesion and biofilm formation. They sustain a large quantity of organisms in prolonged contact with the cornea.

Clinical features

Contact lens-related complications can be divided in five categories depending on the aetiology: infectious, inflammatory, mechanical, hypoxic, and toxic/allergic.

Infectious complications

Microbial keratitis is a major and sight-threatening complication in CL wear.

Overnight, extended wear of CLs and poor hygiene when handling the CLs, increases the risk of microbial keratitis. The commonest pathogen is *Pseudomonas aeruginosa* followed by bacteria (gram positive), fungi, and *Acanthamoeba*.

Clinically, microbial keratitis presents with a stromal infiltrate more centrally located as compared with marginal keratitis, and usually associated with an overlying epithelial defect, conjunctival injection, and anterior chamber reaction.

Fungal keratitis is rare in temperate countries. The commonest pathogens from the non-filamentous species are *Candida spp.* whereas *Fusarium spp.* and *Aspergillus spp.* are the main causes of infection with filamentous fungi. Patients present with redness, photophobia, and pain that can be severe. On slit lamp examination, filamentous infiltrates are usually less dense compared with bacterial infiltrates, grey or white in colour, with indistinct margins and can manifest satellite lesions. Fungal infections are usually slowly progressive.

Acanthamoeba keratitis presents with severe pain, photophobia, limbitis, and a diffuse or focal anterior stromal infiltrate which may present as a ring infiltrate or perineurally. The presence of epithelial pseudodendrites is common and could initially mimic herpetic keratitis resulting in a delay in diagnosis and treatment.

Inflammatory complications

Contact lens-related sterile peripheral corneal infiltrates can be single or multiple, and tend to be localised in the periphery. The epithelium is usually intact and the anterior chamber reaction is minimal or absent. Symptoms are less severe compared with microbial keratitis. These infiltrates are the result of an immunological reaction and are the greatest diagnostic dilemma to early microbial keratitis. Close monitoring, especially early in treatment, should be provided to prevent inappropriate treatment of an early microbial keratitis and to observe for improvement. These infiltrates are thought to represent a hypersensitivity reaction against endotoxins created by the bacteria, the CL material itself, the CL care products, or a combination thereof.

Hypoxic complications

Acute corneal hypoxia is described as a combination of blurry vision, burning sensation, and grittiness of the eyes followed by hyperlacrimation. This condition is often found in patients who have forgotten to remove their CLs before sleeping. Clinically, corneal epithelial microcysts are present; these can lead to macroerosions, stromal oedema, and endothelial bleb formation.

Perhaps the most noticeable effects of CLs are those on the bulbar and limbal vasculature causing increased ocular redness through chronic hypoxia. The prevalence of corneal vascularisation in patients wearing RGP CLs is generally very low, presumably because of the small size of the lenses and the consequent exposure of the limbus and peripheral cornea. Daily wear hydrogel lenses of relatively low oxygen transmissibility are associated with a substantially higher prevalence of corneal vascularisation. Limbal vessel dilation has been identified as the main observable clinical sign preceding the development of corneal vascularisation. Vascularisation alters the immune privilege of the cornea and the anterior chamber which may consequently influence the inflammatory response to trauma or injury.

Mechanical complications

Tight lens syndrome, also known as CLARE (contact lens-induced acute red eye), is defined as an acute inflammatory reaction of the cornea, the conjunctiva, and occasionally the anterior chamber immediately after eye closure. Although most commonly associated with overnight CL wear, it can actually occur at any time of the day upon brief eye closure. The presentation is similar to that of infectious keratitis and includes a mixture of unilateral acute corneal inflammation with mild to moderate blepharospasm, severe conjunctival and limbal hyperaemia, corneal oedema, corneal infiltration (usually multifocal and greatest in the periphery), ocular pain, and severe photosensitivity. The patient may find it difficult to remove the CLs. Examination reveals minimal to no movement of the lens and may show debris trapped underneath the CLs. Epithelial staining, if present, is minimal and coincides with the pattern of debris found under the lens. There is no epithelial defect but a defect or ulcer can be induced following removal of the lens. CLARE is most commonly associated with extended-wear hydrogel lenses due to lens tightening precipitated by hypoxia.

Giant papillary conjunctivitis (GPC) is a condition that has a double aetiology; it represents an immune response against antigenic proteins on the CL and/or it is a mechanical irritation of the tarsal conjunctiva caused by the edge or the surface of the CL. Symptoms include increased ocular itching, mucous discharge in tears, blurred vision, and conjunctival injection. This can be accompanied by decreased CL tolerance and decreased mechanical stability. Clinical presentation is with tarsal hyperaemia, giant papillae, and mucous strands seen in the tears and between the papillae.

Contact lens-induced superior limbic keratoconjunctivitis (SLK) is an inflammatory condition involving the corneal epithelium, stroma, limbus, and the bulbar and tarsal conjunctiva. CL-induced SLK should be differentiated from superior limbic keratoconjunctivitis of Theodore, which has almost identical presentation but is unrelated to CL wear. Examination reveals injection of the superior bulbar conjunctiva, limbal papillary hypertrophy with scattered petechiae, fluorescein staining of the superior cornea, epithelial and subepithelial infiltration of the superior cornea, a papillary reaction on the superior tarsal conjunctiva, and mild superior corneal pannus.

Contact lenses can also cause an alteration of the corneal curvature resulting from a moulding effect produced by long-term CL wear. Treatment consists of making sure there is no irregular astigmatism, CL refitting, and changing the material of the lens.

Toxic and allergic complications

Both toxic and allergic reactions are usually triggered by compounds of the CL care solutions. Conjunctival and limbal injection, diffuse superficial punctate keratopathy, and microinfiltrates are the commonest clinical signs.

All CLs reduce corneal sensitivity. The exact mechanism for corneal hypoesthesia is unknown but may include sensitisation to the mechanical trauma produced by CL and/or corneal metabolic changes that affect the corneal nerves.

Diagnosis

A thorough history taking into account the type and pattern of CL wear along with a slit lamp examination of the anterior segment of the eye, with special attention to the location of the lesions and pattern of signs, is essential. Eyelid eversion is very important where GPC or SLK is suspected. The pattern of punctate staining can give important information and help with the differential diagnosis. Central or peripheral localisation of corneal infiltrates, characteristics of their margins, their size and presence of perineural infiltrates, anterior chamber reaction, and pattern of conjunctival hyperaemia are of great importance for the establishment of the correct diagnosis.

When microbial keratitis is suspected, the nature of the causative organism should be investigated by the collection of samples for microscopy, culture, and sensitivity; multiple samples should be taken. It is not necessary to stop antibiotics already started prior to taking samples for culture. The laboratory should be asked to give antibiotic sensitivities to agents that are available for topical ophthalmic use. Where possible, it is also important to send the CL case and care solution used for laboratory testing.

In vivo confocal microscopy is an extremely useful test when *Acanthamoeba* keratitis is suspected. This test identifies the presence of corneal cysts and irregular trophozoites.

Treatment

- *Microbial keratitis*: Discontinuation of CL wear is essential. Initial treatment should be with a broad-spectrum antibiotic to cover both gram-positive and gram-negative organisms. Topical fluoroquinolones (e.g. ofloxacin, levofloxacin, and moxifloxacin) are still effective in the UK. The topical therapy is subsequently modified

depending on the results of in vitro bacterial sensitivity tests. Treatment is intensive for the first few days to achieve therapeutic tissue concentrations and rapid control of the infection; the frequency can then be reduced depending on the clinical response
- *Sterile peripheral corneal infiltrates*: In the case of doubt, corneal scraping should be performed. Discontinuation of CL wear is essential, followed by the use of topical steroid drops along with prophylactic antibiotic coverage. Close monitoring, especially early in treatment, is essential to prevent inappropriate treatment of an early microbial keratitis and to monitor for improvement
- *Acute hypoxia*: Discontinuation of CL is essential. Once the oedema has resolved, refitting with a high oxygen-permeable lens should be considered
- *Peripheral neovascularisation*: If the neovascularisation does not exceed 1.5 mm radially from the limbus, simple observation is usually sufficient. If the neovascularisation extends more than 1.5 mm into the stroma, CL refitting with a high oxygen-permeable lens should be considered or there should be discontinuation of CL wear altogether
- *Tight lens syndrome*: Immediate cessation of CL wear is advised. Medical treatment consists of intensive lubrication, cycloplegia (if anterior chamber inflammation is present), and a topical steroid in the case of significant inflammation. Prophylactic topical antibiotics should be considered given the similarity in presentation between CLARE and infectious keratitis
- *Giant papillary conjunctivitis and SLK*: Discontinuation of CL for a short period of time and lubrication. The use of combination of mast cell stabilisers and antihistamine ophthalmic medications in GPC generally suffices without the need for potent topical steroids. For both conditions, CL wear can often resume after an improvement in symptoms
- *Toxic or allergic keratitis and conjunctivitis*: CL wear should be discontinued initially and topical unpreserved lubrication should be initiated. Daily disposable (DD) CLs should be considered when possible or a different care solution should be used

Complications

Contact lens-related complications can vary from mild to severe and sight-threatening. Dry eyes, CL intolerance, peripheral corneal neovascularisation and pannus formation represent mild complications and are seldom of functional significance. More devastating complications are usually associated with infectious conditions (e.g. scar formation and need for corneal transplantation) and could potentially cause severe visual impairment and endanger the visual function or the integrity of the ocular globe itself.

Further reading

Alipour F, Khaheshi S, Soleimanzadeh M, et al. Contact lens-related complications: A Review. J Ophthalmic Vis Res 2017; 12:193–204.

Lakhundi S, Siddiqui R, Khan NA. Pathogenesis of microbial keratitis. Microb Pathog 2017; 104:97–109.

The Royal College of Ophthalmologists. (2013). Microbial keratitis. [online] Available from https://www.rcophth.ac.uk/wp-content/uploads/2014/08/Focus-Autumn-2013.pdf [Last accessed October, 2019].

Related topics of interest

- Infectious keratitis (p. 181)
- Corneal ectasia (p. 85)

19 Corneal dystrophies

Key points

- The corneal dystrophies are a group of inherited conditions which are generally bilateral, symmetrical, and slowly progressive
- With the advent of genetic testing the traditional nomenclature and anatomical classification of these dystrophies has been revised
- These dystrophies differ markedly in age of onset and severity; some require no intervention whilst others require multiple corneal transplantations

Epidemiology

The corneal dystrophies are a heterogeneous group of inherited disorders which are usually bilateral, symmetrical, and slowly progressive conditions affecting the structure and/or function of the cornea, and which are unrelated to systemic or environmental factors. However, within the group there are conditions that take exception to each of these general defining characteristics. For example, epithelial basement membrane dystrophy (EBMD) is only rarely inherited, and is more likely a degeneration than a true dystrophy, and posterior polymorphous corneal dystrophy (PPCD) can be clinically unilateral. All of the corneal dystrophies, with the exception of Fuchs endothelial corneal dystrophy (FECD), are rare. FECD itself has been estimated to affect up to 4% of the population over 40 years old in the USA.

Pathophysiology

Most of the corneal dystrophies were described and named before the advent of genetic testing, and some even before the invention of the slit-lamp. Their nomenclature has therefore largely been based on clinical appearance, resulting in phenotype-based or eponymously named dystrophies. Today's ability to genotype these conditions has revolutionised our understanding of their pathophysiology.

Although many different genetic causes have now been identified, one particular gene (located at 5q31), which encodes transforming growth factor beta-induced (TGFBI), has been found to be causative in several previously distinctly classified corneal dystrophies, and now constitutes its own subset of corneal dystrophies (see below). *TGFBI* encodes for keratoepithelin, a protein secreted by corneal epithelium and which acts as an adhesion molecule.

Clinical features

The corneal dystrophies can be classified based on the anatomical layer/s that they predominantly affect. There are currently 22 corneal dystrophy subclassifications; the main ones are described below under their corresponding anatomical subheading.

Epithelial and subepithelial dystrophies

Epithelial basement membrane dystrophy

Most cases of epithelial basement membrane dystrophy (EBMD) (*synonym*: Map-dot-fingerprint dystrophy (**Figrue 19.1**), Cogan's microcystic epithelial dystrophy) have no hereditary basis and present in adult life, and the condition is more likely a corneal degeneration than an inherited disease. As one of its synonyms suggests, it has the appearance of superficial maps, dots and/or fingerprints (best visualised with retro-illumination) in the corneal epithelium. Recurrent corneal erosions can arise from inadequate adhesion of basal epithelial cells.

Meesmann corneal dystrophy

This dystrophy has an autosomal dominant inheritance presenting in childhood, and consists of multiple superficial transparent microcysts, best seen with retro-illumination. Patients are typically asymptomatic but may have mild visual impairment with glare and photosensitivity, and may develop recurrent erosions.

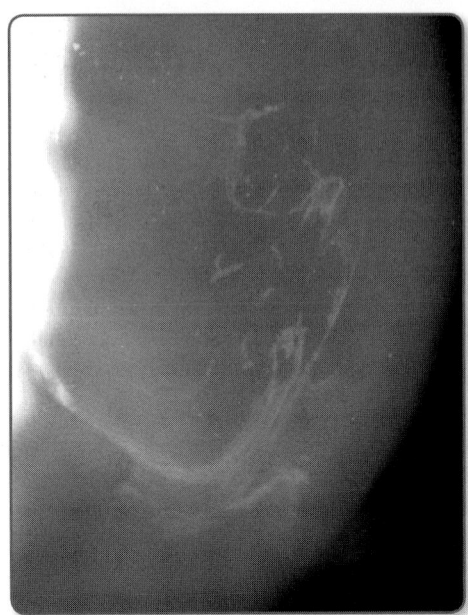

Figure 19.1 Map-dot-fingerprint dsytrophy.

Gelatinous drop-like corneal dystrophy (synonym: Subepithelial amyloidosis)

This autosomal recessive dystrophy, which presents in the first to second decade, can appear like band keratopathy, or with multiple groups of small nodules in a mulberry-like phenotype, which stain with fluorescein. There is often corneal vascularisation and significant stromal opacity with consequent reduction in vision, redness, and photosensitivity. Most patients develop recurrence after surgery such as superficial keratectomy or (lamellar or penetrating) keratoplasty.

Epithelial-stromal *TGFBI* dystrophies (all with autosomal dominant inheritance)

Reis–Bücklers corneal dystrophy (synonym: Corneal dystrophy of Bowman layer type I)

Reis–Bücklers corneal dystrophy (RBCD) presents in childhood with confluent geographic opacities at the level of Bowman's layer and superficial stroma, which progress to deeper stromal layers with time. Patients suffer from recurrent erosions and impaired vision; the erosions tend to reduce with time but the vision tends to decline. Rod-shaped bodies are immunopositive for TGFBI protein.

Thiel-Behnke corneal dystrophy (Synonym: Corneal dystrophy of Bowman layer type II, Honeycomb-shaped corneal dystrophy)

It can be clinically difficult to distinguish Thiel–Behnke corneal dystrophy (TBCD) from RBCD (see heading Investigations). In the early stages, TBCD typically demonstrates multiple flecks with a reticular appearance, whereas RBCD has more irregular diffuse opacities. RBCD tends to follow a more aggressive course than TBCD. Curly collagen fibres are immunopositive for TGFBI protein.

Lattice corneal dystrophy type 1 and variants (synonym: Biber-Haab-Dimmer)

A lattice of ramifying lines spreads deeper and more peripherally with time (sparing the far periphery), along with the development of central haze. Patients present with discomfort and pain as early as the first decade of life, due to recurrent erosions, and they often develop significant visual loss by the fourth decade, necessitating surgery. Abnormal deposits of amyloid characteristically demonstrate birefringence, red-green dichroism under polarised light, and stain with Congo red. In Familial amyloidosis (*synonym*: Meretoja syndrome) there are fewer lattice lines than in lattice corneal dystrophy type 1 (LCD1) and its variants, and the lines start peripherally and spread centrally.

Granular corneal dystrophy type 1 (GCD1)

From early childhood, distinct granular lesions, with clear intervening stroma, increase in number, size and depth with time and gain the appearance of snowflakes. The lesions do not extend to the periphery. Patients experience photosensitivity, erosions and loss of vision as the opacification progresses. Abnormal hyaline deposits stain with Masson trichrome.

Granular corneal dystrophy type 2 (GCD2) (synonym: Avellino dystrophy, combined granular-lattice dystrophy)

Star-like anterior stromal deposits, with deeper dash-like lesions that rarely cross each other (unlike the linear lesions seen in LCD1) (**Figure 19.2**). Usually diagnosed in adolescence or early adulthood, patients experience recurrent erosions and loss of vision as the central axis becomes affected. There are both hyaline and amyloid deposits. Laser refractive surgery is contraindicated as it may exacerbate the opacification.

Stromal dystrophies

Macular corneal dystrophy

Macular corneal dystrophy (MCD) is an autosomal recessive dystrophy whose mutation leads to a defect in the synthesis of keratan sulfate, the major glycosaminoglycan (GAG) in the cornea. It is less common, but more severe than the other stromal dystrophies. The cornea is thinned and its sensitivity is reduced. Severe visual impairment ensues over the first three decades of life. Uniquely to the stromal dystrophies, Descemet's membrane and endothelium are involved, and abnormal GAG deposits are seen throughout the stroma, staining with Hale colloidal iron or alcian blue.

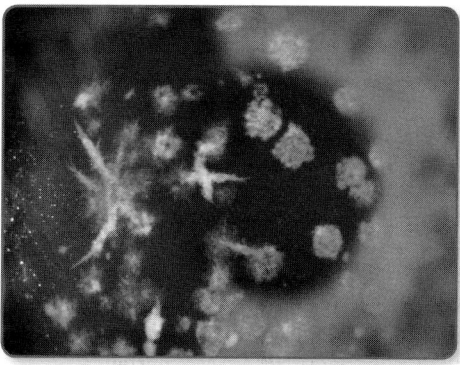

Figure 19.2 Granular dystrophy type 2.

Schnyder corneal dystrophy (synonym: Schnyder crystalline corneal dystrophy)

This autosomal dominant dystrophy results from changes in the gene encoding UbiA prenyltransferase domain-containing protein 1 (UBIAD1). Only about half of cases demonstrate corneal crystals. Patients' photopic vision is increasingly affected with age, whilst scotopic vision is relatively preserved. There are phospholipids and cholesterol deposits throughout the epithelium, Bowman's layer, and the stroma. Send suspected tissue samples as fresh tissue for staining (e.g. using Oil Red O or Sudan black).

Central cloudy dystrophy of François

Central cloudy dystrophy of François (CCDF) is identical to posterior crocodile shagreen (a corneal degeneration), except that CCDF is associated with a family history, although its inheritance is unknown. There are central polygonal stromal opacities separated by linear areas of clear stroma. Patients are generally asymptomatic.

Endothelial dystrophies

Fuchs endothelial corneal dystrophy (FECD)

In Stage 1, corneal endothelial guttata start centrally and progress peripherally (**Figure 19.3**). The condition can advance to endothelial decompensation and corneal oedema (Stage 2), bullous keratopathy (Stage 3), and finally scarring and fibrosis from chronic oedema (Stage 4). Onset is typically in the 4th to 5th decade (except in the rarer early-onset variant), with patients experiencing diurnal variation in vision (worse in the morning) and, later, discomfort and pain from ruptured epithelial bullae. The genetic basis of FECD is complex, and there is a female:male preponderance of approximately 3:1.

Posterior polymorphous corneal dystrophy (PPCD)

This autosomal dominant dystrophy is often asymmetrical, and can be seen in unilateral

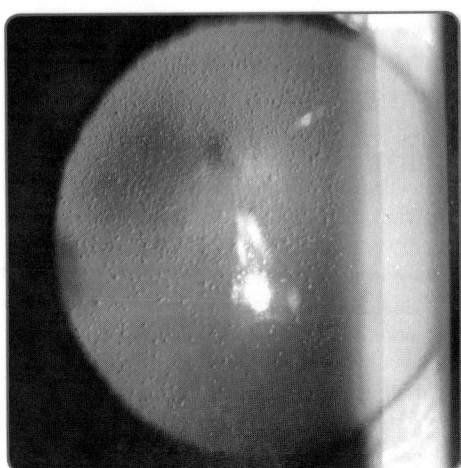

Figure 19.3 Fuchs' endothelial dystrophy.

cases with no heredity. From early childhood there are grey geographic opacities at the level of the endothelium. About 25% of cases require corneal transplantation due to the development of corneal oedema. Endothelial cells affected display ultrastructural features (e.g. desomosomes and microvilli) characteristic of epithelial cells.

Congenital hereditary endothelial dystrophy

From birth, there is bilateral (often asymmetrical) clouding of the cornea, with corneal thickening and a ten-fold reduction in the endothelial cell count. The resultant blurry vision is often associated with nystagmus, although there is little if any progression. There is abnormally increased secretion of a thickened Descemet's membrane by the degenerated endothelial cells and stromal oedema.

Investigations

The principal investigation to enable diagnosis is slit lamp examination, looking for the features described above. Immunohistochemistry is required to definitively distinguish RBCD from TBCD, but a distinguishing feature on optical coherence tomography (OCT) is that TBCD has prominent hyper-reflective deposits at Bowman's layer which extend up into the epithelium in a saw-tooth pattern. OCT also reveals hyper-reflectivity throughout the stroma in MCD.

Specular microscopy of the endothelium in FECD reveals a reduced cell density, polymegathism, and pleomorphism.

Histopathological staining of excised tissues (e.g. during keratoplasty) can aid in the diagnosis of the particular corneal dystrophy, as described in the relevant sections above.

Diagnosis

The phenotype observed on slit lamp examination is still the mainstay of clinical diagnosis. However, this is increasingly being augmented and superseded by genotyping of patients, once the disease causing genetic variant has been identified.

Treatment

Some dystrophies (e.g. CCDF or Stage 1 FECD) do not require treatment. Epithelial and subepithelial dystrophies causing recurrent erosions may be treated by phototherapeutic keratectomy (PTK). Those dystrophies affecting the stroma may be treated with PTK, or, if the lesions are too deep for laser, by superficial keratectomy, deep anterior lamellar keratoplasty (DALK), or penetrating keratoplasty (PKP). Those dystrophies that affect the endothelium, such as FECD, may be treated by targeted replacement of the diseased endothelial layer by Descemet stripping automated endothelial keratoplasty (DSAEK) or Descemet membrane endothelial keratoplasty (DMEK).

Complications

Recurrent corneal erosions, reduced vision, photosensitivity, corneal oedema or decompensation, and recurrence in transplant grafts are all potential complications of corneal dystrophies, as described in the relevant sections above.

Further reading

Klintworth GK. Corneal dystrophies. Orphanet J Rare Dis 2009; 4.

Weiss JS, Møller HU, Aldave AJ, et al. IC3D classification of corneal dystrophies – edition 2. Cornea 2015; 34:117–159.

Related topics of interest

- Corneal ectasia (p. 84)
- Corneal grafts (p. 90)
- Corneal topography (p. 94)
- Dry eye syndrome (p. 122)
- Infectious keratitis (p. 181)

20 Corneal ectasia

Key points

- Corneal ectasia are an important cause of visual limitation in young people
- Keratoconus is the most common corneal ectasia
- Keratoconus early diagnosis and treatment have evolved substantially in the last few years
- The other ectasia, although rare, have specific features that need to be recognised
- Cross-linking has helped to reduce the number of types of ectasia requiring corneal transplantation surgery

Keratoconus

Introduction

Keratoconus is a bilateral (although usually very asymmetric) disorder which is characterised by progressive thinning of the cornea. This corneal thinning leads to corneal steepening resulting in an irregular corneal shape. As a consequence, variable amounts of myopia and irregular astigmatism are usually found.

Keratoconus is the most frequently recognised corneal ectasia. The incidence and prevalence of keratoconus has been underestimated for years due to the lack of accurate technology for its diagnosis. Keratoconus incidence and prevalence depends on ethnics and geographic location, with reported incidences of 19.6-25/100,000 hab/year for Asians compared with 3.3-4.5/100,000 hab/ year for Caucasians. Varying degrees of prevalence among groups of different ethnicities living in the same location suggest some genetic basis for this disease. Both dominant and recessive patterns of inheritance have been described, however, most keratoconus cases are sporadic to date.

Pathophysiology

Keratoconus is thought to be caused by an interplay of genetic and environmental factors. The most important environmental factors are ultraviolet exposure, eye rubbing and allergy. Higher prevalence of keratoconus has been described in very sunny locations such as Saudi Arabia, Israel, or New Zealand. The explanation for this is that ultraviolet light leads to an increased production of reactive oxygen species and keratoconic corneas cannot process this excess, thus causing oxidative stress and corneal thinning. The association with eye rubbing is well known. Recurrent trauma has shown to trigger the release of tumour necrosis factor alpha, interleukin-1 and matrix metalloproteinases 1 and 13 which leads to keratocyte apoptosis, corneal remodelling and thinning.

Keratoconus associations

Keratoconus may be associated with other ophthalmological or systemic diseases. Down syndrome is strongly associated with keratoconus with a prevalence up to 15%. Other associations include Leber congenital amaurosis, some pigmentary retinopathies, connective tissue disorders such as mitral valve prolapse, Ehlers–Danlos syndrome, Marfan syndrome or osteogenesis imperfecta.

Clinical features/diagnosis

The most usual presentation is a patient in their teens or twenties with progressive visual blurring. Photophobia, monocular diplopia and glare are also common symptoms at presentation.

On refraction, significant myopic astigmatism (with loss of corrected vision or not depending on the amount of irregular astigmatism) and scissoring reflex on retinoscopy are typical findings.

On slit lamp examination, keratoconus may be suspected but not in early cases. Typical findings include prominent corneal nerves, vertical posterior stromal striae (Vogt striae), superficial linear scars at the corneal apex due to ruptures of Bowman´s layer, Fleischer ring (yellow annular line at the base of the cone), or Munson sign (angulation of the lower eyelid in downgaze). Acute hydrops which is a spontaneous rupture of the Descemet membrane is usually associated to vigorous eye rubbing and it occurs in 2.5–3% of keratoconus. The patient presents with sudden onset decreased vision, pain and photophobia. Corneal oedema and conjunctival hyperaemia is seen on the examination.

However, nowadays, the main diagnostic methods are computerised videokeratoscopy (reflection-based devices), modern corneal tomography (Scheimpflug-based systems) or the combination of both (**Figure 20.1**).

Placido disk systems use the reflection on the cornea of a series of concentric white and black circles. The reflected image is analysed providing accurate information about the anterior shape of the cornea. However, these devices cannot measure the posterior corneal shape.

Tomographic systems [Scheimpflug, optical coherence tomography (OCT), scanning slit] have advantages over traditional Placido disk-based systems as they allow the measurement of both anterior and posterior corneal surfaces. Posterior corneal distortion is usually the first indicator of corneal ectasia in spite of completely normal anterior surface. Therefore, posterior corneal assessment is mandatory for the early keratoconus diagnosis. Some authors have significantly contributed in the early keratoconus diagnosis by means of analysing both elevation and pachymetric data provided by Scheimpflug imaging (Belin/ Ambrósio enhanced ectasia display for Oculus Pentacam).

Currently, there are some devices that can theoretically assess the cornea biomechanics showing weaker corneas in keratoconic cases. However, this technology is not routinely used in the everyday practice.

Keratoconus grading

Keratoconus is a disease with a wide spectrum of presentation. The most benign form is the subclinical keratoconus

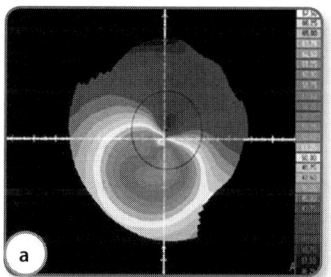

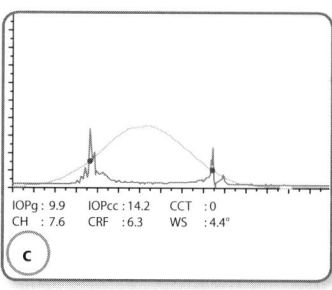

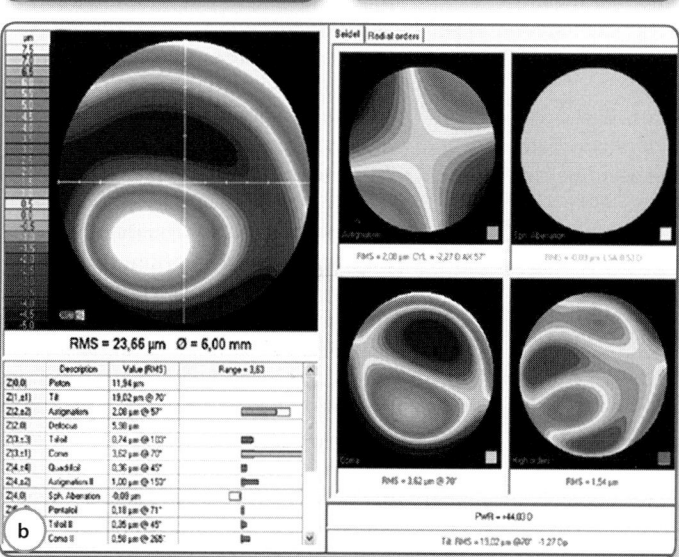

Figures 20.1a to c (a) Modern topography showing a keratoconic anterior corneal shape; (b) Aberrometric analysis showing high corneal aberrations, especially coma; (c) Altered corneal biomechanics.

Topic 20

Table 20.1 Amsler–Krumeich keratoconus grading	
Grade I	**Grade II**
• Eccentric corneal steepening	• Absence of scarring
• Myopia and/or astigmatism < 5 D	• Myopia and/or astigmatism 5–8 D
• Mean central K readings ≤ 48.00 D	• Mean central K readings > 48.00 to ≤ 53 D
	• Minimum corneal thickness 400 μm
Grade III	**Grade IV**
• Absence of scarring	• Central corneal scarring
• Myopia and/or astigmatism 8–10 D	• Not reliable refraction
• Mean central K readings > 53.00 to ≤ 55D	• Mean central K readings > 55 D
• Minimum corneal thickness 300 to 400 μm	• Minimum corneal thickness 200 μm

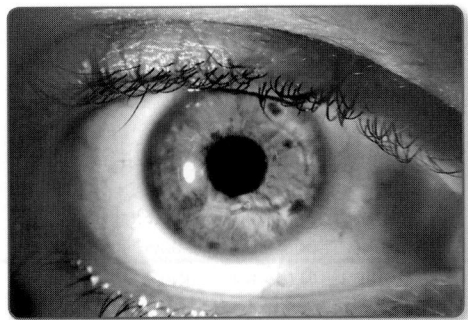

Figure 20.2 Two intracorneal ring segments implanted in a keratoconic cornea.

also known as forme fruste keratoconus or keratoconus suspect. These patients have normal corrected visual acuity with no clinical signs of keratoconus and the diagnosis is only made based on the topographic findings. On contrary, clinical keratoconus or keratoconus is as formerly stated characterised by corneal thinning and steepening leading to irregular astigmatism and different degrees of visual impairment.

Amsler–Krumeich classification is the most extended grading system in keratoconus; it combines refractive, keratometric and clinical signs of keratoconus (**Table 20.1**).

Alió-Shabayek classification, is based on the previous classification but it incorporates the anterior corneal high-order asymmetric aberrations, specifically the coma and its RADIAL orders. Thus, this classification offers more information about the quality of vision of the patients and the degree of irregular astigmatism.

Treatment

Two different treatment approaches are usually necessary in keratoconus.

Treatments aimed to improve the corneal shape and therefore to improve the visual acuity and quality of vision of the patient.

- *Glasses:* Only useful in mild keratoconus cases with low irregular astigmatism. They do not correct irregular astigmatism
- *Contact lenses:* These are usually the best option for those patients who are not able to achieve good vision with glasses. The options are rigid gas-permeable contact lenses (RGP), piggyback lenses, scleral lenses and hybrid contact lenses. All these lenses are rigid, therefore, the irregular surface between the back of the contact lens and the front of the cornea is filled in with tears and creates a lacrimal lens. This masks the regular and irregular astigmatism reducing the high order aberrations
- *Intrastromal corneal ring segments (ICRS):* These are small devices made of polymethylmethacrylate (PMMA) that are implanted within the corneal stroma in order to induce a change in the geometry and power of the tissue (**Figure 20.2**). The best indication is for those patients who having a not very thing and clear cornea, do not achieve good vision with contact lens or fail to tolerate them. Therefore, they sometimes fill the gap between contact lenses and corneal transplantation surgery. The main advantages are that they improve vision with spectacles and contact lens tolerance. For those patients who achieve adequate vision with specs, keratoconus progression

is easier to monitor as contact lens warpage is not an issue
- *Corneal transplantation:* Deep anterior lamellar keratoplasty (DALK)/penetrating keratoplasty (PKP). Approximately, 12–20% of keratoconus patients may need a corneal graft. However, these figures may decrease in the future thanks to corneal collagen cross-linking (CXL). In the UK, the percentage of transplants for keratoconus in which DALK was used increased from 10% in 1999–2000 to 35% in 2007–2008. It is likely that this percentage has further increased currently. In DALK, all the stromal tissue is removed, and a bare Descemet membrane is left

As a result, DALK advantages are the absence of endothelial rejection risk (the patient retains his own endothelium), earlier tapering of steroids, decreased risk of secondary glaucoma and increased wound strength. Thus, it is ideal in patients with mental retardation, phakic patients and in corneas with significant peripheral thinning. In contrast, PKP should be elected when endothelial dysfunction is present or when there is deep corneal scarring affecting the visual axis as it is usually the case after hydrops.

A review that included comparative studies on DALK and PKP concluded that visual and refractive outcomes are comparable when the residual bed thickness in DALK cases is between 25 and 65 microns. Therefore, PKP provides better vision than DALK when residual stroma is left in the latter.

Another remarkable advantage of DALK is a lower rate of endothelial cell loss of 13.9% when compared with PKP 34.6%.

1. *Treatment of acute hydrops:* Conservative treatment includes steroid drops, hypertonic saline drops, cycloplegics and antibiotics drops (if there is an epithelial defect) and sometimes bandage contact lens (BCL) fitting. This treatment provides relief until spontaneous resolution occurs which usually takes 5 to 36 weeks. Surgical interventions such as air/gas intracameral injection or compressing sutures have been also reported. Hydrops resolves leaving a residual scar and flattening of the cone.

2. Treatments which aim to halt the keratoconus progression in those patients with documented progression or even without documented progression but with a very high risk of progression. The only treatment to date that has shown with enough scientific evidence to halt keratoconus progression is the collagen cross-linking of the cornea (CXL). It is a technique that uses ultraviolet-A light and a photosensitiser which is riboflavin (vitamin B2) to strengthen chemical bonds in the cornea. The first described protocol was called Dresden protocol. In this protocol, the epithelium is removed and then riboflavin (vitamin B2) is instilled every 2–3 min for 30 min. Afterwards, the cornea is irradiated with ultraviolet-A for 30 min. During the irradiation period, 1 drop of riboflavin is also instilled every 3–5 min.

Overall and following the Dresden protocol, CXL halts keratoconus progression in around 90% of the cases.

New protocols have been developed in an attempt to shorten the irradiation time by means of increasing the energy (Bunsen-Roscoe law). Accelerated 10 min protocols have shown good efficacy, however, more accelerated than that is probably not effective due to the lack of oxygen.

Also protocols without epithelium removal have been developed (epi-on protocols). The theoretical advantage is a faster and less painful recovery but also much lower risk of infection. However, these protocols are not as effective as epi-off because of 2 reasons. First of all, because riboflavin corneal absorption is worse with intact epithelium, and maybe more importantly, because the epithelium consumes a lot of oxygen thus reducing its availability for the cross-linking photochemical reaction.

CXL+PRK: Some authors advocate to combine these two procedures. While the CXL strengthens the cornea, a low ablation PRK can be performed to reduce patient´s refraction, or much more interestingly, to

Table 20.2 Comparison among ectatic disorders

	Keratoconus	Pellucid marginal degeneration	Keratoglobus
Frequency	Most common	Less common	Rare
Laterality	Bilateral (but asymmetric)	Bilateral	Bilateral
Age at onset	Puberty	20–40 years old	At birth mostly
Protrusion	Inferior paracentral	Superior to area of thinning	Generalised
Thinning	At apex	Inferior band	Peripheral 360°
Hydrops	Possible	Possible	Possible

Source: Modified from Krachmer JH, Mannis MJ, Holland EJ, (Eds). Cornea, 2nd edition, Volume 1. Philadelphia: Elsevier Mosby; 2005. p. 955.

reduce the coma aberration thus improving the quality of vision.

Pellucid marginal degeneration

It is an uncommon, nonhereditary and bilateral ectasia. It is characterised by peripheral inferior thinning. In contrast with keratoconus, protrusion is not located at the point of maximal thinning. In pellucid marginal degeneration (PMD), protrusion is evident above the area of maximal thinning (**Table 20.2**). Most patients are diagnosed when they are 20–40 years old. The examination shows decreased vision as a consequence of high irregular astigmatism.

Treatment

Cross-linking has also shown to be effective in halting this disease. Contact lenses can be fitted to improve vision although it is usually more difficult than in keratoconus. Corneal transplantation surgery may be needed in some patients. Because of the peripheral thinning, grafts tend to be larger and closer to the inferior limbus. This makes the surgery more challenging and also more prone to rejection.

Keratoglobus

It is a rare corneal ectasia characterised by generalised thinning and globular protrusion of the cornea. It is usually not hereditary, bilateral and present at birth. It may be related to a problem in collagen synthesis, and therefore, associated with systemic syndromes as Ehlers–Danlos type VI, Marfan, Rubinstein–Taybi or osteogenesis imperfecta. There are also few anecdotal reports of acquired forms that have been related to vernal keratoconjunctivitis, marginal blepharitis and idiopathic orbital inflammation.

The protrusion is generalised and maximal thinning is located at the corneal midperiphery. Acute hydrops may occur. Due to the extreme thinning traumatic perforation or even spontaneous perforation have been also reported. Patient's symptoms are blurred vision as a consequence of the high myopia and irregular astigmatism. Acute hydrops symptoms are pain, tearing, photophobia and loss of vision.

Treatment is very challenging. Contact lens fitting is difficult and there is also a risk of perforation on contact lens insertion and removal. Counselling about wearing protective glasses is mandatory, especially in children. Conventional penetrating keratoplasty in these patients is also not possible because of the thinned cornea and peripheral graft-host thickness disparity that prevents adequate wound closure. Epikeratoplasty with various modifications has also been described. However, to date, no treatment standard exists.

Iatrogenic ectasia

It is a rare complication after corneal refractive surgery. The estimated incidence is 1 case out of 2,500. It has been described after all the modalities of laser refractive surgery: LASIK, PRK/LASEK and SMILE. However, the vast majority of the reported cases had previous LASIK surgery because it is the most commonly performed procedure and because it has a higher weakening effect on the cornea than the others. The most remarkable characteristic of this ectasia is that it can be prevented in most of the cases.

The most important risk factors in order are: Preop abnormal topography > Residual stromal bed thickness (stromal thickness underneath the flap after the ablation) > Age > Preoperative Pachymetry.

Recently, a new factor called PTA (percentage of tissue altered) has been reported. PTA = flap thickness + ablation depth/central preop pachymetry. It has been shown that the more abnormal the topography is, the lower the PTA value needed for the ectasia. And more important, it has shown that in patients with normal Placido disk topographies, the risk of ectasia is significantly higher when the PTA is ≥ 0.40.

Iatrogenic ectasia treatment follows the same principles of keratoconus treatment. CXL has also shown to be effective in halting the ectasia progression in these patients.

Finally, the incidence of this ectasia is probably much lower currently than what it was formerly stated. The new topographers that incorporate analysis of the back of the cornea help to detect suspicious topographies (that used to be missed before), excluding these patients for surgery.

Further reading

Jorge LAlió. Keratoconus. Recent advances in diagnosis and treatment. Switzerland: Springer International Publishing; 2017.

Krachmer JH, Mannis MJ, Holland EJ (Eds). Cornea, 2nd edition, Volume 1. Philadelphia: Elsevier Mosby; 2005. p. 375.

Santhiago MR, Smadja D, Gomes BF, et al. Association between the percent tissue altered and post-laser in situ keratomileusis ectasia in eyes with normal preoperative topography. Am J Ophthalmol 2014; 158:87–95.

Wallang BS, Das S. Keratoglobus. Eye (Lond) 2013; 27:1004–1012.

Ziaei M, Barsam A, Shamie N, et al. Reshaping procedures for the surgical management of corneal ectasia. J Cataract Refract Surg 2015; 41:842–872.

Related topic of interest

- Corneal grafts (p. 90)

21 Corneal grafts

Key points
- Corneal grafts may be full-thickness or lamellar (i.e. targeting just the pathological layer(s) of the cornea)
- One of the main risks of corneal grafts is graft rejection, which must be recognised and treated promptly to avoid graft failure
- The proportion of lamellar and, in particular, endothelial keratoplasties, has increased markedly over recent years

Epidemiology

Eduard Zirm (1887–1948) performed the first successful corneal transplant in 1905, making it the first solid tissue successfully transplanted in humans, anteceding the first successful kidney transplant by nearly half a century.

In the UK, several thousands corneal transplants are performed each year. The three main indications for corneal graft surgery are: to improve the corneal shape (i.e. in keratoconus); to treat corneal endothelial failure (e.g. from Fuchs' endothelial dystrophy or following cataract surgery); and to treat infection. Other less frequent indications are repair of injury and to remedy corneal opacification.

Pathophysiology

The indication for a corneal graft may be optical (to improve vision), therapeutic (e.g. to remove infected corneal tissue) or tectonic (to maintain the integrity of the globe and replace corneal tissue that has been lost).

Corneal grafts may be undertaken as full-thickness transplants, i.e. penetrating keratoplasty (PKP) (**Figure 21.1**), or lamellar grafts, which aim to replace only the pathological layer(s) of the cornea. Lamellar grafts include Deep Anterior Lamellar Keratoplsty (DALK) (**Figure 21.2**), which leaves the host endothelium in situ and so reduces the risk of rejection, and Endothelial Keratoplasty (EK), of which there are several types; the two most commonly performed

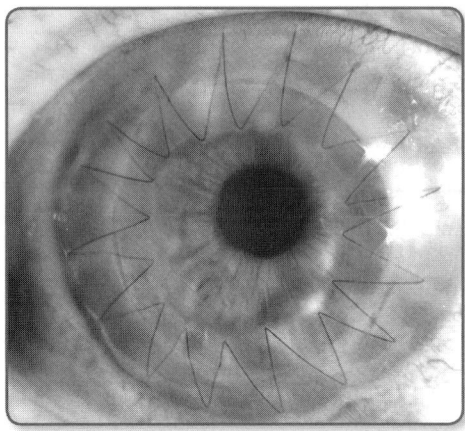

Figure 21.1 Penetrating Keratoplasty with continous suturing.

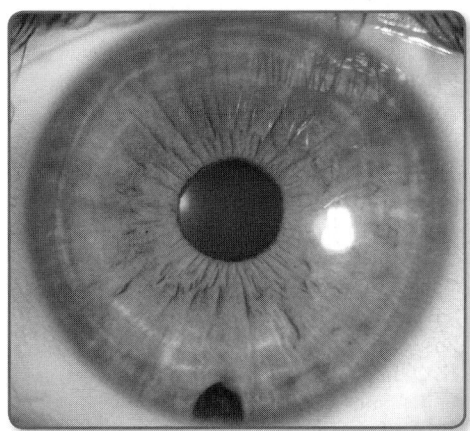

Figure 21.2 Deep Anterior Lamellar Keratoplasty (DALK).

EK sub-types are Descemet's Stripping Automated Endothelial Keratoplasty (DSAEK) and Descemet's Membrane Endothelial Keratoplasty (DMEK). In DSAEK, the corneal endothelial layer along with a thin layer of stroma is transplanted, whereas in DMEK only the corneal endothelial layer on Descemet's membrane is transplanted.

As EK only replaces the inner layers of the cornea, it has several advantages over PKP. These include better structural integrity of the eye, a smaller change in refraction, fewer suture-related problems, a lower risk of graft rejection (as less tissue is replaced), and a faster visual recovery with better final visual acuity. DMEK itself generally has a faster visual rehabilitation and better achievable final visual acuity than DSAEK, as a thinner layer of tissue is transplanted in DMEK.

Risk factors for graft rejection and/or failure include vascularisation, previous grafts/previous graft rejection, inflammation, glaucoma, anterior synechiae, chemical burns and young age of recipient.

Graft allograft rejection mainly occurs via indirect antigen presentation. Tissue matching is generally not required for successful corneal transplantation, due to the immune privilege of the ocular environment into which the graft is transplanted, known as Anterior Chamber-associated Immune Deviation (ACAID). However, many, but not all, studies have shown that Human Leukocyte Antigen (HLA) tissue matching does help increase graft survival, especially in those grafts at high risk of rejection.

Donor tissue should be harvested no longer than 24 hours post-mortem (along with a statutory blood sample being taken within this same time period), and there is a list of exclusion criteria determining those that are ineligible to donate their corneas [e.g. those with human immunodeficiency virus (HIV), hepatitis, or syphilis infection etc].

The type of corneal grafts that are being undertaken has also changed over time. Just over a decade ago, EK accounted for less than 1% of the total number of corneal grafts performed in the UK. This proportion has risen markedly in recent years, so that EK now accounts for over 50% of all corneal grafts undertaken.

The survival of corneal grafts is usually measured in 5-year survival and varies with several factors as described above. The indication for the corneal graft has a large influence on graft survival, with corneal grafts undertaken for keratoconus having some of the best 5-year survival rates (in excess of 90%).

Clinical features

Symptoms of corneal graft rejection include redness, discomfort or pain, light sensitivity, reduced vision and neovascularisation.

Epithelial or subepithelial rejection may manifest as superficial corneal punctate lesions (Krachmer's spots). Stromal or endothelial rejection may manifest as corneal stromal haze and/or oedema with keratic precipitates, an endothelial immune rejection line (Khodadoust line) and anterior chamber (AC) activity such as cells and flare (**Figure 21.3**). The signs of rejection of lamellar grafts such as DALK may be more subtle, given there is no donated endothelium in DALK to which the host immune system can demonstrate its activity.

Investigations

The main investigation of the health of a graft is the slit-lamp examination of the clarity of the cornea. In addition to slit-lamp examination, corneal graft health can be investigated by measuring corneal graft thickness (i.e. pachymetry, which acts as a surrogate marker for endothelial function), refraction and corneal topography/tomography (to assess the refractive properties of the graft), and specular

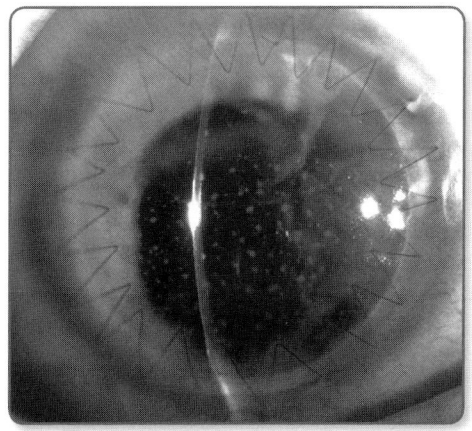

Figure 21.3 Graft rejection, showing Khodadoust line/Krachmer spots in PK.

microscopy of the endothelium (to assess such parameters as endothelial cell density, cell size and cell shape, which can all help indicate the health of the graft). Anterior segment optical coherence tomography (AS-OCT) is also useful, especially in gaining very accurate pachymetry measurements and aiding visualisation of detached EK grafts in the AC.

Diagnosis

The type of corneal graft undertaken depends on the indication for surgery. PKP can be used to replace all layers of the cornea for most indications, and for many years was the only graft type regularly performed. These days, many corneal surgeons prefer to target the corneal layers grafted to just those that are dysfunctional, so, for example, in keratoconus only the corneal stroma is replaced with a DALK, leaving the host endothelium in situ, whereas in Fuchs' endothelial dystrophy, the diseased endothelium alone is effectively replaced with an EK, leaving the host stroma in place. It can be hard to differentiate a PKP from a DALK on slit-lamp examination alone, but the patient should have been told if they underwent a partial thickness or full-thickness graft. DSAEK and DMEK can normally be differentiated by careful slit-lamp examination.

Treatment

The treatment of corneal grafts is generally divided into two phases: the first phase is the immediate post-operative phase wherein the health of the graft is ensured and any early post-operative complications managed. The second phase is the visual rehabilitation phase, usually beginning a few months after surgery, wherein the vision achievable through the graft is optimised. This second phase involves a refraction and corneal tomography/topography, with the use of spectacles, contact lenses, or refractive surgery to optimise the vision.

Complications

Corneal graft surgery can experience general and specific complications. General complications as with other forms of intraocular surgery include infection, haemorrhage, inflammation and changes in intraocular pressure (IOP) and, rarely, loss of sight.

The main specific complication to corneal graft surgery is graft rejection. This causes a targeted host immune response against the donated tissue (usually, but not always, the endothelium), resulting in loss of function of the donated graft and consequent graft failure and loss of optical clarity. Graft rejection can happen any time after surgery but is most common when reducing or stopping post-operative steroid drops, which may be many months after transplant surgery.

Corneal sutures entail their own complications, wherein they may become loose or break; such sutures are a focus for infection and inflammation, which may precipitate graft rejection, and any such sutures must always be removed promptly. When sutures are removed, the graft-host interface in PK or DALK may dehisce and require further surgery to repair. PK and DALK corneal graft sutures are generally interrupted or continuous. A continuous suture has the advantage of reducing surgical time and allowing easier intra- and post-operative suture adjustment, but should generally be avoided in paediatric keratoplasty, and vascularised or infected corneas.

Graft failure can also be primary, wherein the graft fails in the immediate post-operative period; this is usually due to either poor quality of donor tissue or excessive loss of endothelial cells during surgical manipulation.

Recurrence of the original disease may also occur in the graft, such as infections or dystrophy.

There may be considerable post-operative astigmatism present in the graft (especially in PKP), which requires further treatment in order to optimise vision. Approximately, 50% of patients will require a contact lens after a PKP in order to see to UK driving standard in their operated eye (i.e. Snellen 6/12).

Penetrating keratoplasty and DALK grafts may suffer from persistent epithelial defects (ED) and dellen. One must always be cautious of declaring an ED as noninfected in a corneal graft, as many patients will be on topical steroids, and this can mask the normal findings associated with a microbial keratitis, such as redness and corneal infiltrates. If in any doubt, always take a corneal scrape for microscopy, culture and sensitivity, and polymerase chain reaction (PCR) for microbial DNA/RNA where available.

An additional complication of EK is post-operative detachment of the graft, which may require the reinsertion of a gas bubble into the anterior chamber to temporarily tamponade the graft against the posterior surface of the cornea (so-called 're-bubbling'); this occurs in approximately 10% of cases.

Further reading

Hjortdal J. Corneal transplantation. Springer, 2016.
Maguire MG, Stark WJ, Gottsch JD, et al. Risk factors for corneal graft failure and rejection in the collaborative corneal transplantation studies. Ophthalmology 1994; 101:1536–1547.

Related topics of interest

- Corneal dystrophies (p. 79)
- Corneal ectasia (p. 84)
- Corneal topography (p. 94)
- Infectious keratitis (p. 181)

22 Corneal topography

Key points

- Topography (placido disc) measures anterior corneal reflection and can be difficult to interpret
- Tomography (scanning slit/Scheimpflug principle) measures front and posterior cornea elevation and corneal thickness, so giving best overall data
- It provides imaging of the cornea as elevation not curvature for ectasia screening, diagnosis, and surgical treatment

Introduction

Topography is non-invasive imaging of the anterior cornea and measures the surface only using placido-based principles.

Tomography is imaging of the posterior and anterior cornea to give thickness slices using slit scanning beam or Scheimpflug principles. True height maps of elevation can be produced without relying on placido-based assumption of corneal shape.

Elevation maps are a distribution of corneal power in dioptres and normal corneas can fall into one of five general groups of round, oval, symmetrical bow tie, asymmetric bow tie, and irregular corneal topography as shown in **Figure 22.1**.

A symmetrical bow tie is regular astigmatism where principle meridians are 90º apart or perpendicular to each other, the steepest and flattest meridians are shown as K1 and K2 with relevant axes and power (**Figure 22.2**). If the symmetrical bow tie is vertically aligned, it follows with-the-rule astigmatism and if horizontal it is against-the-rule astigmatism. Oblique astigmatism is when the principle axis lies 45° from the horizontal and vertical. The bow tie can also be skewed that is there is angulation between superior and inferior bow tie segments, so they do not lie in the same plane.

An asymmetric bow tie and a cornea with an irregular pattern are both examples of irregular astigmatism where principle meridians are not perpendicular.

Types

Placido disc principle: It is based on the projection of concentric rings on to the cornea's tear film. The pattern of these rings is analysed by computer to give curvature and power readings based on regularity and separation of the reflected rings. The tear film needs to be adequate to avoid distorted rings, so patients are advised to blink pre-imaging.

This reflection-based method of topography assumes the line of sight or visual axis of the patient to be near perpendicular to the corneal apex. This presumption is adequate for the central 1–2 mm zone but beyond can over-diagnose ectasias such as keratoconus (KC).

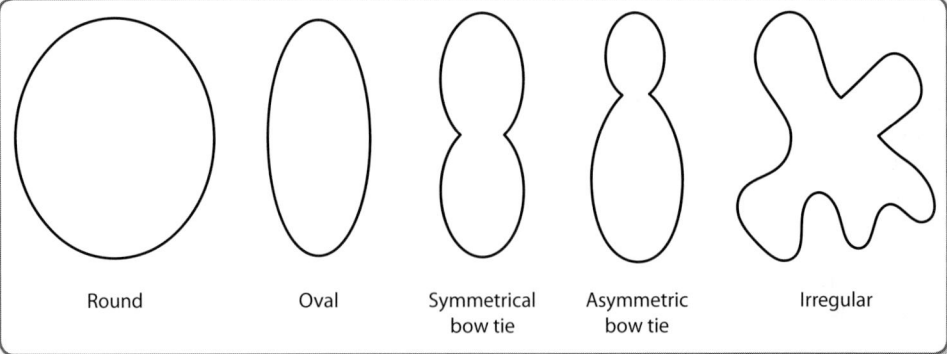

Figure 22.1 Patterns of corneal topography.

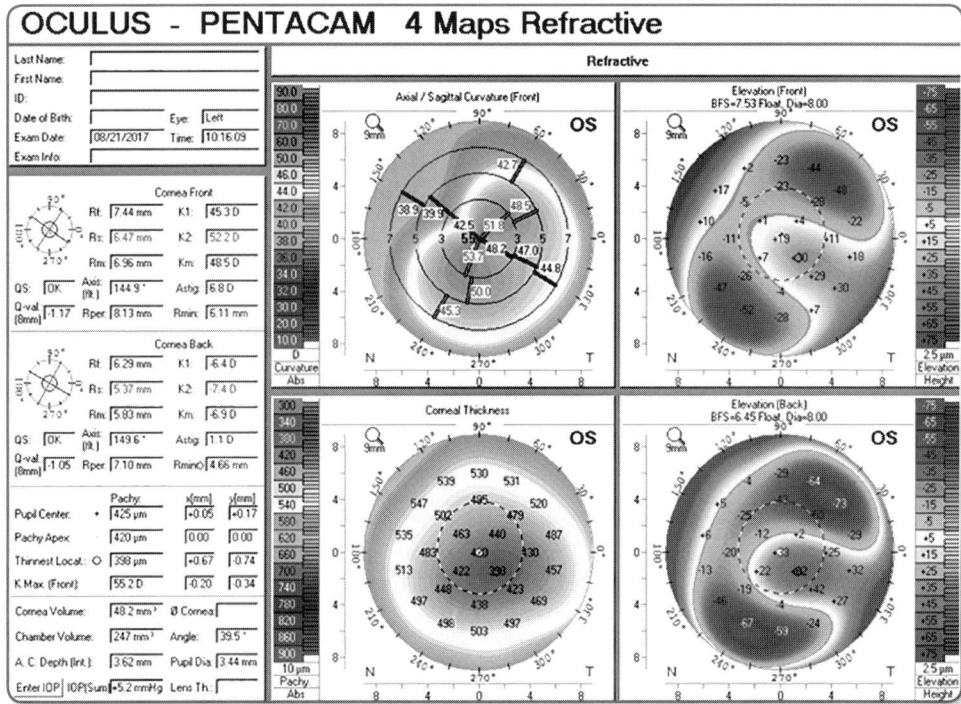

Figure 22.2 4-Map refractive Pentacam corneal tomography scan.

Where reflected mires are close together and thinner, this suggests a steep cornea and those far apart and thicker one of lower power that is a flatter cornea. Images are presented as an anterior sagittal/axial map, a tangential power map, and a mean curvature map. The maps relate the patient's cornea to a best fit sphere.

Scanning slit principle: This is an elevation-based method where multiple slits of light projected on to the cornea are reflected and captured by camera. The difference between the projected and reflected beam is captured as corneal curvature and also corneal thickness to enable mapping of corneal surface power.

The Orbscan (Bausch and Lomb) images the anterior cornea with placido topography, posterior cornea with slit scanning principles, and a posterior elevation map is also mathematically determined

Scanning slit Scheimpflug principle: This method allows for focused and sharp images at oblique tangents given that the cornea is non-planar and images are not necessarily perpendicular to the cornea.

A projected slit at regular intervals is captured by a rotating digital camera and analysed to determine measurements for points on the corneal surface. It formulates a three-dimensional (3D) model of the eye and is the gold standard for data on corneal elevation and pachymetry.

Examples include the Pentacam (Oculus) which is a slit scan and Scheimpflug camera rotating over 180°, Galilei (Ziemer) which is dual Scheimpflug camera and placido based, and also the Sirius (CSO) system.

Uses

The cornea is 70% of the focusing power of the eye. A cornea which is too flat, steep, or uneven will give abnormal vision; topography imaging can detect this and formulate a 3D map to aid diagnosis and plan treatment. Uses for topography are shown in **Table 22.1**

Table 22.1 Uses of corneal topography

Use	Patient groups	Topography aim	Outcome
Screening	Pre-refractive	Exclude KC and forme fruste or subclinical KC	Contraindication to refractive laser correction if signs of KC, forme fruste, or posterior corneal changes suggested
		How much to ablate and what pattern?	Accurate refractive planning
	Pre-cataract surgery	Assess corneal astigmatism as regular or irregular	If regular astigmatism, possibility of toric IOL insertion
Diagnosis	Contact lens fitting	Pooling of tears (cool colours) or lack of tears (warm colours) based on front elevation map	Assess fit for contact lenses Advise to stop lens until corneal map stabilisation
	Ectasia	Corneal warpage – irregular astigmatism/peripheral steepening	Diagnosis, e.g. KC or pellucid marginal degeneration and monitoring of possible progression
Treatment	Post-cataract surgery	Assess corneal astigmatism	Suture removal
	Post-refractive surgery	Ectasia exclusion and unexplained results	Ectasia diagnosis/under-corrected or decentred refractive surgery
	Post-corneal graft surgery	Measure astigmatism irregularity or steep axis based on corneal curvature maps not refraction	Steep-tight suture on same meridian can be removed Flat-compression sutures

IOL, intraocular lens; KC, keratoconus

Steps in interpretation (Pentacam: 4-Maps refractive) (Figure 22.2)

- *Scan quality*: QS scale check reads 'OK'
- *Look at scale*: Colour coding:
  - Steeper: Yellow and red (hotter colours)
  - Flatter: Blue and green (cooler colours)
- *Q value*: Measure of the corneal asphericity at the central 6 mm optical zone. A normal cornea is prolate (flat peripherally, steep centrally) with negative Q indices. An abnormal cornea is oblate (steep peripherally, flat centrally) with positive Q values. Normal Q value is –0.0 to –0.4
- *Map*: Axial/sagittal curvature front (radius of curvature) – this is measured in millimetres or dioptric power (D). Normal is a symmetrical bow tie with equal and aligned inferior and superior (I-S) segments as either round, oval, or bow tied shape. Abnormal patterns are inferior steepening (> 1.5 D difference), superior steepening (> 2.50 D difference), and asymmetrical bow tie or non-specific irregularity such as cone, nipple, oval, crab claw, or globus and these can be central, eccentric, or peripheral with Kmax being the maximum radius of curvature:
  - Steep slope: Small radius of curvature, high dioptric power
  - Flat cornea: Large radius of curvature, low dioptric power
- *Map:* Elevation front/back–compared to best fit sphere (BFS) showing how corneal elevation differs from a known spherical shape. Normal pattern is hourglass. Abnormal pattern is irregular, tongue-like focal change in colour and islands. Also, change in posterior BFS can be sign of subclinical KC:
  - Hot areas: Areas above reference sphere (flatter curvature)
  - Cool areas: Areas lower than the sphere (steeper curvature)

- *Map:* Corneal thickness: Normal is concentric. Abnormal is a bell shape, dome like, or horizontal displaced readings

Corneal topography reporting in examination setting

- Check date taken, patient name, age, and eye laterality
- Type of scan: Name and quality (QS)
- Q value; asphericity: Prolate or oblate
- *Toricity (astigmatism):*
  - *Magnitude:* Amount (difference between K1 and K2 values)
  - *Direction:* With the rule/against the rule
  - *Irregular/regular astigmatism:* Red/blue lines on axial map broken or orthogonal
- Symmetry: Ratio of inferior and superior steepening. Equal bow tie or asymmetry between inferior/superior dioptre readings (I-S symmetry)
- Comment on corneal thickness (thinnest local)
- Compare to other eye

Caution

Beware of unstable tear films and spurious results from corneal artefacts such as dry eye, corneal neovascularisation, and corneal scars. If images are spurious, then look again on slit lamp assessment. Also recommend removal of contact lenses prior to imaging, 3 weeks beforehand in the case of rigid gas permeable hard contact lenses.

Further reading

Klyce SD. (2014). Getting the Most From Topography. [online] Available from https://crstoday.com/wp-content/themes/crst/assets/downloads/crst0714_F5_Klyce.pdf. [Last accessed October, 2019].

Martinez-Abad A, Pinero D. New perspectives on the detection and progression of keratoconus. J Cataract Refract Surg 2017; 43:1213–1227.

Martinez CE, Klyce SD. Keratometry and topography. In: Krachmer JH, Mannis MJ, Holland EJ (Eds). Cornea, 3rd edition. Philadelphia: Elsevier/Mosby; 2011:161–176.

Related topics of interest

- Biometry and lens implant power calculation (p. 22)
- Corneal ectasia (p. 84)
- Refractive surgery (p. 263)

23 Cranial nerve palsy – abducens nerve palsy

Key points
- The most common cranial nerve palsy affecting eye movements
- Approximately, 80% of unilateral isolated adult sixth nerve palsies will spontaneously resolve

Epidemiology

Abducens nerve palsies are the most common ocular motor nerve palsies. The age-adjusted incidence of a sixth nerve palsy is approximately 11.3 cases per 100,000 in the population. The aetiology and incidence of a sixth nerve palsy will vary according to the age group it is affecting; however, the most common causes, accounting for approximately 50% of cases in the adult population, are trauma and ischaemia. Neoplasms were thought to be more common as a cause of a sixth nerve palsy in the adult population but recent studies suggest it only accounts for approximately 5%. However, in children, neoplasms and trauma are the most common causes of abducens nerve palsies. Other causes can include aneurysms (2%), demyelination, and idiopathic (10–25%).

Pathophysiology

The abducens nerve is entirely motor and innervates the ipsilateral lateral rectus muscle; hence, when affected, the resultant deviation is only in the horizontal plane. As with the other cranial nerves, its course from its nucleus to the lateral rectus muscle can be divided into portions, and knowledge of this anatomy together with identification of any associated signs helps to localise the lesion.

These portions include nuclear, subarachnoid, and cavernous, and orbital portions.

Nuclear portion

The sixth nerve nucleus lies beneath the floor of the upper part of the fourth ventricle at the level of the facial colliculus. It contains both motor neurones (supplying the ipsilateral lateral rectus muscle) and interneurons (projecting to the contralateral medial rectus nucleus in the midbrain via the medial longitudinal fasciculus); lesions of the nucleus therefore result in an ipsilateral horizontal gaze palsy, with both eyes tonically deviated to the opposite side. The fascicle of the abducens nerve then passes forwards through the lateral pontine tegmentum to emerge from the brainstem at the pontomedullary junction; infarctions arising from occlusion of the anterior inferior cerebellar artery may therefore result in a sixth nerve palsy associated with ipsilateral fifth, seventh, and eighth cranial neuropathies as well as Horner's syndrome and loss of taste in the anterior part of the tongue (Foville's syndrome). More ventral lesions of the pons can result in a sixth nerve palsy associated with ipsilateral facial palsy (Millard–Gubler syndrome) or contralateral hemiparesis (Raymond's syndrome).

Subarachnoid portion

After leaving the pons, the slender abducens nerve has a long course to the cavernous sinus. It lies within the subarachnoid space as it runs upward, forward and laterally, crossing the upper border of the petrous part of the temporal bone before entering the cavernous sinus. Its long course makes it susceptible to trauma (e.g. head injury) or stretching (e.g. intracranial hypertension). Furthermore, due to its close association to the petrous portion of the temporal bone, untreated middle ear diseases which have spread to the temporal bone commonly affect the sixth nerve (Gradenigo's syndrome).

Cavernous and orbital portions

Within the cavernous sinus, the abducens nerve lies inferolateral to the internal carotid artery and receives a sympathetic branch from the internal carotid plexus before it leaves to join the ophthalmic nerve. The abducens nerve then enters the orbit through the superior orbital fissure and lies within the tendinous ring between the two divisions of the oculomotor nerve.

Clinical features

Lesions of the abducens nerve result in limited or absent abduction (**Figure 23.1**). Since the ipsilateral medial rectus muscle is unopposed, most patients present with horizontal diplopia associated with an esotropia that is worse when looking into the distance or towards the lesion. Some patients will try and compensate for the esotropia with a face turn towards the lesion. It is important to look for signs of any other orbital or neuropathology, including papilloedema.

Investigations

Investigations for a sixth nerve palsy are guided by the history and age of the patient. Basic blood tests include full blood count, glucose and erythrocyte sedimentation rate/C-reactive protein, but in some cases, it may also be appropriate to check acetylcholine receptor antibodies and thyroid function tests. An otoscopic examination to rule out complicated otitis media may be important, particularly in children. Imaging is required in all cases associated with other neurological symptoms or signs, and also if there is excessive pain, a history of progression or failure to spontaneously improve after 3 months.

Diagnosis

The diagnosis of a sixth nerve palsy is suggested by finding an inability to abduct the eye. However other causes of limited abduction ('pseudo-sixth') need to be excluded, including convergence spasm, Duane's retraction syndrome, myasthenia, and orbital pathology.

Treatment

Depending on the aetiology, most (70–80%) adult patients with an isolated unilateral abducens nerve palsy will show some degree of spontaneous recovery. With microvascular (ischaemic) sixth nerve palsies recovery usually begins within 2–3 months and can take up to a year; in approximately 85% cases, the recovery is complete. In contrast, the rate of recovery in traumatic sixth nerve palsies is lower, ranging from 80% with unilateral palsies and 40% with bilateral palsies. In rare cases, recovery from traumatic palsies is associated with aberrant regeneration, with patients exhibiting abducens–oculomotor nerve synkinesis. In general, unilateral incomplete palsies (95%) recover better than severe complete palsies (55%).

Initial treatment can include fogging/patching or prisms. In congenital sixth nerve palsies, the main aim of treatment is to avoid the development of amblyopia. Surgical management is considered if the child begins

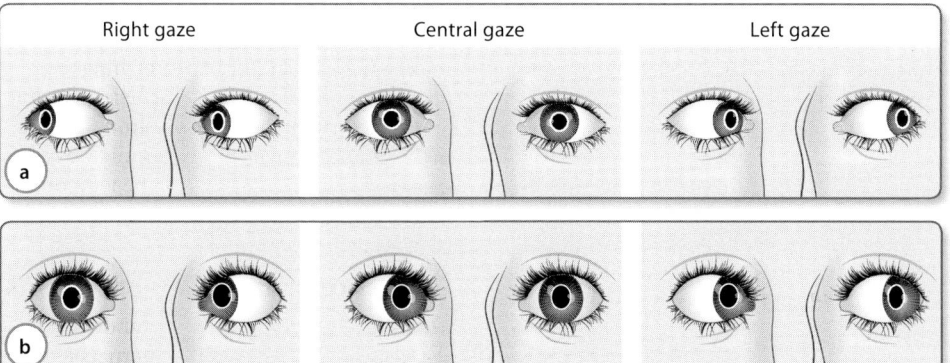

Figure 23.1 Showing right and left gaze in (a) Normal individual (b) Right VI CN palsy (Note: Medial deviation and unable to abduct the right eye).

to develop amblyopia due to the deviation being too large to correct with prisms or when after 9–12 months, an acquired sixth nerve palsy has a large deviation remaining despite prisms. Surgical care can include either botulinum toxin to the medial rectus and/or strabismus surgery. The choice of surgical procedure depends on the degree of remaining function in the lateral rectus muscle – if some function persists then a recess-resect may suffice, whereas patients with little or no remaining lateral rectus function need transposition of the superior and inferior recti, sometimes augmented by botulinum toxin injection into the ipsilateral medial rectus muscle.

Complications

The main complications of a sixth nerve palsy depend on the aetiology and the treatment given. If a patient has a persistent large deviation causing diplopia, they may require strabismus surgery. However, strabismus surgery carries the risk of over-or under-correction; in general, it is better to under-correct and use prisms or botulinum toxin to address any remaining deviation.

Further reading

Al-Zubidi N, Khan R. Sixth nerve palsies. In: Schmidt-Erfurth U, Kohnen T (Eds). Encyclopedia of Ophthalmology. Berlin, Heidelberg: Springer Berlin Heidelberg; 2016:1–5.

Patel SV, Leske DA, Hodge DO, et al. Incidence and etiology of sixth nerve palsy: a population-based study. Invest Ophthalmol Vis Sci 2002; 43:1485.

Shrader EC, Schlezinger NS. Neuro-ophthalmologic evaluation of abducens nerve paralysis. AMA Arch Ophthalmol 1960; 63:84–91.

Yanoff M, Duker JS. Ophthalmology. London: Mosby International Ltd; 1999.

Related topics of interest

- Imaging in ophthalmology (p. 176)
- Cranial nerve palsies – multiple cranial nerves palsies (p. 104)

24 Cranial nerve palsy – facial nerve palsy

Key points
- The facial nerve contains motor, sensory, and parasympathetic nerve fibres
- The facial nerve arises from three nuclei located in the brainstem
- A palsy of the facial nerve can result in inability to close the eye (lagophthalmos)

Epidemiology

Facial nerve (VIIn) palsy may be congenital or acquired. Congenital VIIn palsy accounts for 8–14% of all paediatric facial paralysis cases, and in the majority of these cases (88%), the cause is birth trauma – in particular the use of forceps during delivery. Other causes of congenital facial paralysis include neurodevelopmental conditions such as Moebius syndrome, Goldenhar's syndrome, and DiGeorge syndrome. The incidence of acquired VIIn palsy ranges between 20 and 30 cases per 100,000 people. The main causes are viral infections, trauma, inflammatory conditions of the middle ear or the nerve itself, metabolic diseases, compressive lesions (aneurysms, tumours), and idiopathic. Some studies report that idiopathic VIIn palsy is more frequent in young adults while others find a higher incidence in the elderly.

Pathophysiology

The facial nerve contains motor neurones supplying the muscles of the face, scalp, auricle, posterior belly of digastric, and the stylohyoid and stapedius muscles. It also supplies sensory (taste) fibres to the anterior two-thirds of the tongue and parasympathetic (secretomotor) fibres to the submandibular and sublingual salivary glands and the lacrimal glands. The facial nerve can be injured anywhere along its course from the brainstem to the face, with different clinical features depending on the site of the injury.

The main portions of the facial nerve include:
- *Facial nerve nuclei portion:* The facial nerve has three nuclei – the main motor nucleus, the parasympathetic nuclei, and the sensory nucleus – all of which lie within the pons. The motor nucleus receives input from the precentral gyri of both cerebral hemispheres. Motor neurones supplying the lower part of the face receive contralateral input, whereas motor neurones supplying the upper part of the face receive bilateral input; consequently, upper motor neurone lesions cause weakness only of the lower face, whereas lower motor neurone palsies affect the whole face.

  The parasympathetic nuclei (superior salivatory and lacrimal) receive afferent fibres from the hypothalamus (mediating emotional responses such as crying) and the sensory trigeminal nuclei (mediating reflex tearing from irritation of the ocular surface). The facial nerve then emerges as a motor and sensory root from the anterior surface of the brainstem. Lesions here affect the patient's ability to produce tears and can cause severe keratopathy
- *Facial canal portion:* The facial nerve passes through the facial canal with the vestibulocochlear and intermedius nerves; all three are surrounded by pia mater which becomes a common sheath at the internal auditory canal. In this region the facial nerve takes up 25–50% of the canal diameter leaving it susceptible to injury. The facial nerve then exits the middle ear through the stylomastoid foramen, running lateral to the styloid process before entering the parotid gland and dividing into five main motor branches that innervate the facial muscles

Clinical features

The symptoms and signs of a VIIn palsy depend on the site of the lesion and whether the palsy is complete or partial. Partial injuries tend to have a greater chance of recovery, whereas complete injuries have a poorer prognosis – after 3 years significant facial muscle atrophy can be observed.

The most obvious manifestations of VIIn palsy are motor and include drooping of the eyebrow, lower lid, and lips and lagophthalmos. The pattern of the motor deficit can be classified as partial, hemifacial or complete and allows the clinician to distinguish upper from lower motor neurone lesions. A unilateral isolated lower motor neurone VIIn palsy is also known as Bell's palsy and has a prevalence of approximately 20 cases per 100,000 people. Bell's palsy normally has a sudden onset that can be preceded by facial dysesthesia, hyperacusis, and either epiphora or a dry eye. It is thought that in most cases, the cause is inflammation within the bony facial canal. Lesions elsewhere along the facial nerve are often associated with other symptoms and signs. For example, lesions in the pons may cause a gaze palsy or an abducens nerve palsy since both sixth and seventh nerve nuclei are situated close to one another. If the seventh nerve is affected in the internal auditory meatus, then the vestibulocochlear nerve can be affected giving rise to hearing and balance problems. Other signs of a seventh nerve palsy can include altered or absent taste from the anterior two-thirds of the tongue. Extrinsic lesions such as tumours or ectatic arteries may irritate as well as compress the nerve causing hemifacial spasm as well as facial weakness. Over time, compression of the nerve may lead to aberrant regeneration. From an ophthalmic perspective, the main concern is the impact of VIIn palsy on the ocular surface where exposure (lagophthalmos) and dryness can, in some cases, lead to infective keratopathy and corneal blindness.

Investigations

Appropriate investigations for VIIn palsy are determined from the history and examination. It is particularly important to look for signs of hemifacial spasm or aberrant regeneration (indicating a long-standing and possibly compressive lesion) and other localising features (e.g. fifth, sixth or eighth nerve palsies). Further evaluations of facial nerve function may be useful and include electrophysiological studies (electroneuronography and electromyography), salivary flow, the stapedial reflex, and Schirmer's test. Some patients will need blood tests (full blood count, ESR, glucose and sometimes tests for sarcoid, Lyme etc), and imaging (CT/MRI scans). In general, decisions about whom to investigate and what tests to do for VIIn palsy are taken by ENT surgeons or neurologists, and the main role of the ophthalmologist is to ensure the safety of the ocular surface.

Diagnosis

The diagnosis of VIIn palsy is purely clinical and based on finding evidence of facial nerve dysfunction, usually motor. The examination needs to determine the pattern of the motor deficit, additional motor features (spasm, aberrant regeneration), non-motor features (loss of taste, salivation or lacrimation), and other neurology (other cranial nerve palsies). The degree of facial weakness is gradable using the House-Brackmann scale.

Treatment

Immediate treatment is directed at corneal protection. Patients with poor lid closure need artificial tears or ointment and instructions to tape their eye shut when they sleep. Early ophthalmology evaluation is indicated to ensure there is no development of exposure keratitis. Decisions regarding the frequency of subsequent ophthalmic review and the need for additional measures to protect the cornea are based on an assessment of the risk; poor prognostic factors requiring more intense intervention include a House-Brackmann score ≥ 4, absence of Bell's phenomenon, corneal anaesthesia, and tear deficiency. In refractory cases, botulinum toxin can be injected into the levator muscle to induce ptosis, or a tarsorrhaphy performed.

When a VIIn palsy persists for more than 1 year, it is considered chronic. Careful clinical and electrodiagnostic evaluations over time are needed to establish whether further recovery is expected. If the situation remains stable, and depending on the severity of the VIIn palsy, surgical procedures can be offered to optimise facial symmetry and improve eye closure. With respect to the eye, the relevant surgical procedures include lower lid ectropion repairs (excision wedge procedure and lateral canthopexy), brow ptosis repair (sling), and insertion of a gold weight into the upper lid. Furthermore, any crocodile tears associated with aberrant regeneration can be treated with botulinum toxin injections.

Complications

Seventh nerve palsy can cause disfigurement, facial twitching, pain and loss/altered taste. However, the most important complication of VIIn palsy is lagophthalmos, an issue that is often underestimated by other specialties, so it is incumbent on ophthalmologists to carry out timely evaluations and appropriate interventions to protect the cornea in these patients.

Further reading

Atolini Junior N, Jarjura J, Junior J, et al. Facial nerve palsy: incidence of different ethiologies in a tertiary ambulatory. Intl Arch Otorhinolaryngol 2009; 1313: 175–177.

Elston JS. The management of blepharospasm and hemifacial spasm. J Neurol 1992; 239:5–8.

Evans A K, Licameli G, Brietzke S, et al. Pediatric facial nerve paralysis: Patients, management and outcomes. Int J Pediatr Otorhinolaryngol 2005; 69: 1521–1528.

Falco NA, Eriksson E. Facial nerve palsy in the newborn: incidence and outcome. Plast Reconstr Surg 1990; 85:1–4.

Katusic SK, Beard CM, Wiederholt WC, et al. 1986 Incidence, clinical features, and prognosis in Bell's palsy, Rochester, Minnesota, 1968–1982. Ann Neurol 1986; 20:622–627.

Snell RS. Clinical Anatomy by Regions, 9th edition. London: Lippincott Williams and Wilkins; 2012.

Related topics of interest

- Cranial nerve palsies – multiple cranial nerves palsies (p. 104)
- Imaging in Ophthalmology (p. 176)

25 Cranial nerve palsies – multiple cranial nerves palsies

Key points
- Multiple cranial nerve palsies are a medical emergency and can be caused by a range of sinister conditions
- Ocular symptoms may be the earliest presenting neurological feature
- The ophthalmologist has a key role in recognising and neuro-anatomically localising the lesion which can assist with neuroimaging and further intervention
- Multiple cranial nerve palsies can lead to chronic ocular morbidity

Introduction

Multiple cranial nerve palsies occur when there is simultaneous or serial involvement of two or more cranial nerves from a compressive, ischaemic, inflammatory or infiltrative mechanism. This results in a weakening or complete paresis of those cranial nerves which in turn often cause debilitating symptoms.

Multiple cranial nerve palsies are frequently more challenging to distinguish than isolated cranial nerve palsies and are usually due to a more ominous aetiology. Multiple cranial nerve palsies are variable in their presentation and are not always complete, frequently with an uneven distribution of deficit among the nerves involved. This adds to the diagnostic challenge.

Six out of the twelve cranial nerves have a role in vision (2nd), motility (3rd, 4th, 6th) or neuro-mechanical protection (5th, 7th) and this means that frequently, an episode of multiple cranial nerve palsies is likely to directly involve some form of ophthalmological function. This chapter will look at the clinical manifestations that are of relevance to the ophthalmologist.

Clinical features

A large case series that examined inpatients with multiple cranial nerve palsies has suggested the following (**Table 25.1**):
- *Children:* In children, the most common causes are trauma, followed by tumour, then infection/inflammation. Other rare causes are post-ventriculoperitoneal shunt or in shunt misplacement. Leukaemia may lead to multiple cranial nerve palsies in the event of central nervous system spread of disease.

  Congenital cranial nerve disinnervation syndrome is an umbrella term to describe various congenital oculomotor disorders that can result in single, multiple or aberrantly innervated cranial nerve disorders. It is not completely understood and is complex to treat. It is usually non-progressive
- *Unilateral versus bilateral:* An ipsilateral complex of multiple cranial nerve dysfunction strongly indicates a mass lesion in the cavernous sinus, whereas bilateral involvement of cranial nerves suggests a diffuse process like infiltrative disease, a midline mass lesion that has extended bilaterally, or an inflammatory polyneuropathy

Diagnosis

History is a key in neuro-ophthalmology and it will help narrow down the aetiology and location of the lesion.

When a cranial nerve is suspected to be involved:
- All other cranial nerves should be tested especially the cranial nerves anatomically adjacent to the deficient nerve
- Check the pupil for Horner's syndrome and a relative afferent pupillary defect

Table 25.1 Table of cranial nerve involved, location, and cause

Most likely cranial nerves to be involved	Most likely location of cranial nerve damage	Most frequent causes		
			Adults	Children
6th (Abducens) 7th (Facial) 5th (Trigeminal) 3rd (Oculomotor)	1. Cavernous sinus 2. Brainstem 3. Nerve 4. Clivus and skull base 5. Subarachnoid space 6. Cerebellopontine angle	1. Tumour	Schwannoma Metastases Meningioma Lymphoma	Pontine glioma and other brainstem lesions Lymphoma Metastasis Gliomatosis cerebri
		2. Vascular disease	Lateral pons infarct Medulla infarct Haemorrhage Aneurysm Carotid cavernous fistula Dural sinus fistula	Pituitary apoplexy
		3. Trauma	Road traffic accidents Falls	Basilar skull fracture C-spine fracture Atlanto-occipital subluxation
		4. Infection	Meningitis Mucormycosis	Acute bacterial meningitis
		5. Autoimmune	Guillain–Barré syndrome Miller-Fisher syndrome	Guillain–Barré syndrome
		6. Idiopathic	Tolosa–Hunt syndrome	Congenital: congenital cranial nerve disinnervation syndromes
		7. Inflammation	Multiple sclerosis: Acute disseminated encephalomyelitis (ADEM)	Multiple sclerosis: Acute disseminated encephalomyelitis (ADEM)
		8. Iatrogenic	Surgical complication	

Source: Modified from Keane JR, Mutiple Cranial Nerve Palsies: Analysis of 979 cases. Arch Neurol 2005; 62:1714–1717.

- Check the optic nerves to look for papilloedema
- Check the peripheral nervous system and assess for signs of cerebellar dysfunction

There is also merit in specifically looking for subtle signs of abnormal head posture, conjunctival injection, proptosis, and ocular bruit. This could give a clue to the aetiology.

Note: Testing for the 4th nerve in a patient with a 3rd nerve palsy can be difficult as one usually checks for depression in adduction.

In the case where the oculomotor nerve is involved and there is an abducted eye, ask the patient to depress the eye, make note of a landmark such as a conjunctival vessel and look for 'intorsion'. Intorsion would indicate that the 4th nerve is likely spared.

Common combinations (in order of frequency)

1. 3rd and 6th (Oculomotor and Abducens)
2. 5th and 6th (Trigeminal and Abducens)
3. 5th and 7th (Trigeminal and Facial)

4. 7th and 8th (Facial and Vestibulocochlear)
5. 3rd, 4th, and 6th (Oculomotor, Trochlear and Abducens)
6. 5th, 6th, and 7th (Trigeminal, Abducens, and Facial)
7. 2nd and 3rd and 6th (Optic, Oculomotor, and Abducens)

Note: The 4th nerve is not commonly involved as part of multiple cranial nerve palsies. The 6th nerve on the other hand is the most commonly involved nerve in both isolated as well as multiple cranial nerve palsies.

Localising the lesion

These are four of the most commonly distinguishable anatomical locations based on examination findings (**Table 25.2**). **Figure 25.1** shows how closely the neurovascular structures are in relation to one another.

Table 25.3 details specific features associated with certain conditions.

Investigations

If multiple cranial nerve palsies are clinically suspected, then neuroimaging needs to be arranged urgently. Other ancillary tests are also required depending on the clinical context (**Table 25.4**).

Treatment

Treatment is directed by the clinical findings and the ultimate diagnosis. This topic is beyond the scope of the chapter. Referral to another speciality is often required (e.g. neurology, neurosurgery, ENT, maxillofacial, oncology etc). The following principles apply:
- Treat the underlying cause which may include any of the following:
  - Systemic chemotherapy
  - Immunosuppression

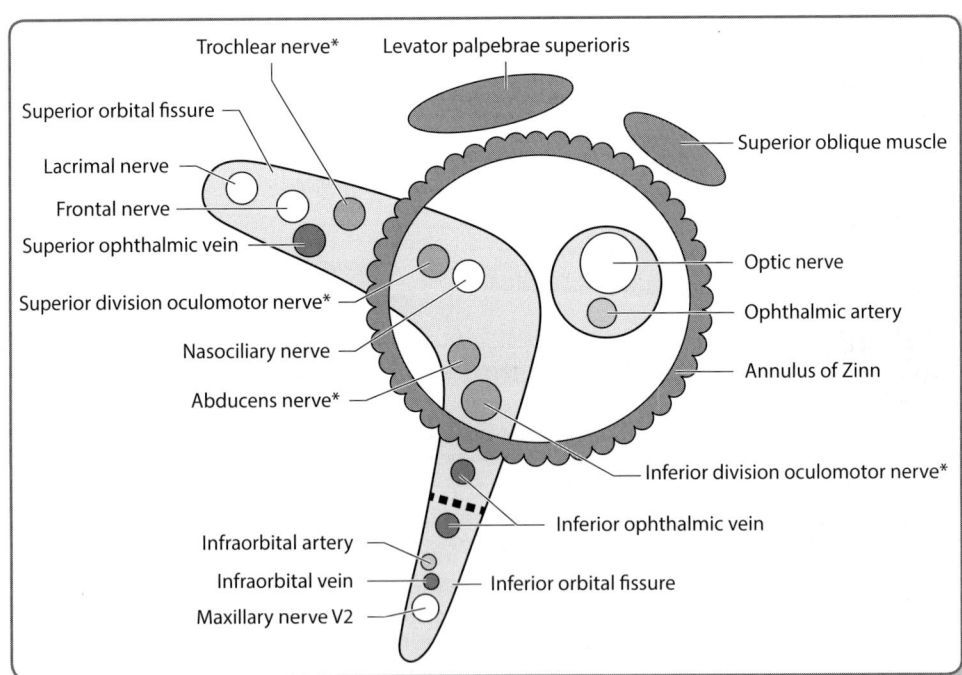

Figure 25.1 The right superior orbital fissure from an anterior view. The nerves with a * are responsible for ocular motility. The cavernous sinus is directly posterior to the superior orbital fissure. These openings are small compartments with vital neurovascular structures arranged in a tight configuration.

Table 25.2 Four clinically distinguishable anatomical locations for multiple cranial nerve palsies

Clinical location	Nerve involved	Description
Spheno-cavernous syndrome	3rd, 4th, 5th (V1 and V2), 6th, Horner's syndrome	This term groups cavernous sinus syndrome and superior orbital fissure syndrome as one entity because clinically, it can be impossible to differentiate due to its close relation
Orbital apex syndrome	2nd, 3rd, 4th, 5th (V1 and V2), 6th, Horner's syndrome	It is similar to a spheno-cavernous syndrome but importantly, the optic nerve can be involved
Cerebellopontine angle syndrome	5th, 6th, 7th, 8th	Causes include: Acoustic neuroma, nasopharyngeal cancers, pontine glioma, and basal skull fractures. In acoustic neuromas, 5th and 8th nerves are involved first followed by 6th and 7th
Lateral medullary syndrome (Wallenberg syndrome)	5th, 8th, 9th, 10th Crossed hemianaesthesia, ipsilateral facial numbness, nystagmus, cerebellar signs, dysarthria, dysphagia, Horner's syndrome	Rare condition caused by stroke or MS. Usually due to involvement of the vertebral artery or the posterior inferior cerebellar artery

Table 25.3 Clinical features of specific conditions

Condition	Other signs/clinical features
Carotid cavernous fistula	Venous congestion, arterialisation of conjunctival vessels, elevated IOP, pulsatile proptosis, ocular ischaemia, choroidal effusions, pain, optic disc swelling and ophthalmoplegia
Leukaemia	Associated with seizures, meningitis, and other focal neurology, occurs due to CNS dissemination of disease
Acoustic neuroma	Hearing loss, known neurofibromatosis type 2
Guillain–Barré/Miller-Fisher	Para infectious
Tolosa–Hunt syndrome	Severe pain, proptosis, responds rapidly to corticosteroid treatment
Gradenigo syndrome	Mastoiditis with secondary Lpsilateral 6th nerve palsy, ipsilateral 7th nerve palsy and ipsilateral facial pain. Corneal sensation may be reduced
Millard-Gubler syndrome (ventral pontine syndrome)	Acquired ipsilateral 6th and 7th nerve palsy and contralateral hemiplegia
Foville syndrome (medial inferior pontine syndrome)	Acquired ipsilateral 6th and 7th nerve palsies. Ipsilateral central Horner syndrome. Ipsilateral analgesia of the face, ipsilateral peripheral deafness, and contralateral weakness
Moebius syndrome	Congenital bilateral 6th and 7th nerve palsy

Table 25.4 Investigations

Investigation	Details
CT scan	Useful when bone detail is required such as in neoplasms with bony involvement or in craniomaxillofacial trauma
Magnetic resonance imaging +/– gadolinium	Evaluating for soft tissue structures in the orbit, cavernous sinus, and brainstem
Magnetic resonance angiography (MRA) or computer tomography angiography (CTA)	Needed if a vascular cause is suspected such as a carotid cavernous fistula, aneurysm, or thrombosis
Blood tests	FBC, U+E, ESR, CRP, ANA, ANCA, RF, ACE, VDRL, Lyme serology
Lumbar puncture	Cytology Cell count and differential Glucose and protein Microbiology PCR studies Serology Opening intracranial pressure Cancer markers
Biopsy of the meninges	Aimed at the regions that are enhancing on MRI. This procedure is reserved for infective and inflammatory causes that cannot be clinically distinguished despite all other investigations

Table 25.5 Treatment for ocular comorbidities

Nerve/type of involvement	Symptom	Treatment
3rd, 4th, 6th	Diplopia/strabismus	Occlusion Prisms Botulinum toxin Surgery when stable: which includes recession, resection or transposition of extraocular muscles
Mass effect	Proptosis	Treat underlying mass Debulking surgery Ocular protection strategies, e.g. lubricants, punctal plugs, glue, Botox to lids, tarsorrhaphy
5th, 7th, Mass effect	Exposure keratopathy	Ocular protection strategies (see above)
2nd	Vision loss	Treat underlying cause
Ocular blood supply compromise	Pain, uveitis, raised IOP	Topical steroids, acetazolamide

- Antibiotics
- Interventional radiology/surgery
- Treat associated comorbidities

Ocular morbidities can include a combination of the ones described in **Table 25.5**.

Differential diagnosis

- Myasthenia gravis
- Thyroid eye disease
- Blowout fracture
- Myopathies

Further reading

Brodsky MC. Ocular motor nerve palsies in children. In: Pediatric neuro-ophthalmology, 2nd edition, New York: Springer 2010:253–295.

Carroll CG, Campbell WW. Multiple cranial neuropathies. Semin Neurol 2009; 29:53–65.

Holmes JM, Mutyala S, Maus TL, et al. Pediatric third, fourth, and sixth nerve palsies: a population study. Am J Ophthalmol 1999; 127:388–392.

Keane JR. Mutiple cranial nerve palsies: Analysis of 979 cases. Arch Neurol 2005; 62:1714–1717.

Related topics of interest

- Cranial nerve palsy – oculomotor (third) nerve palsy (p. 109)
- Cranial nerve palsy – trochlear nerve palsy (p. 113)
- Cranial nerve palsies – abducens nerve palsy (p. 98)
- Myasthenia gravis (p. 212)
- Imaging in Ophthalmology (p. 176)

26 Cranial nerve palsy – oculomotor (third) nerve palsy

Key points

- All acutely presenting oculomotor nerve palsies must be investigated to rule out a life-threatening intracranial aneurysm, even if there is no pain and the pupil is 'spared'
- Ischaemic oculomotor nerve palsy tends to resolve after 6–8 weeks

Epidemiology

Oculomotor nerve palsy is relatively uncommon compared with other neuro-ophthalmic problems. The relative prevalence of oculomotor, trochlear, and abducent nerve palsies has been documented in many large population studies. These studies have found sixth nerve palsies to be the most common followed by oculomotor nerve palsies and then fourth nerve palsies. The most common causes of third nerve palsies include trauma, compressive lesions such as neoplasms and aneurysms of the posterior communicating artery, microvascular/ischaemic (associated with diabetes, hypertension and atherosclerosis) – which account for approximately 20% of cases, and infectious/inflammatory conditions.

Anatomy

The oculomotor nerve supplies all the extraocular muscles except for the superior oblique and the lateral rectus. It also supplies the striated muscle of the levator palpebrae superioris and the smooth muscle of the sphincter pupillae and the ciliary muscle. The anatomical relationships of different regions of the oculomotor nerve account for many different clinical features and patterns of a third nerve palsy.

The regions can be divided into:
- *Nuclear portion*: The third nerve has two motor nuclei: (1) the main motor nucleus and (2) the accessory parasympathetic nucleus (Edinger–Westphal). The main motor nucleus supplies the striated muscles (levator and the extrinsic muscles of the eye) and lies in the anterior part of the deep periaqueductal grey matter of the midbrain at the level of the superior colliculus. The Edinger–Westphal nucleus supplies parasympathetic fibres to the smooth muscles within the eye (constrictor pupillae of the iris and the ciliary muscles) and lies posteriorly to the main motor nuclei. In general, the motor neurones emerging from these nuclei supply ipsilateral muscles, but the supply is contralateral for the superior rectus and bilateral for the levator. This means that in those rare cases of a nuclear third nerve palsy there is bilateral ptosis and also some limited elevation of the contralateral eye
- *Fascicular (intraparenchymal) portion*: Nerve fibres from both the main motor and the accessory nuclei pass ventrally in the dorsal midbrain tegmentum through the red nucleus and medial aspect of the substantia nigra to emerge from the medial aspect of the cerebral peduncle into the interpeduncular cistern. Lesions causing third nerve palsies in this portion are often associated with other neurological findings such as contralateral tremor (Benedikt's syndrome) or contralateral hemiplegia (Weber's syndrome)
- *Subarachnoid portion*: The subarachnoid portion of the oculomotor nerve passes between the posterior cerebral and superior cerebellar arteries and runs ventrally lateral and parallel to the posterior communicating artery. This proximity to arteries within the subarachnoid space renders the third nerve susceptible to compression by aneurysms – most commonly at the junction between the posterior communicating artery and the internal carotid artery

- *Cavernous portion*: The oculomotor nerve pierces the dura on the lateral side of the posterior clinoid process to lie in the lateral wall of the cavernous sinus, above the trochlear nerve. It passes between the petroclinoid ligament above and the interclinoid ligament below. Compression of the third nerve in this segment may arise due to intrinsic lesions in the cavernous sinus (meningioma, internal carotid artery aneurysm) or lateral extension of suprasellar lesions (e.g. pituitary tumours, craniopharyngioma). In many cases, cavernous lesions also cause other neurological deficits, but these may be subtle and overlooked in the examination (e.g. Horner syndrome, trigeminal neuropathy)
- *Orbital portion:* The oculomotor nerve leaves the cranial cavity via the superior orbital fissure adjacent to the fourth cranial nerve but within the tendinous ring. The nerve divides into a small superior division and a larger inferior division

The superior division passes upward lateral to the optic nerve to innervate first the superior rectus and then the levator palpebrae.

The inferior division divides into three branches which supply the medial and inferior recti and the inferior oblique muscles. The branch to the inferior oblique muscles also gives rise to a short, thick branch to supply the preganglionic parasympathetic fibres to the ciliary ganglion. The postganglionic fibres from the ciliary ganglion then supply the sphincter pupillae and the ciliary muscles.

Clinical features

The features of a third nerve palsy can be divided into complete and incomplete lesions.

A complete oculomotor nerve palsy consists of the eye not being able to adduct, elevate or depress, consequently the eye appears abducted and depressed ('down and out') due to the unopposed activity of the lateral rectus and superior oblique muscles. There will also be a complete ptosis due to paralysis of the levator (**Figure 26.1**). The pupil will be dilated and unreactive to light, and accommodation is paralysed.

Incomplete lesions are more common than complete lesions and may spare the extraocular muscles (e.g. only a partial ptosis is present) or the intraocular muscles (the pupil still reacts to light) to varying degrees. The pattern of deficit in incomplete cases depends on the site and nature of the lesion

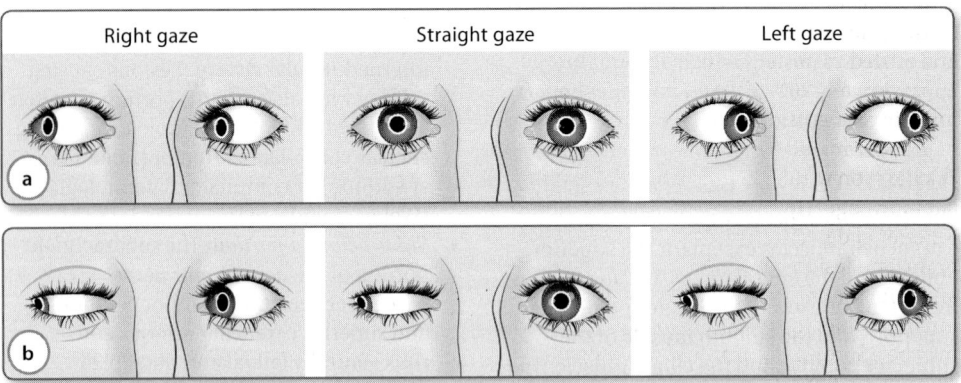

Figure 26.1 Showing right and left gaze in (a) Normal individual (b) Right IIICN palsy (Note: Right lateral and downward deviation and ptosis).

and the stage within its natural history. For example, the parasympathetic fibres travel superficially within the subarachnoid portion of the third nerve so the pupil becomes unreactive relatively early with compressive lesions such as aneurysms, however, this pupil sign cannot be relied on to exclude an aneurysm and imaging studies are still required. Always look for signs of aberrant regeneration (e.g. lid retraction on attempted downgaze) as this indicates that the lesion is compressive or traumatic and has been present for some months or years.

Investigations

The immediate work-up for all third nerve palsies should include vital signs, blood tests (e.g. full blood count, sedimentation rate if age > 50, myasthenic serology if 'pupil-sparing'), and a comprehensive imaging study of the third nerve to exclude compressive lesions such as an aneurysm. Further investigations and management will depend on the patient's age, history, systemic illness, and associated symptoms.

The choice of neuroimaging technique depends on institutional preference/experience and should be discussed directly with the neuroradiologist. Imaging options include computed tomography, magnetic resonance and formal (catheter) angiography In an acute setting, CT angiography (CTA) is regarded as more sensitive than magnetic resonance angiography (MRA) with 90% sensitivity to detect aneurysms 4 mm or greater, and also better demonstrates calcification within lesions and subarachnoid haemorrhage. However, MRI/MRA scanning is better at detecting small intraparenchymal brainstem lesions (tumours, abscesses, and infarctions) and meningeal and dural inflammation. In some equivocal cases, it may be appropriate to proceed to digital subtraction angiography (DSA), the gold standard technique which can reveal aneurysms smaller than 3 mm.

Lumbar puncture can also be done to detect blood in the cerebrospinal fluid (indicating rupture of a posterior communicating artery), inflammation, neoplastic infiltration or infection.

Diagnosis

Diagnosis is dependent on clinical examination while aetiology is suggested by the history/context and confirmed by the investigations.

Treatment

Management of oculomotor palsies is directed at addressing the aetiology. With ischaemic third nerve palsies, they are thought to result from insufficiency of the vasa nervorum or small vessels supplying the nerve. Unfortunately, there is no medical management to directly resolve ischaemic third nerve palsies but luckily most will spontaneously resolve after 6–8 weeks. Treatment is aimed at symptom management while awaiting resolution; this may include occlusion of the affected eye or prisms for the diplopia and pain relief with nonsteroidal anti-inflammatory drugs.

Surgery can be considered for oculomotor palsies when the patient does not recover after 6–12 months and the diplopia and/or ptosis has remained stable. In these cases patients may need strabismus or lid surgery to resolve their remaining deficits.

Complications

Incomplete third nerve palsies tend to have a better prognosis of recovery than complete. Surgical intervention for complete third nerve palsies is challenging (high risk of post-operative diplopia, and ptosis repair often leads to corneal exposure which is exacerbated by the poor Bell's phenomenon) and is rarely attempted.

Further reading

Chaudhary N, Davagnanam I, Ansari S, et al. Imaging of intracranial aneurysms causing isolated third cranial nerve palsy. J Neuro-ophthalmol 2009; 29:238–244.

Miller NR, Walsh FB, Hoyt WF. Walsh and Hoyt's Clinical Neuro-ophthalmology. Philadelphia: Lippincott Williams & Wilkins; 2005.

Vaphiades MS, Roberson GH. Imaging of oculomotor (third) cranial nerve palsy. Neurol Clin 2017; 35:101–113.

Vilensky J, Robertson W, Suarez-Quian C (Eds). The Clinical Anatomy of the Cranial Nerves: The Nerves of "On Olympus Towering Top". Ames, Iowa: Wiley-Blackwell; 2015.

Key topics of interest

- Anisocoria (p. 10)
- Blepharoptosis (p. 35)
- Cranial nerve palsies – multiple cranial nerves palsies (p. 104)
- Imaging in Ophthalmology (p. 176)

27 Cranial nerve palsy – trochlear nerve palsy

Key points
- The trochlear nerve is entirely motor and only supplies the contralateral superior oblique muscle
- Congenital trochlear nerve palsies have a large fusion range with a head tilt

Epidemiology

Trochlear nerve palsies can be divided into congenital and acquired. The true prevalence of congenital fourth nerve palsies is difficult to ascertain because patients have the ability to compensate with the use of a head tilt or large fusional amplitudes (consequently congenital fourth nerve palsies often do not present until adulthood when their fusional control deteriorates). For acquired fourth nerve palsies, there have been several studies commenting on the incidence and aetiology. Most of these studies found trochlear nerve palsy was less common than abducens nerve palsy and was less frequent in the paediatric population.

Congenital trochlear palsy is now classified as one of the congenital cranial dysinnervation disorders (CCDDs) and is thought to arise either because of dysgenesis of the trochlear nucleus or abnormal development of the peripheral nerve. Decompensation of congenital trochlear nerve palsies later in life can occur after cataract surgery because patients lose their ability to compensate while the cataract progresses then become diplopic once their vision is restored. Acquired trochlear nerve palsy is most commonly due to head trauma or microvascular/ischaemic mechanisms in vasculopaths, but rarer causes include inflammatory/infectious conditions and compression by neoplasms.

Anatomy

The trochlear nerve is the longest cranial nerve with the fewest number of axons. It supplies the superior oblique muscle and is entirely motor. Its course from nucleus to the contralateral superior oblique muscle can be divided into the following regions:

- *Nuclear portion:* The nucleus lies inferior to the main oculomotor nucleus in the anterior part of the grey matter at the level of the inferior colliculus in the midbrain. Fibres leave the nucleus and pass posteriorly around the central grey matter to leave the posterior surface of the midbrain. At this point, the nerves decussate with each other, so nuclear lesions (extremely rare) cause a contralateral superior oblique palsy
- *Subarachnoid portion:* The nerve then passes forward and laterally in the subarachnoid space to pierce the arachnoid and dura mater below the free border of the tentorium cerebelli. At this point, the nerve lies in close proximity to the sympathetic pathways in the dorsolateral tegmentum of the midbrain and the pretectal afferent pupillary fibres that run through the superior colliculus. Lesions in this area or trauma to the nerve (bruising or stretching) often result in a fourth nerve palsy associated with a contralateral Horner syndrome or an ipsilateral relative afferent pupillary defect
- *Cavernous portion:* The trochlear nerve lies below the oculomotor nerve in the lateral wall of the cavernous sinus. As it exits the cavernous sinus via the superior orbital fissure, it crosses lateral to the oculomotor nerve. Lesions in this area tend to cause multiple cranial neuropathies
- *Orbital portion:* The trochlear nerve lies above the tendinous ring but medial to the frontal nerve as it passes above the origin of levator palpebrae superioris. It enters superior oblique muscle as a series of small branches

Lesions at any of the above points can cause acquired fourth nerve palsies, either in isolation or with other associated deficits that help localise the lesion.

Clinical features

The superior oblique muscles intort, depress, and abduct the eyes (**Figure 27.1**). If the superior oblique muscle is paralysed, patients complain of vertical, torsional or oblique diplopia which is worse in downgaze and gaze away from the side of the affected muscle. If the problem has been there for more than a few months, then many patients will adapt by adjusting their head position (usually chin depression, face turn away from the lesion and head tilt towards the lesion) a helpful sign indicating that the problem is long-standing. In addition, orthoptic evaluation will demonstrate an enlarged vertical fusion range.

Investigations

Investigations of a trochlear palsy are directed by the patient's history. Most acquired fourth nerve palsies are caused by trauma or ischaemia. Neuroimaging and blood tests are only indicated when the palsy is progressive, non-isolated or there are contextual reasons for suspecting a sinister cause (e.g. recent history of malignancy). In general, blood testing will include vasculopathic causes (diabetes and hypercholesterolaemia), autoimmune conditions (myasthenia gravis and thyroid eye disease), and inflammatory conditions (giant cell arteritis). Neuroimaging such as MRI, CT, and MRA can be useful to help identify inflammatory conditions, neoplastic lesions, and aneurysms.

Diagnosis

Diagnosis is based on clinical findings. Parks-Bielschowsky three-step test can help aid the recognition of a fourth nerve palsy. This test consists of:
- First, determine which eye is hypertropic in primary gaze
- Second, determine in which horizontal direction of gaze the patient's hypertropia increases (worsening their diplopia)
- Finally, determine to which side a head tilt will increase the hypertropia and thus worsen the diplopia

Prisms or Maddox rods are used to quantify the deviations.

Bilateral fourth nerve palsies can be harder to interpret using the Parks–Bielschowsky three-step test since the manifest hypertropic globe will alternate depending on which side the head is tilted (right head tilt – right hypertropia, left head tilt – left hypertropia). In addition, patients with bilateral fourth nerve palsies usually display a V-esotropia pattern and more than 10° of exocyclotorsion.

Ocular torsion can be best identified by fundus examination, photography or OCT imaging. Between 2–8° of ocular torsion measured between the optic disc and fovea compared with the level of the optic disc is found in patients with trochlear nerve

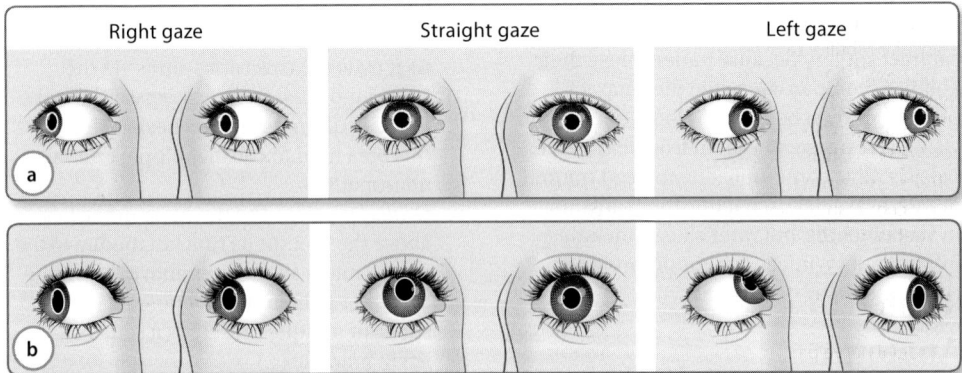

Figure 27.1 Showing right and left gaze in (a) Normal individual (b) Right IV CN palsy (Note: Upward deviation worse on left gaze).

palsies. This test is more sensitive than double Maddox rod testing or Lancaster red-green testing.

Treatment

Treatment of a trochlear nerve palsy depends on the aetiology. Spontaneous recovery is seen in most ischaemic cases and about 50% of idiopathic causes – usually within weeks but in some cases recovery can take 6 months to a year. In traumatic cases, approximately 50% will show some improvement but most will not recover completely. Aneurysms and neoplasms causing trochlear nerve palsies are least likely to recover. In the interim, patients can be given patches or given prisms for their diplopia (note that prisms can only correct deviations that are small and have no torsional component).

After a year, if the patient still has a large deviation causing diplopia, strabismus surgery can be offered. The type of strabismus surgery is dependent on the angle of deviation and if there is a torsional element. Deviations less than 15 prism dioptres will only have one muscle operated on while greater than 15 prismdioptres can have two or three muscles operated on. Some examples of single muscle procedures include inferior oblique myectomy for inferior oblique over-action, superior rectus recession for superior rectus restriction, and superior oblique tendon tuck for laxity.

For deviations larger than 15 prismdioptres, a combination of the previously mentioned muscle surgeries can be done.

For large excyclotorsional deviations seen in bilateral superior oblique palsies, bilateral superior oblique tendons are split so the anterior fibres can be advanced anteriorly and laterally. Thus, the anterior fibres which are responsible for incyclotorsion are stretched/strengthened to increase the power of intorsion (the modified Harada-Ito procedure). Since patients have large vertical fusion ranges, they often have a good post-operative results.

Complications

Complications of a trochlear nerve palsy are related to its treatment. As with any form of strabismus surgery, under and over-corrections can occur. In general, it is better to under-correct than over-correct since long-standing fourth nerve palsies have large fusional ranges; thus, patients can control any small residual deviation. To help minimise the risk of under- or over-correct, some surgeons use adjustable sutures. The most troublesome complication with fourth nerve palsy surgery is iatrogenic Brown syndrome after a superior oblique tuck procedure. In addition, asymmetric bilateral fourth nerve palsies can sometimes be mistaken for unilateral fourth nerve palsies. Hence when surgery is finished, it can unmask the contralateral fourth nerve palsy.

Further reading

Ansons AM, Davis H. Diagnosis and Management of Ocular Motility Disorders, 4th edition. US: Wiley-Blackwell; 2014.
Kowal L, Wong E, Yahalom C.7 Botulinum toxin in the treatment of strabismus. A review of its use and effects Disabi Rehabil 2007; 29:1823–1831.
Roberts C, Dawson Ed Lee J. Modified Harada-Ito procedure in bilateral superior oblique paresis. Strabismus 2002;10:211–214.
Snell RS. Clinical Anatomy By Regions, 9th edition. London: Lippincott Williams and Wilkins; 2012.
Thurtell MJ, Tomsak RL, Daroff RB. Neuro-Ophthalmology. Oxford: Oxford University Press; 2011.

Related topics of interest

- Cranial nerve palsies – multiple cranial nerves palsies (p. 104)
- Imaging in Ophthalmology (p. 176)

28 Diabetic eye disease

Key points
- Diabetic eye disease is a major cause of visual loss in adults
- Optimisation of systemic risk factors is crucial
- Advances in technology and treatment have revolutionised management

Epidemiology

Diabetic retinopathy (DR) is a chronic progressive disease of the retinal microvasculature associated with prolonged hyperglycaemia in diabetes mellitus. It is a leading cause of visual impairment in the working age population. The International Diabetes Federation published data in 2015, showing diabetes affects 415 million people worldwide, predicted to rise to 642 million by 2040. DR affects almost 100 million people worldwide and is set to become an ever-increasing health burden.

Pathophysiology

Hyperglycaemia activates several biochemical pathways including the formation of advanced glycated end-products, activation of protein kinase C and oxidative stress. This leads to microvascular damage with loss of pericytes, disruption of the interendothelial tight junctions, and thickening of the basement membrane. Increased capillary permeability, vascular occlusion, and gradual non-perfusion of the retinal vascular bed lead to ischaemia. Hypoxia advances up-regulation of vascular endothelial growth factor (VEGF), platelet adhesiveness, and fibrinolysis.

Progressive capillary non-perfusion underpins progression from non-proliferative to proliferative DR, with the aberrant formation of new retinal blood vessels. Severe vision loss can result from the fragility and bleeding of neovascular complexes resulting in vitreous haemorrhage or tractional retinal detachment from contraction of fibrous proliferation associated with neovascularisation.

Diabetic macular oedema (DMO) can result in significant visual impairment. It arises from breakdown of the blood-retinal barrier promoting leakage of plasma from the bloodstream into the retina. In recent years, optical coherence tomography (OCT) has revolutionised the diagnosis and monitoring of DMO thus facilitating its management.

Classification

Different approaches to classification have emerged (**Table 28.1**) to include:

1. Designed to cover the full range of retinopathy and aimed for ophthalmologists. It is based on the original Airlie House and subsequent simplified Early Treatment Diabetic Retinopathy Study (ETDRS) classification used in clinical trials.
2. As adopted by the National Screening Committee (NSC) in the UK to reflect vision-threatening risk (**Tables 28.1** and **28.2**).
3. The American Academy of Ophthalmology classification.

The presence of abnormal vessels is the hallmark of proliferative DR. (**Figure 28.1**) Neovascularisation is categorised into arising from or within 1 disc diameter of the optic nerve (NVD) and elsewhere in the retina (NVE). Rubeosis iridis is neovascularisation occurring on the iris (NVI) and in the drainage angle (NVA) and is a manifestation of severe retinal ischaemia heralding the onset of rubeotic glaucoma.

Risk factors for developing retinopathy

Non-modifiable factors
Age, genetics, and duration of diabetes.

Modifiable factors

Poor glycaemic control
Good diabetic control can reduce the risk in both onset and progression of DR. For every percentage point decrease in

Diabetic eye disease

Table 28.1 Classification of diabetic retinopathy

ETDRS	NSC	SDRGS	AAO
10 none	R0	R0	No apparent retinopathy
20 Microaneurysms only	R1 Microaneurysms, retinal haemorrhages, exudates	R1 Mild background	Mild NPDR
35 Mild NPDR			Moderate NPDR
43 Moderate NPDR	R2 Pre-proliferative Multiple blot haemorrhages, IRMAs, venous beading, venous duplication	R2 Moderate BDR	
47 Moderately severe NPDR			
53A-D Severe NPDR		R3 Severe BDR	Severe NPDR
53E very severe NPDR			
61 mild PDR	R3 Proliferative NVD, NVE	R4 PDR	PDR
65 moderate PDR			
71,75 high-risk PDR (vitreous haemorrhage)			
81,85 advanced PDR (tractional RD)			

AAO, American Academy of Ophthalmology; BDR, background diabetic retinopathy; ETDRS, Early Treatment Diabetic Retinopathy Study; IRMA, intraretinal microvascular abnormality; NPDR, non-proliferative diabetic retinopathy; NSC, National Screening Committee; NVE, new vessels elsewhere; NVD, new vessels on disc; PDR, proliferative diabetic retinopathy; SDRGS, Scottish Diabetic Retinopathy Grading Scheme

Table 28.2 Classification of diabetic maculopathy

ETDRS	NSC
CSMO: • Retinal thickening at or within 500 µm of the centre of the macula; • Hard exudates at or within 500 µm of the centre of the macula, if associated with thickening of the adjacent retina • A zone of retinal thickening one disc area in size at least part of which is within one disc diameter of the centre	*M1:* • Macular exudate < or = 1 DD of centre of fovea; • Circinate or group of exudates within macula • Any microaneurysm or haemorrhage < or = 1 DD of centre of fovea only if associated with a best VA of < or = 6/12 • Retinal thickening < or = 1 DD of centre of fovea (if stereo available)

CSMO, clinically significant macular oedema

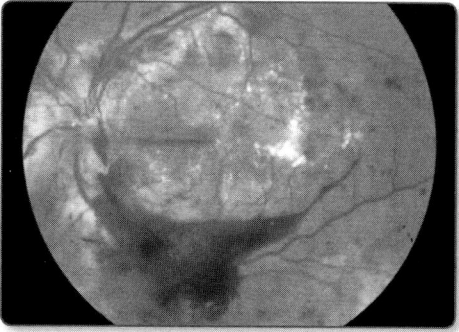

Figure 28.1 Fundus photo of severe diabetic retinopathy and neovascularisation.
(For colour version see plate 1)

glycated haemoglobin (HbA1c) in patients with type 2 diabetes, there can be up to a 35% reduction in the risk of microvascular complications.

Hypertension

Optimisation of blood pressure in patients with hypertension is a major factor in reducing the progression of DR. The UKPDS showed that a reduction of mean systolic blood pressure from 154 mmHg to 144 mmHg demonstrated a 34% reduction in progression of retinopathy and a 47% reduced risk of deterioration in visual acuity in type 2 diabetics.

Hyperlipidaemia

Observational studies suggest that dyslipidaemia increases the risk of DR, particularly DMO. The ACCORD eye study showed a 40% reduction in the odds of having progression of retinopathy over 4 years in patients allocated to fenofibrate in combination with a statin, compared with simvastatin alone.

Fenofibrate likely has more ancillary benefits than are currently understood.

Additional factors

Pregnancy

Progression of retinopathy can occur in pregnancy. A prospective study among type 1 diabetics found DR progression occurred in 27% of patients with laser therapy being required in 6%.

Smoking

No clear association of smoking and retinopathy has been demonstrated. Patients with DR are at higher risk of cardiovascular disease and therefore should be encouraged to stop smoking.

Nephropathy

Nephropathy is an excellent predictor of the presence of retinopathy probably because both conditions are caused by microangiopathies.

Investigations

Systemic investigations are usually carried out under a patient joint care arrangement by a diabetologist, whose investigations will address both modifiable risk factors and end-organ damage.

Ocular investigations using imaging modalities are important for diagnosis and management. These include fundus photography for capturing baseline characteristics and monitoring progression. OCT is essential for a quantitative analysis of the macular thickness and evaluating response to therapy. Fundus fluorescein angiography demonstrates capillary non-perfusion, neovascularisation and the source of macular leakage.

Management

Diabetic retinopathy

Optimisation of systemic risk factors for not only long-term survival but also protection from worsening eye disease is crucial. A personalised HbA1c target, usually between 48 mmol/mol and 58 mmol/mol is set. One should aim for a systolic blood pressure ≤ 130 mmHg in those with established retinopathy and/or nephropathy and a mean systolic blood pressure < 140 mmHg in patients who do not have retinopathy. Statins should also be considered for secondary prevention of macrovascular disease and adding fenofibrate in type 2 diabetics.

Background retinopathy

In the UK, this level of retinopathy is monitored with annual digital photography in population-based screening programmes. All diabetics are invited for screening from the age of 12 years.

Pre-proliferative diabetic retinopathy

It is advised that regular slit lamp biomicroscopic examination by an expert is required for patients with pre-proliferative DR.

Proliferative diabetic retinopathy

Panretinal photocoagulation

The aim of panretinal photocoagulation (PRP) is to destroy the areas of retinal ischaemia which are driving

Diabetic eye disease

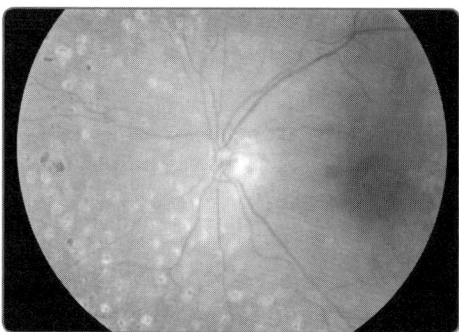

Figure 28.2 Fundus photo showing extensive panretinal photocoagulation (PRP).

neovascularisation (**Figure 28.2**). PRP is administered to all 4 retinal quadrants outside the macular vascular arcade. It is the mainstay of treatment for proliferative DR and reduces the risk of severe visual loss in patients with high-risk characteristics by 50% at 5 years. It may also be considered in severe pre-proliferative DR when for example regular hospital attendance track record is poor, prior to cataract surgery, difficulties examining the patient or in an only eye where the first eye vision was lost to proliferative DR.

The laser targets the retinal pigment epithelium whilst minimising photoreceptor damage. The laser is administered by conventional single shot or multispot laser delivery systems. Multispot laser treatment is less painful and more likely to preserve the central and peripheral visual field. Due to the shorter pulse duration, a larger number of burns are required to achieve full regression of new vessels.

Vitreoretinal surgery
Advanced DR with non-clearing vitreous haemorrhage that may preclude adequate PRP or a tractional retinal detachment should be referred for vitreoretinal surgery.

Intravitreal anti-VEGF
Intraocular VEGF levels are elevated in DR and are important signalling proteins promoting neovascularisation.

Panretinal photocoagulation must be delivered promptly in the presence of NVI. If NVAs are present, then anti-VEGF treatment as an adjunct to PRP has shown favourable results to induce vessel regression more rapidly and reduces the risk of progression to rubeotic glaucoma. For patients with established rubeotic glaucoma, co-management with glaucoma specialists is required.

Anti-VEGF treatment is also known to reduce the severity of DR. The DRCR network compared intravitreal ranibizumab against PRP to treat proliferative DR and found similar visual outcomes at 2 years and the need for fewer vitrectomies and a lower incidence of DMO in the ranibizumab-treated group. This may impact the management of DR in the future as long-term data accumulates.

Diabetic macular oedema

Intravitreal anti-VEGF
The VEGF mediates vascular leakage by affecting tight junction proteins and is an important factor in DMO (**Figure 28.3**). There are two licensed drugs in the UK for centre-involving DMO with a retinal thickness of greater than 400 micrometres.

1. *Ranibizumab (Lucentis):* A humanised recombinant monoclonal antibody fragment that selectively binds to human VEGF-A and prevents it from binding to its receptors. The UK licensed dose is a 0.5 mg/0.05 mL intravitreal injection every month for 3 consecutive months and thereafter guided by response. The minimum period between each injection is 4 weeks.
2. *Aflibercept (Eylea):* The pan-VEGF-A, VEGF-B and placental growth factor blocker, is a humanised recombinant fusion protein. The UK licensed dose is a 2 mg/0.05 mL intravitreal monthly injection for 5 consecutive months, followed by every 2 months. After the first 12 months, the treatment interval may be extended based on visual and anatomic outcomes.
3. *Bevacizumab (Avastin):* The monoclonal antibody inhibits VEGF-A. It is not licensed for intraocular use but is effective in treating retinal vascular disease. It may be considered when there are no licensed alternatives for certain eye conditions

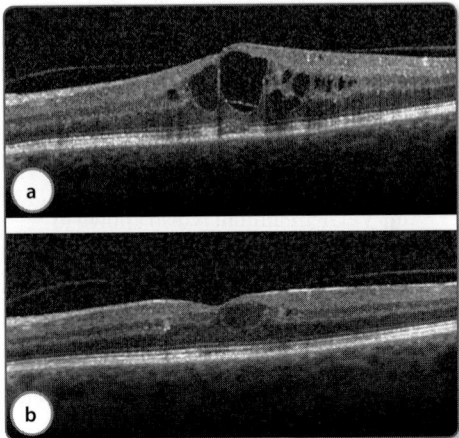

Figure 28.3 (a) OCT of macula showing pre; (b) post-therapy.

RESTORE was a multicentre randomised controlled trial evaluating ranibizumab against ranibizumab with laser and laser alone in DMO. The ranibizumab monotherapy group gained the highest number of letters. This was also captured in the VIVID and VISTA trials showing a significant improvement in vision with aflibercept compared with laser at 1 year.

Intravitreal steroids

The pathogenesis of DMO is complex involving a range of inflammatory markers. Corticosteroids can block the expression of such inflammatory mediators thereby inhibiting leukostasis and improving the barrier function of endothelial cell tight junctions.
- *Dexamethasone 700 μg intravitreal biodegradable implant (Ozurdex)*: This is licensed in the UK for pseudophakic patients, who have been unresponsive or are unsuitable to non-corticosteroid treatment. The drug is released over a period of up to 6 months. An average of 4–5 injections over 3 years provided significant visual and anatomic improvements compared with sham procedure in the MEAD study
- *Fluocinolone acetonide intravitreal non-biodegradable implant (Iluvien)*: This is licensed in the UK for treating chronic DMO in pseudophakic eyes that have not responded to other therapies. There is a sustained release of fluocinolone for up to 36 months. The FAME study showed at 24 months, there was an improvement in vision in 28.7% of the treated group versus 16.2% in controls, which were sustained for the third year

Macular photocoagulation

Before the advent of anti-VEGF treatment, macular laser photocoagulation was the gold standard treatment in DMO. The ETDRS demonstrated that for those eyes with clinically significant macular oedema (CSMO), the rate of moderate visual loss was reduced from 24% to 12% at 3 years in the laser-treated group.

The modified ETDRS macular laser treatment protocol is:
- Focal treatment of leaking microaneurysms (500–3,000 μm from fovea)
- Grid treatment to areas of retinal thickening (500–3,500 μm from fovea)

Recovery of vision is much harder to achieve with laser alone, however, may have a role when other treatments are unsuitable.

Further reading

Duh E, Sun J, Sitt A. Diabetic retinopathy; current understanding, mechanisms and treatment strategies. JCI Insight 2017; 2.pii:93751.

Grading diabetic retinopathy from stereoscopic colour fundus photographs – an extension of the modified Airlie House classification. ETDRS report number 10. Early Treatment Diabetic Retinopathy Study Research Group. Ophthalmology 1991; 98:786.

Public Health England. NHS Diabetic Eye Screening Programme Grading definitions for referable disease, 2017. [online] Available from https://www.gov.uk/government/uploads/system/uploads/attachment_data/file/582710/Grading_definitions_for_referrable_disease_2017_new_110117.pdf [Last accessed October, 2019].

Royal College of Ophthalmologists. (2012). Diabetic Retinopathy Guidelines. [online] Available from https://www.rcophth.ac.uk/wp-content/uploads/2014/12/2013-SCI-301-FINAL-DR-GUIDELINES-DEC-2012-updated-July-2013.pdf [Last accessed October, 2019].

The International Diabetes Federation. (2015). Diabetes Atlas, Seventh Edition 2015. [online] Available from http://www.diabetesatlas.org [Last accessed October, 2019].

Related topics of interest

- Retinal imaging (p. 277)
- Retinal lasers (p. 282)
- Intravitreal injection therapies (p. 193)

29 Dry eye syndrome

Key points
- Dry eye disease has a common prevalence
- Identification of underlying causes is required for satisfactory treatment planning
- The role of anti-inflammatory agents is increasing

Epidemiology
The prevalence reported as high as 50% in some studies of dry eye disease is difficult to ascertain precisely because standardised disease definitions or classifications fluctuate. There is an increased prevalence with age and most studies report it to be more common in women compared with men.

Pathophysiology
The optical quality, of the first refractive elements of the eye, is dependent on the tear film smoothly bathing the corneal epithelium. The corneal epithelium is, at every blink, coated in a replenished layered film consisting of a superficial lipid and underlying aqueous and mucoaqueous layers. The lacrimal glands, meibomian glands and conjunctival goblet cells are some of the elements that are responsible for the production of the tear film. Therefore, on a simplistic level, impairment of these structures or a breakdown in their regulation, contribute to the pathogenesis of dry eye disease.

The current mechanism proposed for the pathogenesis of dry eye disease is proposed by the 'Dry Eye Workshop' as evaporative water loss leading to hyperosmolar tissue damage. It is thought that there is the subsequent creation of a vicious circle of self-perpetuated disease mediated by inflammatory responses and recurrent ocular surface damage.

Clear pathogenic causes for dry eye disease can be attributed to Sjögren's syndrome or ocular graft vs host disease, which involve destruction of the lacrimal gland and subsequent deficiency of the aqueous component of tears. These conditions would, intuitively, lead to aqueous-deficient dry eye disease. Meibomian gland disease can lead to an evaporative dry eye because the resultant deficiency in the lipid layer leads to accelerated tear evaporation.

Clinical features
The symptoms include dryness, burning, stinging, scratchiness, grittiness, tiredness and a feeling of heavy lids. Sometimes, a patient will have associated blurring that may be relieved by blinking. A history should include assessment for associated underlying conditions such as Sjögren syndrome by asking about dry mouth and a history of rheumatoid arthritis. Association of symptom onset in air-conditioned environments, or reflex tearing in windy weather, should be elicited. Contact lens wear and refractive surgery can be risk factors.

A history of allogeneic haemopoietic stem cell transplant surgery would suggest ocular graft vs host disease and this can cause an extraordinarily severe dry eye.

Clinical examination should be methodical; the eyelids must be examined for signs of adequate closure and blepharitis. The tear film breakup time should be measured (< 8 s is abnormal). The corneal surface may demonstrate signs of dry eye, such as punctate epithelial staining. Filaments of mucus may be found in patients with more severe forms of dry eye disease. The superior cornea should be examined for perilimbal hyperaemia, punctate erosions (**Figure 29.1**), and a subtarsal papillary reaction. These signs may indicate superior limbic keratoconjunctivitis.

Investigations
Clinical history and examination assessment are enough to diagnose most cases of dry eye disease. Clinical testing, such as the Schirmer's test, can be employed to detect

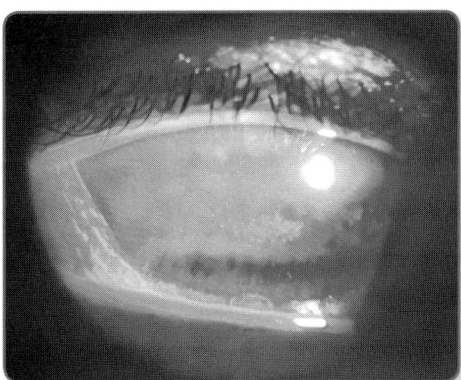

Figure 29.1 Punctate epithelial erosions on the cornea of a patient with dry eye (*For colour version see plate 1*)
Courtesy: M Bizrah Moorfields Eye Hospital.

aqueous deficiency. The Schirmer I test, a test of basal and reflex tear secretion, is performed without the initial instillation of topical anaesthetic. It requires the insertion of the bent tip of a 5 mm × 35 mm strip of no. 41 Whatman filter paper into the inferior fornix. Abnormal wetting would be indicated by progress of < 5 mm in 5 min.

Investigation to confirm a diagnosis is rarely needed outside of research settings. Tear film osmolarity is sometimes of use in such settings.

The presence of anti-Ro and anti-La antibodies can support the diagnosis of primary Sjögren's syndrome.

Diagnosis

Diagnosis should include an attempt to classify the disease into one that is aqueous-deficient, evaporative or mixed.

Evaporative dry eye may be attributed to lid margin disease, impaired eyelid closure or impaired blink. Vitamin A deficiency may be a consideration in some populations. Aqueous-deficient dry eye may be a Sjögren's syndrome dry eye or non-Sjögren's syndrome dry eye. Non-Sjögren's Dry Eye may be associated with, e.g. infiltrative disorders of the lacrimal gland, neurological impairment or cicatricial conjunctival causes.

The severity of dryness can be graded by assessing the amount of corneal and conjunctival staining using the Oxford Grading Scheme as reported by Bron et al.

Treatment

The advantage of attributing a structured diagnosis is that underlying causes can be addressed. For example, effective treatment of blepharitis should be a priority when identified.

The mainstay of treatment for dry eye consists of tear film supplementation, through the use of "artificial tear" drops. Multitudes of examples exist. Some constituent agents, such as carboxymethyl cellulose and hyaluronic acid may promote epithelial healing. Frequent or prolonged use may require the consideration of use of unpreserved forms.

Anti-inflammatories are increasingly considered in the treatment of severe dry eye because they can help manage the inflammatory component of the disease. The use of topical ciclosporin A has become increasingly established in the treatment of severe dry eye.

Autologous serum drops are sometimes required in some cases of dry eye, especially in severe cases such as those associated with Sjögren's syndrome.

Other strategies include temporary or permanent occlusion of puncti in order to conserve tears.

Adjuncts to treatment can include dietary supplementation with oral omega-3 fatty acids.

Complications

Severe dry eye can lead to a filamentary keratitis that prompts patients to 'fish' mucous filaments from their ocular surface. Such behaviour must be discouraged, and treatment of the dry eye can be supplemented with a topical mucolytic such as acetylcysteine. Dry eye can be a significant source of morbidity.

Any preoperative assessment should include an assessment for dry eye. Corneal melting can occur in patients undergoing cataract surgery who have Sjögren's syndrome or rheumatoid arthritis and dry eye is thought to be a risk factor for this rare but devastating complication.

Further reading

Bron A, Evans VE, Smith JA. Grading of corneal and conjunctival staining in the context of other dry eye tests. Cornea 2003; 22:640–650.

Jones L, Downie L, Korb D, et al. TFOS DEWS II management and therapy report. The Ocular Surface 2017; 15;575–628.

Related topics of interest

- Conjunctivitis (p. 72)
- Contact lens-related problems of the eye (p. 75)
- Thyroid eye disease (p. 316)
- Chemical injuries (p. 67)

30 Ectropion

Key points
- Lower lid ectropion is a common problem in the elderly characterised by eversion of the eyelid margin from the globe
- It can lead to ocular surface exposure, dry eye sensation, and tearing both as a reflex phenomenon and also due to punctum ectropion
- It can be classified as congenital, cicatricial, neurogenic or paralytic, involutional, and mechanical
- Treatment is mainly surgical and the surgical technique depends on the cause

Epidemiology

The most common type of eyelid ectropion is involutional which affects the lower lid in about 3% of mainly older adults.

Pathophysiology

There are five main mechanisms causing ectropion as discussed here.

Congenital ectropion
This type of ectropion is rare and when occurring tends to affect the lower lids and is typically caused by a vertical deficiency of the anterior lamella.

Cicatricial
Anterior lamellar shortening may cause cicatricial ectropion. There may be a previous history of injury or surgery in the periocular area with resultant traction from the scar causing an ectropion. Anterior lamellar shortening can also occur in actinic damage to the skin or other dermatological conditions causing skin contraction.

Neurogenic/paralytic
Facial palsy is the main cause of paralytic ectropion. This may be due to pathology or induced by trauma including surgical trauma to the facial nerve. The severity of the condition and the chance of recovery are often related to the aetiology of paralysis.

Involutional
This is the most common type of ectropion which mainly affects the elderly population and is due to the horizontal eyelid laxity.

Mechanical
In mechanical ectropion, a tumour – benign or malignant – causes displacement of the eyelid margin from the globe.

Clinical features

In all types of ectropion, the lid margin is turned away from the ocular surface. Mild cases may be entirely asymptomatic but even a mild medial lower lid ectropion affecting the lacrimal punctum position may be bothersome by causing watering eye. This in turn can cause further periocular skin changes secondary to irritation of tears on the skin. Inflammation of the exposed tarsal conjunctiva causes eyelid and/or ocular surface discomfort. Ectropion due to lower lid laxity may be responsible for watery eye due to lacrimal pump failure.

Eyelid ectropion commonly affects the lower lids. Upper lid ectropion can occur in floppy eyelid syndrome whereby excessive lid laxity leads to the eversion of the upper lid usually during sleep. This tends to cause sore, red, and discharging eye on waking up. There is usually papillary conjunctivitis as a presenting feature. The upper lids would evert easily on lateral traction. There is also associated upper lid lash ptosis. This condition frequently affects the side the patient tends to sleep on. Floppy eyelid syndrome is also associated with higher body mass index and sleep apnoea.

In more severe cases such as in paralytic ectropion, there would be ocular surface exposure and irritation and in most severe cases there would be a risk of keratitis.

Investigations

There are no particular investigations to conform the diagnosis of ectropion apart from direct observation and clinical examination.

Diagnosis

Diagnosis is confirmed by clinical examination and the outward rotation of the lid margin from the ocular surface. In floppy eyelid syndrome, there is usually no obvious upper or lower lid ectropion but there is often a degree of papillary conjunctivitis present and the upper lid would easily evert on gentle horizontal pulling at its lateral aspect.

Treatment

Treatment is mainly surgical and the surgical technique depends on the cause as described below. The principle of treatment is to correct both the horizontal lid laxity (such as in involutional) and the vertical laxity or traction (such as in paralytic and cicatricial) components.

Congenital

In this type of ectropion, there is usually a degree of skin shortage or an increase in the horizontal lid length. Initial treatment is aimed at protecting the ocular surface and the cornea by using frequent topical lubricants and antibiotics. Where surgery is necessary, the choice of intervention depends on the severity and the aetiology of the condition and it includes horizontal lid shortening, full thickness inverting sutures, or a full thickness skin graft.

Cicatricial

In cicatricial ectropion, (**Figure 30.1**) where there is a scar causing the vertical traction, it needs to be released. Milder forms may be treatable with a Z-plasty procedure. Wherever there is a shortage of skin, a full thickness skin graft is necessary. Good donor sites are: upper eyelid, periauricular, retroauricular, subclavicular, and inner aspect of the upper arm. The size of the skin graft needs to be slightly oversized compared with the size of the defect created by a horizontal subciliary incision and creating an appropriately sized space to correct the lid position. Any horizontal laxity needs to be corrected at the same time by a lateral canthal tightening procedure; either canthopexy or lateral tarsal strip.

Paralytic

In paralytic ectropion, the main concern is the lagophthalmos causing ocular surface exposure. Topical lubricants and antibiotics need to be used frequently before and after any surgical treatment and it is often necessary to be continued for long term. The aim of the treatment is to protect the cornea and the ocular surface by reducing the degree of the lagophthalmos. This requires reducing the exposed ocular surface both horizontally and vertically. Depending on the severity of orbicularis weakness, one or more of the following procedures may be required – lateral tarsal strip with higher than normal attachment of the strip to the lateral orbital rim, lateral tarsorrhaphy, Lee medial canthoplasty, and lower lid suspension using a sling (using fascia or synthetic materials). In longstanding paralytic ectropion, skin contracture may occur needing full thickness skin graft.

Involutional

This is the most common type of ectropion and is usually caused by horizontal lid laxity (**Figure 30.2**). Treatment is aimed to correct the degree and the position of the laxity. In medial ectropion, the punctum position needs to be corrected and a medial spindle procedure may be necessary. It

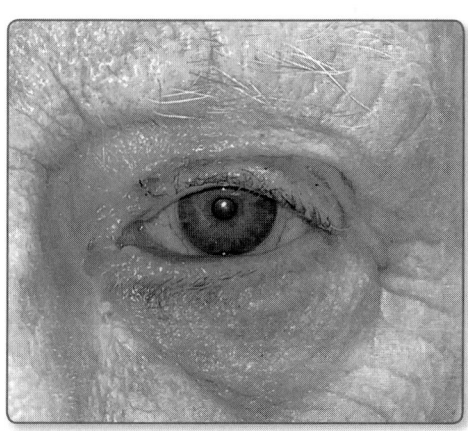

Figure 30.1 Lower lid cicatricial ectropion.

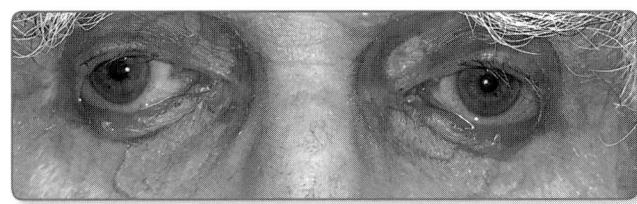

Figure 30.2 Lower lid involutional ectropion.

is worth noting at this point that chronic punctum ectropion often causes punctum stenosis which needs to be addressed too (see Chapter 32). Horizontal lid laxity can be corrected by either lateral canthopexy or lateral tarsal strip depending on the degree of laxity. In more severe cases where there is tarsal eversion, lower lid retractor reattachment is necessary which is performed through a subtarsal conjunctival incision. Prior to surgical treatment of chronic cases of severe ectropion, it is often beneficial to treat the condition with topical steroid ointments at night for a period of around a month. This will reduce the degree of inflammation of the exposed tarsal conjunctiva and will improve and optimise the condition prior to surgery. Ectropion correction in these cases can be very uncomfortable due to positioning of an inflamed tarsal conjunctiva over the globe.

The treatment of floppy eyelids is included in this section as although the aetiology of the condition is believed to be related to a decrease in tarsal elastin, the condition is characterised by excessive laxity of the eyelid. The conservative treatment includes regular topical lubricants particularly using ointment as well as wearing a patch at nights to prevent nocturnal eversion of the eyelid (mainly upper lid). The surgical treatment is essentially aimed to shorten the horizontal length and for the upper lid a full thickness lateral wedge excision is very effective although an upper lid lateral tarsal strip procedure is also possible.

Complications

Common complications of the surgery are bleeding, infection, and scar tissue formation. Suture granuloma formation can occur depending on the type of suture material used. In case of using skin graft there is further risk of graft failure and donor site wound healing complications.

Further reading

Collin JRO (ed). A Manual of Systematic Eyelid Surgery, 3rd edition, illustrated. Elsevier Health Sciences; 2006.
JA Nerad. Techniques in Ophthalmic Plastic Surgery. Elsevier Health Sciences; 2012.

Tyres AG, Collin JRO. Colour Atlas of Ophthalmic Plastic Surgery, illustrated edition. Butterworth-Heinemann; 2008.

Related topics of interest

- Entropion (p. 128)
- Epiphora (p. 131)

31 Entropion

Key points
- Lower lid entropion is a common problem in the elderly characterised by inwards rotation of the eyelid margin towards the globe
- It can lead to ocular surface irritation, photophobia, watery eye, and corneal scarring particularly if affecting the upper lid
- Causes of entropion can be classified as congenital, cicatricial, spastic, and involutional
- Treatment is mainly surgical and the surgical technique depends on the cause

Epidemiology

The most common type of eyelid entropion is involutional which affects the lower lid in about 3% of mainly older adults.

Pathophysiology

There are four main mechanisms causing ectropion as discussed here.

Congenital entropion

This is a very rare condition and can affect both the upper and the lower eyelids. Pathophysiology of this condition includes pretarsal orbicularis hypertrophy or inferior retractors attachment abnormalities.

Involutional

This is the most common type of entropion which mainly affects the elderly population. It only affects the lower eyelid and any upper lid entropion is usually due to a cicatricial cause. The three main mechanisms for lower lid involutional entropion act both at a vertical and a horizontal vector and involve laxity of the inferior retractors, overriding of preseptal orbicular, and horizontal lid laxity.

Cicatricial

This type of entropion is caused by a shortening of the posterior lamella and the subsequent inwards rotation of the eyelid margin. It can affect both the upper and the lower eyelids. Main causes of cicatrisation are: trauma including previous surgery, ocular cicatricial pemphigoid (OCP), alkali burns, Steven–Johnson syndrome, trachoma, recurrent chalazia, and blepharitis.

Spastic

In this condition, a subtle degree of involutional entropion can become manifest by orbicularis spasm. This is often initiated by local or ocular surface irritation.

Clinical features

In all types of entropion, the lid margin is turned towards the globe with eyelashes in contact with the ocular surface. Mild cases may be intermittent and only become apparent when there is ocular surface irritation or during forceful eye closure. It is important to assess cases of trichiasis for eyelid margin rotation and correct the lid position where indicated.

In early stages, there may be occasional irritation, photophobia, and watering of the affected eye. In addition, in more chronic cases, there may be conjunctival and/or corneal scarring due to chronic abrasion of eyelashes against the ocular surface. This is more likely to occur in upper lid entropion.

In involutional entropion, there is commonly some horizontal lid laxity of the lower lids. In cicatricial cases, there would be scarring of palpebral conjunctiva, adhesion bands between the tarsal and bulbar conjunctiva, and in more severe cases foreshortening of the fornix. Corneal pannus or scarring may be present in chronic cases of upper lid cicatricial entropion.

Investigations

There are no particular investigations to confirm the diagnosis of entropion itself apart from direct clinical examination. In suspected cases of OCP, however, direct immunofluorescence testing and conjunctival biopsy may be necessary.

Diagnosis

Diagnosis is confirmed by clinical examination and observation of the lid margin position. In mild cases, forceful lid closure may make the subtle entropion more obvious. In cicatricial cases, there would be signs of scarring, adhesion bands, and foreshortening of the fornix. Corneal scarring and vascularisation may be present due to chronic rubbing of eyelashes.

Treatment

Treatment is mainly surgical and using ocular surface lubrication to alleviate the ocular surface irritation while waiting for the surgical correction of entropion. Temporary measures also include applying a tape to the lower eyelid and botulinum toxin injection to weaken the lower lid orbicular muscle in spastic cases.

The surgical technique is aimed to correct the cause as outlined below.

Congenital

In congenital entropion where there is overriding of orbicularis muscle, an ellipse of the anterior lamella (skin and muscle) is excised in the medial aspect of the lower lid and the lid retractors are sutured to the inferior border of the tarsus (Hotz procedure). Not all cases of congenital entropion require surgery, and an operation is only necessary if there is irritation and persistent photophobia and recurrent conjunctivitis. In milder cases of epiblepharon, everting sutures are often adequate to correct the condition.

Cicatricial

In cicatricial entropion, where there is an underlying autoimmune condition, it needs to be treated medically first. The cicatrisation process may be exacerbated by surgery without adequate immunosuppression treatment in OCP. In nonactive cases or nonprogressive disease such as trachoma or Steven–Johnson syndrome surgery can be performed where necessary. Surgical treatment involves release of the conjunctival scars and eversion of the lid margin to achieve normal anatomical position. There is often a need to address the shortening of the posterior lamella by using a graft. The choice of the graft material depends on the tarsus shortage and stability and the degree of conjunctival scarring. The common donor sites to address lid stability are hard palate, nasal septal chondromucosa, and ear cartilage grafts. Buccal or labial mucous membrane can be used where there is a need to lengthen the fornix.

In mild cases of lower lid cicatricial entropion, tarsal fracture and outward rotation of the lid margin may be adequate.

Upper lid entropion requires anterior lamella repositioning in mild cases and posterior lamella advancement in moderate cases. This usually requires a grey-line split to achieve dissociation between the anterior and posterior lamellae in order to allow adequate repositioning. Everting sutures are placed at the superior border of the tarsus to emerge on the skin above the lash line to reposition the anterior lamella. More severe cases of upper lid entropion are treated by posterior lamella graft, tarsal fracture, rotation of the terminal tarsus or tarsus excision. Good donor sites for mucous membrane graft are buccal and labial mucosa. Auricular cartilage is a good donor tissue for upper lid reconstruction where there is unstable eyelid margin due to tarsus loss.

Spastic

Spastic entropion in the absence of any horizontal lid laxity can be treated by everting sutures. This is usually performed by using three double armed, absorbable sutures passed through the fornix and exiting below the lash line to achieve a slight overcorrection. Temporary treatment with injection of botulinum toxin in the orbicularis muscle is also an effective method of addressing spastic entropion.

Involutional

In this type of entropion, (**Figure 31.1**) the horizontal lid laxity must be corrected alongside with any other contributing factors which are usually laxity of the lower lid retractors and overriding of the preseptal orbicularis. In mild cases, a lateral tarsal strip

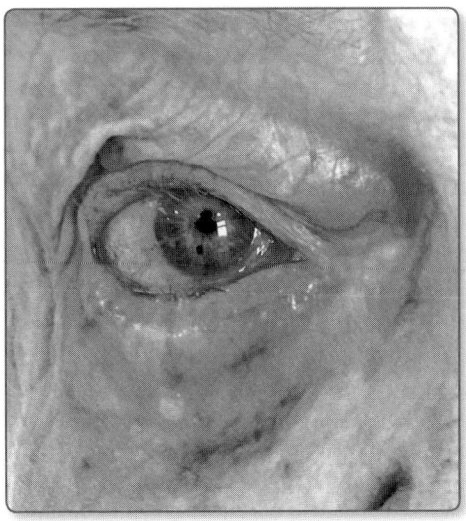

Figure 31.1 Lower lid involutional entropion.

procedure may be adequate but everting sutures or inferior retractor reinsertion is usually necessary in other cases. Inferior retractors are sutured to the inferior tarsus plate through a subciliary skin incision to achieve better stability of the lower lid. Everting sutures on their own are usually only a temporary treatment but it is a useful procedure if other definitive surgical options are not possible.

Complications

Common complications include bleeding, infection, scarring, and suture granuloma. There is also risk of under- or overcorrection of the lid margin position. In case of using a graft, there is a risk of graft failure and donor site wound healing issues.

Further reading

Collin JRO (ed). A Manual of Systematic Eyelid Surgery, 3rd edition, illustrated. Elsevier Health Sciences; 2006.

JA Nerad. Techniques in Ophthalmic Plastic Surgery. Elsevier Health Sciences; 2012.

Tyres AG, Collin JRO. Colour Atlas of Ophthalmic Plastic Surgery, illustrated edition. Butterworth-Heinemann; 2008.

Related topics of interest

- Blepharitis (p. 32)
- Conjunctivitis (p. 72)
- Epiphora (p. 131)
- Chemical injuries (p. 67)

32 Epiphora

Key points

- Watery eye could be due to tear hypersecretion, abnormal tear distribution or insufficient tear drainage (or a combination of these factors)
- Hypersecretion is often a reflex phenomenon secondary to ocular surface irritation, ocular inflammation or allergy
- Abnormal tear distribution is often due to eyelids abnormality
- Outflow obstruction may be congenital or acquired
- Acquired obstruction may be primary or secondary

Epidemiology

There are wildly different figures of up to 6% reported regarding the incidence of congenital nasolacrimal duct obstruction (NLDO).

Acquired NLDO has an average annual incidence rate of approximately 30 per 100,000.

Pathophysiology

Watery eye tends to occur where there is an imbalance of tear production and tear outflow (**Figure 32.1**). It is worth noting that there are patients with outflow obstruction who have reduced tear production and remain asymptomatic.

Hypersecretion as a reflex phenomenon is often secondary to ocular surface irritation. Common causes include dry eyes, ocular inflammation (uveitis, dacryoadenitis), corneal or subtarsal foreign bodies, trichiasis, blepharitis, and entropion. Corneal epithelial defect (including recurrent corneal erosion) or ulcer also causes a watery eye.

Lid malpositions cause epiphora by direct ocular surface irritation such as in entropion and ectropion or by reduced tear outflow. Lower lid laxity affects the efficiency of the lacrimal pump, e.g. in paralytic ectropion. Lacrimal punctum ectropion causes epiphora due to failure of the tear reaching the drainage system. The exposed punctum in medial ectropion often becomes stenotic over time. There is a special case of abnormal lower lid punctum position in a condition called Centurion syndrome. In this condition, there is anterior displacement of the medial canthus tendon leading to the punctum's position being anatomically more anterior than normal and not in contact with the globe.

Lacrimal gland hypersecretion can also occur in gustatory lacrimation following recovery from seventh nerve palsy and aberrant regeneration of the seventh nerve.

Epiphora caused by outflow obstruction can be at various levels along the drainage system. This includes conjunctivochalasis with a redundant fold of the conjunctiva

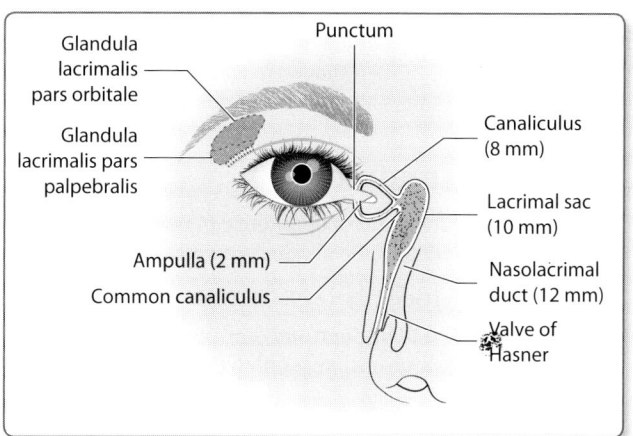

Figure 32.1 Schematic diagram of the nasolacrimal duct system.

interfering with the normal flow of the tear to the punctum, punctum stenosis, canalicular stenosis, common canalicular stenosis, lacrimal sac obstruction, and nasolacrimal duct obstruction. In congenital NLDO, the most common site of obstruction is at the distal end of the nasolacrimal duct due to the failure of perforation of valve of Hasner.

There are inflammatory causes secondary to systemic disease that can cause lacrimal duct obstruction including: Wegener, sarcoidosis, ocular cicatricial pemphigoid, sinus histiocytosis, and scleroderma.

Systemic chemotherapy with docetaxel and 5-fluorouracil is known to cause punctum and canalicular stenosis in a proportion of patients undergoing treatment.

Trauma, including surgery, can cause canalicular or nasolacrimal duct damage and subsequent scarring leading to epiphora.

Clinical features

Watering eyes can be identified clinically on direct examination. There is often a raised tear line or tear running on the cheek. This can cause periocular skin changes with skin excoriation due to chronic irritation by the tear overflow. Further clinical features would identify the cause of the epiphora.

Ocular surface or intraocular inflammation may cause hypersecretion. In dry eyes, corneal fluorescein staining may be present. There is usually a raised tear line regardless of the cause.

Eyelid abnormalities including meibomian gland dysfunction, trichiasis, entropion, and ectropion are easily identifiable on clinical examination. The punctum position and its stenosis can be identified clinically.

In cases of NLDO, there may be an expressible mucocele on direct pressure on the lacrimal sac. In cases of dacryocystitis, beware of the position of the enlarged, inflamed lacrimal sac. If it is above the medial canthus tendon, there should be a suspicion of medial canthus mass not consistent with dacryocystitis and this must be investigated further to exclude neoplasms.

Investigations

Most cases of epiphora do not require any investigations and the cause is often evident by clinical examination. In cases of outflow obstruction, syringing of the tear duct in the clinic would provide adequate information regarding the patency or obstruction of the canaliculi and the nasolacrimal duct. Where there is an expressible mucocele, syringing is not required as expression of mucus from the puncture on direct pressure on the mucocele confirms both the patency of the canaliculus and the obstruction of the nasolacrimal duct.

Dye disappearance test is a useful test carried out during clinical examination using 2% fluorescein to assess if the dye freely drains into the tear drainage system and disappears from the ocular surface. In cases of overflow, it is useful to note if this occurs from the medial or the lateral aspect of the eyelid. In cases of eyelid laxity and lacrimal pump failure, there is some lateral overflow of tear on the cheek.

In select cases of unusual presentation with suspected tumour, history of previous nasal surgery or a CT scan with or without dacryocystogram (DCG) may be indicated. A DCG outlines the nasolacrimal system and demonstrates any obstruction site and irregularity along the pathway but is not commonly required in majority of cases. Lacrimal duct scintigraphy is used to assess cases of functional epiphora.

Diagnosis

Tear overspill on the cheek confirms a diagnosis of epiphora. In milder cases, a raised tear line is present. The cause of epiphora is diagnosed on basis of clinical features and investigations as outlined above.

Treatment

Treatment of epiphora can be divided into medical and surgical, as described here.

Medical treatment

- Lid hygiene and oral antibiotics where appropriate for blepharitis

- Lubricating drops for dry eyes to prevent reflex hypersecretion
- Anti-allergy drops or tablets to treat allergic conjunctivitis
- Oral nonsteroidal anti-inflammatory drugs for treatment of dacryoadenitis
- Steroid drops to treat ocular inflammation
- Botox injection into the lacrimal gland for treatment of gustatory lacrimation

Surgical treatment

- Excision of conjunctivochalasis
- Lid tightening for lower lid laxity
- Lid position correction in entropion and ectropion
- Disinsertion of the anteriorly positioned medial cantonal tendon's anterior limb in Centurion syndrome
- Punctoplasty or insertion of perforated punctum plugs to treat punctum stenosis
- Probing in congenital NLDO
- Dacryocystorhinostomy (DCR) for NLDO
- Lester-Jones tube and DCR for canalicular stenosis

Treatment is targeted to the cause which may be multifactorial such as in blepharitis causing eyelash misdirection and punctum stenosis requiring lid hygiene, electrolysis or epilation of the misdirected lashes and punctoplasty. Similarly several surgical procedures may be required to correct puncture ectropion and puncture stenosis and NLDO.

Complications

Common complications of surgery including bleeding, bruising, infection, and scarring apply here. In punctoplasty there is a risk of restenosis and further scarring. In DCR surgery, the major risk is the nose bleed during and in the early post-operative period. There is a risk of common canalicular scarring post-operatively causing failure. In cases of Lester-Jones tube insertion, there is a risk of tube extrusion. This can be reduced by using tubes that have an intranasal silicone flange which would prevent the tube loss.

Complications of syringing and probing in treatment of congenital NLDO include nose bleed, restenosis of the obstruction, and creating false passage.

Complication of botulinum toxin injection into the lacrimal gland includes temporary ptosis and diplopia.

Further reading

Collin JRO. A Manual of Systematic Eyelid Surgery, 3rd edition, illustrated. Elsevier Health Sciences; 2006.
Nerad JA. Techniques in Ophthalmic Plastic Surgery. Elsevier Health Sciences; 2012.
Olver J. Colour Atlas of Lacrimal Surgery, illustrated edition. Butterworth-Heinemann; 2002.

Related topics of interest

- Ectropion (p. 125)
- Entropion (p. 128)

33 Episcleritis

Key points

- Episcleritis is a benign condition that presents commonly to eye casualty departments
- Care must be taken to differentiate episcleritis from scleritis, its more serious counterpart. This is commonly done with simple instillation of a drop of 2.5% phenylephrine
- Treatment is seldom required but, if needed, consists of a stepwise treatment ladder of ocular lubricants, weak topical steroids, stronger topical steroids, and oral nonsteroidal agents

Epidemiology

The estimated incidence of this condition is approximately 41/100,000 per year with the limited course of the condition being such that the overall prevalence is only slightly higher at 52.6/100,000 per year. It is common to see this condition in eye casualty departments and therefore knowledge of what it is and how to diagnose it is essential mainly to ensure it is either not mistaken for another more serious condition and inappropriately treated, or another more serious condition is mistaken for episcleritis and therefore undertreated. The main differential diagnosis is scleritis.

Pathophysiology

The episclera is a thin layer of connective tissue that is deep to the bulbar conjunctiva but overlies the much denser sclera coat of the eye. Its purpose is to assist the movement of the globe inside the orbit by allowing the conjunctiva a certain degree of travel, which it achieves through being split into two layers which are only loosely associated, therefore, allowing them to pass over each other unimpeded. Inflammation of the episclera is termed episcleritis and is idiopathic in two-thirds of cases. The remaining third are associated with meibomian gland dysfunction, dry eye, allergic eye disease and blepharitis, and rarely systemic conditions such as systemic lupus erythematosus. Local insults to the episclera via chemical injuries, burns or trauma, can also result in episcleritis.

Clinical features

The patient is commonly a young female who is otherwise fit and well. Older patients who present are more likely to have some of the associated conditions mentioned above. There is typically little if any pain, though if present, this is seldom very significant and more of a mild ache. Commonly, the patient has been told by close friends of a patch of redness in the eye and it is this constant mentioning by friends that impels the sufferer to seek help. If the area of injection is flats it is termed 'simple' episcleritis (**Figure 33.1**); and if it is raiseds it is termed 'nodular' (**Figure 33.2**). The nodule itself, if present, is usually only raised by a millimetre or two at most and light from the slit lamp, if shone at it, will classically pass through the nodule rather than stop at the surface due to the very low density of the mass itself. 'Simple' episcleritis is further subdivided into sectoral, in which the injected area is limited to one place, or 'diffuse', in which it involves the entire episclera of the affected eye. It is very unusual

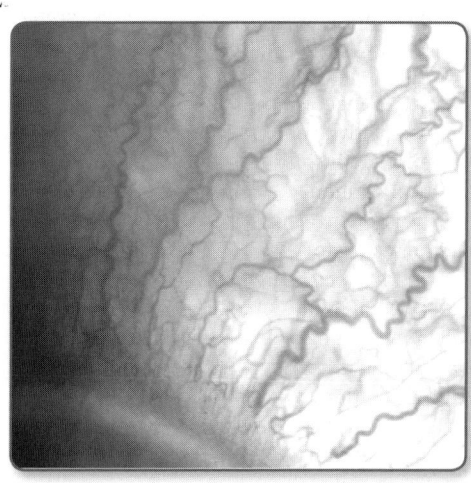

Figure 33.1 Simple episcleritis.

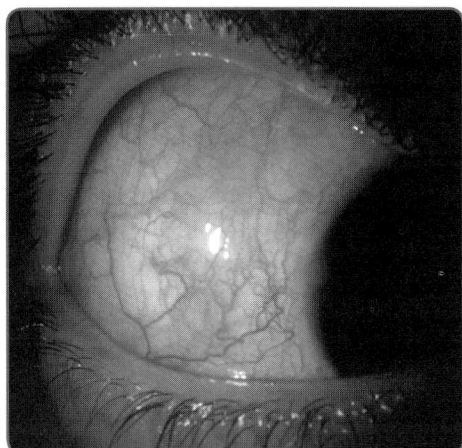

Figure 33.2 Nodular episcleritis.

for both eyes to be affected simultaneously and should this be the case, the diagnosis should be questioned. The redness itself is caused by dilated plexuses of small vessels at the level of the episclera which is deep to the conjunctiva but above the sclera. Sometimes ascertaining the level of the dilated vessels can assist diagnosis although in practice this can be difficult clinically.

Investigations

The first and most important assessment is to eliminate scleritis from the list of differential diagnoses. Scleritis, an inflammation deep to the episclera, can present in a very similar fashion, at least initially, where there is a sectoral patch of redness or a nodule present with the affected layer of blood vessels being only slightly deeper. A simple clinic test for doing exactly this is the vasoconstrictor test. A drop of phenylephrine 2.5% instilled into the conjunctival sac of the affected eye can either cause total resolution of the area of injection by constricting the blood vessels, or it cannot. If it does this is one more piece of evidence for episcleritis as the blood vessels affected in scleritis are too deep and the inflammation too severe for phenylephrine to make any significant difference. This is the most important test than can be performed in clinic and rarely further investigation is needed unless the diagnosis is in doubt.

In rare cases, after the diagnosis of episcleritis has been made, further investigations will need to be undertaken to look for systemic conditions associated with this. As mentioned, these are far less important than with scleritis but should the patient admit to other undiagnosed connective tissue pathology such as skin, joint, cartilage or respiratory symptoms, then prompt referral to a rheumatologist may be the order of the day.

Diagnosis

The diagnosis is almost always arrived at clinically, with the aid of the helpful vasoconstrictor test. A simple history of a red patch in the eye with perhaps a mild ache should prompt examination for other causes of injection and should none be found, a diagnosis of episcleritis can then be made. Beware of bilateral injection and always look for signs of anterior segment disease such as dry eyes, meibomian gland dysfunction, conjunctivitis, thyroid eye disease, and all other conditions that can cause injection. It is also important to ensure that the anterior chambers are quiet, thereby excluding anterior uveitis. Asking about previous surgery is also essential as mistaking problems with prior buckle operations perhaps performed in the distant past for retinal detachment and forgotten by the patient, for nodular episcleritis or nodular scleritis, has indeed been described. As scleritis is the main differential diagnosis it is important to understand the nature of the pain as any symptoms severe enough to wake the patient during sleep or to significantly impact on the comfort of day-to-day activity must be considered scleritis until proven otherwise. Once other conditions have been confidently excluded, episcleritis can then be diagnosed.

Treatment

Most of the time no treatment is needed beyond simple reassurance. Episcleritis is commonly self-resolving and usually disappears of its own accord over a 2 to 4-week period. Usually, the patient can be reassured that the condition is self-limiting. That said, if there is mild pain present or if the course is longer than the usual 4 weeks, then there is a role for treatment.

The first step on the ladder is a simple ocular lubricant of any variety which can be used four times a day for 2–6 weeks. This can be effective at tackling pain though patients can then be made culturally dependent on needing treatment for any flare-ups no matter how mild they may be. Should ocular lubrication not suffice, the next step is a weak topical steroid agent such as fluorometholone (FML) four times a day for a week followed by twice a day for a week. This usually settles things though the risk is that, as with all steroid-based treatments, therapy cessation may result in rebound episcleritis which then induces a vicious cycle of treatment. For this reason, graduation to the next step on the ladder, topical dexamethasone 0.1% should be resisted as much as possible. Beyond this, oral nonsteroidal agents such as flurbiprofen 100 mg three times a day for a few days can be used. As the ladder is ascended, the response to treatment and the need for stepping up should alert the ophthalmologist to the possibility of another condition, classically scleritis, being present. Topical nonsteroidal anti-inflammatory drugs are sometimes used. They have the benefit of being very safe and have a low incidence of side effects but are probably no more efficacious than lubricants.

Complications

Complications can occur through misdiagnosis, classically misdiagnosing anterior non-necrotising scleritis as episcleritis, as well as those that occur from any treatment prescribed. Steroid drops, among other things, can cause intraocular pressure elevation, contribute towards cataract formation and foster dependency. The patient should also be warned about the possibility of flare-ups of the condition in future, which is particularly the case should treatment in the form of topical steroids be used.

Further reading

Akpek EK, Uy H, Christen W, et al. Severity of episcleritis and systemic disease association. Ophthalmology 1999; 106:729–731.

Gwyn Samuel Williams, Mark Westcott. Practical Uveitis: Understanding the Grape. Taylor and Francis; 2017.

Honik G, Wong IG, Gritz DC. Incidence and prevalence of episcleritis and scleritis in Northern California. Cornea 2013; 32:1562.

Related topic of interest

- Scleritis (p. 302)

34 Esotropia

Key points
- Convergent squints often occur at an early age
- There is a high risk of amblyopia
- Refractive errors (hypermetropia) may be associated with childhood esotropia

Epidemiology

Esodeviation is an inward turn and misalignment of the eyes (convergent squint). It is the most common type of strabismus in western populations, with prevalence of 2% in children under 6 years.

Esodeviations are either latent (esophoria) or manifest (esotropia). In esophoria, the ocular misalignment is controlled by fusional mechanisms, and decompensation can occur in certain situations, e.g. fatigue and illness.

Pathophysiology

Common causes of esotropia in children and adults are listed in **Table 34.1**. As with other forms of strabismus, esotropia can be primary (childhood forms) or secondary. Causes of secondary esotropias are sensory, restrictive, or paretic. Accommodative esotropia results from stimulation of the accommodation convergence mechanism to compensate for the uncorrected hypermetropia stimulates convergence. Sensory esotropia is due to reduced vision from media opacity, e.g. congenital cataract, retinal or optic nerve pathology. Restrictive esotropia is due to extraocular muscle or orbital pathology, e.g. thyroid orbitopathy or medial orbital fracture. Lateral rectus weakness from abducens (CN VI) paresis can result in esotropia.

Clinical features

Esotropia in children

Pseudoesotropia (appearance of convergent strabismus when there is no true misalignment on cover testing) must be ruled out. It is usually due to a broad nasal bridge or prominent epicanthal folds, more apparent in lateral gaze.

Newborns and young infants can exhibit small-angle intermittent esotropia until 6 months of age when the child's vision and fixation ability improve. Infantile esotropia is a constant, moderate to large angle alternating esotropia (> 30 Δ) that presents after birth but before 6 months of age. Most children are in good general health and have no significant refractive error, or amblyopia. Due to the early disruption to binocular visual development, infantile esotropia is associated with dissociated vertical deviation, inferior oblique overaction and manifest latent nystagmus.

Accommodative esotropia usually presents after 18 months of age. It is the most common form of strabismus in children, often appearing when the child is tired or ill, and eventually becomes constant. Accommodative esotropia is usually refractive, i.e. associated with hypermetropic refractive error, and responds to spectacles, but can also be non-refractive due to a high accommodative convergence/accommodation (AC/A) ratio. The angle of deviation is usually greater at near. Prolonged accommodative esotropia may lead to amblyopia and loss of binocular vision.

Table 34.1 Common causes of esotropia in children and adults

Children	Adults
Pseudoesotropia	Untreated or residual childhood esotropia
Infantile esotropia	Lateral rectus (cranial nerve VI) palsy
Accommodative esotropia	Thyroid orbitopathy
Sensory esotropia	Decompensating esophoria
Congenital cranial disinnervation disorders (e.g. Duane syndrome)	Myasthenia gravis
	Myopic esotropia
Microtropia	Age-related distance esotropia

An uncommon cause for esotropia in children is congenital cranial disinnervation disorders, the most common of which is Duane syndrome. There is almost complete abduction deficit due to absent/hypoplastic abducens nucleus, minimal esotropia in primary position, and globe retraction on adduction due to co-innervation of the medial and lateral rectus from the oculomotor nucleus.

A *microtropia* is an esotropia less than 10 Δ and is a common finding (1% prevalence). It is usually the result of anisometropia or post-strabismus surgery. There is motor fusion and abnormal retinal correspondence. Microtropia can decompensate into a manifest esotropia.

Rare causes of esotropia in children are convergence spasm (esotropia, pseudomyopia, and miosis), cyclical esotropia, and lateral rectus [cranial nerve VI (CN VI)] palsy. Esotropia can also occur in the presence of nystagmus, as convergence dampens nystagmus resulting in improved vision ("nystagmus blockage syndrome"). Finally, consecutive esotropia may occur following strabismus surgery for exotropia.

Esotropia in adults

A common cause of esotropia in adults is untreated or residual childhood esotropia.

Lateral rectus (CN VI) *palsy* can occur with microvascular insult, raised intracranial pressure or other intracranial pathology. A full cranial nerve and neurological examination is required to exclude other focal neurological signs. The esotropia is larger at distance than near, and abducting saccades are weak. Most cases will require neuroimaging with MRI brain to exclude intracranial space-occupying lesions.

Thyroid eye disease often involves the medial rectus and inferior rectus, resulting in esotropia. Management involves strabismus surgery after controlling active disease, and following orbital decompression if necessary.

Decompensating esophoria occurs when fusional mechanisms cannot control esophoria, particularly in fatigue or ill health. Present with intermittent diplopia and asthenopia symptoms toward the end of the day.

Myasthenia gravis is a neuromuscular junction disorder which can affect all extraocular muscles, resulting in variable and fatiguable strabismus which is usually accompanied by ptosis. Esotropia, exotropia, and vertical strabismus can occur.

High myopia may be associated with instability of the extraocular muscle pulley system, resulting in inferior displacement of the lateral rectus muscles causing esotropia. Similarly, age-related distance esotropia occurs due to involution of these connective tissue pulleys.

Investigations

All patients with esotropia need a full examination at the initial visit including visual acuity, cycloplegic refraction, and dilated fundus examination. The presence or absence of binocular function is helpful in decision-making. Tests for binocular function include red filter test, Bagolini's striated glasses test, worths 4 dot test, after image test and Synaptophore.

Any child presenting with acute-onset constant strabismus requires careful clinical assessment and neuroimaging with MRI to exclude intracranial pathology. In addition, diplopia in children is a red flag for acquired strabismus, as infantile strabismus conditions are not associated with diplopia. Reduced abduction and the presence of nystagmus are also red flags for acquired strabismus.

In adults, neuroimaging is necessary for patients suspected of having CN VI palsy unless there are strong microvascular risk factors and no associated clinical signs. If thyroid eye disease is suspected, serum thyroid function and antibodies as well as orbital imaging are required. Patients with variable strabismus and suspected of having myasthenia gravis should undergo serum antibodies and single-fibre EMG testing.

Diagnosis

The diagnosis of esotropia is based on clinical examination including cover testing and eye movement testing.

Esotropia

Treatment

As with other forms of strabismus, the treatment of esotropias can be:
- Observation
- Spectacles
- Prisms (temporary Fresnel prism or ground-in)
- *Occlusion*: In adults for symptomatic relief of diplopia where prism correction is not possible, i.e. particularly for large angle and incomitant strabismus
- Orthoptic exercises
- *Chemodenervation*: Botulinum toxin injection into overacting muscle or antagonist of paretic muscle
- *Strabismus surgery*: Usually recession of medial rectus, resection or plication of lateral rectus, or transposition of vertical recti

Recommended treatment for childhood strabismus depends on the cause. Refractive error and amblyopia if present need to be managed simultaneously.

- *Infantile esotropia*: Early strabismus surgery, i.e. before 12–18 months of age, with the aim of restoring binocular vision, usually bimedial rectus recession. The aim of surgery is 5–10 Δ esotropia, which can allow some peripheral fusion. Surgery can be augmented with injection of botulinum toxin. Associated inferior oblique overaction can be managed with inferior oblique recession. There is a risk of amblyopia developing postoperatively and children need to be followed up closely to monitor for this. Up to 30% of children develop consecutive exotropia in later life
- *Accommodative esotropia*: Glasses with the full hypermetropic correction are prescribed to remove the accommodative component (**Figure 34.1**). If there is no residual deviation, this is termed fully accommodative esotropia. Atropine

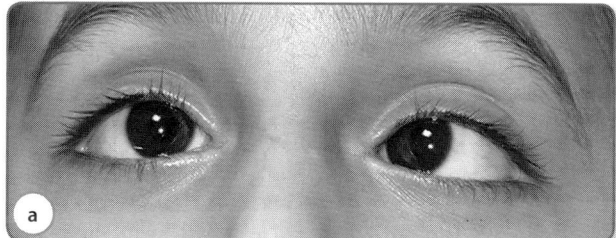
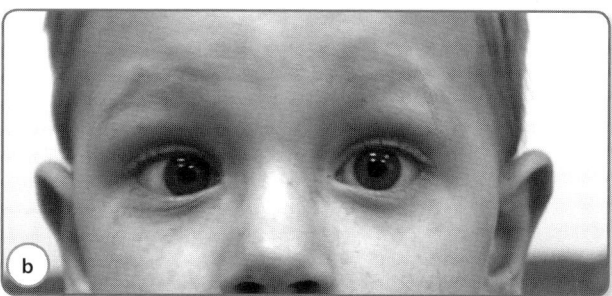
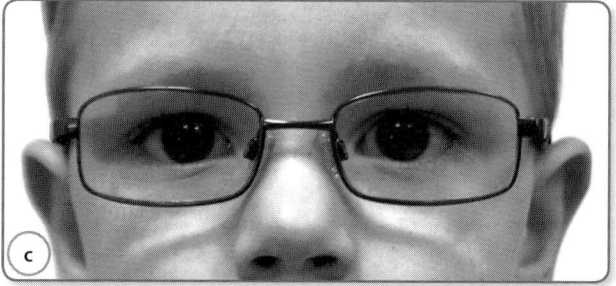

Figure 34.1a to c Left esotropia with amblyopia.

refraction may be necessary to uncover the full amount of latent hypermetropia. A residual esotropia after full hypermetropic correction (part accommodative esotropia) requires strabismus surgery to restore binocular vision, or for cosmesis in older children
- Nonrefractive accommodative esotropia can be managed with executive bifocal glasses or surgery (**Figure 34.2**)
- *Duane syndrome*: Usually observation unless there is a significant head turn to compensate for the esotropia in primary position

Considerations in the management of adult strabismus include:
- Underlying diagnosis
- Presence or absence of binocularity, i.e. if there double vision?
- Cosmesis.

Any underlying cause, e.g. thyroid eye disease, needs to be treated first. Patients with double vision should have therapeutic occlusion or prisms until definitive treatment can be given. Esotropia in adults is generally managed with prisms, botulinum toxin, and strabismus surgery.

Complications

Constant esotropia in childhood can be associated with loss of binocular function and amblyopia. Adults with esotropia may experience troublesome double vision.

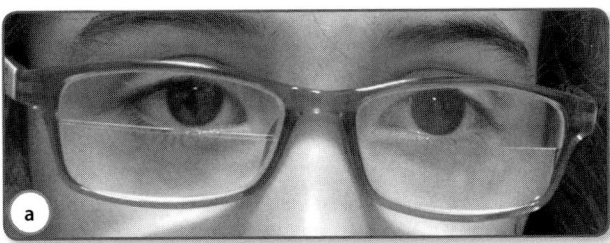
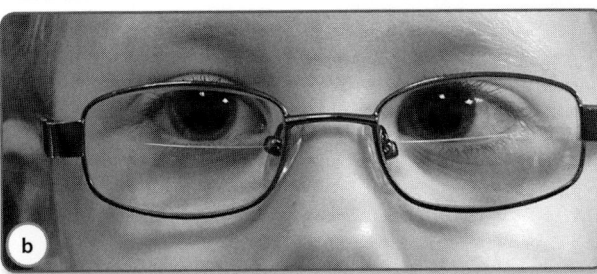
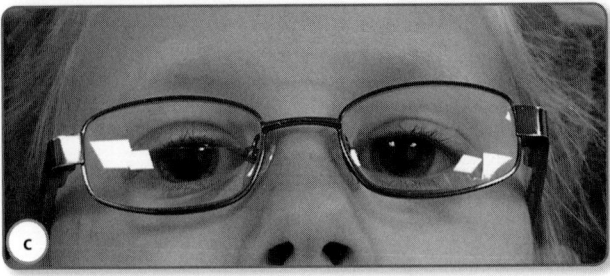

Figure 34.2a to c Patient with executive bifocal glasses.

Further reading

Greenberg AE, Mohney BG, Diehl NN, et al. Incidence and types of childhood esotropia: a population-based study. Ophthalmology 2007; 114:170–174.

Hutcheson KA. Childhood esotropia. Curr Opin Ophthalmol 2004; 15:444–448.

Lambert SR. Accommodative esotropia. Ophthalmol Clin North Am 2001; 14:425–432.

Related topics of interest

- Cranial nerve palsies – abducens nerve palsy (p. 98)
- Cranial nerve palsies – multiple cranial nerves palsies (p. 104)
- Strabismus surgery (p. 312)

35 Exotropia

Key points
- Divergent squints rarely result in amblyopia
- They may be a result of poor vision in one or both eyes

Epidemiology

An exodeviation is an outward turn and misalignment of the visual axes and represents the most common type of strabismus in Asian populations and the second most common strabismus in Western populations. Studies in the USA suggest a prevalence of 1% in children aged < 11 years.

Exodeviations can be latent (exophoria) or manifest (exotropia). In exophoria, the ocular misalignment is controlled by fusional mechanisms, decompensating with fatigue and illness.

Pathophysiology

The common causes of exotropia in children and adults are listed in **Table 35.1**. As with other forms of strabismus, exotropia can be primary (childhood forms) or secondary. Secondary exotropias include sensory, restrictive, and paretic pathologies.

Intermittent exotropia is a large phoria controlled intermittently by fusional convergence, typically breaking down into exotropia intermittently on distance fixation, when the child is unwell or tired. There is hemiretinal suppression, no asthenopia or reported diplopia. Consecutive exotropia can occur months or years following surgery for esotropia. Sensory exotropia is due to reduced vision in one or both eyes from media opacity, retinal or optic nerve pathology. Medial rectus weakness can occur secondary to oculomotor [cranial nerve III (CN III)] palsy, resulting in exotropia.

Clinical features

Pseudoexotropia is uncommon but can occur due to large angle kappa, or dragged macula in cicatrising conditions, e.g. retinopathy of prematurity.

Exotropia in children

Intermittent exotropia
It account for the majority of exodeviations in children and adults. It presents between 18 months and 5 years of age. Parents may report that the child closes one eye in bright sunlight, or exotropia noticed when the child is tired or looking at distance targets. If the angle measures the same for distance and near, it is termed basic intermittent exotropia. If the angle is greater for distance than near, it is termed divergence excess exotropia. It may be true divergence excess (no change with +3D lenses), or simulated divergence excess (the near angle increases to the same as distance when tested wearing +3 D lenses) where accommodative or fusional convergence provides partial control of the exotropia at near. Refractive error and amblyopia are uncommon, and ocular rotations are full. The Mayo Clinic control score (**Box 35.1**) can be used to monitor the control over time.

Consecutive exotropia
It can occur in up to 30% of patients undergoing surgery for childhood esotropia. It can occur any time following surgery and may manifest in adulthood. Diplopia is uncommon due to suppression or abnormal retinal correspondence. There may be restriction of adduction due to medial rectus underaction (**Figure 35.1**).

Table 35.1 Common causes of exotropia in children and adults	
Children	**Adults**
Pseudoexotropia	Untreated or residual childhood exotropia
Intermittent exotropia	Oculomotor (CN III) palsy
Consecutive exotropia	
Congenital exotropia	Convergence insufficiency
	Sensory exotropia
	Decompensating exophoria
	Myasthenia gravis

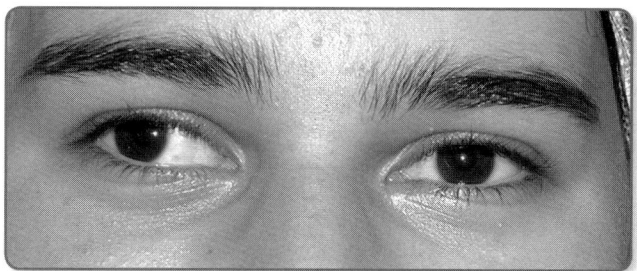

Figure 35.1 Right exotropia (consecutive following childhood esotropia surgery).

Box 35.1 Mayo Clinic control scale for intermittent exotropia

5 = Constant exotropia
4 = Exotropia > 50% of the exam before dissociation
3 = Exotropia < 50% of the exam before dissociation
2 = No exotropia unless dissociated, recovers in > 5 seconds
1 = No exotropia unless dissociated, recovers in 1–5 seconds
0 = No exotropia unless dissociated, recovers in < 1 second (phoria)

Note: Tested for both distance and near to give an overal score out of 10.

Source: From Mohney BG, Holmes JM. An offcie-based Scale for Assessing Control in Intermittent Exotropia. Strabismus 2006; 14:147–150.

Congenital exotropia

It is usually associated with an underlying neurological condition, craniofacial syndrome or congenital CN III palsy.

Exotropia in adults

Common causes of exotropia in adults include untreated or residual childhood exotropia, or consecutive exotropia following childhood esotropia surgery. The angle can be large, with limitation of adduction.

Oculomotor (CN III) palsy

It must be considered in adults presenting with new onset exotropia and diplopia. It is usually accompanied by a hypotropia, ptosis and in some cases, mydriasis. A full CN and neurological examination is required to exclude other focal neurological signs. The exotropia can be of variable angle and is incomitant.

Convergence insufficiency

It is characterised by exotropia mainly for near fixation. It can be precipitated by illness or prolonged near work. The patients report asthenopia or 'eye strain' and diplopia during periods of near work, usually later in the day. Convergence near point and motor fusional amplitudes are poor.

Sensory exotropia

It occurs in older children and adults with unilateral or bilateral poor vision. Depending on the level of vision, diplopia or abnormal retinal correspondence can be present.

Decompensating exophoria

It is a divergent strabismus kept latent by the presence of motor and sensory fusion, but becomes manifest due to deterioration in vision, or with fatigue (e.g. drugs, alcohol, head injury). The patients retain good binocular function, and report diplopia only when the deviation is manifest. Symptoms are more common with increasing age.

Myasthenia gravis

It is a neuromuscular junction disorder that can affect any extraocular muscles, with variable and fatiguable strabismus, often accompanied by ptosis. Esotropia, exotropia, and vertical strabismus can occur.

Investigations

All patients with exotropia need a full examination at the initial visit including visual acuity, cycloplegic refraction, and dilated fundus examination. The presence or absence of binocular function is helpful in decision-making. A synoptophore may be used to check for this if a manifest deviation is present.

Any child presenting with acute onset constant strabismus requires careful clinical assessment and neuroimaging with MRI to exclude intracranial pathology. In addition, diplopia in children is a red flag for acquired strabismus, as infantile strabismus conditions are not associated with diplopia.

Although microvascular CN III palsies can occur, all patients should have urgent CT angiography to exclude life-threatening aneurysm.

Diagnosis

The diagnosis of exotropia is based on clinical examination, including cover testing and ocular rotations (**Figure 35.2**).

Treatment

As with other forms of strabismus, the treatment of exotropias can be:

- Observation
- Spectacles
- Prisms (temporary Fresnel prism or ground-in) (**Figure 35.3**)
- *Occlusion*: In adults for symptomatic relief of diplopia where prism correction is not possible, i.e. particularly for large angle and incomitant strabismus
- Orthoptic exercises
- *Chemodenervation*: Botulinum toxin injection into overacting muscle or antagonist of paretic muscle
- *Strabismus surgery*: Usually recession of lateral rectus, resection of medial rectus, re-advancement of previously recessed medial rectus or transposition of vertical recti

Recommended treatment for childhood strabismus depends on the cause. Refractive error and amblyopia if present need to be managed simultaneously.

The management of intermittent exotropia is challenging. Unlike childhood esotropia, the role of surgery is less defined. In the majority of children with good control, observation is sufficient. Orthoptic exercises that promote fusional convergence, e.g.

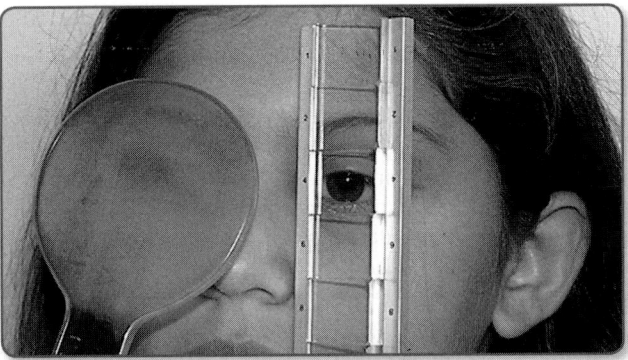

Figure 35.2 A cover test showing patient with exotropia.

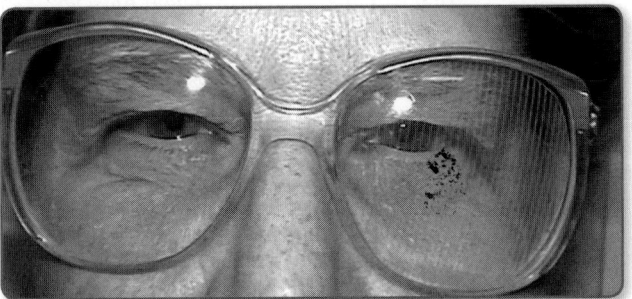

Figure 35.3 Patient with Fresnel prims in their glasses.

pencil push-up, may be helpful. Alternate occlusion and over-minus glasses do not work in the long term. Strabismus surgery may be recommended to preserve binocular function if there is evidence of deteriorating control with reduced stereopsis, especially for distance fixation. There is a risk of overcorrection and inducing amblyopia with surgery, which is therefore often deferred until older age when the indication is purely cosmetic. The surgical target is based on the largest measured angle, i.e. far distance following prolonged occlusion. Bilateral lateral rectus recession and unilateral recess or resect procedure are both used, with similar results.

Considerations in the management of adult strabismus include:
- Underlying diagnosis
- Presence or absence of binocularity, i.e. is there double vision?
- Cosmesis

Any underlying cause of exotropia, e.g. CN III palsy needs to be investigated and treated first. The patients with double vision should have prisms or therapeutic occlusion until definitive treatment can be given.

Surgical correction of consecutive exotropia can be challenging due to altered anatomy from previous surgery, with unpredictable results. The use of adjustable sutures for adults improves outcomes. The risk of diplopia following correction of consecutive exotropia is small, but must be discussed with the patients.

Convergence insufficiency is best treated with orthoptic exercises and surgery is rarely indicated.

Decompensating exophoria can be treated by optimizing visual acuity (e.g. glasses and cataract surgery).

Complications

Constant exotropia in childhood can be associated with loss of binocular function and amblyopia. Adults with exotropia may experience troublesome double vision.

Further reading

Donahue SP. Clinical practice. Pediatric strabismus. N Engl J Med 2007; 356:1040–1047.
Govindan M, Mohney BG, Diehl NN, et al. Incidence and types of childhood exotropia: a population-based study. Ophthalmology 2005; 112:104–108.
Hatt SR, Gnanaraj L. Interventions for intermittent exotropia. Cochrane Database Syst Rev 2013:CD003737.
Joyce KE, Beyer F, Thomson RG, et al. A systematic review of the effectiveness of treatments in altering the natural history of intermittent exotropia. Br J Ophthalmol 2015; 99:440–450.
Rubin SE. Management of strabismus in the first year of life. Pediatr Ann 2001; 30:474–480.

Related topics of interest

- Imaging in ophthalmology (p. 176)
- Cranial nerve palsy – oculomotor (third) nerve palsy (p. 109)
- Strabismus surgery (p. 312)

36 Eyelid trauma

Key points
- Always carry out a full ophthalmic examination including dilated fundus examination and ocular motility to check for damage to other ocular structures
- In any injuries medial to the puncta, one must suspect canalicular injury
- Consider photographic documentation for medicolegal reasons

History

In any case of trauma, it is important to establish the mechanism of injury. This allows one to ascertain the risk of associated injuries, such as the risk of injuries to other ocular structures other than the lid, the potential for a foreign body, risk of infection (for example; cases of human or animal bites/scratches), and possible organisms.

Epidemiology

Eyelid traumas are an important subtype of facial trauma with ocular injury accompanying up to two-thirds of cases.

Pathophysiology

The nature of trauma is that the mechanism and presentation can vary and often with complex combinations. Effective management of eyelid trauma calls for a thorough understanding of the surrounding anatomy including the nasolacrimal system.

Clinical features

Clinical features may include:
- Tissue disruption around the eyelid
- Displacement of the punctum
- Protruding preseptal fat
- Rounding, displacement or abnormal laxity of the medial canthus (indicating medial canthal tendon avulsion)
- Damage to the nasolacrimal system
- Ptosis (indicating damage to the levator aponeurosis)

Examination and investigations

All lid lacerations must be carefully examined and explored to ensure the extent of the injury is known. In particular, one must ensure a visual acuity is assessed and clearly recorded. Any possibility of globe rupture must be excluded. A full dilated ophthalmic examination is recommended to rule out the involvement of other ocular structures. The potential for retained foreign body and the need for imaging [computed tomography (CT) of brain or orbit] must be considered, and guided by the mechanism of injury. The depth of the wound may be determined by using toothed forceps or cotton bud to gently open one edge of the wound. Check for any evidence of bony injury to the orbit by examining for obvious deformity, bony steps and crepitus. In all lid lacerations or avulsions nasal to the puncta, canalicular involvement must be suspected and the nasolacrimal system should be syringed to check for patency. It is also important to consider photographic documentation as the injury and outcome may have medicolegal implications.

Treatment

For all lid traumas, do not forget to ensure the cornea is protected with adequate lubrication and that the patient's tetanus immunisations are up to date. If they are not, then consider the need for tetanus vaccination, or immunoglobulin if indicated. The technique for repair depends on the location and depth of the laceration, alongwith whether there is any tissue loss or not. Post-repair chloramphenicol ointment three times a day to the wound and the eye for 1 week should be applied.

For lacerations that are small, partial thickness (restricted to the anterior lamellar) and not involving the lid margin, consider whether healing by secondary intention (laissez faire) may be most appropriate. If not, then close the defect with 6-0 silk, nylon or polypropylene, with suture removal after 1 week.

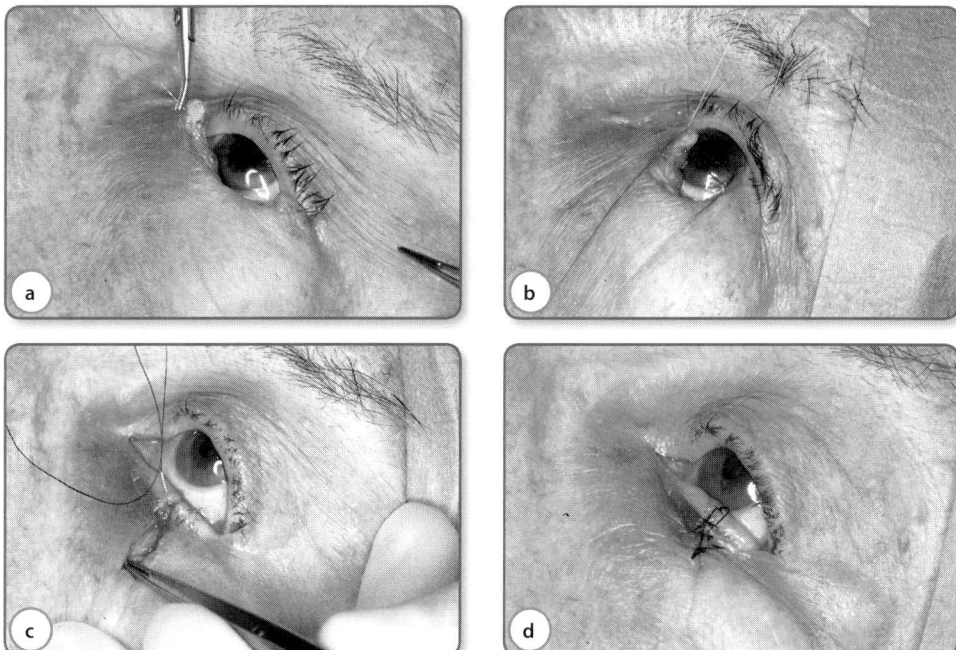

Figures 36.1a to d Photographs showing stages of repair of lower lid. (a) The initial tarsal is placed (6-0 vicryl). Alignment of the tarsal suture is paramount to prevent wound notching/misalignment; (b) Second tarsal suture is placed lower down tarsus (6-0 vicryl). In the lower lid two to three tarsal sutures are usually sufficient, whereas three to four are often required in the upper lid; (c) Grey line suture placed (6-0 silk). Leave suture ends long; (d) Skin closed with interrupted sutures (6-0 silk). Ends are also left long and tied into lowermost suture along with the grey line suture ends to keep the suture ends from touching the cornea.

For full-thickness lacerations, first debride and freshen up the wound edges. They must generally be closed with a layer to tarsus (interrupted 6-0 vicryl sutures to tarsus), then 1 layer to orbicularis (6-0 vicryl) and finally to the skin (interrupted 6-0 silk or nylon). For full-thickness lacerations, one must ensure that the injury is indeed isolated to the lid and not involving the globe or other orbital structures. Primary closure is generally possible in injuries resulting in a small amount of tissue loss from the lid (0–25% tissue loss). For injuries causing tissue loss in excess of 25%, it is recommended that the patient is referred to specialist oculoplastic services as they may require reconstructive procedures to close the defect. Studies have shown that there is no increased complication rate or impact on long-term outcome by waiting up to 48 hours before the repair is performed. In the meantime, ensure the wound is kept moist (ointment and cover with saline-soaked gauze pads).

For lacerations involving the lid margin it is important that the contour of the margin is preserved to prevent notching and margin malposition (**Figures 36.1a to d**).

For lacerations involving the canaliculus, early repair within 48 hours has often been recommended, but recent literature has shown similar outcomes between early (< 48 hours) and late (> 48 hours). The most challenging part of these repairs is often locating the distal (nasal) canalicular end. It is recommend that these cases are performed under a general anaesthesia (GA) and that topical phenylephrine drops are applied to decongest the area, as this can help one visualise the distal canalicular end. If it is still not possible to find the canalicular ends, a viscoelastic can be administered through the other canaliculus to dilate the lacrimal system which help visualisation of the cut canaliculus. Once you have located the canaliculus, a monocanicular stent (e.g. Mini Monika) should be placed and will need to be left in situ for at least 2 weeks.

Further reading

Chu YC, Wu SY, Tsai YJ, et al. Early versus late canalicular laceration repair outcomes. Am J Ophthalmol 2017; 182:155–159.

Tyres AG. Colour Atlas of Ophthalmic Plastic Surgery, 4th edition. Amsterdam, Netherlands: Elsevier; 2017.

Related topics of interest

- Lacrimal surgery (p. 201)
- Trauma – globe rupture (p. 319)

37 Femtosecond laser-assisted phacoemulsification

Key points

- The femtosecond laser uses a neodymium: glass laser with a 1053-nm wavelength of light
- Complication rates are similar between femtosecond laser-assisted phacoemulsification (FLACS) and conventional phacoemulsification surgery
- Current evidence does not show any significant differences in the visual outcomes of FLACS compared to conventional phacoemulsification surgery
- FLACS can produce an accurate and reproducible capsulorrhexis
- FLACS has both logistical and cost implications for the management of theatre

Introduction

Femtosecond laser-assisted cataract surgery (FLACS) uses the predictable accuracy of the femtosecond laser to perform a number of steps of cataract surgery including corneal incisions, capsulorrhexis and lens fragmentation prior to phacoemulsification.

The femtosecond laser

The femtosecond laser is an infrared 1053 nm wavelength neodymium: glass laser. This allows the energy to be focused to a 3-μm spot size, which has high accuracy (within 5 μm) in the anterior segment. Energy is delivered as high frequency ultra-short pulses (10^{-15} seconds) and eliminates collateral damage to surrounding tissues.

Laser tissue interactions result in photo-disruption of tissue through formation of plasma. Plasma is free of electrons and ionised molecules so rapidly expands and results in a cavitation bubble. The force of this expanding bubble results in discrete focal tissue disruption. Accurate spatial arrangement of laser energy delivery allows predictable dissection of tissues on a microscopic level.

Imaging

An important element of FLACS is the necessity for accurate spatial imaging of the cornea, iris, pupil, and lens to allow laser energy to be delivered to the correct structure. Current FLACS systems use either spectral domain optical coherence tomography or ray tracing reconstruction to image anterior segment anatomy and map the treatment with in-built image analysis that detects interfacial relationships. Factors such as the position of the anterior capsule, posterior capsule, lens thickness and tilt are incorporated into treatment planning to avoid complications caused by incorrect laser delivery.

The cornea needs to be clear to allow adequate visualisation of the anterior segment. Scarring, edema or corneal folds decrease the quality of the image of the anterior segment and can result in incomplete laser dissection.

Current FLACS systems either have direct contact (applanating) or avoid direct contact (non-applanating) with the cornea. Non-contact applanation with water immersion decreases the possibility of developing corneal folds which can distort laser energy delivery, resulting in incomplete capsulotomies.

Patient positioning

The patient must be able to lie flat and remain still for a short duration. Local anaesthetic drops are instilled into the eye prior to positioning the applanation cone between the lids. Gentle suction is applied via the cone. Rapid OCT imaging is followed by application of the laser.

Treatment planning

- The diameter of capsulorhexis is determined to precisely overly the lens optic and can be limbus or pupil centred

- The lens can be divided into 2, 4, 6, or 8 segments dependent on surgeon preference
- Fragmentation of the lens allows softening, which can be performed in a grid or cylinder pattern
- There is a predetermined safety zone to protect the posterior capsule. The laser avoids this zone
- Clear corneal entry incisions and relaxing incisions to address corneal astigmatism can be preset
- Any of the above parameters can be excluded. Many surgeons simply perform capsulorrhexis and lens division

Femtosecond laser-assisted phacoemulsification

An intraocular pressure (IOP) increase of 10 mmHg occurs with docking of the applanation cone. Subconjunctival haemorrhages can arise from suction on the conjunctiva. Patients with advanced glaucoma or retinal vascular disease may not be suitable for FLACS.

The surgeon must confirm the treatment plan on the OCT image and ensure that the posterior capsule is correctly identified before authorising laser application (**Figure 37.1**).

The capulorrhexis is performed first, then lens fragmentation and finally corneal incisions. Duration of laser depends on the number of steps and degree of cataract.

If intraoperative suction loss occurs the laser automatically stops and docking is repeated allowing the procedure to be completed (unless there are gas bubbles within the anterior chamber that prevent imaging).

Conventional phacoemulsification then follows. This can occur 1–2 hours later. However, progressive pupillary miosis occurs following femtosecond laser due to prostaglandin release and, hence, uses non-steroidal anti-inflammatory agents as an adjunct to dilating drops has been advocated. Corneal incisions remain closed due to tissue bridges that require blunt separation before entry into the eye.

Difficult cases

Patients with back or neck issues can struggle with positioning required for the FLACS. Unlike conventional laser, the table cannot be adjusted to allow improved positioning of the head. Deep set eyes, large noses and obesity can also prevent effective docking of the applanation cone.

Small pupils

The pupil size needs to be at least 5 mm to allow an adequately sized caspulorrhexis.

Suction loss

The patient must be able to lie still for the duration of the treatment or there can be a suction loss.

Incomplete capsulotomy

An incomplete capsulotomy can occur but this has decreased with improvements in the software designs and accurate imaging.

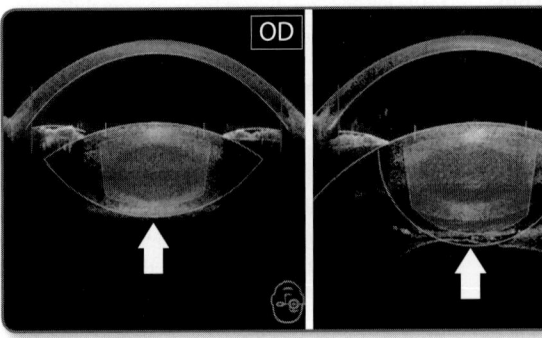

Figure 37.1 Intraoperative optical coherence tomography imaging (OCT) of the anterior segment of the right (OD) and left eye (OS) of the same patient demonstrates the importance of correctly identifying intraocular structures. OD OCT analysis correctly identifies the posterior capsule of the lens (white arrow) allowing safe completion of FLACS. Intrinsic software analysis of the OS OCT image incorrectly identifies the anterior vitreous face as the posterior capsule resulting in an unplanned posterior capsulotomy.
Courtesy: Mr Bruce Allan, Consultant Ophthalmologist, Moorfields Eye Hospital, London.

Patients with steep corneas and keratometry above 47 D or significant lens tilt are at a higher risk of incomplete capsulotomy.

Computer failure

There can be instances of complete system failure. Patients should be made aware that due to this risk there may be a need to revert to conventional phacoemulsification.

FLACS versus conventional phacoemulsification

There is currently no evidence from any studies that FLACS is superior to conventional phacoemulsification.

Capsulotomy

Capsulotomies created with femtosecond laser are more precise in size, position and reproducibility. There is no evidence that this results in better refractive results, lens position or lens tilt compared to manual capsulorrhexis.

Lens fragmentation

The FLACS requires less phacoemulsification energy compared to conventional surgery. This causes less endothelial cell damage during surgery.

Macular oedema

There is no significant difference in the occurrence of macular oedema.

Incisions

Femtosecond laser assisted corneal incisions have been demonstrated to have good stability and reproducibility. There is no evidence that they are better than standard clear corneal incisions.

Visual acuity

As yet there is no statistically significant difference in the outcome between conventional phacoemulsification surgery and femtosecond laser assisted cataract surgery. Both techniques have very good outcomes.

Theatre time

The FLACS is a 2-step procedure and the time required to complete the case is longer then the time required for conventional surgery.

In centres where femtophaco is utilised, modifications to the theatre logistics can be made to increase efficiency. This may include a separate room with a technician performing femto-laser and surgeon completing the case to increase productivity.

Cost

Femtophaco is more costly than conventional phacoemulsification as purchasing costs can be between $400,000 to $500,000. There is ongoing maintenance/servicing cost as well as the costs of disposable interfaces that are needed per case.

Future directions

Lenses that clip onto the capsulorrhexis are available and may aid lens centration and prevent lens tilt. The results of randomised controlled studies of FLACS versus phacoemulsification are keenly anticipated. Adjustment of intraocular lens power and multifocality using the femtosecond laser has been shown to be possible and may provide a new direction for femtosecond lasers in cataract surgery.

Further reading

Abell RG, Darian-Smith JBK, Allen PL, et al. Femtosecond laser-assisted cataract surgery versus standard phacoemulsification cataract surgery: Outcomes and Safety in more than 4000 cases at a single centre. J Cataract Refract Surg 2015; 41:47–52.

Day AC, Gore DM, Bunce C, Evans JR. Laser-assisted cataract surgery versus standard ultrasound phacoemulsification cataract surgery. Cochrane Database Syst Rev 2016; 2016; 7:CD010735.

Dick HB, Scultz T. A review of laser-assisted versus traditional phacoemulsification after cataract surgery. Ophthalmol Ther 2017; 6:7–18.

Donaldson KE, Braga-Mele R, Cabot F, et al. Femtosecond laser-assisted cataract surgery (Review). J Cataract Refract Surg 2013; 39:1753–1763.

Related topics of interest

- Cataract – acquired (p. 43)
- Corneal topography (p. 94)

38 Full-thickness macular holes

Key points

- Full-thickness macular holes (FTMHs) result from centrifugal displacement of the neural retina with separation of the fovea resulting in visual disturbance
- The natural history of most FTMHs is poor for central visual function
- Surgery with pars plana vitrectomy (PPV) results in over 80% successful closure with marked improvement in visual acuity and function

Introduction

Full-thickness macular holes are an anatomic defect in the fovea featuring interruption of all neural retinal layers from the internal limiting membrane (ILM) to the retinal pigment epithelium. They represent a specific end of the spectrum of diseases of the vitreomacular interface.

Epidemiology

Reported FTMH prevalence varies between 0.1% and 0.8% in adults aged > 40 years, while age-adjusted incidence has been reported at 7.8 per 100,000 of the general population per year.

Incidence increases after 65 years of age, with women affected almost three times as much as men. The condition is unilateral in 80% of cases.

Other risk factors include high myopia and ethnicity. South Asian and Afro-Caribbean patients present with larger FTMH than Caucasians. In addition, Afro-Caribbean ethnicity is an independent risk factor for surgical failure.

The risk of FTMH development in the fellow eye without posterior vitreous detachment has been estimated at around 17% at 10 years.

Pathophysiology

Ultrasound and optical coherence tomography (OCT) data have suggested that perifoveal posterior vitreous detachment (PVD) and vitreomacular traction (VMT) are associated with the earliest macular hole stages. Anteroposterior (perifoveal PVD) and dynamic (ocular movements), anterior or oblique vitreous tractional forces have been shown to be the primary cause of idiopathic FTMH formation.

Secondary FTMHs are caused by other pathologic conditions and do not have concurrent VMT. They have been reported in cases of blunt ocular trauma, macular schisis, macular telangiectasia type 2, central retinal vein occlusion, diabetic macular oedema, uveitis, age-related macular degeneration, and after PPV.

Clinical features

Gass defined the different stages of FTMHs based on clinical appearance.
- *Stage 1*: Impending hole (a yellow spot at the fovea)
- *Stage 2*: Full-thickness defect < 400 μm in diameter
- *Stage 3*: Full-thickness defect > 400 μm in diameter
- *Stage 4*: Stage 3 with a complete PVD

Most stage 1 and 2 lesions are asymptomatic. In later stages, metamorphopsia and micropsia precede loss of central vision with a central scotoma.

Clinical examination has classically suggested the Watzke–Allen test for diagnosis of FTMH. A narrow slit beam is projected across the macular hole. The test is considered positive if the patient reports distortion or a gap in the slit. However, the introduction of OCT has made it apparent that the sensitivity of the Watzke–Allen test is only around 60%.

Investigations

Although the Gass classification is still in clinical use, OCT-based data has added significantly to our understanding of FTMHs. The International Vitreomacular Traction Study (IVTS) Group has proposed an OCT-based classification system for the spectrum of diseases of the vitreomacular interface (**Table 38.1**).

An important consideration is the choice of scanning protocol; the lowest line spacing protocol available through the fovea is suggested.

Optical coherence tomography also permits accurate follow-up of patients undergoing surgical or other procedures, or over a period of observation.

Diagnosis

Detection of the full-thickness defect on OCT scans through the fovea is an unequivocal sign of FTMH. OCT can also distinguish between FTMH, macular pseudohole, or lamellar macular hole.

Optical coherence tomography is also used to accurately measure various characteristics of FTMH including base width, minimum linear diameter (MLD) (**Figure 38.1**), height, and a variety of macular hole ratios. These can be useful in predicting the success of surgical or pharmacological treatment, and counselling patients on outcomes. FTMH can be classified as small (MLD < 400 µm) or large (MLD > 400 µm).

More accurate prognosis for vision recovery may be possible by assessing other OCT signs, including structural integrity of the photoreceptors at the site of the inner and outer segments (IS/OS) junction defect and the integrity of the external limiting membrane (**Figure 38.2**).

Treatment

In cases of vitreomacular adhesion (VMA) or vitreomacular traction (VMT), observation for a few months is a valid initial approach, especially if patients are still asymptomatic or mildly symptomatic. Complete and spontaneous resolution of traction is seen in approximately 53% of eyes.

Approximately, 30–50% of stage 1 lesions resolve spontaneously often with resolution of symptoms. Spontaneous closure may also occur in stage 2 or 3 lesions in less than 10% of cases.

Pharmacologic vitreolysis with ocriplasmin has been licensed for treatment of symptomatic VMA/VMT, including when associated with small FTMHs. Ocriplasmin induces liquefaction of the vitreous and vitreoretinal separation. A Cochrane Library Systematic Review concluded however that up to 20% of treated eyes still require additional surgical treatment within 6 months. In the UK, 92%

Table 38.1 The IVTS classification for vitreomacular adhesion, traction and full-thickness macular hole

Clinical Stages	Appearance on SO-OCT
VMA	Vitreous adhesion to central macula without any structural changes
VMT	Vitreous adhesion and traction of the macula without a FTMH Possible cystoid changes, cavitation and elevation of fovea from RPE
Small FTMH	MLD ≤ 250 µm
Medium FTMH	250 < MLD ≤ 400 µm
Large FTMH	MLD > 400 µm Full PVD more likely

IVTS, International Vitreomacular Traction Study; SD-OCT, spectral domain optical coherence tomography; VMA, vitreomacular adhesion; VMT, vitreomacular traction; FTMH, full thickness macular hole; RPE, retinal pigment epithelium; MLO, minimal linear diameter; PVD, posterior vitreous detachment.

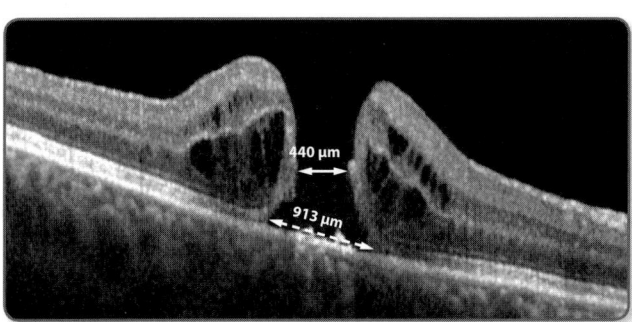

Figure 38.1 Large FTMH characteristics measured with spectral-domain optical coherence tomography (SD-OCT). Dotted line: Maximum base width of FTMH is 913 µm. Thick Line: Minimum linear diameter (MLD) is 440 µm.

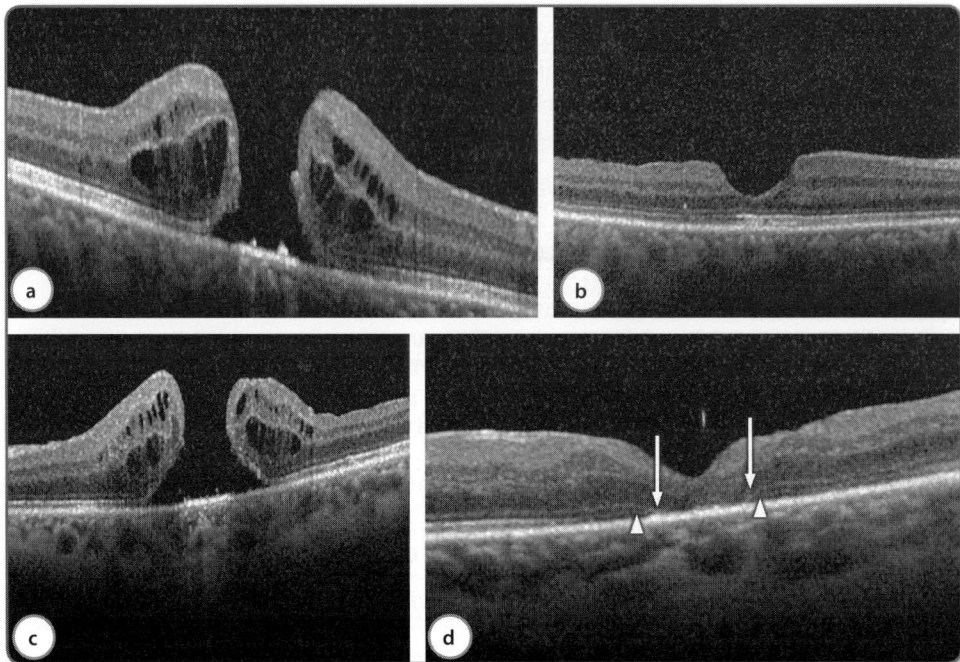

Figures 38.2a to d Two patients with successful anatomic outcomes but different visual prognosis following surgery for FTMH. (a and b) SD-OCT shows large FTMH preoperatively and hole closure with intact outer retinal structure postoperatively; (c and d) SD-OCT shows large FTMH preoperatively and hole closure with disruption of the photoreceptor layer (IS/OS junction) (arrowheads) and external limiting membrane (arrow) postoperatively. Visual prognosis is worse in this patient despite macular hole closure.

of vitreoretinal surgeons do not routinely use ocriplasmin for the treatment of small FTMH.

The standard treatment for FTMH today is PPV with intravitreal gas tamponade. ILM peeling during surgery has also been shown to increase FTMH closure rates. The proposed mechanism of effect is the release of the tangential traction allowing for approximation of the hole edges. Moreover, in light of the hypothesis that FTMHs are closed by glial cell proliferation, it is also thought that ILM peeling induces a relatively consistent degree of trauma to facilitate this gliosis. Additionally, removal of ILM also reduces epiretinal membrane formation.

There is controversy over the role of face-down posturing postoperatively. Minimal or no posturing for small macular holes is acceptable. However, for larger holes, there may be a role. Reported success rates in terms of closure are 85–100%.

Failure to close FTMH after primary surgery reduces the prognosis for successful closure after reoperation or visual improvement. Different techniques have been used to attempt to close persistent FTMH following standard repair, including additional gas injection, ILM re-peeling, use of silicone oils, autologous transplantation of a free ILM flap or detachment of the macula with balanced salt solution. There has been however no data to date suggesting a definitive method as best.

Complications

Randomised control led trials reported vitreous floaters, photopsia, and injection-related eye pain as common complications of ocriplasmin treatment. Blurred vision, visual impairment, and increased or new macular hole were also reported with greater incidence compared with placebo or sham injection.

The UK National Ophthalmology Database Study for FTMH showed that almost 88% of PPV procedures reported no complications. The most common complications were iatrogenic retinal tears and lens touch.

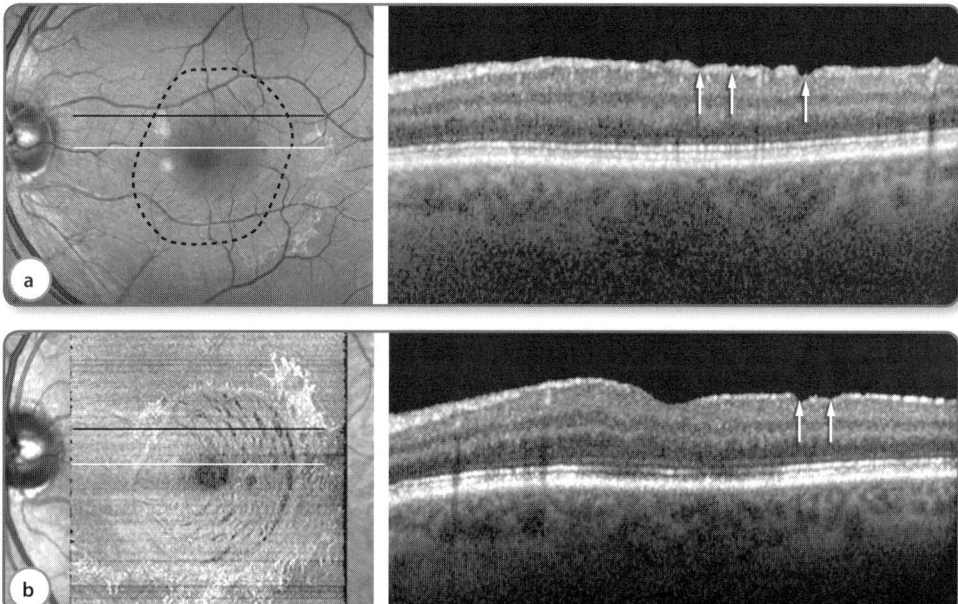

Figures 38.3a and b Dissociated nerve fibre layer (DNFL) appearance following ILM peeling. Infrared (a) and enface (b) imaging with corresponding optical coherence tomography scanning of the characteristic dimples (arrows) along the course of the nerve fibres. The depth of these dimples is limited to the retinal nerve fibre layer thickness.
Courtesy: Professor David Steel, Sunderland Royal Eye Infirmary, UK.

Cataracts are the commonest secondary effect of vitrectomy, especially when gas tamponades are used. Progression of existing cataracts has been reported in 34% of patients at 12 months following the procedure.

The use of indocyanine green for ILM staining is associated with potential toxicity, therefore membrane blue dyes are used in most countries.

Despite its proven efficacy and relative safety, ILM peeling is a traumatic procedure that has acute effects on the underlying retinal nerve fibre layer. ILM peeling often results in temporary swelling of the arcuate nerve fibre layer (SANFL). This may be the earliest manifestation of dissociated optic nerve fibre layer (DONFL) which occurs later in the post-operative period (**Figure 38.3**). However, it is probably a transient feature that does not affect visual recovery.

Infectious endophthalmitis is very rare, occurring in 0.02–0.07% of cases after PPV.

Further reading

Chandra A, Lai M, Mitry D, et al. Ethnic variation in primary idiopathic macular hole surgery. Eye (Lond) 2017; 31:708–712.

Duker JS, Kaiser PK, Binder S, et al. The International Vitreomacular Traction Study Group classification of vitreomacular adhesion, traction, and macular hole. Ophthalmology 2013; 120:2611–2619.

Jackson TL, Donachie PHJ, Sparrow JM, et al. United Kingdom National Ophthalmology Database study of vitreoretinal surgery: report 2, macular hole. Ophthalmology 2013; 120:629–634.

Steel DHW, Lotery AJ. Idiopathic vitreomacular traction and macular hole: a comprehensive review of pathophysiology, diagnosis, and treatment. Eye (Lond) 2013; 27(Suppl 1):S1–21.

Related topics of interest

- Retinal imaging (p. 277)
- Vitreoretinal surgery (p. 350)

39 Giant cell arteritis

Key points

- Giant cell arteritis (GCA) is a chronic vasculitis of large and medium vessels
- Giant cell arteritis is the most common form of vasculitis affecting people over 50 years of age
- Giant cell arteritis is an ophthalmic emergency as when the ophthalmic artery is affected, it can lead to irreversible visual loss
- The most common ocular manifestation of GCA is anterior ischaemic optic neuropathy (AION), though the range of clinical presentation is vast
- Immediate management involves a high dose of glucocorticoid which is tapered according to symptoms and signs

Epidemiology

Giant cell arteritis, previously referred to as temporal arteritis, is the most common form of vasculitis affecting people aged over 50 years. Its incidence peaks between the ages of 70 years and 80 years. GCA predominantly affects Caucasians of Northern European descent. The highest incidence rates have been reported in Norway affecting 32.4/100,000 people > 50 years of age. Women are affected ~2.5 times more than men.

Pathophysiology

The pathoaetiology of GCA remains poorly understood. It is likely that the combination of both genetic and environmental risk factors contributes. The variance in racial susceptibility and the association of *HLA-DRB1*04* in genetic studies support a genetic contribution to GCA. There is overlap between GCA and polymyalgia rheumatica (PMR). Although there are distinct differences, these diseases share genetic risk factors. Environmental factors, including infective aetiologies, have been implicated, but no study has conclusively demonstrated a link between GCA and a pathogen.

The immunopathogenesis of GCA is highly complex. It is presumed to be an autoimmune disease. Advancing age is the strongest risk factor for GCA and likely contributes to the dysfunction of the immune and vascular systems. Ischaemic tissue injury in GCA is the result of a process that likely begins within the walls of susceptible arteries in which local vascular dendritic cells (vasDCs) embedded in the adventitia, act as endogenous immune sentinels, recruit and subsequently activate CD4+ T cells. These then direct the activity of effector macrophages, causing a granulomatous inflammation, luminal compromise and vessel occlusion, resulting in ischaemia. The antigen responsible for this cascade of events remains unknown.

Clinical features

Symptoms

Giant cell arteritis can produce a wide range of ischaemic symptoms including headaches, scalp tenderness and jaw claudication. The most common visual symptoms are amaurosis fugax, visual loss and diplopia. Scalp tenderness and jaw claudication are strongly suggestive of disease. The odds of having a temporal artery biopsy (TAB) positive result have been reported to be 9 times greater when a patient experiences jaw claudication. Jaw claudication is also found more commonly in patients with ocular involvement.

The patients may experience constitutional symptoms including fatigue, general malaise, fever, anorexia, and weight loss. The non-specific nature of these constitutional symptoms often causes delay in diagnosis. Approximately 20% of patients present with only ocular symptoms or signs and experience no constitutional symptoms (occult GCA). The heterogeneity of GCA presentation makes it a challenging diagnosis.

Signs

Although GCA is a systemic disease, the organ most commonly affected is the eye. The range of ocular manifestations is vast. GCA most commonly affects the optic nerve vasculature which results in ischaemic optic neuropathy

(ION), both anterior and rarely posterior (AION and PION). Acute arteritic-AION (A-AION) from GCA classically manifests as a chalky white disc at fundoscopy and represents up to 80% of the ocular findings seen in GCA. Other common presentations, which may occur individually or with other signs, include central retinal artery occlusion, cilio-retinal artery occlusion, cotton wool spots and cranial nerve palsies. Rarer manifestations include choroidal ischaemia, anterior segment ischaemia, and ocular ischaemic syndrome.

Investigations

Commonly performed blood tests to identify an inflammatory state include erythrocyte sedimentation rate (ESR) and C-reactive protein (CRP) but neither are specific and may be elevated in other inflammatory or infective conditions. ESR and CRP values can be normal in patients with GCA. Hence, both markers need to be interpreted within clinical context. Platelet count has shown to be beneficial at predicting a positive TAB.

The gold standard for diagnosis is histological analysis of a TAB. GCA is characterised by mononuclear infiltration of the vascular wall (granulomatous panarteritis), often in the presence of accompanying Langhans giant cells, and fragmentation of the elastic lamina.

The role of colour Doppler ultrasonography (USG), magnetic resonance angiography, computed tomographic angiography and positron emission tomography have all been investigated in diagnosing GCA. USG of the temporal artery (typically revealing dark hypoechoic circumferential wall thickening around the artery lumen, the so-called 'halo sign') may, in some cases, be a good alternative diagnostic technique. Imaging studies are yet to supersede TAB in the diagnosis of GCA, though they may have a role in screening for large vessel involvement.

Diagnosis

The diagnosis of GCA remains largely clinical. In practice, in the acute setting, the clinician relies on clinical features consistent with GCA and the interpretation of the available blood test to determine GCA probability. An acute-phase response characteristic of GCA includes raised ESR and CRP, anaemia, and thrombocytosis. A TAB is performed ideally within a week of presentation. The results of the TAB should not delay clinical diagnosis or treatment initiation in the acute setting. Upon receiving the results, a negative TAB, in the setting of a high-risk patient with clinical features and blood markers suggestive of disease, does not preclude diagnosis as the presence of skip lesions may result in sampling error.

Treatment

The main treatment modality of GCA is glucocorticoids. The management of GCA largely depends on disease stage. The main stages of treatment are: (1) the initiation of therapy in acute disease, (2) maintenance therapy to bring disease to quiescence, and (3) management of relapses.

The British Society of Rheumatology (BSR) guidelines recommend immediate high-dose glucocorticoid therapy when clinical suspicion of GCA is raised. Patients presenting with 'uncomplicated GCA', i.e. patients with no jaw claudication or visual disturbance, should be started on 40–60 mg prednisolone daily. In cases of evolving visual loss or amaurosis fugax, 'complicated GCA', they recommend 500–1,000 mg intravenous methylprednisolone should be administered for 3 days followed by oral glucocorticoids. In those with established visual loss, the main reason for prompt treatment is to protect the contralateral eye and prevent large-vessel complications. However, on occasions, patients have recovered some vision with steroid treatment. Despite successful treatment, GCA relapses in 20–30% of patients. Longitudinal studies have shown that one of the most common causes of disease flare-ups (>50%) is quick tapering of steroid dose or withdrawal of therapy.

Other immunosuppressants tested to date in the treatment of GCA provide limited benefits. Common adjunctive steroid-sparing agent such as azathioprine, methotrexate and anti tumour necrosis factor (TNF) agents may be used although these have not been proven superior to steroids. However, tocilizumab, a humanised monoclonal antibody against the interleukin-6 (IL-6) receptor may have a role, as it improves both induction and maintenance of remission in patients with GCA for up to 12 months and allows for less cumulative steroid exposure.

Complications

Complications can either be disease-related or associated with treatment. Non-ocular complications of GCA include stroke and aortic aneurysm.

Glucocorticoid treatment is effective but side effects can affect up to 90% of those with GCA. Prolonged corticosteroid therapy is associated with weight gain, diabetes, hypertension, peptic ulceration and osteoporosis. As such, patients on long-term steroids, should be prescribed medication to protect their stomach and bones. Prolonged steroid treatment can also affect vision by causing cataracts, glaucoma and macular oedema.

Further reading

De Smit E, O'Sullivan E, Mackey DA, et al. Giant cell arteritis: ophthalmic manifestations of a systemic disease. Graefes Arch Clin Exp Ophthalmol 2016; 254:2291–2306.

Hayreh SS. General characteristics of giant cell arteritis. In: Hayreh SS (Ed). Ischemic Optic Neuropathies. Dordrecht: Springer; 2011. pp. 163–178.

Mackie SL, Dejaco C, Appenzeller S, et al. British Society for Rheumatology guideline on diagnosis and treatment of giant cell arteritis.. Rheumatology (Oxford). 2020. pii: kez672. doi: 10.1093/rheumatology/kez672.

Related topics of interest

- Headache (p. 172)
- Retinal arterial occlusion (p. 267)
- Optic neuropathies (p. 239)

40 Glaucoma – inflammatory

Key points
- Glaucoma is one of the serious complications of uveitis, being more common in chronic than in acute cases and in anterior than in posterior uveitis
- Timing of surgical intervention requires careful consideration as the fluctuating nature of the inflammatory episodes is associated with considerable variation in intraocular pressure (IOP)
- Success rates for surgical intervention in inflammatory glaucoma may be less than those for primary disease

Epidemiology
Approximately 20% of uveitis patients develop glaucoma. However, there is considerable variation depending on the type of uveitis:
- Fuchs heterochromic uveitis – the prevalence of secondary glaucoma has been reported to be between 9% and 59%
- Juvenile idiopathic arthritis – between 14% and 48% of children are reported to develop glaucoma
- Herpes-simplex keratouveitis – a retrospective study of 50 patients reported that all had recurrent herpes simplex virus (HSV) disease prior to presenting with elevated IOP, and none had increased pressure on initial presentation of ocular herpetic disease. In addition, patients who presented with elevated IOP had either stromal keratitis disease (96%) or a metaherpetic ulcer (4%). In a separate study of patients with HSV and varicella zoster virus (VZV) stromal keratitis, the total incidence of ocular hypertension was 47% during the period of active uveitis, and there was a 13% incidence of persistently elevated IOP during the remission period

Pathophysiology
Uveitis associated raised IOP may be in the context of either an open or a closed angle mechanism some of which are outlined below.
- Three main mechanisms of open angle glaucoma are as follows:
  - Inflammatory cells causing mechanical obstruction at the level of the trabecular meshwork
  - Trabeculitis – inflammation of the trabecular meshwork itself
  - Iatrogenic pressure rise due to a steroid response – the exact mechanism is poorly understood but thought to be due to the reduced trabecular meshwork outflow. It is reported that 5% of the population are high steroid responders exhibiting ≥ 15 mmHg rise in IOP above baseline
- Three main mechanisms of angle closure glaucoma are as follows:
  - Formation of peripheral anterior synechiae or neovascularisation eventually leading to synechial angle closure
  - Formation of posterior synechiae eventually leading to 360 adhesions around the pupillary border (seclusio pupillae) blocking flow from the posterior to the anterior chamber
  - Forward rotation of the ciliary body such as is seen in Vogt–Koyanagi–Harada disease

Clinical features
Specific clinical features may point to certain aetiologies are as follows:
- *Behçet's, sarcoidosis, and toxoplasmosis:* Possible iris bombe
- *Fuchs uveitis syndrome:* Hypochromia, nodules on pupillary margin (Koeppe) or iris surface (Busacca), small stellate keratitic precipitates, and microhyphaema with gonioscopy, tonometry or paracentesis (Amsler sign)
- *Herpetic uveitis:* Diffuse or sectoral iris atrophy, stromal keratitis, and dendritic ulcer

- *Posner-Schlossman syndrome:* Recurrent unilateral episodes of raised IOP, typically in the range of 40–60 mmHg in a white eye with minimal flare and occasional cells and/or keratitic precipitates
- *Sarcoidosis:* Lacrimal gland swelling
- *Subluxed or malpositioned IOL:* Iris atrophy and pigment dispersion seen following cataract surgery
- *Vogt–Koyanagi–Harada syndrome:* Systemic signs of poliosis and vitiligo

Investigations and diagnosis

Ultrasound biomicroscopy (UBM) and anterior segment optical coherence tomography (AS-OCT) can both be used to determine angle configuration as an adjunct to gonioscopy. Both investigations are helpful when the angle anatomy is obscured, e.g. by heavy pigmentation. UBM is able to image ciliary body and lens.

Optical coherence tomography of the optic disc and retinal nerve fibre layer (RNFL), Heidelberg retinal tomography (HRT) and optic disc photography may all have a role in monitoring for progressive optic disc damage. However, RNFL measurements must be interpreted with caution as RNFL measurements have been shown to be thicker in active uveitis and changes in measured RNFL thickness may reflect fluctuations in uveitic activity rather than a glaucomatous process.

Treatment

Medical management

Management of uveitic glaucoma involves treating the inflammation as well as lowering pressure. In some scenarios, e.g. Posner-Schlossman syndrome, adequate control of inflammation will also facilitate reduction of IOP. Steroids should be used at a dose that adequately suppresses the inflammation. Whilst some patients may manifest a steroid response, in general, it is preferable to treat the inflammation and then manage any steroid response appropriately. There may be a role for agents such as loteprednol or rimexolone which produce less steroid response than more potent topical steroids such as dexamethasone. Consideration should be given to sharing care with a uveitis specialist with experience in using steroid-sparing agents.

Beta-blockers should be used first line in uveitic glaucoma. Carbonic anhydrase inhibitors can be used as second-line agents but should be avoided in endothelial failure. Prostaglandin analogues should be used with caution, as there are reported cases of these agents causing anterior uveitis, cystoid macula oedema, and reactivation of herpes simplex keratitis. There is evidence of reduced IOP lowering efficacy if prostaglandin analogues are used in conjunction with topical nonsteroidal anti-inflammatory agents. Alpha-2 agonists should similarly be used with caution due to the possibility of inducing or reactivating anterior uveitis. Miotics should generally be avoided as they affect the integrity of the blood-aqueous barrier, can potentiate inflammation and increase the risk of posterior synechiae formation.

Surgical management

The ciliary body may be compromised in uveitic eyes and as such these eyes are at greater risk of hypotony compared to non-uveitic eyes and intraoperative antimetabolites should, therefore, be used with caution.

Trabeculectomy augmented with antimetabolites has been extensively used in inflammatory glaucoma although may be less successful in aphakic eyes or eyes with neovascularisation. In cases with active inflammation, preoperative topical steroids should be used. In eyes with particularly aggressive inflammation, consideration should be given to preoperative course of systemic steroids such as prednisolone. Flap sutures should be tied tight to mitigate against the risk of early hypotony with close follow-up and careful suture manipulation/removal as indicated.

Aqueous shunt surgery also has an important role and may be the procedure of choice in aphakic eyes and in eyes with significant conjunctival scarring, neovascularisation or uveitis associated with juvenile idiopathic arthritis.

Nonpenetrating surgery has been used in inflammatory glaucoma with some success. This may be more appropriate in eyes that do not require a low target IOP. The absence of anterior chamber entry and iris manipulation reduce the risks of hypotony and exacerbation of intraocular inflammation, respectively.

Eyes with pupil block and secondary angle closure should be managed by intensive dilatation to break the posterior synechiae and surgical iridectomy. Intracameral tissue plasminogen activator can be used in eyes where a fibrinous membrane is occluding the pupil.

Complications

Inflammatory glaucoma is a potentially blinding condition. Complications may arise from the inflammatory process, e.g. peripheral anterior synechiae, posterior synechiae, iris bombe, and seclusio pupillae. Glaucomatous optic neuropathy can lead to visual loss; surgical interventions for raised pressure/glaucoma are associated with a higher incidence of postoperative complications including hypotony.

Further reading

Kulkarni A, Barton K. Uveitic glaucoma. In: Shaarwy TM, Sherwood MB, Hitching RA, Crowston JG, (Eds). Glaucoma. Medical Diagnosis and Therapy. London, UK: Elsevier Saunders; 2015. pp. 410–424.

Muñoz-Negrete FJ, Moreno-Montañés J, Hernández-Martínez P, et al. Current Approach in the Diagnosis and Management of Uveitic Glaucoma. Biomed Res Int 2015; 2015:742–792.

Siddique SS, Suelves AM, Baheti U, et al. Glaucoma and uveitis. Surv Ophthalmol 2013; 58:1–10.

Related topics of interest

- Angle closure glaucoma (p. 6)
- Glaucoma – medical management (p. 162)
- Secondary open angle glaucoma (p. 305)

41 Glaucoma – medical management

Key points
- Topical ocular hypotensives remain the mainstay of glaucoma treatment worldwide
- Patient compliance is an important factor in effectiveness of treatment and this may be improved by the use of fixed combination drops
- Established drops work by reduction of aqueous production or improvement in outflow mechanism
- Future research and emerging medical therapies include sustained release preparations/devices as well as neuroprotective agents

Introduction

The only current effective medical treatment for glaucoma is lowering the intraocular pressure (IOP). This is usually achieved topically, although in certain emergency situations, systemic carbonic anhydrase inhibitors or osmotic agents may be used. One of the most common reasons for topical therapeutic failure is patient compliance, reasons for which, amongst many, include forgetfulness, inconvenience and side effects. In recent years, several fixed combination and preservative-free have been introduced in an attempt to facilitate convenience and hence adherence to treatment. Research is currently being carried out on implantable sustained release preparations including periocular rings, punctal plugs, canalicular inserts, intracameral rods, subconjunctival depot/inserts, and scleral anchored implants. Established agents include parasympathomimetics, prostaglandin analogues, selective sympathomimetics (α_1- and α_2- receptor) sympatholytics (β-blockers), carbonic anhydrase inhibitors and hyperosmotic agents. Some of the current investigational chemicals include nitric oxide agents, adenosine receptor agents and RHO-associated protein kinase inhibitors. A point to note when considering side effects to topical therapy is that as well as symptoms associated with the active agents, some patient may have adverse reactions to the preservatives (e.g. benzalkonium chloride, polyquaternium-1, and stabilised oxychloro complex) contained within these drops. A final thought when considering prescribing topical treatment is the patients' manual dexterity which may be limited by conditions such as arthritis, and the use of drop applicator aids may be helpful in such circumstances.

Prostaglandin analogues

- *Pharmacology:* Increase in uveoscleral outflow, 20–40% IOP reduction
- *Peak effect:* 10–14 hours
- *Washout:* 4–6 weeks
- *Contraindications:* May incite inflammation (use in caution in uveitis or secondary glaucoma)
- *Side effects:*
  - Ocular: Hyperaemia, foreign body sensation, hypertrichosis, increased pigmentation of iris and lashes, cystoid macular oedema, and reactivation of herpes keratitis
  - Systemic: Flu-like symptoms, muscle and joint aches, caution advised in pregnancy
- *Drug interactions:* Pilocarpine reduces flow through uveoscleral outflow by contracting ciliary muscles and has an antagonistic effect to prostaglandin use
- *Examples:* Latanoprost (Xalatan), travoprost (Travatan), and bimatoprost (Lumigan) which is a prostanoid, tafluprost, and Monopost (preservative-free latanoprost)

Beta-blockers

- *Pharmacology:* Suppress aqueous production, 20–30% IOP reduction

- *Peak effect:* 2–3 hours
- *Washout:* 1 month
- *Contraindications:* Precipitates bronchospasm and is potentially dangerous in pre-existing airway disease, cardiac conduction defects and acute or decompensated heart failure
- *Side effects:*
  - *Ocular:* Well tolerated and local side effects generally not significant. It may include dry eyes, punctate keratopathy, and cornea anaesthesia
  - *Systemic:* Bradycardia, heart block, bronchospasm, central nervous system (CNS) depression, anxiety, confusion, sexual dysfunction, and fatigue
- *Drug interactions:* May make oral beta-blockers less efficacious, may mask hypoglycaemia in diabetics on hypoglycaemic medication
- *Examples:* Timolol (includes Timoptol and Tiopex-preservative free) and betaxolol (Betoptic)

Carbonic anhydrase inhibitors

- *Pharmacology:* Decrease aqueous production, 15–20% IOP reduction
- *Peak effect:* 2–3 hours
- *Washout:* 48–72 hours
- *Contraindications:* Sulphonamide allergy, severe renal impairment, and premature new-borns (may lead to acidosis)
- *Side effects:*
  - *Ocular (topical preparation):* Induced myopia, keratitis, periocular contact dermatitis, and conjunctivitis
  - *Systemic:* Hypersensitivity (Stevens-Johnson syndrome), blood dyscrasia (agranulocytosis, aplastic anaemia, thrombocytopaenia), paraesthesia, renal stone formation, taste perversion (bitter taste), hypokalaemia. and acidosis
- *Drug interactions:* May increase toxicity with co-administration of ciclosporin, digitalis, lithium, aspirin, diuretics. Reduces the effects of oral hypoglycaemic agents and cholinesterase activity
- *Examples:* Dorzolamide (Trusopt), brinzolamide (Azopt), and acetazolamide (Diamox) – taken orally

Alpha agonists

- *Pharmacology:* Reduction of aqueous production, increased uveoscleral outflow (brimonidine) and reduction of episcleral venous pressure (apraclonidine), 20–30% IOP reduction
- *Peak effect:* 2 hours
- *Washout:* 7–14 days
- *Contraindications:* CNS depression in paediatric population as it may penetrate the blood–brain barrier, caution with hepatic, and renal impairment
- *Side effects:*
  - *Ocular:* Foreign body sensation, eyelid oedema, allergy, follicular conjunctivitis, periocular dermatitis, mild eyelid retraction, and tachyphylaxis
  - *Systemic:* Hypotension, vasovagal, dry mouth and nose, fatigue, and depression
- *Drug interactions:* Synergistic hypotensive effect when used with monoamine oxidase inhibitors and may cause cardiovascular collapse
- *Examples:* Brimonidine tartrate (Alphagan) and apraclonidine

Parasympathomimetics

- *Pharmacology:* Contract ciliary muscle to increase outflow of aqueous, 15–25% IOP reduction
- *Peak effect:* 1.5–2 hours
- *Washout:* 48 hours
- *Contraindications:* Breakdown of blood–aqueous barrier and should be avoid in uveitic or neovascular glaucoma. Ciliary muscle contraction reduces anterior chamber depth by causing axial thickening of the lens and is contraindicated in angle closure, phacomorphic glaucoma, and malignant glaucoma
- *Side effects:*
  - *Ocular:* Miosis, accommodative spasm, brow ache, myopic shift, retinal tears or detachments, angle closure, endothelial toxicity, conjunctival hyperaemia, cataractogenesis, dimming of vision, and constriction of visual fields
  - *Systemic:* Salivation, bronchial mucus secretion, sweating, bradycardia,

hypotension, bronchospasm, abdominal cramps, vomiting, nausea, and diarrhoea
- *Drug interactions:* Antagonises effects of prostaglandin analogues
- *Examples:* Pilocarpine (includes Pilopine), carbachol, and echothiophate iodide

Hyperosmotic agents

- *Pharmacology:* Increases plasma osmotic pressure leading to absorption of fluid from vitreous and reduces vitreous volume
- Usually reserved for short-term acute situations due to potentially serious side effects
- *Side effects:*
  - Mainly systemic: Severe headache, back pain, diuresis, pulmonary oedema, heart failure, circulatory overload, seizure, and cerebral haemorrhage
- *Examples:* Glycerine (oral or intravenous), isosorbide (oral), and mannitol (intravenous)

Table 41.1 Glaucoma eye drop combination preparations

Combination preparations	Components
Cosopt	Timolol + dorzolamide
Xalacom	Timolol + latanoprost
DuoTrav	Timolol + travoprost
Ganfort	Timolol + bimatoprost
Taptiqom	Timolol + tafluprost
Combigan	Timolol + brimonidine
Azarga	Timolol + brinzolamide
Simbrinza	Brinzolamide + brimonidine

Combination therapy

Treatment regiments can be redesigned to avoid multiple medications and doses (**Table 41.1**). Advantages include allowing fewer doses, reducing exposure to preservatives and possible improvement in patient adherence.

Further reading

Adams CM, Stacy R, Rangaswamy N, Bigelow C, Grosskreutz CL, Prasanna G. Allingham RR, Damji KF, Freedman S, et al. Management of Glaucoma. In: Shields Textbook of Gluacoma, 6th ed. Philidelphia: Lippincott Williams and Wilkins 2011:389–433.
Cheema A, Chang R, Shrivastava A, et al. Update on the Medical Treatment of Primary Open-Angle Glaucoma. Asia Pac J Ophthalmol 2016; 5:51–58.

Glaucoma–Next Generation Therapeutics: Impossible to Possible. Pharm Res 2018; 36:25.
Steven DW, Alaghband P, Lim KS. Preservatives in glaucoma medication. Br J Ophthalmol 2018; 102:1497–1503.

Related topics of interest

- Angle closure glaucoma (p. 6)
- Glaucoma – primary open angle (p. 165)
- Normal tension glaucoma (p. 219)
- Ocular hypertension (p. 226)
- Secondary open angle glaucoma (p. 305)

42 Glaucoma – primary open angle

Key points
- Primary open angle glaucoma (POAG) is a blinding disease with significant morbidity, associated healthcare costs, and is increasing in prevalence
- POAG is an optic neuropathy typically demonstrating optic disc cupping and a characteristic pattern of visual field loss (**Figure 42.1**)
- There are several key landmark studies that have demonstrated the benefit of lowering intraocular pressure and this is the goal of surgical and medical treatment
- There are multiple imaging modalities that can be employed for assessing optic disc and angle features

Epidemiology

Primary open angle glaucoma (POAG) is increasing in prevalence and incidence worldwide as is primary angle closure glaucoma. This is thought to be predominantly due to demographic changes. Open angle and closed angle disease have regional differences in prevalence that are well established with higher rates of closure found in Asian populations and open angle disease in Caucasian and African populations in general. In 2013, the number of people (aged 40–80 years) with glaucoma worldwide was estimated to be 64.3 million and is projected to increase to 111.8 million in 2040. The incidence of POAG is reported to be

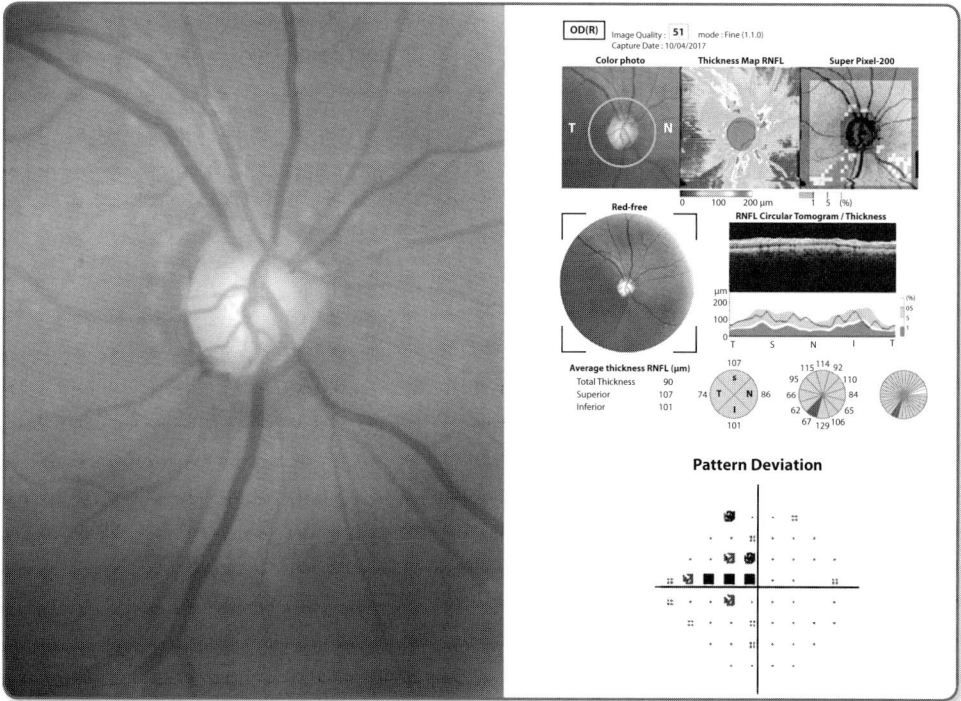

Figure 42.1 Typical findings in primary open angle glaucoma (POAG), showing optic disc photo (note the inferotemporal disc haemorrhage and neuroretinal rim thinning with an associated nerve fibre layer defect), optic disc optical coherence tomography (OCT) and corresponding visual field defect. (*For colour version see plate 1*)

greater in men, those of African ancestry and people living in urban areas.

Risk factors for the development and progression of glaucoma include age (the prevalence of glaucoma increases significantly with age). Race has also been found to contribute with increased incidence and morbidity in African populations. Elevated IOP is a significant risk factor and central corneal thickness was shown in Ocular Hypertension Treatment Study (OHTS) to be a significant risk in conversion from OHT to glaucoma (see Ocular Hypertension Chapter). In patients with a family history of glaucoma, there is an increased prevalence of glaucoma. Several studies have identified multiple potential genetic markers and genes that are associated with higher rates of glaucoma, but definitive causative relationship is yet to be demonstrated and there are no screening tests. Myocilin mutation on TIGR gene is one such potential example and ever expanding list includes CDKN2B-AS1, CAV1 and CAV2, TMCO1, ABCA1, AFAP1, GAS7, TXNRD2, ATXN2, the chromosome 8q22 intergenic region, and SIX1 and SIX6. Central corneal thickness (CCT) is an independent risk factor for the conversion of OHT to POAG and influences Goldmann tonometry readings. The Goldmann tonometer is calibrated for a CCT of 555 μm and thinner corneas will read artificially lower.

Pathophysiology

Glaucoma is a term referring to a family of conditions with characteristic visual field losses and associated optic disc damage. POAG has been defined by the International Society of Geographical and Epidemiologic Ophthalmology (ISGEO) as presence of typical visual field defect and characteristic optic disc changes. Elevated eye pressure is not required for a diagnosis of POAG but when the eye pressure is less than 21 mmHg, it is termed as normal tension glaucoma (NTG).

No single cause of POAG has been identified but there are several postulated pathophysiological mechanisms. Intraocular pressure is controlled by the production of aqueous from the ciliary body and the outflow of aqueous from the trabecular meshwork and uveoscleral route, and a disruption to this flow (without an obvious primary cause – see secondary open angle glaucoma chapter) is thought be the underlying cause. Increased pressure may interact with the biomechanical stresses experienced by the optic nerve, specifically at the level of the lamina cribrosa. In POAG and NTG, the nerve may also be comprised by vascular issues and cerebrospinal fluid pressure may also play a role leading to further susceptibility to damage from raised intraocular pressure.

Clinical features

A good history to identify risk factors for glaucoma and exclude other optic neuropathies is essential in diagnosing and assessing the potential risk of developing a primary or secondary glaucoma. It is also important to assess for possible side effects to any potential treatment thus asking about asthma or cardiac history is important. POAG is typically asymptomatic until moderate to advanced disease unless central fixation has been affected early. If the central field is affected, patients will often describe blurring and report difficulties in adjusting from light to dark.

Clinical assessment and subsequent reviews are informed in the UK by the National Institute for Health and Care Excellence (NICE) guidelines; the assessment of the patient involves:

- *Intraocular pressure (see OHT chapter):* Greater than 24 mmHg has been suggested as the level for referral but not based on eye pressure alone. NTG is not a rare condition, so the absence of a high pressure should not rule out pathology
- Biomicroscopy and/or ophthalmoscopy – to identify any structural abnormality or evidence of a secondary glaucoma. Disc cupping can be localised or widespread and occasionally is preceded by a flame haemorrhage at the optic disc. Additionally, the nerve fibre layer can be assessed to identify any clinically evident nerve fibre retinal layer thinning. Larger, myopic eyes tend to have larger nerves and

Glaucoma – primary open angle

larger cup disc diameters, there are also racial variations
- Corneal thickness is an independent risk factor and pachymetry is an ultrasound-based measure of corneal thickness
- Gonioscopy of the disc angle to identify any evidence of angle closure, angle recession, or neovascularisation
- A simple colour vision assessment (e.g. using Ishihara test plates) to exclude potential non-glaucomatous (although can be affected in advanced glaucoma) optic nerve disease
- Imaging of the disc and retinal nerve fibre layers can help to identify disc damage and if this correlates with a visual field deficit, a greater significance may be attributed to it

Investigations

Investigations for POAG centre around two specific goals: the diagnosis of glaucoma and the determination of progression of glaucoma. Progression describes a worsening of the patient's glaucomatous disease but it is important to be aware that such terminology can cause patient's consternation as progression has a positive implication. In POAG, multiple imaging techniques have been utilised to assess the optic nerve structure. OCT is the most commonly used aside from disc photography. It possibly has greater flexibility being able to assess angle and macular abnormalities. However, the fast developments in glaucoma imaging have left issues with legacy data; disc photography for ongoing monitoring does not have this problem.

Gonioscopy is an essential part of the assessment. Visualisation of angle structures is important to exclude secondary glaucoma and angle closure as well as to evaluate potential treatment options such as SLT laser.

Visual field assessment – commonly by static perimetry from, e.g. Humphrey's Visual Field machine or in those unable to perform well. Goldmann visual fields (dynamic visual field testing) can be performed.

Diagnosis

The diagnosis of POAG can be complicated by unreliable visual fields or simultaneous alternative pathology such as macular degeneration or significant myopia. Structural changes do not always predate functional changes but around 30% nerve fibre loss is required to produce a defect in standard automated perimetry. If the structural and functional losses occur in correlating locations then greater significance is given to this evidence.

The assessment of a patient with suspected glaucoma must begin with a good history as with other conditions. It is important to clinically exclude secondary causes of glaucoma as indicated by the history and clinical assessment. There are several additional areas that must be addressed in the history such as their prior eye pressures, family history, systemic medications, systemic enquiries, and social history such as driving status.

Treatment

All treatment goals currently revolve around the reduction of IOP. This is based on evidence from Early Manifest Glaucoma Trial (EMGT) and others demonstrating a clear benefit to lowering eye pressure in preventing development of and reducing the risk from the progression of glaucoma.

The options for intervention are: medications, laser, and surgery. Medications involve five major categories of drugs (see Glaucoma-medical management chapter): prostaglandin analogues such as Latanoprost that increases uveoscleral outflow, beta-blockers such as Timolol that reduces aqueous production, carbonic anhydrase inhibitors such as acetazolamide and brinzolamide, and α_2- antagonists such as apraclonidine. Occasionally, osmotic agents may be used such as mannitol or miotic agents such as pilocarpine.

Laser treatment

Laser can be applied to the trabecular meshwork by argon laser (much less frequently used now) or selective transmission laser (SLT) in POAG, both procedures can result in inflammation and significant pressure spikes, thus follow-up is important especially in more pigmented angles. Endoscopic cyclophotocoagulation is direct visualisation and destruction of the ciliary processes and can be effective in IOP control. Cyclodiode photodestruction to the ciliary body laser is externally applied laser also targeting the ciliary body to reduce aqueous formation.

Surgery (trabeculectomy, aqueous shunts, MIGS, etc.)

Surgical options include trabeculectomy, deep sclerectomy, and aqueous shunt procedures that work on creating alternative aqueous drainage pathways. There are also 'minimally invasive' devices, termed as MIGS, that can be used (see Chapter 53). These typically involve bypassing traditional outflow mechanisms and consist of small shunts or spacing devices, e.g. iStent and Hydrus implants.

Complications

Primary open angle glaucoma is a potentially blinding lifelong disease that cannot be cured and once present, the damage to the optic nerve cannot be remedied.

Further reading

GOV.UK. driving requirements for glaucoma. [online] Available from https://www.gov.uk/glaucoma-and-driving. [Last accessed October, 2019].

National Institute for Health and Care Excellence. (2017). Glaucoma: diagnosis and management. [online] Available from https://www.nice.org.uk/guidance/ng81. [Last accessed October, 2019].

Tseng VL, Coleman AL, Chang MY, et al. Aqueous shunts for glaucoma. Cochrane Database Syst Rev 2017; 7:CD004918.

Related topics of interest

- Glaucoma – medical management (p. 162)
- Minimally invasive glaucoma surgery (p. 208)
- Optic disc imaging (p. 232)
- Perimetry (p. 248)

43 Glaucoma in children

Key points
- Glaucoma is an uncommon but important cause of vision impairment in children
- Primary congenital glaucoma (PCG) is the most common glaucoma in infancy
- The mainstay of treatment is surgery

Introduction

Glaucoma is a rare but important cause of childhood vision impairment. PCG is the most frequent cause of childhood glaucoma, occurring in approximately 1 in 20,000 live births in the UK. The most common cause of secondary glaucoma in children is following congenital cataract surgery. Controlling intraocular pressure (IOP) is achieved in the majority of children by surgical intervention but managing associated ocular abnormalities, such as successful management of ametropia and amblyopia is vital to achieve an optimal visual outcome.

Classification

Childhood glaucoma is classified into primary and secondary causes:
- *Primary childhood glaucoma:*
    - Primary congenital glaucoma
    - Juvenile open-angle glaucoma (JOAG)
- *Secondary childhood glaucoma:*
    - Glaucoma associated with non-acquired ocular anomalies (anterior segment dysgenesis, aniridia)
    - Glaucoma associated with non-acquired systemic disease or syndrome (Down syndrome, Sturge–Weber syndrome)
    - Glaucoma associated with acquired condition (uveitis, trauma related and steroid induced)
    - Glaucoma following cataract surgery (aphakia and pseudo-phakia)

Pathophysiology

The underlying pathophysiology of childhood glaucoma is highly variable, particularly for secondary causes of the disease. The elevated IOP in PCG is due to outflow resistance. Dysgenesis of the angle structures (trabeculodysgenesis) leads to a disruption of aqueous drainage. Angle surgery (goniotomy or trabeculotomy) aims to restore the physiological outflow pathway, which allows control of the IOP. The pathophysiology of the most common secondary glaucoma, which occurs after cataract surgery, is ill-defined but may have multiple factors, including dysgenesis of the anterior segment structures, trauma to the developing eye during cataract surgery and the prolonged effects of steroids or low-grade inflammation post-operatively. Other pathological causes of glaucoma in children include raised episcleral venous pressure, which may be involved in Sturge–Weber syndrome.

Clinical features

Childhood glaucoma is always a pressure-dependent disease and the clinical features relate to the elevated IOP in the developing eye. The classical triad of symptoms in PCG is photophobia, epiphora, and blepharospasm. Other presenting features include buphthalmos (enlarged cornea) and a cloudy cornea. Signs that can develop later include squint, nystagmus, reduced vision, and increasing myopia (caused by an increase in globe size).

Buphthalmos and corneal changes are unique to childhood glaucoma and are a sign that the elevation in IOP occurred under the age of 3 years. Elevated IOP beyond this age does not usually result in these signs, which can make the diagnosis more challenging. As the IOP rises, splits occur in Descemet's membrane (Haab's striae), which can be orientated in any direction. As the endothelium splits, aqueous inflow into the cornea can cause sudden cloudiness.

Diagnosis

A high index of suspicion, urgent onwards referral, and an adequate clinical examination are essential for the diagnosis of childhood glaucoma. It is also important to document the age at clinical onset of the disease (which can determine prognosis), associated systemic problems (although PCG is usually an isolated finding), a family history of glaucoma, and consanguinity.

Examination is often very challenging due to the photophobia in infants and an examination under anaesthetic (preferably with intravenous ketamine, which does not lower IOP) is often required. The confirmation of glaucoma in children is a clinical decision, based on the presenting symptoms and the constellation of signs on clinical examination.

The gold standard for IOP measurement is Perkins tonometry, under ketamine anaesthesia. Other important clinical findings are as follows:

- *Cornea:* Note oedema and opacity, signs of anterior segment dysgenesis and horizontal corneal diameter (> 11 mm in a newborn, > 12 mm in infants and > 13 mm at any age is suspicious, as is any asymmetry), and Haab's striae
- *Gonioscopy:* Note the typical angle appearance in PCG (a flat, high iris insertion, with 'scalloped' insertion, along with iris hypoplasia and prominent iris blood vessels). Also, look for signs of anterior segment dysgenesis [posterior embryotoxon with iris adhesions (Axenfeld anomaly), corectopia, and full-thickness iris holes]
- *Optic disc assessment:* Look for any optic disc asymmetry, or enlarging cup-to-disc ratio (CDR). Optic disc cupping can be reversible in children when there has been an adequate reduction in IOP
- *Refraction:* Progressive myopia or reducing hypermetropia in aphakes can be an indirect sign of uncontrolled IOP. Ultrasonography is an essential tool to assess changes in axial length, particularly in younger children and also in looking for co-existent disease
- *Systemic evaluation:* The examination under anaesthesia (EUA) can be used for a systemic examination and provide a useful time to obtain blood samples for genetic studies

Treatment

Childhood glaucoma is usually said to be a 'surgical disease', in that almost all cases of PCG require surgery, along with the majority of cases of secondary glaucomas. However, in secondary glaucoma, medical treatment is usually instigated as first-line treatment and surgery is reserved for progressive glaucoma, when medical therapy is sub-optimal or not tolerated by the child. In all cases of childhood glaucoma, it is important not to persist with sub-optimal control of medical therapy. Equally, also be aware that children are at a higher risk of adverse effects of drugs and poor tolerance. Due to the expected long-term use of topical agents, it is also preferable to use non-preserved drops, which are better tolerated in children and have a less toxic effect on the ocular surface, which may be important in any future glaucoma surgery. Beta-blockers and prostaglandin analogues are frequently used in both primary and secondary glaucomas but α_2- agonists (brimonidine) should be avoided in children below the age of 6 years, due to their serious and sometimes life-threatening side effects, such as respiratory depression, cardiovascular abnormalities, and lethargy.

Glaucoma surgery in children is more complex, technically difficult and has a higher rate of complications than in adults, so it should be performed in tertiary centres, with an adequate surgical volume. Repeat surgery is often required and, therefore, needs continuity of care by familiar surgeons, to instil both rapport with the child and confidence from the family.

Surgical options

- *Angle surgery (goniotomy or trabeculotomy):* First line in PCG but can be successful in JOAG, Sturge–Weber syndrome, and aphakic glaucoma. Circumferential (360º trabeculotomy) increasingly performed with good results, by opening all drainage channels
- *Filtering surgery (trabeculectomy or glaucoma drainage devices):* Following failed angle surgery or first line in secondary glaucomas
- *Cyclodestruction:* It can be used for poorly sighted eyes, high-risk eyes or first line

in aphakic glaucoma. Cyclodiode laser treatment can be repeated but often limited to a maximum of two treatments, due to the risks of hypotony and phthisis with repeated treatments

Complications

The choice of filtering surgery after failed angle surgery is debatable and good outcomes have been reported for both trabeculectomy (augmented with mitomycin-C) and glaucoma drainage devices (particularly Baerveldt tube implants). Trabeculectomy surgery requires much greater post-operative surveillance and intervention and involves frequent EUAs and control of post-operative scarring, which can be challenging, even with high-dose mitomycin-C. Tube surgery requires much less post-operative intervention but has an increased risk of tube exposure and endophthalmitis, along with corneal complications, such as decompensation but can have excellent long-term control of IOP, with less risk of conjunctival thinning, bleb avascularity and achieves good, diffuse posterior drainage of aqueous humour. Surgeon preference is important in deciding which technique is the most appropriate in each individual case.

Further reading

Hoyt C, Taylor D. Pediatric Ophthalmology and Strabismus, 4th edition. New York: Elsevier Saunders 2012:353–367.

Papadopoulos M, Cable N, Rahi J, et al. The British Infantile and Childhood Glaucoma (BIG) Eye Study. Invest Ophthalmol Vis Sci 2007; 48:4100–4106.

Weinreb RN, Grajewski A, Papadopoulos M, et al. Childhood Glaucoma. Netherlands: Kugler Publications; 2013.

Related topics of interest

- Glaucoma – inflammatory (p. 159)
- Glaucoma – medical management (p. 162)
- Secondary open angle glaucoma (p. 305)

44 Headache

Key points

- Migraine is severe, common, has a myriad of presentations and a major societal impact
- Although rare, cluster headache is so severe that it should be treated as an emergency
- Thunderclap and high-pressure headache are important to identify as they may have very serious underlying causes
- Some meningitides can mimic migraine
- Giant-cell arteritis must always be considered in new-onset headaches in the elderly

Epidemiology

There are many types of headache. **Table 44.1** provides a list of those that are common, severe, or cause clinical concern. Tension-type headache is very common in the general population (prevalence 86%) but mild and rarely presents to secondary care services. Migraine has a prevalence of around 12% in the general population, with a female preponderance, and is significantly over-represented in patients referred to specialist services.

Cluster headache has a general population prevalence of <1% and a male preponderance. Rarer still is giant-cell arteritis which nevertheless represents the most common systemic vasculitis and needs to be considered in the differential for new-onset headache in the elderly; it virtually never occurs in individuals younger than 50 years and peaks in incidence in the 70s. The epidemiology of other secondary headaches follows that of their underlying aetiologies.

Table 44.1 Classification of headaches

Primary headaches	Migraine
	Tension-type headache
	Cluster headache
	Primary headache associated with sexual activity
	Primary thunderclap headache
	Primary stabbing headache
	New daily persistent headache
Secondary headaches	Thunderclap headache
	Giant-cell arteritis
	Cervical artery dissection
	High-pressure headache
	Low-pressure headache
	Medication overuse headache
	Meningitis associated headache
	Cervicogenic headache
	Sinus-related headache
Painful cranial neuropathies and other facial pains	Trigeminal neuralgia
	Occipital neuralgia
	Painful ocular nerve palsy
	Optic neuritis

Pathophysiology

Cortical spreading depression is important in migraine. This wave of cellular depolarisation spreading across the cortex often lasting 10–30 minutes gives rise to the aura of migraine, activation of trigeminal nerve afferents and alteration in blood–brain barrier permeability. These cause inflammatory changes in the pain-sensitive meninges. Much interest is currently focussed on the role of calcitonin gene-related peptide (CGRP), found in the trigeminal ganglion, which is thought to serve as a relay between peripheral and central pain mechanisms in migraine. Genetic factors are important in migraine. Many patients have a family history and exhibit 'migraine biology' with a tendency to suffer from attacks from a young age triggered by such factors as alcohol and menstruation, a propensity towards travel-sickness, and childhood cyclical vomiting and abdominal pain.

The pathophysiology of cluster headache is poorly understood but may have to do with hypothalamic activation resulting in a secondary trigeminal-autonomic reflex. Giant-cell arteritis is a chronic granulomatous vasculitis of medium to large blood vessels which although is generalised, tends to affect those arteries arising from the aortic arch, clinically relevant arterial involvement in the superficial temporal, ophthalmic and vertebral arteries.

There are many causes of thunderclap headache which can be primary or secondary to other processes such as subarachnoid haemorrhage, cranial vessel dissection, and venous sinus thrombosis. Any space-occupying lesion can present as a high-pressure headache, but this can also be seen in idiopathic intracranial hypertension and venous sinus thrombosis. Diabetes often underlies painful ocular motor nerve palsies, but investigations for other processes are often necessary.

Clinical features

Migraine is a severe throbbing or vice-like pain (unilateral or bilateral) and can even extend to the face, neck, and shoulders. It is commonly episodic but can become chronic. A typical migraine attack lasts hours unless treated. It may be preceded by a prodrome of irritability, low or elevated mood and food cravings. The migraineur often reports aversion to light (photophobia), sound (phonophobia), and less commonly smell (osmophobia). Nausea and occasional vomiting occur due to gastroparesis. Migraineurs are very motion sensitive and will prefer to lie still.

The migraine aura develops over 10–30 minutes presenting commonly with visual phenomena (zig-zag lines in a hemifield (fortification spectra), a central black spot spreading slowly into the hemifield (scintillating scotoma), kaleidoscopic patterning in a hemifield and other phenomena such as dots, spots, and shimmering). These visual phenomena are usually black and white. Other auras present with spreading tingling in face and limbs, loss of speech (dysphasia) or less commonly hemiparesis, ophthalmoplegia, and vertigo. The aura may occur without headache (acephalgic migraine).

Patients with cluster headache experience strictly unilateral agonising pain around or behind the eye lasting 15–180 minutes associated with trigeminal autonomic symptoms (eyelid oedema and ptosis, conjunctival injection and lacrimation, nasal congestion and rhinorrhoea, pupillary meiosis and facial redness and sweating) and marked physical agitation. Patients may have several attacks a day often at the same time each day (circadian periodicity) and although cluster headache can be chronic, it more often presents episodically where it demonstrates circannual periodicity of bouts which can last weeks to months.

Giant-cell arteritis should always be considered in a new-onset headache in the elderly. It is characterless and although may localise to the temple, where a thickened, pulseless and tender temporal artery is palpable, it may wax and wane in other cranial locations. Constitutional symptoms, joint, muscle pain and stiffness (polymyalgia rheumatica), and jaw claudication are often reported.

Thunderclap headache is often occipital, builds up to maximum intensity in seconds (< 1 minute) and dramatically severe. Many such patients have other signs such as confusion, loss of consciousness, meningismus, seizures, and focal neurology. High-pressure headache is worse when supine and therefore at night and in the morning. Marked and prolonged exacerbation following coughing, bending, straining, and sneezing is suggestive, although migraine can also be exacerbated transiently by these triggers. In contrast to migraine, vomiting is profuse and effortless owing to pressure on the area postrema of the medulla. Pulsatile tinnitus and visual obscurations may also be reported. These latter phenomena of transient loss of vision with changes in posture are seen in patients with papilloedema and represent episodic ischaemia of the optic nerve head.

Investigations

Classic presentations of migraine and cluster headache do not require further investigations in the face of a normal neurological examination. Suspected giant-cell arteritis is suggested by a very elevated erythrocyte sedimentation rate and sometimes C-reactive protein (rarely values can be normal) and confirmed by a positive temporal artery biopsy (although the granulomatous inflammation can be patchy). Thunderclap headache necessitates exclusion of subarachnoid haemorrhage with computed tomography (CT) of brain and lumbar puncture. If subarachnoid haemorrhage is excluded and CT brain imaging fails to demonstrate an obvious cause, then further tests visualising brain arteries (dissection) and veins (sinus thrombosis) may be necessary to try to establish the underlying cause. Features of high-pressure headache with papilloedema would prompt urgent brain imaging and if normal, further tests may include imaging of cerebral veins (sinus thrombosis) and lumbar puncture (idiopathic intracranial hypertension). Painful ocular motor nerve palsies and visual loss (optic neuritis) should prompt onward neurological referral.

Diagnosis

Migraine can mimic thunderclap headache and high-pressure headache. Bacterial and viral meningitis can mimic migraine but a high-temperature, obtundation and true neck rigidity is not seen in migraine. Cluster headache can give rise to a Horner's syndrome sometimes necessitating vascular imaging to rule out carotid dissection. A high index of suspicion is needed to successfully diagnose giant-cell arteritis.

Treatment

Table 44.2 gives an overview of options available for the management of migraine and cluster headache. Treatment strategies are decided based on headache frequency and severity, patient choice and side-effects of treatment. Most recently, the development of drugs and monoclonal antibodies blocking the effect of CGRP promises to change the migraine management landscape. Giant-cell arteritis and its symptoms are exquisitely responsive to glucocorticoid treatment. Where this fails, there is evidence for other immunosuppressive drugs including methotrexate, leflunomide and cyclophosphamide. Treatment of high-pressure and thunderclap headaches is dependent on their underlying aetiology.

Table 44.2 Management strategies for some primary headache syndromes

	Episodic	Chronic
Migraine	Lifestyle measures * Analgesics and triptans Antiemetics Preventatives can be considered in severe cases	Lifestyle measures* Analgesics and triptans (avoid medication overuse)** Antiemetics *Preventatives:* • Beta-blockers (e.g. propranolol) • Tricyclics (e.g. amitriptyline) • Angiotensin II blockers (candesartan) • Calcium channel blockers (flunarizine) • Anticonvulsants (e.g. topiramate and sodium valproate) Botulinum toxin
Cluster headache	High-flow 100% oxygen Sumatriptan injections Greater occipital nerve block† Glucocorticoids Preventatives can be considered in long bouts	High-flow 100% oxygen Sumatriptan injections Greater occipital nerve block*** *Preventatives:* • Verapamil • Topiramate • Lithium

* Avoidance of stress, regularisation of sleeping and eating patterns and occasionally avoidance of triggers may help.

** Frequent use of analgesics (especially opioid-based) may precipitate a chronic low-grade medication overuse headache.

† Infiltration of methylprednisolone and lignocaine around the greater occipital nerve may help cluster headache but also migraine, cervicogenic headache, and occipital neuralgia.

Complications

Migraine has a significant societal financial impact owing to work-days lost. Cluster headache is so severe that it must be managed promptly; rarely suicide has been reported with this headache. Very high rates of morbidity and mortality are associated with bacterial meningitis and subarachnoid haemorrhage. Giant-cell arteritis can cause blindness (retinal artery occlusion, anterior ischaemic optic neuropathy) but also devastating posterior circulation strokes.

Further reading

Headache. Continuum 2018; Vol.24, No.4. (https://journals.lww.com/continuum/toc/2018/08000) [last accessed February 2020]

Related topics of interest

- Giant cell arteritis (p. 156)
- Optic neuritis (p. 236)

45 Imaging in ophthalmology

Key points

- Imaging in ophthalmology should be targeted to the location of suspected pathology
- Computed tomography (CT) is rapid and effective as a first-line investigation, particularly in orbital trauma, infection or inflammation, and in assessing orbital masses
- Magnetic resonance imaging (MRI) is useful for problem solving in the orbit and for the investigation of the retro-orbital visual and eye movement pathways

Introduction

The main modalities available for the investigation of ophthalmic disease are ultrasound (US), CT and MRI, supplemented by CT and MR angiography (CTA and MRA) and digital subtraction angiography (DSA). In oncological contexts nuclear imaging, particularly positron emission tomography (PET), is also useful.

For specific indications, fluoroscopic studies (i.e. dacryocystography) and plain radiographs (for potential orbital foreign bodies) may be indicated, but these are less commonly used. Ocular US is covered in a separate chapter so it will only be referred to here briefly, and similarly optical coherence tomography (OCT) is important in retinal assessment but beyond the scope of this chapter.

An overview of the imaging modalities used for investigation of different parts of the visual pathway is given in **Table 45.1**.

Computed tomography

Computed tomography makes use of the differential absorption of X-rays by different tissues in the body to build an image. Modern helical scanners allow the patient to move through the scanner quickly as multiple X-ray sources and detectors rotate around them, building up a volume of cross-sectional information, which can then be reconstructed in any plane.

This is a rapid process which produces high-resolution images and with the administration of iodine-based contrast agents, the vessels and any focal pathology can be highlighted. Images can also be post-processed to enhance the visualisation of specific tissues and the contrast between them (known as 'windowing'), increasing the information provided by the study.

Advantages and disadvantages

In the context of ophthalmology, CT provides excellent assessment of the bony orbit and good soft tissue in detail, and the orbital fat and extra-ocular muscles can be evaluated.

Table 45.1 Imaging modalities in ophthalmology. Ideal modality is according to location of pathology (supplementary/second-line investigations in brackets)

Location of pathology	Investigation of choice
Globe	Ultrasound (MRI, CT orbits)
Orbital vessels	Ultrasound (CTA, MRA, DSA)
Retina	OCT (Ultrasound)
Extraocular muscles	CT orbits – non-contrast (MRI orbits)
Intra-orbital mass	CT, MRI orbits – with contrast
Anterior visual pathway	MRI orbits/brain
Posterior visual and eye movement pathways	MRI brain (CT brain)
Bone	CT orbits – non-contrast
Foreign body	X-ray/CT non-contrast
Lacrimal apparatus	Dacryocystography (MR/CT)
Systemic metastases from ocular/orbital tumour	PET-CT

PET-CT, positron emission tomography–computed tomography; OCT, optical coherence tomography

Multiplanar, thin-slice imaging is essential and has become the norm in the majority of centres for investigation of orbital pathology. The speed of acquisition makes CT the perfect first-line investigation, particularly in cases of orbital trauma, and is also ideal in the setting of potential orbital foreign bodies.

The drawbacks are the radiation dose (particularly relevant for the eyes) and potential adverse reactions to iodine-based contrast agents.

Uses

The major uses of CT in ophthalmology are:
- Assessment of the orbit in trauma, particularly for evaluation of bone and foreign bodies
- Suspected thyroid eye disease, where the size of the muscles is easily appreciated
- Follow-up of previously treated orbital pathology
- Infective and inflammatory conditions of the orbit
- Localisation and characterisation of intra- or peri-orbital mass lesions (**Figure 45.1**)

The latter two indications should prompt the administration of contrast.

Magnetic resonance imaging

Magnetic resonance imaging draws its name from the magnetic properties of hydrogen ions, which behave differently depending on the body tissue in which they reside. Using a sequence of magnetic gradients and pulses of radio waves, which can be changed depending on the sequence used, these ions can be aligned and energised. The energy they release as they relax can be used to generate images.

Advantages and disadvantages

Magnetic resonance images have exquisite soft tissue contrast and depending on the parameters used, the contrast between different tissues can be highlighted and specific properties of tissues can be investigated. This makes MRI a more complex tool, but ideal for problem solving. The soft tissue contrast is particularly useful for delineating pathology in the brain where

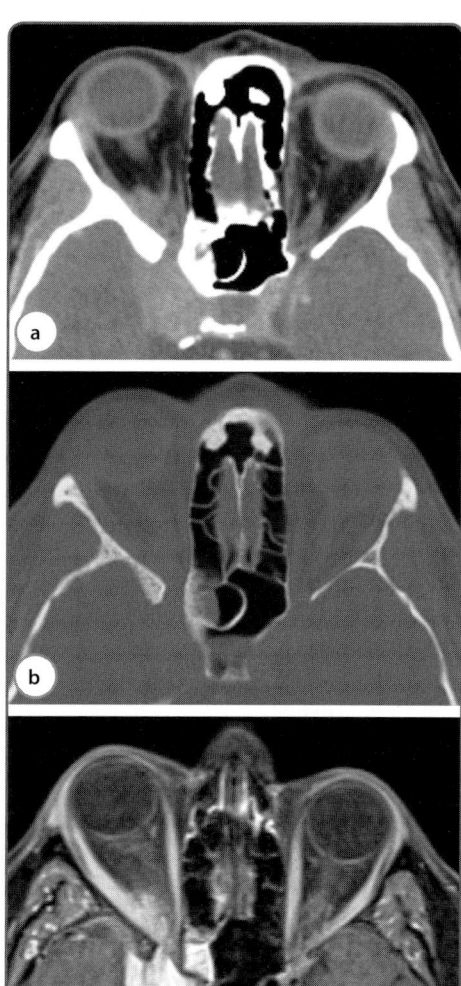

Figure 45.1 CT and MRI examples in a case of a cavernous sinus meningioma with orbital extension. Axial CT with contrast through the orbits and cavernous sinuses (a) demonstrates expansion of the right cavernous sinus with a hyperintense mass that extends through the orbital apex, with consequent right-sided proptosis. The same section on bone windows (b) demonstrates hyperostosis of the right sphenoid bone (compatible with a meningioma), and on contrast-enhanced T1-weighted MRI (c) the mass can be seen with additional enhancement of the dura overlying the right temporal lobe and mild mass effect on the adjacent brain with sulcal effacement.
Note: The superior bone detail on CT but the increased soft tissue resolution on MRI.

the level of detail provided far exceeds that of CT.

The drawbacks associated with MRI are the much longer acquisition time when compared to CT, the potential discomfort of the patient in the narrower bore of the scanner, and the problems associated with the magnetic field; pacemakers and other medical devices have to be carefully screened before scanning and the presence of metallic foreign bodies can preclude entry to the scanner entirely. In the case of implanted medical devices, these should always be declared and discussed with the MRI radiographers; many new devices are MRI compatible but require careful safety checking before entering the scanner. The website HYPERLINK "http://www.mrisafety.com" www.mrisafety.com provides a useful resource for checking compatibility. There is also the risk of adverse reactions to the Gadolinium-based contrast agents. Finally, there are a number of artefacts which can degrade images and in particular, ocular implants and dental amalgam can cause significant artefact affecting orbital images.

Sequences

The multiple sequences available in MRI can be confusing; a brief summary is included below of the primary sequences used in ophthalmic and neuroimaging.
- *T2*: Fluid and fat appear bright on this sequence; as increased water content/oedema is often a sign of pathology, this is a useful sequence for detection of abnormalities
- *T1*: Fat is best assessed on this sequence, and assessment of contrast enhancement is performed using T1 sequences before and after contrast administration. Fluid appears dark on this sequence
- *Fat-saturated sequences/short tau inversion recovery (STIR)*: T1- and T2-weighted imaging can be acquired with fat saturation, which makes fat appear dark and can help to highlight pathology in the orbit. STIR performs a similar function
- *Diffusion-weighted imaging (DWI) and the corresponding apparent diffusion coefficient (ADC)*: DWI and the corresponding ADC map demonstrate the degree to which water can move freely within a tissue. This can act as an indirect marker of cellularity, so

for example, orbital lymphoma, as a very cellular tissue, demonstrates abnormally increased diffusion restriction. Abscess formation is another important cause of increased diffusion restriction in the orbit, and, within the brain, ischaemia is a key cause
- *Fluid-attenuated inversion recovery (FLAIR)*: Used when imaging the brain, FLAIR cancels out the signal from water, causing it to appear dark, which can highlight other areas of pathology which may be masked on T2 imaging

Uses

The major context in which MRI is a first-line investigation is in the assessment of the retro-orbital pathways for vision and eye movement, as the superior soft tissue contrast is crucial for detecting abnormalities in the optic nerve and chiasm and within the brain parenchyma. However, MRI is also often useful in problem solving within the orbit; for example, in further characterisation of mass lesions identified on CT or US. It is also useful for assessing concurrent brain involvement in infective and inflammatory pathology of the orbit. A summary of common clinical indications for CT or MRI is provided in **Table 45.2**.

Angiographic imaging and intervention

Often US is best for assessing local vascular anomalies within the orbit, but CT or MR angiography is useful when the abnormality

Table 45.2 Imaging modality (CT or MRI) for specific clinical indications	
Computed tomography	Magnetic resonance imaging
Orbital trauma	Optic neuropathy: • Compressive (intrinsic/extrinsic) • Inflammatory • Degenerative
Orbital infection	Cranial nerve palsy
Foreign bodies	Gaze palsy
Thyroid eye disease Orbital mass	

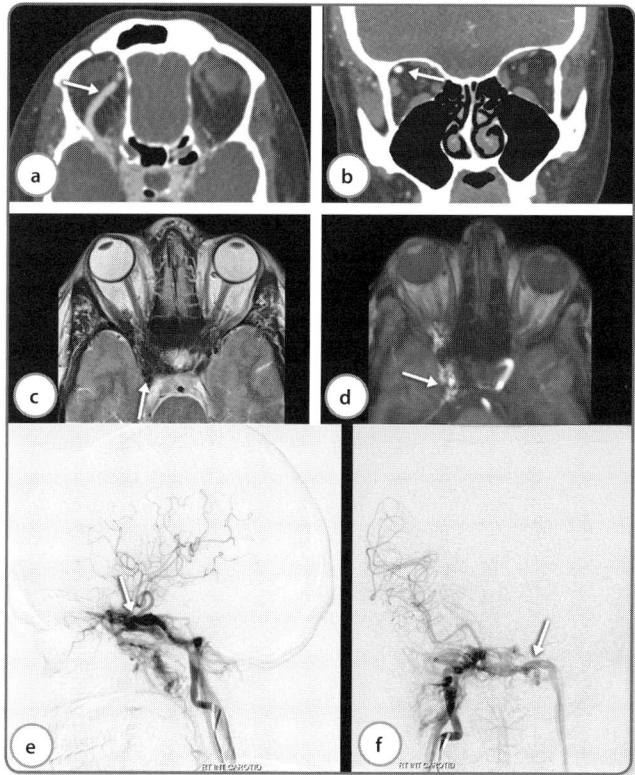

Figure 45.2 Endovascular treatment of a caroticocavernous fistula (CCF). (a) Axial T2 MRI demonstrates dilated right superior ophthalmic vein (arrow) and right proptosis; (b) Digital subtraction angiogram (lateral view) demonstrates arteriovenous shunting at the cavernous sinus (arrow) compatible with a CCF; (c) Guidewire positioned adjacent to the CCF; (d) CCF embolised with glue, resulting in closure of the fistula; (e, f) demonstrates a fistulous connection in the cavernous sinus (e, arrow) with early venous filling, including on the contralateral side (f, arrow).

involves the more proximal vessels [e.g. in the case of aneurysms causing cranial nerve palsies, or a caroticocavernous fistula (CCF)] (**Figures 45.2a** to **f**). To further characterise these abnormalities, a digital subtraction angiogram, which is an invasive procedure involving arterial puncture, can be performed and necessary intervention can be undertaken via this endovascular route. Examples of potential interventions relevant to ophthalmology include:

- Coiling or embolisation of aneurysms or CCFs
- Embolisation of tumours
- Stenting: For example, of the transverse sinuses in idiopathic intracranial hypertension, which may present as papilloedema
- Direct local administration of medication (e.g. chemotherapy for retinoblastoma)

Nuclear imaging

Nuclear imaging techniques make use of radioactive tracers – a component which emits radioactivity coupled to a component, i.e or mimics an endogenous molecule in the body. This molecule is 'labelled', so that when placed in a machine that can detect the emitted radioactivity, a picture of the location and amount of the molecule can be built up. The most commonly used in ophthalmology is 18F-fluorodeoxyglucose (FDG) PET-CT, which labels glucose in order to detect areas of increased metabolic activity, and couples the nuclear imaging (FDG-PET) with more detailed structural imaging (CT) to improve the localisation. FDG PET-CT is useful in a number of contexts:

- Ocular tumours (particularly melanoma) and detecting distant metastases
- Primary orbital or secondary lymphoma
- Orbital tumours and orbital metastases from other primary tumours
- Infections and granulomatous disease (e.g. tuberculosis)

Further reading

Aviv RI, Miszkiel K. Orbital imaging: Part 2. Intraorbital pathology. Clin Radiol 2005; 60:288–307.

Baert AL, Sartor K, Müeller-Forell WS, et al. Imaging of Orbital and Visual Pathway Pathology, 1st edition. New York: Springer-Verlag; 2002.

Swienton DJ, Thomas AG. The visual pathway—functional anatomy and pathology. Semin Ultrasound CT MR 2014; 35:487–503.

Related topics of interest

- Headache (p. 172)
- Trauma – globe rupture (p. 319)
- Tumours – eye lid (p. 323)
- Tumours of the choroid (p. 329)
- Tumours – conjunctival neoplasia (p. 336)
- Tumours of the uvea (p. 340)
- Tumours of the retina (p. 345)

46 Infectious keratitis

Key points

- Bacterial, viral, fungal, or protozoal infections can affect the cornea
- Prompt initiation of correct therapy is essential
- Suspicion for atypical organisms should remain high, if improvement is not rapid

Epidemiology

In the UK and US, infectious keratitis is most often associated with contact lens wear. In developing countries, ocular trauma, often associated with agricultural work, is the most common cause.

Pathophysiology

Defects in the corneal epithelium are required for most pathogenic mechanisms associated with bacterial and fungal infection. An intact corneal epithelium can be penetrated by *Neisseria gonorrhoeae* and *Haemophilus influenzae*. *Pseudomonas* and staphylococcal infection account for most infections in contact lens wearers. *Moraxella* is often the cause of infections in those with systemic comorbidity such as diabetes or alcohol abuse.

Acute infection prompts collagenase and matrix metalloproteinase production by inflammatory cells. These can lead to corneal melting and put the cornea at risk of perforation. Corneal tissue heals with scarring, of varying degree, and this, combined with irregular astigmatism, is the main cause of impaired vision following resolution of an acute episode of keratitis.

Viral keratitis normally follows a subclinical primary infection with the herpetic virus. Herpes simplex type 1 is the most common causative virus. Varicella zoster is a less common cause. Viral replication transport to the peripheral nerve endings of the sensory trigeminal nerve axons leads to clinical re-activation.

Clinical features

Pain is the main presenting feature of a microbial keratitis. Contact lens wear or trauma is likely to feature in the history. Other risk factors should be sought, including overnight wear of contact lenses and contact lens hygiene.

On examination, especially, if the underlying cause is not obvious, care should be taken to examine for a possible nidus of infection, such as a dacryocele, lid malposition, neuropathy or immunosuppression. Pain out of proportion to signs in the context of contact lens wearers should invoke suspicion of *Acanthamoeba* infection.

Documentation, which can be supplemented by photographs (**Figure 46.1**), should include measurements of infiltrates,

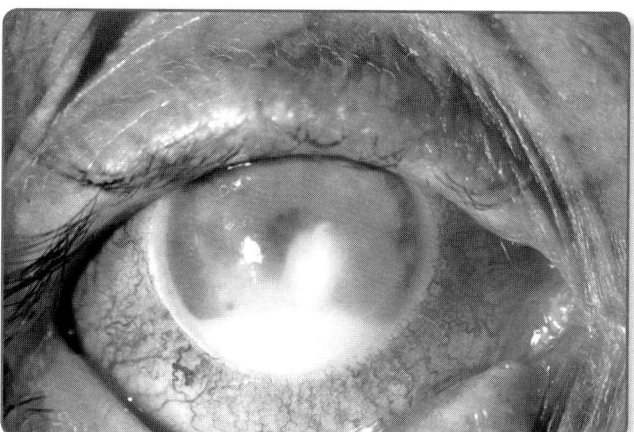

Figure 46.1 A patient with corneal infiltrate and hypopyon due to bacterial keratitis.
Courtesy: M Bizrah Moorfields Eye Hospital.

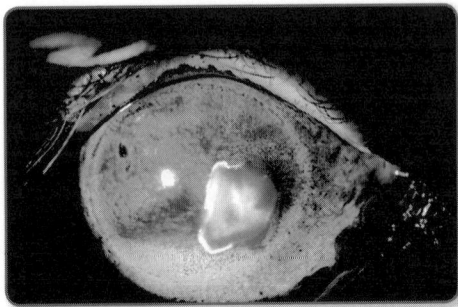

Figure 46.2 Epithelial defect, demonstrated by fluorescein staining, overlying an infiltrate caused by bacterial keratitis. (*For colour version see plate 2*) *Courtesy:* M Bizrah Moorfields Eye Hospital.

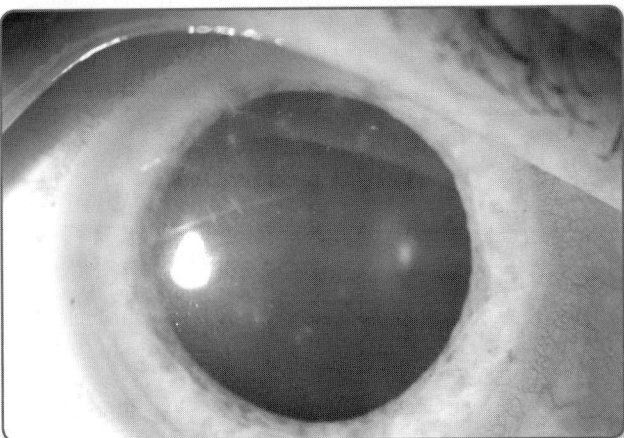

Figure 46. 3 Patient with perineural infiltrates in a case of Acanthamoeba keratitis. *Courtesy:* M Bizrah Moorfields Eye Hospital.

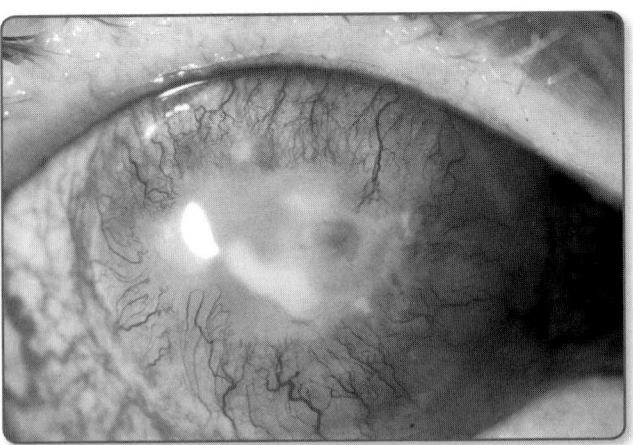

Figure 46.4 Fungal keratitis with satellite lesions. (*For colour version see plate 2*) *Courtesy:* M Bizrah Moorfields Eye Hospital.

epithelial defects (**Figure 46. 2**) and percentages of corneal thinning compared to normal. Associated features, such as perineural infiltrates (indicative of *Acanthamoeba*, see **Figure 46.3**) and feathery margins or satellite lesions (indicative of fungal keratitis, see **Figure 46.4**), should be documented.

Dendrites are characteristic of a herpetic epithelial keratitis and are caused by actively replicating virus forming epithelial vesicles. Immunocompromise or immunosuppression can facilitate the development of a very large epithelial defect (geographic ulcer). Viral particles can elicit an immune-mediated response causing a stromal, endothelial keratitis or keratouveitis.

In contact lens wearers, pseudodendrites may mislead the examiner away from a true diagnosis of an *Acanthamoeba* infection.

Investigations
Corneal scrape
A scrape should be taken for gram staining and culture. A blood agar plate and nutrient broth should provide suitable adequate support for the most common organisms to be cultured. Specialist media can be considered, if atypical organisms are suspected. *Acanthamoeba* growth is supported by plating an epithelial biopsy on a non-nutrient agar plate with an *Escherichia coli* overlay. Fungi can be cultured on Sabouraud's dextrose agar.

Polymerase chain reaction
The use of polymerase chain reaction (PCR) is emerging, especially in the diagnosis of atypical organisms such as *Acanthamoeba* and fungi. It is useful in the diagnosis of viral causes. The limitations of this technique are that non-pathogenic or ocular flora can lead to false positives.

Confocal microscopy
Patients with suspected *Acanthamoeba* can be examined for the presence of double-walled cysts on confocal microscopy. This technique is also useful for picking up fungal hyphae and filaments in suspected fungal keratitis.

Diagnosis
The diagnosis of a microbial keratitis is invariably a clinical one. Pain, combined with the clinical examination findings of an infiltrate, is highly suggestive of a microbial keratitis (although sterile infiltrates can occur). There may be an overlying epithelial defect.

Diagnosis of a microbial keratitis may be inadvertently delayed, if there is steroid use at presentation of an epithelial defect. Topical steroid use can prevent the normal leucocyte inflammatory response that manifests as a classic infiltrate, so such defects may require early consideration of scraping for organism detection.

Response to antimicrobial therapy helps to confirm the diagnosis; a poor response should prompt a search of atypical organisms.

Treatment
Bacterial keratitis requires the rapid commencement of intensive, broad-spectrum antibiotics. Local sensitivities will guide antibiotic choice. Studies suggest that single-agent empirical therapy for an initial sterilisation phase is sufficient. The use of chloramphenicol in contact lens-related keratitis is associated with a worse outcome and should be avoided as it fails to sufficiently cover against *Pseudomonas* infection. Close follow-up should be maintained. A review at 1-day post-commencement of treatment may not be useful, as clinically *Pseudomonas* infections may appear worse. Instead, pain and worsening vision should be emphasised as reasons for the patient to return sooner than a proposed 2-day follow-up.

The use of steroid drops in the healing phases of microbial keratitis has been controversial; however, the Steroids for Corneal Ulcers Trial has helped to provide some rationale for their adjuvent use. The trial found that overall there was no difference from the adjuvent use of steroids with regards to 3-month visual acuity outcomes, scar size, or progression to perforation. This may reassure some with regards to 'safety'. Subgroup analysis demonstrated limited benefit to their use on deep or central ulcers. However, *Nocardia* ulcers had a worse outcome when randomised to steroids versus placebo.

Fungal keratitis requires prolonged treatment, and the findings of the Mycotic Ulcer Treatment Trial support the use of topical Natamycin. Steroid use in fungal infection can lead to adverse outcomes.

Superficial herpetic disease can be treated effectively with topical trifluridine, acyclovir or ganciclovir.

The treatment of viral keratitis has been guided by the results of the Herpetic Eye Disease Studies. The important findings are summarised as follows.

In epithelial disease, the addition of oral acyclovir does not reduce the risk of development of stromal keratitis or iridocyclitis.

However, long-term, oral acyclovir 400 mg twice a day reduced by almost half the probability of recurrence of any form of herpetic eye disease.

Patients with stromal keratitis benefit from treatment with topical steroid in addition to a topical antiviral. There is no benefit from the addition of an oral antiviral.

The treatment of Acanthamoeba keratitis often requires a prolonged course of multiple agent regimens such as guttae polyhexamethylene biguanide (PHMB) 0.02%, guttae propamidine isethionate (Brolene) or guttae chlorhexidine 0.02%.

Pain may be controlled with simple oral analgesics and a short course of a topical cycloplegic. Pain can be particularly difficult to manage in cases of severe *Acanthamoeba* keratitis.

Complications

Perforation can occur requiring corneal gluing or tectonic grafting. In the longer term, visual rehabilitation will depend on the location and extent of scarring. It is modulation of the scarring that provides scope for future research direction.

Further reading

Allan BD, Dart JK. Strategies for the management of microbial keratitis. Br J Ophthalmol 1995; 79:777–786.

Dart JK, Radford CF, Minassian D, et al. Risk factors for microbial keratitis with contemporary contact lenses: a case-control study. Ophthalmology 2008;115:1647–1654.

Srinivasan M, Mascarenhas J, Rajaraman R, et al. The steroids for corneal ulcers trial (SCUT): secondary 12-month clinical outcomes of a randomized controlled trial. Am J Ophthalmol 2014; 157:327–333.

Related topics of interest

- Blepharitis (p. 32)
- Conjunctivitis (p. 72)
- Contact lens-related problems of the eye (p. 75)
- Corneal graft (p. 90)

47 Intermediate uveitis

Key points

- Inflammation involving the vitreous body (vitritis) and ciliary body with less anterior segment inflammation and minimal chorioretinal or retinovascular involvement
- The severest end of the spectrum is termed as 'pars planitis' with vitritis, retinal vasculitis in the periphery, and pars plana exudation
- New onset vitritis in an older person should raise the possibility of a masquerade syndrome (primary vitreoretinal lymphoma)
- Up to 15% of patients with 'idiopathic' intermediate uveitis will go onto develop multiple sclerosis on long-term follow-up

Epidemiology

Intermediate uveitis can be idiopathic but also secondary to several infectious or non-infectious aetiologies described herein. It is most common in young adults of either sex, with a female preponderance due to the association with multiple sclerosis. Asymmetry of the disease is common but usually on careful examination of the second eye, there is evidence of bilateral involvement. Approximately 15% of all uveitis cases are described as intermediate in nature.

Pathophysiology

As with the other forms of uveitis, there is a presumed, but unknown, antigenic trigger that leads to a maladaptive immune response occurring to host tissue. The far peripheral retina and pars plana are the primary target in intermediate uveitis with inflammatory exudate and immune cells extravasating into the vitreous humour.

Clinical features

Symptoms

Some patients may be asymptomatic or have chronic presentations, they are often sent in from optometrists who have detected vitreous floaters on routine examination. Patients principally complain of dot-like floaters and blurred vision with very little pain.

Examination

By definition, there should be little anterior segment inflammation in comparison to the vitreous component. There may be some peripheral retinal vascular sheathing but significant retinal vasculitis should be treated differently (see retinal vasculitis chapter) and there should not be retinochoroidal lesions to suggest a posterior uveitis. However, cystoid macula oedema (CMO) due to diffusion of inflammatory cytokines is common (and a major reason for visual loss).

The hallmark of the disease is the vitreous changes, which include inflammatory cells in the posterior vitreous (in contrast to spill over from anterior uveitis where the cells are in anterior vitreous). 'Snowballs' are round fluffy pale aggregates of inflammatory material sitting above the inferior retina and casting a shadow (**Figure 47.1**). 'Snow banking' is exudation of material sitting directly on the far peripheral retina at the ora serrata and a sign of severe disease. The amount of vitreous 'haze' produced by these changes can be graded with the indirect ophthalmoscope and used to assess severity and measure response to treatment (**Table 47.1**).

Investigations

All forms of the disease should be investigated, as it may result from a serious

Table 47.1 Binocular indirect ophthalmoscopy (BIO) score–grading of the severity of vitreous haze

BIO score	Fundus details
0	Clear view
1	Haze, but vessel details visible
2	Vessels visible but no detail
3	Disc visible but not vessels
4	No view of disc or vessels

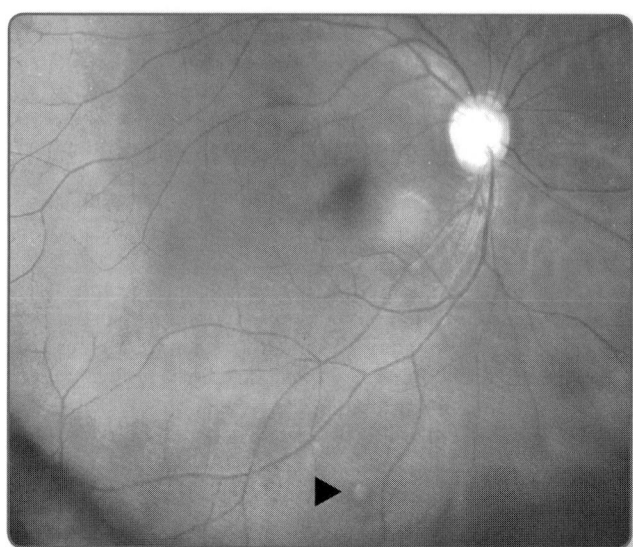

Figure 47.1 Wide field fundus photograph of a right eye showing (black arrowhead) a 'snowball' sitting just above the retina in the posterior vitreous. (*For colour version see plate 2*)

systemic condition or potentially curable infectious agent. The investigations can be targeted as for anterior uveitis but with a lower threshold to check for infections such as TB or Lyme disease. If retinal vasculitis is predominant then investigate as suggested in the "Retinal Vasculitis" Chapter. Beware new onset vitritis in an older patient which is poorly responsive to treatment, this could represent initial presentation of primary vitreoretinal lymphoma (PVRL), a masquerade syndrome.

Initial investigations

- *Blood testing*: Full blood count (FBC), urea and electrolyte (U and E), erythrocyte sedimentation rate (ESR), C-reactive protein (CRP), angiotensin-converting enzyme (ACE), and treponemal (syphilis) serology
- *Chest X-ray:* Sarcoid and tuberculosis (TB)
- Optical coherence tomography (OCT) may be normal or may show cystoid macula oedema

Imaging – fundus fluorescein angiogram) (wide field, if possible)

- *Posterior pole features*: 'Hot' disc with leakage, cystoid macula oedema
- *Peripheral features*: Similar to retinal vasculitis but less severe and more diffuse–look for capillary non-perfusion and ferning (leak from the capillary bed)

Targeted investigations-based on results above/suspicions

- *Tuberculosis testing*: Mantoux skin testing or interferon gamma release assay on blood
- Serology for HIV an, Lyme disease
- Brain imaging for demyelinating lesions but consider referral to a neurologist who may counsel against this, if it is unlikely to change the patient's diagnosis and instead leads to anxiety
- If PVRL is suspected then a vitreous biopsy is required and careful histopathology/cytology by a pathologist able to handle the small samples produced (may require referral to a national specialist centre)

Diagnosis

The essential principle for diagnosis in intermediate uveitis is ensuring before a decision is made to observe or reassure the patient that infections, masquerade uveitis, retinal vasculitis, and posterior uveitis are ruled out as detailed above.

Differential diagnosis

- Vitreous spill-over in severe anterior uveitis

- Vitreous detachment or haemorrhage with red blood cells or pigment floating in the vitreous
- Primary vitreoretinal lymphoma
- Fuch's' heterochromic cyclitis with prominent vitreous debris and cells

Treatment

If there is good visual function and minimal symptoms then observation in mild cases is warranted. It is unclear that what are the long-term effects of mild far peripheral activity or vascular leak on visual function. It is probable that after several decades, there is a marked reduction in peripheral retinal function; however, uveitis specialists are split as to whether it is worth decades of potentially toxic medication to prevent this. When central vision is affected by cystoid macula oedema or severe floaters then the reasons to treat are clearer.
- *Corticosteroids:* As with all inflammatory diseases, these are the mainstay of treatment
  - *Topical* may be worth trying a trial of dexamethasone 0.1% four times a day, to see if there is a beneficial effect
  - *Periocular* or intravitreal beneficial for unilateral disease or where there is significant asymmetry in activity
  - *Oral* required in severe sight-threatening disease, consider in bilateral disease
- *Steroid-sparing medication:* Used to allow oral steroids to be tapered or in severe cases as an adjunct. In contrast to posterior uveitis, the weaker antimetabolites azathioprine has a role here alongside cyclosporine, methotrexate, etc.

- Surgical treatment of complications, e.g. vitrectomy for epiretinal membrane (ERM) or vitreous haemorrhage

Complications

As with other forms of uveitis, there is a risk of secondary cataract and glaucoma development from both the disease and steroid treatments. The risk of glaucoma is less in intermediate than chronic uveitis or panuveitis however. Cystoid macula oedema is common with intermediate uveitis and is the main cause of vision loss.

As with retinal vasculitis, there is a risk of capillary non-perfusion with resulting ischaemia and then neovascularisation. Treating the inflammation is the first line in managing these new vessels followed by laser therapy to the ischaemic areas alone guided by FFA. The vitreous haemorrhages and vitritis result in fibrotic changes in the vitreous body, which can lead to retinal tears, retinal detachments, further haemorrhages, but more commonly ERM, which can affect vision and requires surgical treatment.

Prognosis

Although patients may complain about floaters, the cause for severe visual loss is involvement of the macula with ERM and CMO. Mild cases without visual loss can be observed but severe cases lead to visual loss in 20% of eyes. Some long term cases can enter remission either with treatment or spontaneously, conversely around 15% will develop multiple sclerosis after 10 years due to the high correlation between the two diseases.

Further reading

Nussenblatt RB, Palestine AG, Chan CC, et al. Standardization of vitreal inflammatory activity in intermediate and posterior uveitis. Ophthalmology 1985; 92:467–471.

The Standardization of Uveitis Nomenclature (SUN) Working Group. Standardization of uveitis nomenclature for reporting clinical data. Results of the first international workshop. Am J Ophthalmol 2005; 140:509–516.

Related topics of interest

- Anterior uveitis (p. 14)
- Posterior uveitis (p. 259)
- Retinal vasculitis (p. 286)

48 Intraocular lenses

Key points

- Acrylic intraocular lenses (IOLs) are the most widely used in the developed world
- Posterior capsule opacification rates are lower with sharp edge designs and highest with hydrophilic acrylic material
- Intraocular lenses can be implanted 'in the bag' (intracapsular), sulcus, or anterior chamber (**Figure 48.1**)
- Intraocular lenses are available in both pseudophakic and phakic designs
- Astigmatism and presbyopia correction require non-standard IOLs

Introduction

Cataract surgery has moved from a visually rehabilitative procedure to one that aims to reduce spectacle dependence by eliminating refractive error and, increasingly, presbyopia. Intraocular lens technology is the most important aspect of this objective.

Basic IOL design

Intraocular lenses are composed of a central optic that delivers the refractive power of the lens and either two or four haptics, which anchor the IOL in position. Optics and haptics may be constructed of a single material (single piece IOL) or different materials that are later fused (multiple piece IOL).

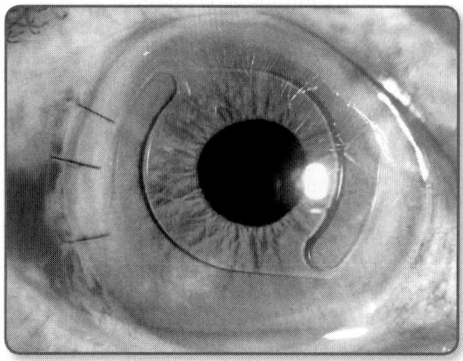

Figure 48.1 Anterior segment showing anterior chamber lens.
Courtesy: Ali Mearza, Ophthalmic Consultants of London.

Optic edge design

Square or sharp edge optics have lower rates of posterior capsule opacification (PCO) due to increased inhibition of lens epithelial cell migration. However, they can be associated with more positive dysphotopsias such as glare, particularly when combined with high-refractive index materials.

Light filtration

Essentially all IOLs filter ultraviolet light to protect the retina. Newer IOLs incorporate yellow chromophores to block short wavelength blue light. There is some evidence of benefit in patients with macular degeneration. Acuity and colour vision are similar between blue light filtering IOLs and clear IOLs, although glare may be less with the former. The same type should be used for both eyes as some patients may report differences in colour perception between the two eyes.

Intraocular lens material

Poly(methyl methacrylate)

Poly(methyl methacrylate) (PMMA) IOLs are ubiquitous in the developing world. They are highly biocompatible, rigid, and of relatively low refractive index. They are non-foldable and require a large incision for insertion, which makes them suitable for manual small incision cataract surgery and extracapsular cataract extraction. They are ideal when a rigid material with a low inflammatory profile is required, such as anterior chamber lenses.

Silicone

Silicone IOLs have a higher refractive index than PMMA and fold easily. Although anterior capsule contraction is brisk, posterior capsule opacification (PCO) rates are relatively low. Once inserted, these IOLs tend to unfold rapidly in an uncontrolled manner. They should be avoided in silicone-tamponaded eyes as silicone oil has a propensity to adhere to the optic, which can reduce vision, even after removal of the oil.

Hydrophobic acrylic

Acrylic is currently the most widely used IOL material in the developed world. Hydrophobic acrylic IOLs are flexible, fold easily, and unfold slowly. PCO rates are generally low and IOLs are resistant Nd:YAG (neodymium-doped yttrium aluminum garnet) laser pitting. The main concern with these lenses has been the incidence of dysphotopsias relating to the high-refractive index, of which glare in mesopic conditions is the most commonly reported. However, alterations to the edge design of newer models have significantly reduced the incidence. Glistenings or small fluid-filled vacuoles on the optic were also previously common (**Figure 48.2**) although newer IOLs have an increased water content to resist glistening formation.

Hydrophilic acrylic

These lenses flex and unfold in a similar fashion to hydrophobic acrylic IOLs. Additionally, the hydrophilic surface of these lenses provides excellent biocompatibility, which makes them ideal in uveitic eyes. They are also the preferred lens in silicone oil-filled eyes as they have less tendency to attract oil. PCO rates, however, are amongst some of the highest of any material, which may be related to the rounder edge of these lenses rather than the material itself. Older models were also associated with optic opacification due to calcium deposits, which occasionally required IOL explantation.

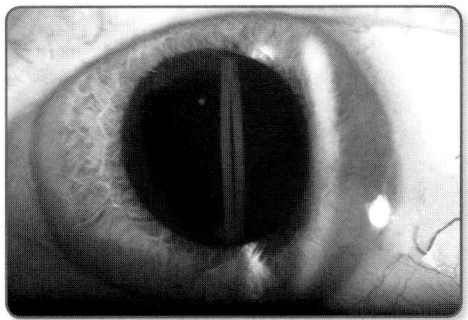

Figure 48.2 Anterior segment showing example of glistening. (*For colour version see plate 3*)
Courtesy: Romesh Angunawela, Moorfields Eye Hospital, London.

Collamer

These relatively new lenses are composed of collagen and a copolymer. Theoretically, they are the most biocompatible lens material as the collagen attracts fibronectin that forms a layer around the IOL thereby reducing a potential foreign body reaction and PCO rates.

Pseudophakic IOL implantation position

The physiological crystalline lens position is most accurately approximated with intracapsular IOL implantation. This is also the most stable position for the lens as the capsular bag enwraps the lens. Posterior capsule rupture with vitreous loss usually necessitates IOL positioning in the ciliary sulcus. A three-piece foldable IOL with thin haptics should be used to reduce iris chaffing and the risk of uveitis-glaucoma-hyphaema-syndrome. The IOL power should be reduced by 0.5–1.0 dioptres depending on the magnitude of the power. Providing the anterior capsule is intact, optic capture can be attempted by prolapsing the optic through the anterior capsule opening. This improves stability and centration and gives similar refractive outcomes to intracapsular placement meaning that the IOL power need not be adjusted.

Damage to both the anterior and posterior capsule or significant zonular dialysis will require an anterior chamber lens (angle supported or iris fixated) or scleral fixed posterior chamber IOL. The iris fixated IOL (Artisan) is a rigid PMMA IOL that employs an enclavation system with claw haptics that attach the optic to the iris. It can be attached to the anterior or posterior (retropupillary) iris surface. The angle supported IOL (Kelman Multiflex) is also a PMMA IOL and may be associated with more secondary glaucoma and corneal endothelial cell loss, although there are similar concerns regarding the latter with the Artisan IOL. Peripheral iridotomy should be performed for all anterior chamber IOLs to prevent pupil block.

Scleral fixed IOLs can be glued or sutured and probably cause less endothelial disturbance but are difficult to insert and associated with a higher rate of cystoid macular oedema, lens tilt, and lens decentration.

Intraocular lens and ocular aberrations

Aberrations are the presence of imperfections within the optical system of the eye that prevent light being focused on a single retinal point.

Spherical aberration

Throughout life the cornea maintains positive spherical aberration (excessive convergence of peripheral rays) which varies little with age. This is neutralised by the young crystalline lens, which produces negative spherical aberration (under convergence of peripheral rays). As the crystalline lens matures, spherical aberration increases, which may contribute to reduced contrast sensitivity. Modern aspheric IOLs are neutral or negatively aspheric to simulate the crystalline lens in youth. Small amounts of residual positive or negative spherical aberration in pseudophakes may enhance depth of focus.

Astigmatism

Toric IOLs (**Figure 48.3**), which neutralise corneal astigmatism, are available in most materials, single piece and multipiece, and in monofocal and multifocal designs. Intracapsular, sulcus, and anterior chamber (iris fixed) versions are available. Rotational stability is critical and a 10° misalignment post-operatively causes around 33% loss of astigmatic correction. Axis marking should be carried out pre-operatively on the slit lamp with patient upright. There are also computerised systems available, which use iris or vessel landmarks to orientate the axis. Lens-bag adhesions reduce rotation post-operatively and are probably strongest with acrylic materials. Outcomes are more predictable with regular bow-tie corneal astigmatism, which can be assessed using Placido-disc videokeratoscopy or Scheimpflug imaging.

Presbyopia-correcting IOL

These lenses attempt to address the loss of accommodation that occurs with monofocal IOLs. Small amounts of residual ametropia and astigmatism can degrade image quality significantly with multifocal and accommodating IOLs.

Multifocal IOLs

These IOLs fall into two broad categories: refractive (e.g. ReZoom) and diffractive (e.g. ReSTOR). Refractive IOLs build concentric zones of different refractive powers into the optic to produce near and distance bifocality. Diffractive IOLs use a series of concentric steps cut into the optic to achieve bi- or trifocality across the entire optical zone (**Figures 48.4** and **48.5**). Hybrid IOLs combine the two technologies. For refractive IOLs, the convergence of light will depend on which zone it enters and vision is therefore pupil size dependent. Reduced contrast sensitivity, halos, and glare are more common with both types of IOLs. Intermediate distance vision is generally compromised with multifocal compared with monofocal IOLs but newer diffractive IOLs come in trifocal [(e.g. AT LISA (Trifocal)] and quadrifocal (PanOptix) designs, which attempt to address this issue. Rotationally asymmetric multifocal IOLs (Lentis Mplus and SBL-3) are bifocal IOLs with a small sector shaped near vision segment blended into a larger distance vision segment. Early results suggest that contrast sensitivity may be better with these lenses than other multifocals.

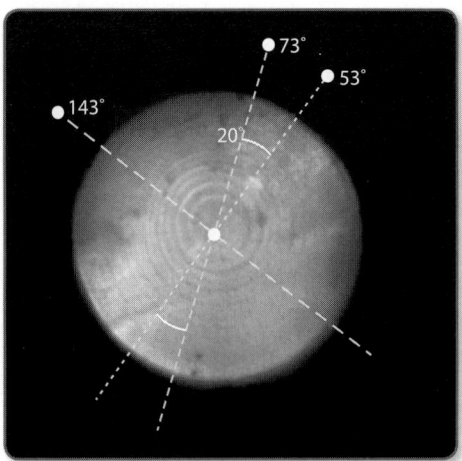

Figure 48.3 Anterior segment, showing a toric lens in situ.
Courtesy: Romesh Angunawela, Ophthalmic Consultants of London.

Intraocular lenses

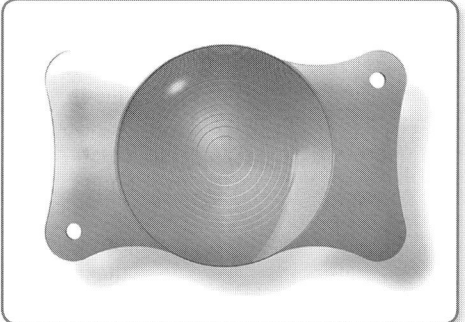

Figure 48.4 Diffractive trifocal lens manufactured by Zeiss Meditec, Germany is an example of one of the many multifocal lenses available for achieving glasses independence at the time of cataract surgery
Courtesy: Carl Zeiss Meditec company.

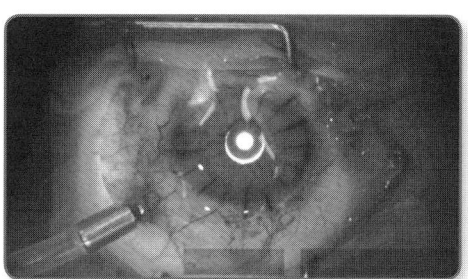

Figure 48.6 Retro-illumination image showing a small aperture IC8 (Acufocus, California) lens in an eye with a corneal transplant.
Courtesy: Romesh Angunawela.

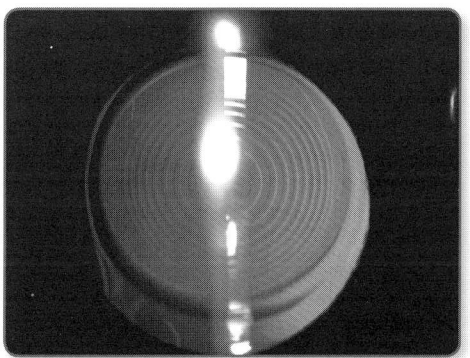

Figure 48.5 Anterior segment showing a trifocal lens in situ.
Courtesy: Allon Barsam, Ophthalmic Consultants of London.

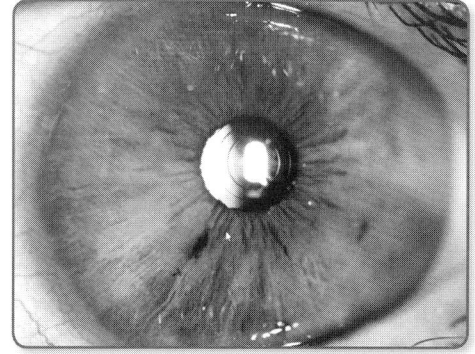

Figure 48.7 Anterior segment showing a phakic IOL.
Courtesy: Mearza, Ophthalmic Consultants of London.

Accommodating IOLs

These IOLs alter their refractive power by anterior–posterior movement in response to ciliary muscle contraction. The true amplitude of accommodation achieved is likely to be small with single optic designs (e.g. Crystalens). Dual optic designs (e.g. Synchrony IOL) connect two lenses of different refractive powers by a spring mechanism, which may confer a larger accommodative amplitude.

Small aperture IOLs

A small aperture can be integrated into a monofocal IOL (IC-8) or inserted into the ciliary sulcus as a secondary procedure following intracapsular IOL implantation (Xtrafocus). They use an opaque annular mask to mimic the pinhole effect (**Figure 48.6**), which extends depth of focus and can correct small degrees of ametropia, astigmatism (both regular and irregular), and higher order corneal aberrations.

Phakic (piggyback) IOL

These lenses can be used to treat large amounts of ametropia and astigmatism in younger patients (generally under 50) who are unsuitable for laser refractive surgery (**Figure 48.7**). They are available in iris fixated (Verisyse), sulcus (Visian internal collamer lens or Zeiss phakic refractive lens) versions, and both spherical and toric designs. Myopia of around −23.00 dioptres can be corrected with these lenses and the iris fixed version can correct up to +12.00 dioptres, but they should be used with caution in shallow anterior chambers of less than 3 mm depth. These lenses are associated with the same problems as their pseudophakic counterparts including endothelial cell loss and may induce cataract formation.

Further reading

Bellucci R. An introduction to intraocular lenses: material, optics, haptics, design and aberration. Cataract, volume 3. Berlin, Germany: Karger Publishers; 2013. pp. 38–55.

de Silva SR, Evans JR, Kirthi V, et al. Multifocal versus monofocal intraocular lenses after cataract extraction. Cochrane Database Syst Rev 2016; 12:CD003169.

Kessel L, Andresen J, Tendal B, et al. Toric intraocular lenses in the correction of astigmatism during cataract surgery: a systematic review and meta-analysis. Ophthalmology 2016; 123:275–286.

Related topics of interest

- Biometry and lens implant power calculation (p. 22)
- Cataract – complications of surgery (p. 50)

49 Intravitreal injection therapies

Key points

- Intravitreal injection therapies are most commonly used to manage neovascular age-related macular degeneration (AMD), diabetic macular oedema (DMO), and macular oedema associated with retinal vein occlusion (RVO)
- Intravitreal injection therapies currently licenced for intraocular use include ranibizumab, aflibercept, dexamethasone implants, fluocinolone acetonide implants, and ocriplasmin. Unlicensed intravitreal therapies are also commonly used. Newer drugs will also soon be available
- Patients receiving intravitreal injections should be informed about potential procedure-related and drug-related adverse events during the consent process

Introduction

Intravitreal drug delivery allows the protective ocular surfaces to be circumvented and high concentrations of drug delivered to the desired site of action. Pivotal clinical trials (**Table 49.1**) have identified significant visual benefits of this approach over the previous standard of care for a number of retinal diseases. This has led to regulatory authorities such as the European Medicines Agency (EMA) granting licenses for intravitreal drugs for several indications (**Table 49.1**). The National Institute for Health and Care Excellence (NICE) assesses cost-effectiveness of medications in England and Wales and makes recommendations for when public funding should be used for these medicines, often with inclusion criteria that are more restrictive than the EMA license. Other countries may come to different conclusions depending on the health economic model used. The potential procedure-related (**Table 49.2**) and drug-related (**Table 49.1**) adverse events of intravitreal therapy are summarised below.

Drug classification

Anti-vascular endothelial growth factor

Intravitreal anti-vascular endothelial growth factor (anti-VEGF) therapies are beneficial in treating the vasogenic response associated with the conditions described below.

Licensed indications

- Neovascularisation secondary to:
- Neovascular AMD, including retinal angiomatous proliferation (RAP) and idiopathic polypoidal choroidal vasculopathy (IPCV):
    – Ranibizumab was approved by NICE in 2008 for neovascular AMD provided best corrected visual acuity was between 6/12 and 6/96, lesion size ≤12 disc areas, there was no permanent structural damage and evidence of recent disease progression
    – Aflibercept was similarly approved by NICE in 2013
- Pathological myopia associated choroidal neovascular membrane (CNVM):
    – Ranibizumab was NICE approved in 2013
    – Aflibercept was NICE approved in 2017
- Macular oedema (MO) associated with:
- Diabetic maculopathy:
    – Ranibizumab was NICE approved in 2013 for centre-involving diabetic macula oedema (DMO) with central retinal thickness ≥400 μm
    – Aflibercept was similarly approved by NICE in 2015
- RVO consisting of central retinal vein occlusion (CRVO), branch retinal vein

Table 49.1 Summary of dosing, indications, key clinical trials, and potential side-effects of common intravitreal drug therapies. *Continues opposite...*

Medication	Dosage	Indication and key clinical trials		Potential drug-related adverse events
Anti-VEGFs				
Ranibizumab (Lucentis)	0.5 mg in 0.05 mL	CNVM	ANCHOR (2006), MARINA (2006)	Systemic thromboembolic events
		DMO	RISE and RIDE (2011), RESTORE (2012)	
		BRVO	BRAVO (2009)	
		CRVO	CRUISE (2009)	
		Myopic CNV	REPAIR (2013), RADIANCE (2014)	
		PDR	DRCR.net Protocol S (2015)	
Aflibercept (Eylea)	2 mg in 0.05 mL	CNVM	VIEW 1 and VIEW 2 (2012)	
		DMO	VIVID and VISTA (2015)	
		BRVO	VIBRANT (2016)	
		CRVO	COPERNICUS (2012), GALILEO (2012)	
		Myopic CNV	MYRROR (2013)	
		PDR	CLARITY (2017)	
Bevacizumab (Avastin)	1.25 mg in 0.05 mL	Neovascular AMD	CATT (2012), IVAN (2013), LUCAS (2015)	
		DMO	BOLT (2012), DRCR.net Protocol T (2016)	
		CRVO	SCORE2 (2017) LEAVO (2019)	
Corticosteroids				
Dexamethasone implant (Ozurdex)	700 µg	DMO	MEAD (2014), BEVORDEX (2016)	Cataract formation in phakic eyes Raised IOP
		BRVO and CRVO	GENEVA (2010)	
		Non-infectious posterior uveitis	HURON (2011)	
Fluocinolone implant (Iluvien)	190 µg	DMO	FAME (2010)	
Triamcinolone	1–2 mg in 0.05 mL to 4 mg in 0.1 mL	DMO	TDMO (2006), DRCR.net Protocol I (2010)	
		RVO	SCORE (2009)	

Table 49.1 Continued...

Antimicrobials			
Vancomycin	1 mg in 0.1 mL	Bacterial endophthalmitis Gram-positive organisms	Retinal toxicity
Amikacin	0.4 mg in 0.1 mL	Bacterial endophthalmitis Gram-negative organisms (alternative to ceftazidime in patients with penicillin allergy)	
Ceftazidime	2 mg in 0.1 mL	Bacterial endophthalmitis Gram-negative organisms	
Amphotericin B	10 µg in 0.1 mL	Fungal endophthalmitis	
Clindamycin	1.0 mg in 0.1 mL	Ocular toxoplasmosis	
Foscarnet	2.4 mg in 0.1 mL	Viral retinitis	
Vitreolytic agents			
Ocriplasmin	125 µg in 0.1 mL	Vitreomacular traction	MIVI-TRUST TG-MV-006 and TG-MV-007 (2012)	Risk of increased vitreous floaters Significant photopsia

BRVO, branch retinal vein occlusion; AMD, age-related macular degeneration; CRVO, central retinal vein occlusion; DMO, diabetic macular oedema; PDR, proliferative diabetic retinopathy; RVO, retinal vein occlusion

Table 49.2 Potential peri-operative and post-operative complications of intravitreal procedures

Peri-operative	Post-operative
Ocular pain	Endophthalmitis
Subconjunctival haemorrhage	Retinal detachment
	Vitreous haemorrhage
Corneal abrasion	Vitreous floaters
Lens contact	Cataract
Temporary raised intraocular pressure	Intraocular inflammation
Central retinal artery occlusion	Persistent raised intraocular pressure
Hypotony	Vision loss
Vitreous floaters	
Vision loss	

Note: Caution should be exercised so as not to deliver intravitreal injections in an elective setting if there is concurrent ocular infection.

occlusion (BRVO), and hemiretinal vein occlusion (HRVO):
- Ranibizumab was NICE approved in 2013 for MO following CRVO. It was also NICE approved for BRVO if macular laser had failed or was not suitable
- Aflibercept was NICE approved for MO following CRVO in 2014. It was also NICE approved for BRVO in 2016 as a primary therapy

Unlicensed indications

Neovascularisation secondary to:
- AMD:
  - Bevacizumab was reported to have benefit in CATT (2012), IVAN (2013) and LUCAS (2015).
- Acquired macular disease including angioid streak associated CNVM, presumed ocular histoplasmosis syndrome (POHS) associated CNVM, and other miscellaneous macular diseases

MO associated with:
- Diabetic maculopathy:
  - Bevacizumab was reported to have benefit in treating DMO in BOLT (2012) and DRCR.net Protocol T (2016)

Retinal vein occlusions:
- Bevacizumab was reported to have benefit in SCORE2 (2017) and LEAVO (2019)
- Radiation retinopathy, retinal artery microaneurysm, and macular telangiectasia type 1

Ischaemic retinopathy secondary to:
- Proliferative diabetic retinopathy (PDR):
  - Ranibizumab was reported to have a favourable safety and efficacy profile compared with panretinal photocoagulation (PRP) in patients able to attend regularly at 2 years in DRCR.net Protocol S (2015)
  - Aflibercept was reported to have a favourable safety and efficacy profile compared with PRP in patients able to attend regularly at 12 months in CLARITY (2017)
- Retinopathy of prematurity:
  - Reduced dose intravitreal ranibizumab (RAINBOW 2019)
- Idiopathic retinal vasculitis, aneurysms and neuroretinitis (IRVAN) syndrome and ocular ischaemic syndrome
- Neovascular glaucoma

Corticosteroids

Intravitreal steroid therapies are frequently used to treat the conditions described below.

Licensed indications

- MO associated with:
  - Diabetic maculopathy:
    - Dexamethasone implant (Ozurdex) was NICE approved in 2015 for DMO in pseudophakic eyes that are unresponsive to or unsuitable for non-corticosteroid treatment
    - Fluocinolone acetonide implant (Iluvien) was NICE approved in 2013 for chronic DMO in pseudophakic eyes that are unresponsive to available therapies
  - Retinal vein occlusion:
    - Dexamethasone implant (Ozurdex) was NICE approved in 2011 for MO secondary to CRVO and BRVO when laser had failed or was not suitable
- Inflammation associated with non-infectious posterior uveitis
  - Dexamethasone implant (Ozurdex) was NICE approved in 2017 for eyes with active non-infectious posterior uveitis and worsening vision with a risk of blindness

Unlicensed indications

- MO associated with:
  - Diabetic maculopathy:
    - Triamcinolone was reported to improve visual acuity particularly in pseudophakic eyes in TDMO (2006) and DRCR.net Protocol I (2010)
  - Retinal vein occlusion:
    - Triamcinolone was reported to improve visual acuity in SCORE (2009)
  - Triamcinolone has been used in the management of post-operative cystoid macular oedema (Irvine-Gass syndrome)

Antimicrobial therapies

Unlicensed intravitreal antimicrobial therapies are frequently used in the treatment of acute post-operative endophthalmitis, penetrating eye injury, intraocular foreign body, chronic post-operative endophthalmitis, and endogenous endophthalmitis. Intravitreal clindamycin can be used in the management of ocular toxoplasmosis. Intravitreal foscarnet can be used acutely for viral retinitis secondary to herpes simplex virus (HSV), varicella zoster virus (VZV) or cytomegalovirus (CMV). Intravitreal amphotericin B following formal vitrectomy can be used for fungal endophthalmitis that has invaded the vitreous.

Vitreolytic therapies

Ocriplasmin was NICE approved in 2013 for vitreomacular traction in stage II full-thickness macular holes with a diameter of ≥400 μ and/or severe symptoms in the absence of an epiretinal membrane.

Further reading

Mehta H, Tufail A, Daien V, et al. Real-world outcomes in patients with neovascular age-related macular degeneration treated with intravitreal vascular endothelial growth factor inhibitors. Prog Retin Eye Res 2018; 65:127–146.

National Institute for Health and Clinical Excellence. Guidelines on macular degeneration, diabetic macular oedema and retinal vein occlusion. Available from https://www.nice.org.uk/guidance/conditions-and-diseases/eye-conditions [Last accessed October, 2019].

The Royal College of Ophthalmologists. (2018). Ophthalmic service guidance. Intravitreal injection therapy. [online] Available from https://www.rcophth.ac.uk/wp-content/uploads/2018/02/Intravitreal-Injection-Therapy.pdf [Last accessed October, 2019].

Related topics of interest

- Age-related macular degeneration (p. 1)
- Diabetic eye disease (p. 116)
- Retinal vein occlusion (p. 290)

50 Lacrimal infections

Key points

- Acute dacryocystitis is characterised by the rapid onset of pain, erythema, and swelling below the medial canthal tendon and can lead to a medical emergency
- Endoscopic dacryocystorhinostomy (en-DCR) is an effective treatment for acute dacryocystitis, with good short- and long-term success rates
- Dacryocystectomy (excision of the lacrimal sac) can be a safe alternative to DCR in some frail, elderly patients
- Canaliculitis is frequently missed as a cause of recurrent conjunctivitis – look for an inflamed, pouting lacrimal punctum

Epidemiology

Lacrimal sac infections (dacryocystitis) most commonly occur in people over 40 years of age, although rarely can affect infants (congenital). Acute dacryocystitis in newborns is rare, occurring in less than 1% of births.

Pathophysiology

The underlying cause of dacryocystitis is thought to be a distal nasolacrimal duct obstruction (NLDO). As fluid collects within the obstructed lacrimal sac it leads to its distension, which at some point may then occlude (or kink) the common canaliculus, effectively creating an abscess space. Systemic antibiotics penetrate this cavity poorly, leading to progression of the acute infection despite treatment. This is evidenced by studies which find a majority of cultures sent at the time of drainage still result in positive bacterial growth, despite the patient being on systemic antibiotics at the time.

Staphylococcus aureus is the most commonly isolated organism (35% of cases), with coagulase-negative *Staphylococcus* (12%) and streptococcal species (specifically *Streptococcus pneumoniae*) also commonly isolated. Rare isolates include *Haemophilus influenzae* and *Candida* species.

The bacteria associated with canaliculitis tend to form granules, which increase their virulence and make them largely resistant to topical antibiotics. *Actinomyces israelii* is the most common causative organism.

Clinical features

Acute dacryocystitis (**Figure 50.1**) typically presents with pain, erythema, and swelling, below the medial canthal tendon. The patient may have a history of pre-existent epiphora, but this may not always be elicited.

This abscess of the lacrimal sac can lead to orbital cellulitis, an orbital abscess, superior ophthalmic vein thrombosis, osteomyelitis, cavernous sinus thrombosis or meningitis.

Chronic dacryocystitis is associated with chronic tearing, mucus discharge, conjunctival inflammation, and infection.

Canaliculitis (**Figure 50.2**) is often misdiagnosed. Primary disease is the result of an infection of the canaliculus and proximal lacrimal duct which is associated with eyelid thickening, erythema, and the presence of a classic pouting punctum.

Investigations

- A full ocular examination to assess for orbital involvement, specifically visual acuity, ocular motility, and assessment of optic nerve function
- Culture of purulent material, either through a pre-existent fistula or during surgical drainage

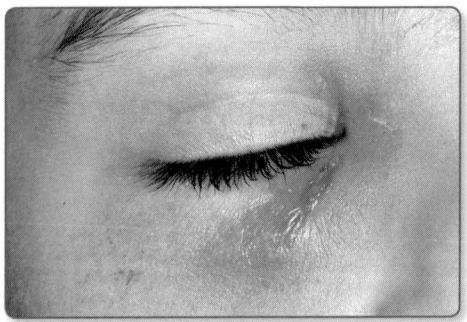

Figure 50.1 Photo of acute dacryocystitis.

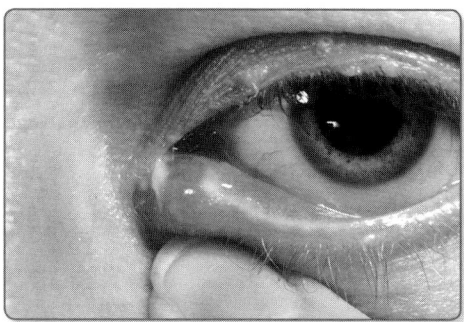

Figure 50.2 Photo of canaliculitis. (*For colour version see plate 3*)

- If the mass spreads above the medial canthus further investigation (e.g. imaging) is warranted

Diagnosis

Patients present with epiphora, and a mucocele that has become secondarily infected due to tear stasis (acute or chronic dacryocystitis) or a chronic discharging fistula to the skin. There is redness and swelling, with a firm mass centred over the lacrimal fossa. If syringing of the nasolacrimal system is attempted (generally to be avoided as it will be painful in this setting), it will confirm a complete occlusion.

Treatment

Despite the poor penetration of antibiotics into the abscess cavity, empirical systemic antibiotics are usually initiated in the hope that they may help to control the acute infection.

Prior to the development of DCR surgery, dacryocystitis was managed by dacryocystectomy, whereby the lacrimal sac and any fistulae present were excised.

Historically, external DCR (ex-DCR) surgery was performed several weeks after the onset of the infection, in order to reduce the likelihood of recurrent dacryocystitis and to deal with the patient's epiphora. Surgical management during the acute phase was generally avoided, in order to reduce the risk of spread of infection, fistula development, and surgical difficulties of operating through inflamed, oedematous tissues.

Performing en-DCR in an acute setting provides advantages by avoiding the concerns faced with an ex-DCR. En-DCR converts an anaerobic abscess cavity into an aerobic cavity through non-infected tissue planes. Abscess drainage allows a rapid recovery and resolution of symptoms. En-DCR is advocated by many surgeons who perform this type of surgery. Long-term functional success has been demonstrated in 90% of cases when carried out by experienced surgeons.

Canaliculitis is treated by surgical removal of the canalicular contents by punctoplasty with retrograde expression, simple curettage or canaliculotomy. Medical treatment alone will fail a large percentage of patients.

Complications

If untreated or inadequately managed, dacryocystitis can lead to complications such as orbital cellulitis, orbital abscess, superior ophthalmic vein thrombosis, and meningitis.

In infants, congenital dacryocystitis can be a very serious disease associated with significant morbidity and mortality. If not treated promptly and aggressively, the infection can progress to orbital cellulitis (because of a poorly formed orbital septum in infants), brain abscess, meningitis, sepsis, and death. Congenital dacryocystitis can be associated with an amniotocoele, which may lead to airway obstruction.

Transcutaneous drainage of the lacrimal sac can lead to a persistent fistula in 5% of cases. A DCR is required to correct the associated nasolacrimal duct obstruction.

Dacryocystectomy differs from DCR surgery in that there is no osteotomy or breaching of the nasal mucosa. There is less risk of nasal haemorrhage, with less surgery time and anaesthesia required. It may, therefore, be a safer procedure to perform on frail, elderly patients.

Further reading

Chisty N, Singh M, Ali MJ, et al. Long-term outcomes of powered endoscopic dacryocystorhinostomy in acute dacryocystitis. Laryngoscope 2016; 126:551–553.

Freedman JR, Markert MS, Cohen AJ. Primary and secondary lacrimal canaliculitis: A review of literature. Surv Ophthalmol 2011; 56:336–347.

Wu W, Yan W, MacCallum JK, et al. Primary treatment of acute dacryocystitis by endoscopic dacryocystorhinostomy with silicone intubation guided by a soft probe. Ophthalmology 2009; 116:116–122.

Related topics of interest

- Lacrimal surgery (p. 201)
- Orbital cellulitis (p. 242)

51 Lacrimal surgery

Key points

- Watery eye (epiphora) is a common symptom, but only a minority of persons will require a surgical intervention
- Dacryocystorhinostomy (DCR) can be performed via an endonasal approach (usually endoscopic) or externally through a skin incision (en-DCR or ex-DCR)
- DCR has a high success rate, although some pros and cons of the different approaches still exist
- Lacrimal sac infection (dacryocystitis) benefits from prompt surgical drainage by means of an en-DCR
- Lacrimal gland disorders are less common and require specialist input

Lacrimal surgery encompasses tear outflow disorders (watery eyes), some dry eye treatments (e.g. punctal occlusion, canalicular excision) as well as rarer surgery for pathology of the lacrimal gland itself. These latter points are beyond the remit of this chapter.

Epidemiology

An intermittently watery eye whilst outside, in the cold or wind is not abnormal. It is almost universally experienced at times and patients should be reassured this, unless there is an unusually marked impact upon them.

Lacrimal gland lesions are estimated to affect just over 1 per million individuals per year, with an incidence of neoplastic lesions estimated to be 0.7 per million individuals per year. The low incidence of lacrimal gland carcinoma means treatment is isolated to a few specialist centres.

Pathophysiology

Epiphora, or the overflow of tears, is a very common concern which can compromise both quality of life and cause discomfort. Tearing can have many causes, which broadly falls into either a hypersecretive (lacrimation) or outflow obstruction mechanism. The former is more common and can include patients experiencing a normal physiological response (to any ocular surface irritant), ocular surface disease, or even simple blepharitis with a secondary lipid deficient tear film.

In patients with outflow obstruction, lacrimal secretion is thought to be normal, but blockage or hold up of tear drainage causes spill over of tears. In the majority of cases, this is attributed to an obstruction of unknown cause. Obstruction secondary to a pathological process is less commonly encountered, and can be due to benign or neoplastic disease intrinsic to the lacrimal outflow pathways, or extrinsic disease causing secondary compressive nasolacrimal sac or duct obstruction. Secondary obstructive causes should be investigated and treated in their own right, with lacrimal drainage surgery withheld until a diagnosis is reached and appropriate treatment initiated. Where there is evidence for local neoplastic disease, lacrimal drainage surgery may even be contraindicated.

Clinical features

Gentle pressure over the lacrimal sac can sometimes cause reflux of mucus into the tear film which is indicative of a mucocele. Likewise, mucus reflux during syringing is also suggestive. As a general rule, it is worth noting that even large mucoceles only rarely cause globe displacement. This should, therefore, prompt investigation to exclude a space-occupying lesion.

In the setting of dacryocystitis, en-DCR offers a rapid resolution of symptoms, converting an anaerobic abscess cavity into an aerobic cavity through non-infected tissue planes with associated drainage and long-term control of epiphora.

Owing to the superotemporal location of the lacrimal gland within the anterior orbit, disorders of the lacrimal gland typically cause inferior and nasal displacement of the globe. Proptosis can develop. Blepharoptosis, ocular motility disturbance, and diplopia are more likely to occur with malignant tumours.

Investigations

A full ocular examination to exclude other treatable causes of epiphora is required. Often treatment requires a stepwise process, where the most obvious or simplest treatable cause is addressed first. Careful syringe and probe by the treating clinician is necessary. A subset of patients will appear freely patent to syringe but still manifest an outflow obstruction, as demonstrated by physiological testing (such as lacrimal scintigraphy) (**Figure 51.1**). Even 5–10% regurgitation or reflux of tears during syringing can be significant and easily missed if it is not specifically observed for.

Additional investigation (e.g. CT or the orbits/sinuses) should be performed if something is atypical with the expected clinical findings or history. In a larger lacrimal practice, more sinister pathology of the lacrimal sac/fossa will be encountered regularly over the year.

Lacrimal scintigraphy is mainly useful for those rare cases where a patient has significant symptoms but an entirely normal examination; whilst apparently being completely patent to syringe. In this group, a 'functional block' is suspected. Provide patient information regarding the likely need for a DCR and use the test to justify the need for tear duct surgery once the results/images are available. This results in a quick consultation at the second visit, as the patient has had time to consider the surgery and is expecting the earlier recommendation to be confirmed. A scintigram will, however, rarely point the clinician away from DCR ('good news!') towards simpler eyelid surgery as a possible cure.

Diagnosis

- No other clinically discernible cause for epiphora
- Delayed fluorescein clearance
- Raised tear film
- Demonstrable outflow obstruction (either partial or complete)

Treatment

The principles of surgery for blockage of the lacrimal outflow tract probably dates back 1000 years, when 12th century Andalusian oculists described a small spear-shaped instrument perforating the lacrimal bone in a nasal direction until blood flows through the nose and mouth. The probe was then wrapped in cotton (either dry or soaked in ox fat) and would be exchanged every day in order to maintain the patency of the created fistula.

This principle remains the same to date, with modern DCR dating back to the dawn of the 20th century. In terms of anatomic goals, the aims of surgery are simple: the lacrimal sac is connected directly to the nose by removal of the separating bone and mucosa. A fistula is formed that allows tears to pass directly into the nasal vault through the lateral nasal wall. This must occur at a level above the mechanical obstruction in order to bypass it. The traditional method has been through an external (skin) approach as described by Toti and modified by Dupuy-Dutemps (Ex-DCR).

Although the endonasal approach was perhaps described prior to this, it is only in recent decades that attention has turned to En-DCR for both primary procedures and to revise failures. En-DCR was first described by Caldwell in 1893, but failed to gain popularity due to the difficulty in accessing the lacrimal sac via the nasal cavity. With the advent of improved endoscopic instrumentation, en-DCR surgery was re-described in the 1990s and has continued to evolve.

DCR surgery can be performed under local or general anaesthesia. For both ex-DCR and

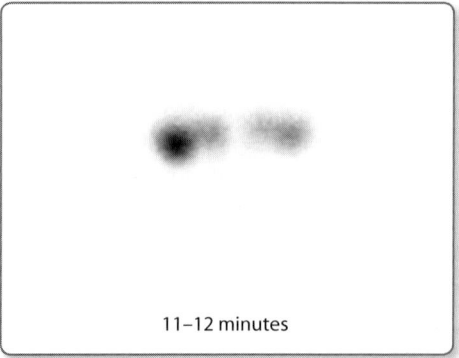

Figure 51.1 A lacrimal scintigraphy showing NLD obstruction.

en-DCR, additional local anaesthetic (with adrenaline) administration is recommended. This will help the anaesthesiologist, aid surgical visualisation through improved haemostasis as well as minimise post-operative pain (to the level where only a couple of paracetamols should suffice). Nasal packs soaked in cocaine 4%, adrenaline 1:1000 or a mixture (e.g. Moffett's solution) should be applied via packing, swabs or cotton buds.

External dacryocystorhinostomy

- Performed through a cutaneous incision, 10–12 mm long, sitting medial to the medial canthus on the flat of the nose. Smaller incisions and other locations are common practice
- A skin flap is formed to reveal the anterior limb of the medial canthal tendon, which is divided and the periosteum opened
- The periorbita is elevated to displace the lacrimal sac and duct laterally
- A 3-mm up-biting right-angled Kerrison rongeur is used to break through the thin bone of the lacrimal fossa and a bony osteotomy is formed, proceeding initially anteriorly, inferiorly and finally posteriorly. An osteotomy at least 15 mm in diameter is created ('large enough to place one's thumb into')
- The lacrimal sac is probed and opened longitudinally. Any suspicious mucosa should be biopsied and submitted for pathology
- The nasal mucosa is incised in a similar longitudinal fashion, with relieving incisions at either end, forming a 'H' shape
- A silicone stent is usually inserted and tied loosely over an artery clip to prevent cheese-wiring of the canaliculi
- The posterior lacrimal sac flap is sutured to the posterior nasal flap, typically with three bites of a continuous 6/0 Vicryl suture
- Three sutures are then used to oppose the anterior nasal mucosal and anterior lacrimal sac flaps. Where possible, these are suspended by attachment to the overlying orbicularis
- The anterior limb of the medial canthal tendon is re-approximated and the skin is typically closed with a 6-0 polypropylene suture

Endonasal dacryocystorhinostomy

- Performed either by direct visualisation, or more commonly, with the use of an endoscope
- Mechanical or 'powered' are the most common current forms
- After decongestion, an elliptical or inferiorly-based tramline nasal mucosal incision down to bone is made. This leads from close to the roof of the nose, down past the axilla of the middle turbinate to the mid-point of the maxillary line, where it will overly the nasolacrimal duct
- The mucosa is stripped from underlying bone and peeled away with a Freer elevator
- An osteotomy is fashioned with an attempt to rongeur sufficient bone superiorly and anteriorly to easily visualise the entire width and most of the length of the lacrimal sac and duct (a forward-biting up-cutting 40° Kerrison rongeur is useful for this)
- Sufficient bone must be removed superiorly, as up to a third of the lacrimal sac will lie above the level of the axilla of the middle turbinate. The agger nasi air cells (the anterior most anterior ethmoidals) serve as a useful landmark
- The medial wall of the sac is tented with a probe to ensure that all bone at least 5–10 mm above the common canalicular opening has been removed
- The lacrimal sac can then be 'opened like a book' and the lacrimal system is usually intubated

Complications

Risks common to all forms of DCR surgery include bleeding, wound infection, and damage to the lacrimal puncta if silicone stents are used. Cerebrospinal fluid leaks occur exceptionally rarely in DCR, with only a few case reports worldwide.

Until recently, ex-DCR was considered the 'gold-standard'. However, the reported success rate of both procedures in the modern literature is now similar when ex-DCR is compared to en-DCR procedures that remove adequate bone for full lacrimal sac exposure, marsupialisation, and mucosal flap apposition. With both en-DCR and ex-DCR, subjective success can be achieved in 95% (or more) of cases, with objective success close to 100%. A lack of agreed or standardised outcome measures or even duration of follow-up highlights how difficult comparisons actually are.

Skin scarring is a potential complication unique to ex-DCR, with up to 10% of patients describing them to be cosmetically significant. Damage to the facial nerve during ex-DCR can also occur.

Further reading

Ali MJ, Psaltis AJ, Murphy J, et al. Powered endoscopic dacryocystorhinostomy: A decade of experience. Ophthal Plast Reconstr Surg 2015; 31:219–221.

Rose GE. The lacrimal paradox: Toward a greater understanding of success in lacrimal surgery. Ophthal Plast Reconstr Surg 2004; 20:262–265.

Related topics of interest

- Lacrimal infections (p. 198)

52 Leucocoria

Key points
- Leucocoria means 'white pupil' and refers to an abnormal white pupil reflex when light reflects off a pale lesion posterior to the iris
- Leucocoria can be the presenting sign of a wide range of ocular and systemic diseases, which may be life-threatening (e.g. retinoblastoma) or sight-threatening (e.g. cataract)
- Leucocoria should be viewed as a 'red flag' sign, and when seen in children without a known cause should be referred urgently to a paediatric ophthalmologist for a full assessment

Epidemiology

Leucocoria is a non-specific sign. Incidence and prevalence depends on the aetiology and varies between countries. UK data is presented here:
- Between 50–60 cases of retinoblastoma (RB) are diagnosed every year and leucocoria is the presenting sign in 56% of cases
- Childhood cataract is thought to affect 3–4 in 10,000 children
- The incidence of retinopathy of prematurity (ROP) requiring treatment is 4% amongst neonates of birth weight less than 1,500 g. Leucocoria in this group is a late sign indicating retinal detachment (RD) and poor prognosis. Screening aims to identify ROP before RD occurs
- Coats' disease affects around 1 in 100,000 children

Pathophysiology

The normal red reflex occurs when light is reflected back out of the eye from the orange-red choroid underlying the transparent retina. Leucocoria is a white pupil reflex which occurs when light is reflected from a pale lesion within the eye. An anatomical approach ('front to back') can help establish a differential diagnosis (**Table 52.1**). Pseudo-leucocoria refers to transient leucocoria in the presence of a normal ocular examination, and is typically caused by reflection of light from the optic disc. It is also caused by anisometropia or strabismus.

To increase utility and reduce false positives, the red reflex should be tested in a darkened room using a bright light source such as a direct ophthalmoscope. If the pupils are small and the red reflex diminished, the test should be repeated 30 minutes after dilating the pupils with 1% tropicamide.

Table 52.1 Causes of leucocoria

Lens	Cataract (congenital or infantile, isolated or with systemic associations), lens capsule opacification
Vitreous	Persistent foetal vasculature (PFV), familial exudative vitreoretinopathy (FEVR), retrolental fibrosis, organised vitreous haemorrhage, endogenous endophthalmitis
Retina	Retinoblastoma (RB), retinopathy of prematurity (ROP), Coats' disease, optic disc or chorioretinal coloboma, myelinated retinal nerve fibre layer, toxoplasmosis, toxocariasis, retinal detachment (RD), retinoschisis, retinal dysplasia (e.g. incontinentia pigmenti or Norrie's disease), medulloepithelioma, retinal astrocytic hamartoma
Pseudo-leucocoria	Anisometropia, strabismus, non-axial flash photography (projecting onto optic disc)

Clinical features

A comprehensive history can help to diagnose the underlying cause of leucocoria:
- *Age of onset*: Leucocoria presenting at or soon after birth is suggestive of congenital cataract, persistent foetal vasculature (PFV), ROP, or retinal dysplasia; leucocoria presenting in infancy or older children is suggestive of RB, Coats' disease, toxocariasis or tuberous sclerosis (TS)
- *Associated ocular symptoms*: Blurred vision, redness, pain, photophobia, or strabismus
- *Associated non-ocular symptoms*: Facial skin changes such as butterfly distribution

angio-fibromas and behavioural problems (TS), developmental delay (Norrie disease, ROP)
- *Past ocular history*: Trauma (leucocoria secondary to cataract, RD or vitreous haemorrhage), prior ROP (leucocoria secondary to RD or retrolental fibrosis)
- *Past medical history*: Prematurity, birth weight and other co-existing syndromes
- *Family history:* Important in hereditary conditions such as RB (which may also occur spontaneously), familial exudative vitreoretinopathy (FEVR), and coloboma

A thorough examination usually reveals the diagnosis:
- Binocular and uniocular visual acuity should be assessed in an age-appropriate manner, e.g. response to light (newborns), preferential looking (infants), Kay picture test (toddlers), Keeler logMAR (pre-school)
- Bruckner test is performed using the direct ophthalmoscope at a distance looking at the red reflex simultaneously in both eyes, and can quickly identify opacities in the visual axis, as well as significant anisometropia or strabismus
- Prior to instillation of mydriatic drops, pupils must be assessed for the presence of a relative afferent pupillary defect, which indicates unilateral (or asymmetrical) optic nerve or severe retinal disease
- Cycloplegic retinoscopy should be performed to identify refractive errors (in order to prevent amblyopia) and to rule out anisometropia as a cause of pseudo-leucocoria
- Anterior segment examination may reveal a cataract, lens capsule opacification (**Figure 52.1**) anterior chamber inflammation, neovascularisation (RB or Coats), or signs of abnormal anterior segment development such as microphthalmia or microcornea (PFV)
- Dilated fundus examination may reveal vitritis (toxocariasis, endophthalmitis), vitreous haemorrhage, vitreous seeds (endophytic RB), hyaloid vascular complex remnant (PFV), a colobomatous or dysplastic optic disc, abnormal retinal vasculature (RB, Coats, ROP, FEVR), a retinal lesion (RB, Coats, toxocariasis, astrocytic hamartoma), chorioretinal coloboma, or a retinal detachment
- Examination under anaesthesia may facilitate ultrasound biomicroscopy and retinal imaging in infants

Investigations

Although the aetiology is usually apparent following history taking and examination, some further investigations may be useful:
- Ultrasonography may show an intra- or subretinal mass with calcification (RB, astrocytic hamartoma), subretinal fluid (Coats' disease, RD), hyaloid vascular complex remnant (PFV), or granuloma (Toxocara lesion)
- Optical coherence tomography (OCT) provides detailed anatomical information about the macula such as intra or subretinal fluid or fibrosis
- Fundus fluorescein angiography (FFA) may show abnormal retinal vessels and leakage (Coats' disease), hyperfluorescence (RB, toxocariasis) or peripheral avascularity (ROP, FEVR)
- Retinal imaging is useful in documenting disease progression or response to treatment
- Magnetic resonance imaging (MRI) may be useful in RB if there is a suspicion of extraocular spread
- Serology for Toxoplasma or Toxocara antibodies
- Genetic investigations are performed in conditions with a known or possible hereditary aetiology such as

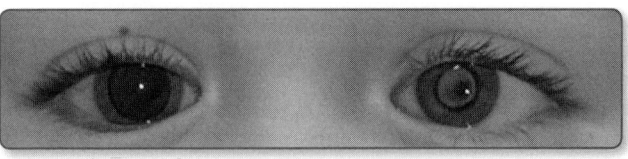

Figure 52.1 Leucocoria in the left eye due to lens capsule opacification following cataract surgery. (*For colour version see plate 3*)

retinoblastoma, FEVR, Norrie's disease or retinal astrocytic hamartoma (TS)

Diagnosis

Retinoblastoma is a life-threatening condition if untreated and therefore the most important diagnosis to make amongst those which might present with leucocoria. The diagnosis following leucocoria is still largely a clinical one based on the features above, in order to allow prompt and appropriate treatment. Confirmation of a pathogenic mutation (RB1 on chromosome 13) in heritable instances informs screening programmes for the index case and relatives and is absent in non-heritable cases.

Treatment

Treatment depends on the underlying cause of the leucocoria:
- Retinoblastoma treatment depends on the stage of the tumour and may include transpupillary laser thermotherapy, cryotherapy, chemotherapy or enucleation. Newer therapies (intravitreal and intra-arterial chemotherapy) are increasingly allowing eye preservation
- Congenital cataract (particularly if unilateral) is highly amblyogenic and necessitates surgical extraction around 6 weeks of age
- Conditions associated with abnormal retinal vasculature, e.g. ROP, FEVR and Coats' disease typically require retinal laser photocoagulation (with an emerging role for anti-VEGF injections) to reduce complications such as retinal detachment
- Infectious aetiologies, e.g. toxoplasmosis and toxocariasis may require systemic treatment in active instances with anti-microbials and steroids
- As with all paediatric eye conditions, particular attention should be given to the identification and management of refractive error and amblyopia

Complications

Complications may result from late presentation, delayed referral or misdiagnosis, and can be associated with poorer outcomes or even increased mortality. Specific complications include:
- Disease progression, e.g. extraocular spread of RB (associated with a poorer prognosis) or exudative retinal detachment in Coats' disease
- Amblyopia, which may develop quickly, especially in young children with a unilateral lesion in the visual axis
- Poor surgical outcomes

Further reading

Dimaras H, Kimani K, Dimba EA, et al. Retinoblastoma. Lancet 2012; 379:1436–1446.

Hartnett ME. Advances in the understanding and management of retinopathy of prematurity. Surv Ophthalmol 2017; 62:257–276.

Shields JA, Shields CL, Honavar SG, et al. Clinical variations and complications of Coats' disease in 150 cases: the 2000 Stanford Gifford Memorial Lecture. Am J Ophthalmol 2001; 131:561–571.

Related topics of interest

- Cataract – congenital (p. 55)
- Retinoblastoma (p. 294)
- Retinopathy of prematurity (p. 298)

53 Minimally invasive glaucoma surgery

Key points

- Minimally invasive glaucoma surgery (MIGS) is a rapidly evolving field that aims to offer a safer and less invasive alternative to traditional glaucoma surgery
- Research is required on the long-term clinical and economical efficacy of MIGS to determine how MIGS can best complement the current armamentarium of glaucoma treatment
- In advanced glaucoma requiring a low target intraocular pressure (IOP), trabeculectomy and tube surgery remain the gold standard of treatment

Introduction

Minimally invasive glaucoma surgery (MIGS) aims to offer a safer and less invasive alternative to traditional glaucoma surgery. There is no single definition of MIGS but it is widely accepted to have the following characteristics: ab interno approach, minimal trauma, good safety profile, and rapid patient recovery. MIGS can be categorised based on their mechanism of action: enhancing trabecular/Schlemm canal outflow, increasing uveoscleral outflow (the only available device has recently been withdrawn), creating subconjunctival outflow pathway, or reducing aqueous production. MIGS procedures can generally be performed alone or in conjunction with cataract surgery. Most are targeted at patients with early to moderate glaucoma. Here, we discuss a few of the commonly performed MIGS.

Enhancing trabecular/ schlemm canal outflow

The juxtacanalicular trabecular meshwork (TM) is believed to be the greatest resistance to aqueous outflow in open angle glaucoma. Therefore, procedures and devices in this category, aim to improve intraocular pressure (IOP) by reducing the resistance of or removing a part of the anterior wall of the trabecular meshwork. These include, shunts to facilitate flow of aqueous humour across the TM (iStent, Glaukos Corp; Hydrus, Ivantis Inc.), incisions in the TM [Trabectome, Neomedix Corporation; Trab360, Gonioscopy-assisted transluminal trabeculotomy (GATT)], dilation of the Schlemm canal [Ab interno canaloplasty (ABiC) and VISCO360, Sight Sciences], goniotomy, and excision of a strip of TM (Kahook Dual Blade).

Stents that bypass the trabecular meshwork reduce the resistance by providing more direct access to Schlemm canal and thereby the collector channels. The efficacy of these stents may in part be influenced by where the stent is placed relative to active collector channels, which is difficult to predict. Postoperative IOPs of these procedures are limited by the episcleral venous pressure.

iStent (glaukos corporation)

This is a heparin-coated, nonferromagnetic titanium L-shaped stent measuring approximately 1.0 by 0.3 mm that is inserted into Schlemm canal. In a prospective randomised controlled trial (RCT) of patients with mild-to-moderate glaucoma, the proportion of patients with IOP of 21 mmHg or less without medications was significantly higher in the combined cataract surgery plus single istent arm (61%) compared to the cataract surgery alone arm (50%) ($p = 0.036$). There was no statistical difference in the proportion of patients with an IOP reduction of at least 20% without medications in the two groups (53% vs. 44% respectively, $p = 0.09$). There was no reported difference in complications. Multiple istent implants may achieve greater the IOP-lowering effect.

iStent inject (glaukos corporation)

This second-generation trabecular bypass device from Glaukos measuring 360×230 μm

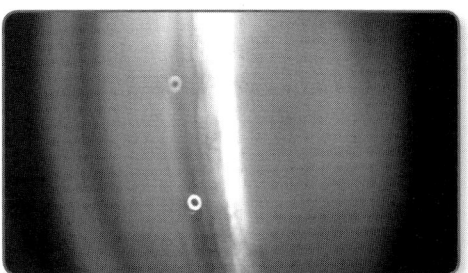

Figure 53.1 Gonioscopic view of two istent injects. *Courtesy: Mr Keith Barton, Moorfields eye Hospital.*

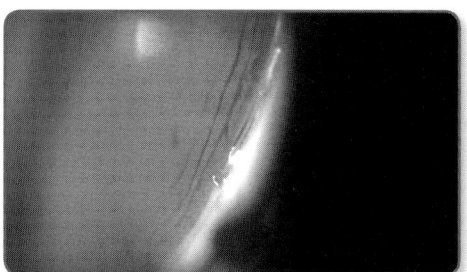

Figure 53.2 Gonioscopic view of Hydrus. (*For colour version see plate 3*) *Courtesy: Mr Keith Barton, Moorfields eye Hospital.*

is made with the same material as the original istent. There are two stents in each injector and the stents are typically injected 30–60° apart through the nasal trabecular meshwork into Schlemm canal (**Figure 53.1**). In a prospective RCT of primary open-angle glaucoma (POAG) patients not controlled on a single topical medication, implantation of two iStent injects was found to be at least as effective as a fixed combination of latanoprost and timolol at the 12-month follow-up. A recent second-generation of iStent Inject (iStent Inject W) with a wider flange has recently been introduced.

Hydrus (Ivantis Incorporation)

This is an 8-mm long nickel-titanium alloy that is injected into the Schlemm canal and acts as a scaffold to dilate the canal for approximately 3 clock hours, providing access to multiple collector channels. 1–2 mm of the inlet is left in the anterior chamber to drain fluid into Schlemm canal (**Figure 53.2**). In a prospective RCT of POAG patients with visually significant cataracts (HORIZON Study), a higher proportion of patients in the combined cataract surgery plus Hydrus implant arm had at least 20% reduction of unmedicated IOP compared to the cataract surgery alone arm at 2 years (77.3% vs. 57.8% group, $p < 0.01$). Focal peripheral anterior synechiae were found in 18% of the Hydrus implant group, but were not found to be associated with an increase in IOP.

Ab interno canaloplasty (ABiC)

In ABiC, a microcatheter is used to cannulate Schlemm canal though an ab interno small incision of the trabecular meshwork. Viscoelastics is then injected through the catheter to viscodilate Schlemm canal and the proximal the collector channels, aiming to break any obstructions and adhesions. One of the devices used for ABiC is the iTrack microcatheter (*Ellex*), a 250-μm microcatheter with an illuminated tip. The manufacturer reported a 37% reduction in mean IOP and 67% reduction in mean number of medications at 1 year in 98 patients who underwent the procedure. No serious adverse events were noted.

Trabectome (NeoMedix Incorporation)

This device uses electrocautery to achieve ab interno goniotomy. A hand piece is introduced through a clear corneal incision and with a combination of irrigation, aspiration, and ablation a thin strip of TM is removed. There is currently no randomised prospective studies available but there have been reports of reduction in both IOP (>30%) and post-operative number of medications. The most common complications associated with the procedure are hyphaema, corneal injury, peripheral anterior synechiae, and transient IOP spikes.

Increasing uveoscleral outflow

There is currently no commercially available MIGS device in this category. Supraciliary stents would be placed in the potential space between the sclera and the ciliary body. This creates a controlled cyclodialysis cleft, with the dimensions of the cleft limited by the size of the stent. These stents would have the advantage over the trabecular bypass stents in that their effect is not limited by how close they are to active collector channels or by the episcleral venous pressure. The only commercially available device in this category, Cypass Micro-Stent (*Alcon Inc.*), was recently (August 2018) withdrawn globally by the manufacturer following the results of a 5-year follow-up trial.

Creating a subconjunctival filtration pathway

The subconjunctival pathway is a non-physiological pathway that has been the route of aqueous drainage for traditional glaucoma surgery. This method of aqueous drainage produces a subconjunctival bleb, therefore, can be associated with bleb-related complications that are seen in trabeculectomy and tube surgery.

XEN gel stent (*allergan plc.*)

The XEN45 gel stent is a 6-mm stent with an internal diameter of 45 μm (**Figures 53.3a and b**). It is made from porcine collagen cross linked with glutaraldehyde and becomes pliable when hydrated. The stent creates a channel from the anterior chamber to the subconjunctival space to form a bleb. Mitomycin C (MMC) is frequently applied subconjunctivally prior to the procedure. The gel stent works on the basis of Poiseuille's law – the length and inner diameter of the tube control the flow rate to prevent hypotony. Bleb needlings may enhance the function of fibrosed blebs but there is currently no long-term data. Serious complications of XEN implant such implant exposure and endophthalmitis are rare but have been reported.

Reducing aqueous production

Endocyclophotocoagulation (iridex oculight)

In endocyclophotocoagulation (ECP), the anterior ciliary processes are treated with an 810-nm diode laser while under direct visualisation using an endoscopic laser probe. In a retrospective nonrandomised matched-control study of POAG patients, there was a greater proportion of patients with combined cataract surgery plus ECP who had IOP < 21 mmHg and > 20% IOP reduction compared to cataract surgery alone at 1 year (69.6% vs. 40%, p = 0.004). The former group also had a greater reduction in number of medication (0.73 ± 0.71 vs. 0.23 ± 0.56; p = 0.001). Reported complications include intraocular inflammation, raised intraocular pressure, and cystoid macular oedema, which resolved with medical treatment.

Discussion

Minimally invasive glaucoma surgery has the potential to provide less invasive and lower risk surgical interventions to patients with drop intolerances and non-compliance issues who may otherwise have to undergo traditional

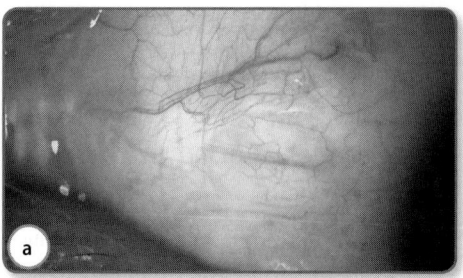
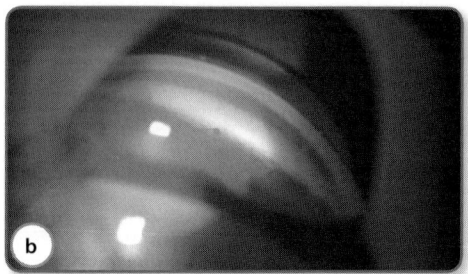

Figures 53.3a and b (a) Subconjunctival portion of XEN implant with a shallow diffuse bleb. (b) Gonioscopic view of the intraocular portion of the XEN implant. (*For colour version see plate 3*)
Courtesy: Mr Keith Barton, Moorfields eye Hospital.

surgery. However, the current published data on MIGS are of variable quality and lack standardisation, which makes it difficult to compare the devices and to identify the ideal patient population for each device. There also needs to be more study on the long-term clinical and economic efficacy of MIGS so that we can understand how MIGS can best complement the current armamentarium of glaucoma medication and traditional surgery.

Further reading

Agrawal P, Bradshaw SE. Systematic Literature Review of Clinical and Economic Outcomes of Micro-Invasive Glaucoma Surgery (MIGS) in Primary Open-Angle Glaucoma. Ophthalmol Ther 2018; 7:49–73.

Fingeret M, Dickerson JE Jr. The Role of Minimally Invasive Glaucoma Surgery Devices in the Management of Glaucoma. Optom Vis Sci 2018; 95:155–162.

Richter GM, Coleman AL. Minimally invasive glaucoma surgery: current status and future prospects. Clin Ophthalmol 2016; 10:189–206.

Related topics of interest

- Glaucoma – primary open angle (p. 165)

54 Myasthenia gravis

Key points

- Myasthenia gravis is a potentially life-threatening condition
- Ninety percent of patients with ocular myasthenia will develop systemic disease within 2 years
- Fifty percent of patients with ocular myasthenia are seronegative – negative blood tests do not exclude the diagnosis
- Patients with myasthenia gravis require radiological imaging (CT or MRI) to exclude a thymoma
- Myasthenia gravis is an autoimmune condition and many patients require long-term immunosuppression

Epidemiology

Myasthenia gravis affects all races and ages with an annual incidence of 150–250 per million. Overall, females are more often affected. Amongst younger patients, women predominate and amongst older patients, men predominate. Juvenile myasthenia gravis is defined as onset before the age of 15 years.

Pathophysiology

Myasthenia gravis is an autoimmune disease in which antibodies bind to acetylcholine receptors (AChRs) or functionally related molecules on the post-synaptic membrane of the neuromuscular junction. The result is impaired neuromuscular transmission leading to muscle weakness and fatigability. Antibodies against AChR, muscle-specific kinase (MUSK), and lipoprotein receptor-related protein 4 (LRP4) are sensitive and specific for the diagnosis of myasthenia. 10–15% of all patients are seronegative and 50% of patients with ocular myasthenia are seronegative. In seronegative patients, the diagnosis is secured by electrophysiological testing and response to therapy. In approximately 10% of patients, the condition is associated with a tumour of the thymus gland (thymoma). Congenital myasthenic syndrome is a distinct condition.

It is related to gene abnormalities that cause changes to the proteins which play a role in transmission at the neuromuscular junction.

Myasthenia gravis can be subdivided into the following categories:

- Generalised myasthenia (66%):
  - Late onset: Age > 50
  - Early onset: Age < 50 (including juvenile myasthenia)
- Ocular (10–15%)
- Seronegative (10–15%)
- Thymoma (10%)
- MUSK (1–10%)
- LRP4 (1–3%)

Clinical features

Myasthenia gravis is characterised by variable, fatigable, muscle weakness.

Ocular myasthenia may involve the levator palpebrae superioris, the extraocular muscles (EOM), and the orbicularis oculi. Ptosis may be isolated or seen in combination with extraocular muscle involvement. Ptosis often begins unilaterally but in most cases will become bilateral. Often, ptosis is absent on waking and more evident in the evening. Myasthenic ptosis will become more pronounced with manual elevation of the opposite lid although this is not pathognomic. Cogan lid twitch is suggestive of myasthenia. This is elicited by asking the patient to look down for 10 seconds and then to make a vertical saccade into primary position. During a positive test, the upper lid will elevate and then gradually become ptotic, or the lid will twitch.

Involvement of the extraocular muscles is common and often coexists with involvement of the levator palpebrae superioris. Any combination of muscle involvement can occur and myasthenia may mimic a cranial nerve palsy, internuclear ophthalmoplegia or a gaze palsy. Saccades will be of normal velocity contrasting with neurologic ophthalmoplegia which will have reduced saccadic velocity.

Patients with myasthenia often have weakness of the orbicularis muscle. This can be tested by attempting to manually open the patients' eyes during forced lid closure. Some patients may develop scleral show following a period of complete lid apposition during voluntary lid closure. This is caused by muscle fatigue.

Myasthenia does not cause clinically noticeable pupillary abnormalities.

Systemic clinical features of myasthenia include bulbar involvement – dysarthria, dysphagia, dyspnoea, and masticatory weakness. Limb muscles may also be involved. Proximal, symmetric weakness is most common with arms affected more frequently than legs. Axial muscle involvement may lead to weakness of neck flexion and extension. Respiratory muscle involvement can cause exertional dyspnoea, orthopnoea, tachypnoea or respiratory failure. This is a potentially life-threatening complication. The term myasthenic crisis is used for patients requiring intubation and ventilation due to the severity of the respiratory muscle involvement. Often this is associated with severe oropharyngeal weakness which can result in upper respiratory tract obstruction or severe dysphagia with aspiration.

Investigations

Ice test

- The strength of myasthenic muscles improves with cooling. This is thought to be due to a reduction in the effect of acetylcholinesterase. The ice test can be used in suspected myasthenic patients with ptosis and has a sensitivity of 90% and 100% specificity. The test is performed as follows – the size of the palpebral aperture in the primary position is measured. The patient is asked to close their eyes for 2 minutes and the palpebral aperture is measured again. Crushed ice, wrapped in a surgical glove is applied to the ptotic lid for 2 minutes. The palpebral aperture is then measured again. If the ptosis improves more than 2 mm after the application of the ice compared with eye closure alone then the test is considered positive

Sleep test

- In the majority of patients, ptosis and diplopia are better on waking and worsen over the course of the day. This is thought to be related to resting of these muscles overnight. A similar principle can be employed as a clinical test. The patient's ocular alignment and palpebral aperture are measured and they are then asked to close their eyes. After 30 minutes of eyelid closure, the ocular alignment and palpebral aperture are measured again. Patients with myasthenia should show a significant improvement in their measurements

Autoantibodies

- Acetylcholine receptor antibodies are highly specific for myasthenia gravis. AChR antibodies are directly pathogenic via crosslinking of AChRs leading to accelerated degradation of these receptors through complement binding and activation and by inducing AChR conformational changes or blocking acetylcholine binding
- Muscle-specific kinase antibodies are associated with more severe generalised disease. Facial and bulbar muscles are frequently affected. MUSK antibodies are not associated with the pure ocular subgroup, however, ocular signs are sometimes observed in conjunction with generalised features of disease
- *Lipoprotein receptor-related protein 4 (LRP4):* Patients tend to have mild disease. It has been reported as positive in some patients within the ocular subgroup
- Agrin, collagen Q, and cortactin autoantibodies have been detected in some patients
- Titin and ryanodine antibodies have been proposed as markers of severe disease

Pharmacologic testing

- A short-acting (edrophonium) or longer acting (neostigmine) anticholinesterase can be administered intravenously/intramuscularly to assess improvement of suspected myasthenia signs, e.g. ptosis or extraocular motility abnormalities.

These two tests are rarely used now due to the risk of associated systemic side effects related to over-stimulation of the parasympathetic nervous system, e.g. bradycardia, asystole, syncope, and seizures. If the test is to be performed, IV atropine, resuscitation equipment, and trained personnel, e.g. an anaesthetist should be available

Nerve stimulation tests

- *Repetitive nerve stimulation:* Repetitive supramaximal motor nerve stimulation (2–3 Hz). If there is a 10% reduction in amplitude between the 1st and 5th response to stimulation, then this is abnormal. There is a wide sensitivity range (50–100%), therefore a negative test does not exclude the diagnosis
- *Single fibre electromyography:* Useful to help secure a diagnosis in patients who are antibody-negative. It is positive in 88–99% of all patients with myasthenia gravis. Myasthenic patients have increased 'jitter' and 'blocking'. Single fibre EMG abnormalities are also found in other neuromuscular transmission disorders including Lambert–Eaton syndrome, botulism and congenital myasthenic syndromes. Oculopharyngeal dystrophy and amyotrophic lateral sclerosis can also cause increased jitter

Other tests

- CT/MR of the thymus (chest X-ray lacks sensitivity to detect thymomas)
- FBC, ESR, ANA, and TFTs should be performed in all patients diagnosed with myasthenia due to the association with thyroiditis and systemic lupus erythematosus (SLE)

Diagnosis

A diagnosis of myasthenia gravis is not based on one test alone but is made with reference to the clinical symptoms and signs, the results of the above-mentioned investigations and response to treatment.

Treatment

Drugs

- All subgroups of myasthenia gravis respond to inhibition of acetylcholinesterase. The most effective drug is generally pyridostigmine. If patients respond well to pyridostigmine, then additional medication may not be required. Propantheline can be given for gastrointestinal side effects
- The MUSK subgroup tends to respond poorly to acetylcholinesterase inhibition
- Immunosuppression is required if patients fail to have a satisfactory response to inhibition of acetylcholinesterase. Prednisolone or prednisolone in combination with azathioprine is most often used as the first line. Prednisolone has been reported to reduce the risk of progression to generalised disease in patients presenting with ocular features
- Azathioprine has a synergistic effect with prednisolone and helps to reduce the dose of steroid required. Thiopurine methyltransferase (TPMT) activity should be tested before treatment commences as low or absent levels are associated with toxicity
- Mycophenolate mofetil, methotrexate, cyclosporine, and tacrolimus have been used for second-line immunosuppression
- Rituximab has shown potent effects in severe myasthenia gravis that is refractory to prednisolone and azathioprine

Thymectomy

- Patients with myasthenia gravis and a thymoma should undergo thymectomy. Early thymectomy in early onset myasthenia gravis has been shown to be beneficial. Most of these patients have thymic hyperplasia

Myasthenic crisis

- Intravenous immune globulin or plasma exchange are the treatments of choice. Immune globulin is often more easily administered
- Intensive care admission
- Treatment of exacerbating factors, e.g. infections

Further reading

Gilhus NE. Myasthenia gravis. N Engl J Med 2016; 375:2570–2581.

Gilhus NE, Verschuuren JJ. Myasthenia gravis: subgroup classification and therapeutic strategies. Lancet Neurol 2015; 14:1023–1036.

Related topics of interest

- Imaging in ophthalmology (p. 176)
- Cranial nerve palsies – multiple cranial nerves palsies (p. 104)

55 Neovascular glaucoma

Key points

- Neovascular glaucoma leads to a secondary angle closure often associated with severe vision loss
- Treatment of the underlying retinal ischaemia remains key to achieving disease control
- Panretinal photocoagulation and anti-vascular endothelial growth factor (VEGF) treatments offer synergistic treatment benefits
- The long-term need for incisional glaucoma surgery is high

Epidemiology

Neovascular glaucoma (NVG) poses a significant management challenge, but when present, the visual outcome is often poor. The disease is multifactorial in its aetiology, and evidence reporting the overall disease prevalence is sparse.

For the majority of cases, retinal ischaemia is the common pathway leading to NVG. The common causes of retinal ischaemia are central retinal vein occlusion, proliferative diabetic retinopathy (PDR), each accounting for one-third of cases, ocular ischaemic syndrome (OIS), reportedly 13%, and less commonly also after central retinal artery occlusion (CRAO)–both OIS and CRAO are typically associated with carotid artery disease.

The overall risk of an ischaemic CRVO leading to NVG is thought to be 45%; the risk of an ischaemic hemiretinal vein occlusion leading to NVG is small, 3% in one series.

In PDR, the probability of developing NVG exceeds 20%.

Pathophysiology

In NVG, the following events must occur in sequence:
- Hypoxia associated with retinal ischaemia is known to drive the release of VEGF, key to the process of angiogenesis–primarily VEGF-A. There is also some evidence to support the role of inflammatory cytokines
- Angiogenic factors accumulate anteriorly, leading to the development of neovascularisation of the iris (NVI) and iridocorneal angle (NVA). An associated fibrovascular membrane develops over the iris and subsequently also over the angle, leading to an outflow obstruction
- Progression to the formation of peripheral anterior synechiae will occur as this membrane contracts, giving rise to secondary angle closure and also the formation of ectropion uveae

The stage at which neovascularisation is identified, will determine the likelihood of the presence of glaucoma, and also aides in predicting whether its management will be refractory to medical management.

In addition to the common vascular causes outlined, NVG also presents in association with the following groups of diseases:
- Uveitis – both anterior and posterior; including Behçet's, sarcoidosis, sympathetic ophthalmia and Vogt-Koyanagi–Harada syndrome
- Tumours – iris, ciliary body and choroidal melanoma; retinoblastoma; ocular lymphoma
- Radiation of ocular malignancies – external/proton beam, plaques – leading to retinopathy and ischaemia
- Other retinopathies – Coats' disease; Sickle cell retinopathy; Eales disease; chronic retinal detachment +/– proliferative vitreoretinopathy

Clinical features

Symptoms
- Will vary with the stage, severity and cause of the disease, but can include recent loss of vision, photophobia, pain or headache often corresponding with raised intraocular pressure. Patients may also be asymptomatic in the early stages of the disease

Signs
- Should include evidence of NVI, fine peripupillary new vessels extending peripherally, and/or NVA; associated

hyphaema; presence of anterior chamber flare and cells
- Gonioscopy is essential to stage the disease – look for angle new vessels; if open, observe for a fibrovascular membrane. Membrane proliferation and contraction will lead to peripheral anterior synechiae, and also ectropion uveae
- Intraocular pressure (IOP) may be normal in the earlier stages, but typically rises with disease evolution to a high level; glaucomatous optic neuropathy may be found at presentation or develop; visual field loss may also be elicited
- Corneal oedema may preclude a clear fundus view; fundoscopy, if possible, may identify the event leading to retinal ischaemia – including signs of CRVO, PDR or OIS, or supportive evidence of the less common causes

Investigations

- A detailed undilated anterior segment slit-lamp examination + gonioscopy (as above) are key initial investigations
- Where the media view permits, dilated fundoscopy may be supported by fundus fluorescein angiography to establish the presence and extent of retinal ischaemia, or of other retinal pathology. For example, Choroidal mass lesions or retinal detachment
- Anterior segment fluorescein angiography– useful to detect the early presence of NVI, or where the slit-lamp findings are equivocal
- Carotid Doppler ultrasound – useful in support of a suspected case of OIS
- B-scan ultrasound – if media are unclear, an important exam to exclude mass lesions of the retina or choroid, retinal detachment; also, to assess the vitreous for haemorrhage or vitritis

Further appropriate systemic investigations may stem from any of the above.

Diagnosis

Early diagnosis of neovascularisation, and its effective treatment, is thought to limit or delay the onset of NVG. Therefore, effective surveillance of high-risk cases is essential.

A relevant history, including systemic disease profile, and a thorough anterior and posterior segment examination, including IOP, are likely to lead to a high diagnostic yield. The above auxiliary investigations may also be useful, particularly in the context of media opacity, in order to understand the aetiology of a particular case.

In the presence of established retinal ischaemia, and evidence of anterior segment neovascularisation with elevated IOP, and either an open angle or synechial angle closure, NVG is the likely diagnosis.

If marked cornea oedema is present, anterior segment details and retinal status may not be assessable, this can introduce initial diagnostic uncertainty until the media is clear. Effective medical control of the IOP can improve the clinical detail.

Treatment

There are two related main elements to the effective management of NVG:
- Reduction of the ischaemic drive
  - Treating the underlying systemic/local disease process
  - Treating the resultant neovascularization (Laser/anti-VEGF)
- Control of IOP
  - Topical/systemic ocular antihypertensives
  - Surgical [glaucoma drainage devices (GDD)/cyclophotocoagulation)

Reduction of the ischaemic drive

In the presence of NVG, evidence supports panretinal photocoagulation (PRP) targeted at areas of retinal ischaemia to reduce VEGF production as a key treatment, also reducing the demand for oxygen.

Having established the role of VEGF in neovascularisation, intravitreal anti-VEGF treatment has emerged as an important treatment option, effective in achieving rapid NVI/NVA regression within 3 days of injection. Bevacizumab has been used off-label widely in this context, but ranibizumab and aflibercept have also been shown to be effective alternatives.

If used in isolation, regression is thought to last 8–10 weeks. Evidence supports their use as an adjunct to PRP rather than in isolation, often improving media clarity, thereby allowing effective application of PRP to achieve prolonged neovascular regression.

Success in achieving NVI/NVA regression is thought to delay progression through the stages of NVG to the sequelae of refractory synechial angle closure glaucoma.

Control of intraocular pressure

The threat of severe, irreversible vision loss from advanced glaucomatous optic neuropathy is as important as the visual sequelae of the retinal ischaemic disease that is the pathological drive. Control of the IOP also facilitates management of the retinal ischaemic disease by maintaining clarity of media, particularly the cornea.

In the presence of open angles and early neovascularisation, IOP may be normal or medically manageable (using all tolerated classes of topical/systemic ocular antihypertensives). Topical steroid in the presence of inflammation may be used.

As synechial angle closure evolves, NVG typically becomes refractory to medical management, requiring surgical control. In one study only 17% of open angle compared to 93% of closed angle treated NVG eyes required surgical control of IOP.

Both Ahmed valves and Baerveldt tubes, appear more successful in achieving surgical IOP control than bleb-dependent trabeculectomy, where the marked inflammation associated with NVG is thought to lead to their failure.

Augmenting surgery with intravitreal anti-VEGF treatment appears to reduce the rate of perioperative complications such as hyphaema, which can compromise GDD function in the early postoperative period, and some evidence also supports better visual outcome success compared to unaugment surgery.

If despite achieving IOP control vitreous haemorrhage or lens opacity still precludes an adequate fundus view to perform PRP, then vitrectomy + endolaser may be indicated.

Cyclodiode laser may be considered in eyes with low visual potential, but at the risk of developing hypotony or progressing to phthisis.

If a modifiable underlying cause of retinal ischaemia is identified (e.g. Carotid stenosis in OIS, or chronic retinal detachment), then appropriate treatment should be explored.

Complications

Severe vision loss from the glaucomatous sequelae of neovascularisation of the anterior segment is of greatest concern in this condition. In the presence of the severe retinal ischaemia required to drive this disease process, the visual potential may already be guarded. If glaucoma existed prior to neovascularisation, the visual outcome is typically poorer.

Glaucoma surgery itself can give rise to complications. Neovascular vessels are friable; spontaneous hyphaema can arise, or complicate surgery peri- or postoperatively. If non-resolving vitreous haemorrhage is present, vitrectomy may be required.

The intravitreal administration of bevacizumab itself has a good safety profile from the experience of its use in treating choroidal neovascularisation, however, in eyes that are ischaemic as is the case here, there are isolated rare case reports of severe loss of vision immediately after its administration.

Further reading

Andrés-Guerrero V, Perucho-González L, García-Feijoo J, et al. Current Perspectives on the Use of Anti-VEGF Drugs as Adjuvant Therapy in Glaucoma. Adv Ther 2017; 34:378–395.

Hayreh SS. Neovascular glaucoma. Prog Retin Eye Res 2007; 26:470–485.

Wakabayashi T, Oshima Y, Sakaguchi H, et al. Intravitreal bevacizumab to treat iris neovascularization and neovascular glaucoma secondary to ischemic retinal diseases in 41 consecutive cases. Ophthalmology 2008; 115:1571–1580.

Related topics of interest

- Glaucoma – medical management (p. 162)
- Retinal vein occlusion (p. 290)
- Retinal lasers (p. 282)

56 Normal tension glaucoma

Key points

- Intraocular pressure (IOP) reduction remains key to management of normal tension glaucoma (NTG)
- High index of suspicion is needed to exclude nonglaucomatous optic neuropathy
- A large proportion of patients with NTG remain stable for 5 years even without treatment, and the risk of progression should be taken into account before treatment is initiated

Epidemiology

The prevalence of NTG varies across populations. Predominantly western population-based studies report the prevalence NTG to be 20–39% of patients diagnosed with a glaucomatous visual field defect, whereas 92% of Japanese patients with primary open angle glaucoma (POAG) were found to have IOP of <21 mmHg. The disease is more common in females and typically presents at an older age compared to patients with POAG.

Pathophysiology

The pathophysiology of NTG remains unclear. Trials, such as the Collaborative Normal Tension Glaucoma study (CNTGS) have shown that IOP reduction reduces the risk of NTG progression by two-thirds. However, a reduction in IOP alone does not appear to reduce progression in all cases. Furthermore, the CNGTS found that 40% of patients did not progress without treatment. Where the disease process of glaucoma is a multi-faceted combination of IOP-dependant and IOP independent factors, IOP-independant influences may be more significant in NTG.

IOP independent causes include vascular dysregulation and upregulation of inflammatory cytokines from oxidative stress leading to localised inflammation, resulting in compromised optic nerve head perfusion.

Other proposals for the presence of glaucoma in the context of 'normal pressures' include altered structural integrity at the lamina cribosa, cornea/scleral biomechanical factors causing erroneously low IOP measurements, and NTG being a result of a primarily central nervous system (CNS) neurodegenerative disorder manifesting in a glaucoma-like condition.

Some of the associations with systemic IOP-independent factors that have been identified to be involved in the onset and progression of NTG are shown in **Table 56.1**.

Clinical features

Apart from having IOP consistently less than 21 mm Hg in NTG, there are subtle features to distinguish this entity from POAG. Careful examination of the optic disc in NTG may reveal a thinner neuroretinal rim compared POAG eyes with similar visual field defects. Optic disc haemorrhages and b-zone peripapillary atrophy are also more frequently reported in NTG eyes. Peripapillary halos, seen as an area of absent retinal pigment epithelium (RPE) with localised cupping, may represent acquired optic nerve pits, are

Table 56.1 Risk factors for normal tension glaucoma

Ocular factors	Elevated intraocular pressure (IOP)
	Nocturnal IOP spikes
	Optic disc haemorrhage
	Myopia
Nonocular factors	Abnormal vasoregulation • Migraines • Raynaud's phenomenon • Anaemia
	Cardiovascular dysregulation • Systemic hypertension • Systemic hypotension • Nocturnal hypotension • Cardiac arrhythmias
	Obstructive sleep apnoea

usually located inferiorly and associated with disc haemorrhages and an increased risk of progression in NTG.

Visual field defects in NTG tend to occur closer to fixation and are often deeper and more focal as compared to POAG. Field losses in NTG may be greater than expected based on examination of the optic disc alone.

Investigations

Potential causes of secondary glaucoma such as previous steriod response, burnt-out pigmentary glaucoma or uveitis with previous high intraocular pressure should be excluded through comprehensive history and ocular examination. As a single clinic measurement of IOP may not be representative, phasing can be useful to differentiate high versus normal tension glaucoma due to diurnal variation in IOP.

Systemic investigations should be considered with the help of an internist to diagnose IOP independent risk factors such as nocturnal hypotension and obstructive sleep apnoea, especially when disease progression is refractory to IOP-lowering. In the event where progression continues despite optimisation of IOP and IOP independent risk factors, the diagnosis should be revisited.

Nonglaucomatous optic neuropathies, such as compressive, infiltrative or ischaemic aetiologies, can mimic NTG, and distinction between the two are important. Atypical examination findings should prompt neuroophthalmic evaluation and include neuroimaging (**Box 56.1**). However, there may be overlaps in examination findings. In the setting of advanced glaucomatous damage, reduced vision and dyschromatopsia may be found, and a relative afferent pupillary defect may be elicited in asymmetric glaucoma.

Treatment

Reduction of IOP is the only treatment effective in slowing disease progression. The CNTGS demonstrated that a 30% reduction in IOP reduced the risk of progression from 35–12%.

Lowering of IOP can be achieved medically, with laser trabeculoplasty (may not be as effective as in reducing IOP compared POAG/OHT cases but may alter diurnal IOP fluctuations) or filtration surgery. Prostaglandin analogues have been accepted to be first-line agents for IOP lowering.

Use of timolol to lower IOP is controversial. The Low-Pressure Glaucoma Treatment Study (LoGTS) comparing timolol with brimonidine (which is usually less tolerated due to side effects) as monotherapy showed greater rates of progression in timolol users, despite similar IOP reductions in both groups. It has been proposed that beta-blockers may aggravate systemic nocturnal hypotension leading to glaucoma progression and there has been a suggestion that the effects of brimonidine may also be in part due to neuroprotective effects. Given the reduction in aqueous production at night, aqueous suppressants (e.g. topical carbonic anhydrase inhibitors) may in theory have little effect on nocturnal IOP and hence ocular perfusion pressure, whilst lowering IOP during the daytime.

Some of the current research on the treatment of NTG is focused on neuroprotective agents as well as nutritional supplements and phytochemicals, which may have a role as adjunctive therapy in the future.

In patients who deteriorate despite reduction to single-digit IOP, optimisation of systemic risk factors for NTG (e.g. alteration in timing/dosage of systemic beta-blockers based on nocturnal dips, as demonstrated with 24-hour blood pressure monitoring) to maximise optic nerve head perfusion may help to slow disease progression.

> **Box 56.1 Clinical features suggesting nonglaucomatous optic neuropathy**
> - Optic disc neuroretinal rim pallor
> - Visual field defects along the vertical meridian
> - Visual field defect out of proportion to severity of disc excavation
> - Unexplained visual loss
> - Relative afferent pupillary defect
> - Abnormal colour vision

Prognosis

The CNGTS and the Early Manifest Glaucoma Trial (EMGT) reported similar findings that 40% of enrolled patients did not progress over 5 years without treatment. In the event of progression, the rate of visual field loss is generally slow. However, given the starting level of IOP, target pressures that may be adequate in POAG may not be appropriate and would need to be lowered in NTG patients. As further evidence becomes available, the significance of the potential suggested underlying mechanisms and theories in NTG pathogenesis will become clearer, which will hopefully result in better targeted treatment.

Further reading

Anderson DR, Drance SM, Schulzer M, et al. Natural history of normal-tension glaucoma. Ophthalmology 2001; 108:247–253.

Razeghinejad MR, Lee D. Managing normal tension glaucoma by lowering the intraocular pressure. Surv Ophthalmol 2019; 64:111–116.

Shaarawy T, Sherwood M, Hitchings R, et al. Normal-Tension Glaucoma. In: Glaucoma – Medical Diagnosis & Therapy (Vol. 1), 2nd edition. London: Elsevier 2015: 378–386.

Related topics of interest

- Glaucoma – medical management (p. 162)
- Glaucoma – primary open angle (p. 165)

57 Nystagmus

Key points
- Nystagmus is a rhythmical involuntary movement of the eyes
- Understanding different forms of nystagmus is essential for appropriate management

Epidemiology
The incidence of nystagmus in the UK has been reported to be between 1 and 2.4 per 1,000.

Pathophysiology and classification
The prerequisite for the development of a normal visual system is the integration of information from the afferent sensory system and ocular motor system during brain maturation in early childhood. Any eye condition that can cause sensory deprivation and poor vision which leads to interruption of stable ocular fixation has potential to cause nystagmus. Traditionally, this type was known as sensory deprivation nystagmus. If no underlying cause could be found, it was labelled as motor or idiopathic. Some of previously idiopathic types of nystagmus were explained by gene mutations, e.g. it was found that certain types of horizontal and periodic alternating nystagmus are caused by mutations in gene *FRMD7* on chromosome X. This gene is responsible for establishing asymmetric connections between starburst amacrine cells and ganglion cells in the retina.

Onset of nystagmus after the maturation of visual system will be considered as acquired and in contrast to infantile nystagmus it almost always causes oscillopsia – sensation of movement of visual world and decreased visual acuity.

Etiological classification of acquired nystagmus:
- Loss of vision (pre-chiasmal, chiasmal and post-chiasmal lesions)
- Peripheral vestibular input (Vestibular neuritis, Meniere's disease, and benign paroxysmal positional vertigo)
- Central nervous system disease (cerebellar and brainstem lesions)
- Metabolic causes, medication, and drugs

Clinical features
Nystagmus originates from dysfunction of the slow eye movement stabilising system responsible for maintaining steady fixation in the primary position, in eccentric gaze and while moving. The eye first drifts away (slow phase) which is followed by corrective saccadic movement aimed for refixation. This type is known as jerk nystagmus. The direction of nystagmus is by convention defined by its fast phase, even though the slow phase is pathological. Other features that are described are amplitude and velocity. In pendular nystagmus, there is no fast phase, eyes drifting back and forth with the same velocity. Infantile nystagmus is commonly the combination of jerk and pendular eye movements.

Nystagmus can be physiological – clinically relevant form is end point nystagmus, present only in extreme gaze, fatigable (dampens after a few beats), often low amplitude and symmetrical.

Pathological form of gaze-evoked nystagmus – present immediately on attempting eccentric gaze, it is sustained, often higher amplitude and asymmetrical. It is usually induced by intoxication (alcohol, sedatives, anticonvulsants, hypnotics) or structural CNS lesions.

Infantile nystagmus
There are three main forms of infantile nystagmus.

Infantile nystagmus syndrome
- Unifying diagnosis for nystagmus previously known as congenital motor and sensory nystagmus
- Usually occurs in first 3–6 months

- Compensatory head posture to bring the eyes in position with minimal or no nystagmus (Null point)

Fusion maldevelopment nystagmus syndrome
- Previously known as latent/manifest latent nystagmus
- Usually caused by strabismus or significant cataract which interrupts fusion
- Usually occurs later than infantile nystagmus syndrome (INS)

Spasmus nutans syndrome
- Idiopathic, asymmetrical, multiplanar pendular nystagmus with small amplitude
- Usually associated with head nodding and head tilt, occasionally strabismus
- Occurs between 4 months and 12 months, resolves by 5 years of age
- Diagnosis is made retrospectively

Acquired nystagmus

Peripheral vestibular nystagmus
- Horizontal jerk nystagmus, same direction in all positions of gaze, dampens with fixation
- Can be associated with hearing loss, tinnitus, vertigo, nausea, and vomiting

Central vestibular nystagmus
- Jerk or pendular, changing direction with different gazes, does not dampen with fixation
- Usually accompanied with acute onset of vertigo, nausea and dizziness

Other clinical types of acquired nystagmus:
- *Upbeat nystagmus:*
  - Focal lesions of pons and medulla
  - Lesions of anterior cerebellar vermis
  - Meningitis
  - Wernicke's encephalopathy
  - Tobacco, barbiturate intoxication
  - Organophosphate poisoning
- *Downbeat nystagmus:*
  - Vestibulocerebellar and cervicomedullary junction lesions (spinocerebellar degeneration, Arnold-Chiari malformation)
  - Metabolic disorders
  - Multiple sclerosis
  - Encephalitis
  - Paraneoplastic
  - Alcohol, medication intoxication (anticonvulsants, lithium, etc.)
  - Idiopathic.
- *Pendular nystagmus:*
  - Multiple sclerosis
  - Oculopalatal tremor – degeneration of olivary nucleus, asymmetric dissociated nystagmus, rhythmic movement of eyes, palate, face and larynx, persists in sleep
  - Oculomasticatory myorhythmia – pathognomonic for CNS Whipple disease
  - Complete loss of vision – monocular or binocular
  - Toluene toxicity
- *Periodic alternating nystagmus:*
  - Cerebellar (nodulus, uvula) and cervicomedullary junction lesions
  - Change of direction in regular cycles, each one can last for up to 4 minutes
- *Rebound nystagmus:*
  - Chronic cerebellar or brainstem disease
  - Gaze-evoked nystagmus which changes direction once back in primary position
- *Brun's nystagmus:*
  - Large cerebellopontine angle tumour
  - Combination of high amplitude and low frequency in the direction of gaze ipsilateral with the lesion and low amplitude and high frequency in contralateral gaze
- *Internuclear ophthalmoplegia:*
  - Lesions of medial longitudinal fasciculus in pons and midbrain
  - Combination of unilateral jerk horizontal oscillation of the abducting eye with adduction deficit of ipsilateral eye (which determinates the side of INO). This phenomenon resolves with patching of adducting eye
- *Pure torsional nystagmus:* Usually medullary lesions, often seen with ocular tilt reaction
- *See-saw nystagmus:*
  - Chiasmal lesion – pendular nystagmus, midbrain lesions – jerk nystagmus

– Intorsion and elevation of one eye and simultaneous extorsion and depression of the other eye

Nystagmoid movements, saccadic oscillations

These ocular movements are caused by dysfunction of the fast eye movement system. One of the postulated mechanisms is dysfunction of omnipause neurons in pons which then generates saccades that interrupt fixation.

- Square-wave jerks consist of a small amplitude saccade that interrupts fixation and a corrective saccade usually separated by 200-msec intervals. It may be normal to some extent, but if large or frequent, this could be a sign of Parkinson's disease, progressive supranuclear palsy, dementia, schizophrenia, and cerebellar disease
- Psychogenic (functional) saccadic oscillations are voluntarily induced rapid horizontal saccades which usually last for 5–10 seconds and cannot be sustained for longer than 30 seconds. Such individuals use strong convergence effort to initiate these episodes. Eyelid flutter, squinting and strained facial expression are common associated features. It can be interrupted by distraction or fixation on a target
- Ocular flutter refers to horizontal saccades and opsoclonus to multidirectional random saccades without an intersaccadic interval most common causes are viral encephalitis and paraneoplastic
- Induced convergence-retraction is a syndrome associated with dorsal midbrain lesions. Attempts to initiate upward saccade causes bilateral fast horizontal convergent movement oscillation and retraction of the globe. Vertical gaze palsy and light-near dissociation are other features of this syndrome
- Superior oblique myokymia is usually idiopathic episodic high-frequency monocular torsional oscillation that typically lasts for up to 10 seconds. It can be provoked by looking into the field of action of involved superior oblique. Occurs in healthy individuals, but rarely it can also be a sign of brainstem lesions

Investigations

Eye movements can be recorded with different methods. Analysing waveforms can reveal characteristic features and help in distinguishing certain types of nystagmus.

In most of the patients with acquired nystagmus, imaging techniques, like MRI scan, will be used to look for structural lesions (tumours, demyelination, stroke). Blood tests are done when suspecting inflammatory aetiology, vitamin deficiency, paraneoplastic syndrome, etc.

Diagnosis

Thorough history and clinical features will help to direct further diagnostic workup. In many types of nystagmus, specific features would help to localise lesion which can then be confirmed with imaging methods.

Treatment

The mainstay treatment for acquired nystagmus is to treat the underlying cause. For infantile and some selected cases of acquired nystagmus, there are five different modalities of treatment aimed to improve vision and correct compensatory head posture:

- Optical correction with prisms to bring the eyes to null position
- Contact lenses
- Medication – depending on type of nystagmus; gabapentin, memantine, baclofen, and valproate
- Botulinum toxin injections
- Surgery: Two types – four-muscle tenotomy and reattachment to reduce proprioceptive feedback, and Kestenbaum procedure aimed at shifting the null point

Further reading

Liu G, Volpe N, Galetta S. Neuro-ophthalmology: Diagnosis and Management, 2nd edition. US: Saunders 2010:587–610.

Miller NR, Subramanian P, Patel V. Walsh & Hoyt's Clinical Neuro-Ophthalmology: The Essentials, 3rd edition. Netherlands: Wolters Kluwer 2016;402–422.

Pane A, Miller N, Burdon M. The Neuro-Ophthalmology Survival Guide, 2nd edition. US: Elseviers 2017:253–273.

Related topics of interest

- Imaging in ophthalmology (p. 000)
- Headache (p. 172)
- Strabismus surgery (p. 312)

58 Ocular hypertension

Key points
- 'Landmark trials' have identified risk factors for progression of ocular hypertension
- Ocular hypertension (OHT) only requires treatment if visual impairment within the patients' lifetime is a risk
- A significant body of the population may have ocular hypertension

Epidemiology

The definition of OHT is one borne of epidemiology and is commonly specified as over 21 mmHg intraocular pressure (IOP), which is 2 standard deviations above the mean found in several large population-based studies. However, a single intraocular pressure measurement of 21 mmHg does not provide a suitable IOP to consider screening for glaucoma. Indeed, no single IOP level has been found to have adequate sensitivity and specificity when taken in isolation. OHT is only diagnosed in the absence of glaucomatous damage, open angles on gonioscopy and when there have been no prior episodes of angle closure. The prevalence of OHT varies with ethnicity and age.

Pathophysiology

The flow, production, and drainage of aqueous humour is in a fine equilibrium and disturbance to this can result in the variety of pathologies seen in this chapter. Aqueous is produced at the ciliary body at a rate estimated at 2.2–2.9 µL/min depending on age; the two drainage pathways are via the trabecular meshwork into episcleral veins and via the uveoscleral route. In OHT, it is thought that both pathways have reduced outflow.

There are several landmark papers that have identified the main risk factors for the development of glaucoma from OHT and the progression rate is around 1–2% annually. The main risk factors for conversion are race, age, central corneal thickness (CCT), vertical cup/disc ratio, IOP, and mean VF defect. OHTS study found that African Americans were more at risk of progression. However, larger cup/disc ratios are also found more commonly in African American population. Eyes with thinner corneas were also more at risk of progression as were larger C/D ratios and larger mean VF deficits.

Investigations

The assessment of a patient with OHT or referred for assessment of OHT begins in a similar way as for the assessment of a patient with primary open-angle glaucoma as this is a significant differential (see Chapter 42).

Current NICE guidelines state that the following tests must be offered at initial assessments:
- Visual field assessment using standard automated perimetry (central thresholding test), repeated, if necessary, to establish severity at diagnosis (e.g. Humphy Visual Field)
- Optic nerve assessment and fundus examination using stereoscopic slit lamp biomicroscopy, with pupil dilatation
- IOP measurement using Goldmann applanation tonometry (slit lamp mounted)
- Peripheral anterior chamber configuration and depth assessments using gonioscopy or Van Herrick peripheral anterior chamber depth assessment where unable to perform gonioscopy
- Central corneal thickness measurement (these can be performed with optical or ultrasound pachymeter)
- Disc imaging must be performed as a baseline assessment

When assessing the patient with OHT, Humphrey visual fields are commonly performed with a 24-2 pattern that tests the central 48°. 30-2 and 10-2 are commonly used as well but in certain situations rather than routinely. The fields are assessed for any evidence of glaucoma or alternate optic neuropathy. It is important that the reliability indices are also considered, these often improve in capable patients due to a learning effect. Automated perimetry can be tiring for patients and sometimes faster testing times or even manual Goldmann perimetry can obtain more reliable information. SITA (Swedish interactive threshold algorithm) may decrease testing time and increase reliability.

Central corneal thickness is an independent risk factor for the progression of OHT to glaucoma but also affects the reading of intraocular pressure by devices such as non-contact tonometer (NCT) and Goldmann applanation tonometry with thinner corneas reading a lower pressure.

Disc imaging may be performed by a multitude of technologies including glaucoma diagnostics (GDx) and Heidelberg retinal tomography (HRT) (replaced by OCT mostly), OCT and disc photography. Each has strengths and weaknesses and OCT is currently one of the more popular modalities. An ever-present risk with new technologies is with regards to legacy data. Often old scans are not able to be incorporated into new machines or alternate modalities making comparisons with historic data challenging in this is especially challenging as changes may take years to manifest increasing the likelihood of systems becoming replaced. Disc photographs are a useful way of circumventing this issue.

Treatment

Not all ocular hypertensives require treatment. The need for treatment must be based on the risk of visual impairment within that patient's lifetime taking account of IOP, CCT, family history, and life expectancy.

A generic prostaglandin analogue is recommended by NICE as a cost-effective first-line drug if treatment is required. If no treatment is required, then the patient may be monitored in the primary care community setting. The current IOP threshold in the UK for hospital/specialist monitoring of OHT is 24 mmHg. If treatment has been commenced, then review intervals are based on the risk of progression from the results of the assessment and risk of progression.

Combinations of medications are sometimes required to lower the pressure satisfactorily to reduce the risk of vision loss. Topical medication can cause a range of side effects from redness, conjunctivitis, swelling, dizziness, and allergy. Thus switching medications to avoid systemic or local problems is recommended. NICE guidelines suggest an alternate prostaglandin then a beta-blocker should be the first change, but if these are not tolerated, then carbonic anhydrase inhibitors, sympathomimetics or miotics may be considered.

Preservatives are additives in drops to improve the shelf-life of the drug and they may also play some role in bioavailability. Sadly they are also responsible for some of the ocular surface disease problems that can occur with topical glaucoma medications, additionally some individuals may be allergic to these preservatives. Preservative-free drops are now commonplace in the market and indicated in ocular surface disease or in patients with allergies.

Due to increasing demands on glaucoma services, cost-effective strategies for managing low-risk OHT patients and stable POAG have been developed including virtual and optometry-delivered services. At virtual clinics, patients have their tests performed by technicians and then these results are reviewed at a later time.

Complications

Glaucoma is an increasingly prevalent disease and blindness is a great concern to patients. For patients with a low-risk for progression to glaucoma, it is important that they are reassured that blindness is very unlikely and advised to maintain regular reviews. There is a significant potential morbidity associated with anxiety.

Topical medication has the potential for side effects and if these occur, the risk of progression to glaucoma must be considered before considering other options. Close monitoring is sometimes an appropriate option for elevated pressures in an at-risk patient who has no evidence of glaucoma but is troubled by significant side effects of treatment.

Commonly OHT is detected by optometrists via NCT. Ideally before referral to a secondary service, repeat measurements on separate occasions via NCT should be performed if a Goldmann applanation tonometer is unavailable. NICE guidelines state that a decision to refer should not be based on IOP alone. It has been highlighted by studies such as the EPIC-Norfolk Eye Study that there is a large potential healthcare burden; the incidence of OHT was found to be 10% and suspect glaucoma 7% in a healthy volunteer cohort. Mechanisms to manage this body of patients in a cost-effective manner is set to become an increasingly important aspect in the delivery of care.

Further reading

Brubaker RF. Flow of aqueous humour in humans. Invest Ophthal Mol Vis Sci 1992; 32:3145–3165.

National Institute for Health and Care Excellence. External validation of the OHTS-EGPS model for predicting the 5-year risk of open-angle glaucoma in ocular hypertensives. [online] Available from https://www.nice.org.uk/guidance/ng81 [Last accessed October, 2019].

Takwoingi Y, Botello AP, Burr JM, et al. Surveillance for ocular hypertension study group. Br J Ophthalmol 2014; 98:309–314.

Related topics of interest

- Glaucoma – primary open angle (p. 165)
- Optic disc imaging (p. 232)
- Perimetry (p. 248)

59 Ophthalmia neonatorum

Key points
- The commonest infection in the first month of life
- Timely treatment is highly effective and economical
- A lifetime of blindness can result, if untreated

Epidemiology

The incidence of ophthalmia neonatorum (ON) is reported as 1–24% of all neonates, varying between and within countries according to socioeconomic risk factors. In Africa, between 1,000 and 4,000 are blinded by ON each year.

Prevalence of chlamydial disease is 2–20% amongst pregnant women. Gonococcal cervical disease prevalence is approximately 22% in developing economies (1% in affluent countries). Rates of gonococcal ON are around 5% in sub-Saharan Africa and 100 times less in Europe.

Pathophysiology

Ophthalmia neonatorum is synonymous with neonatal conjunctivitis; conjunctival inflammation in the first month of life, typically due to infection though not exclusively so. Aetiology depends on the complex interplay between geographical, socioeconomic, and healthcare-related factors, amongst others.

Sexually acquired cervical *Neisseria gonorrhoea* or herpes simplex (HSV) may transfer to a neonate during vaginal delivery. An untreated mother with *Chlamydia* will pass the infection, intrapartum, to the infant in a third of cases.

Non-gonococcal neonatal bacterial conjunctivitis can be caused by *Staphylococcus aureus*, *Streptococcus pneumoniae*, and various gram-negative organisms. Congenital blockage of the nasolacrimal system may cause recurrent cases.

Herpes simplex virus has important systemic consequences; neonates have an immature immune system and ocular surface infection can result in disseminated disease, encephalitis, pneumonitis, and hepatitis and profound comorbidity. Transmission, to the baby, of primary maternal herpetic disease, occurs at far higher rates (60%) than reactivated disease (2%).

In some countries, neonates receive universal prophylactic topical treatment, especially where ON is highly prevalent and access to microbiological testing is limited. Prophylactic therapies can cause a chemical conjunctivitis. Therapies include 1% silver nitrate, 2.5% povidone iodine, and 0.5% erythromycin ointment. Advantages of povidone iodine (vs silver nitrate) include:
- Reduced incidence of ON by 44% (vs. 24%)
- Greater efficacy in treating *Chlamydia* and non-inferiority against *Gonococcus*
- Single treatment is effective and inexpensive

Clinical features

A history of recent maternal sexually transmitted infection (STI) may suggest the candidate pathogen. There is commonly co-contraction of more than one STI.

Chlamydial infection can be indicated by pneumonitis, rhinitis, and otitis. Pseudomembrane formation may be present. If untreated, the conjunctivitis will resolve however, corneal scarring and visual loss can occur. Onset is often after babies have left hospital so presentation is commonly initially to primary care (**Table 59. 1**).

Table 59.1 Clinical syndrome descriptors related to microbiological cause of ophthalmia neonatorum

Pathogenic organism	Onset	Discharge characteristics
Chlamydia	4–28 days	Mucopurulent
Gonococcus	1–3 days	Hyper-purulent
Bacterial (non-gonococcal)	2–5 days	Purulent
Herpetic	1–14 days	Watery
Chemical	Within 48 h of topical therapy	Watery

The hallmark of gonococcal disease is early onset and profuse purulent discharge.

Other bacterial causes are more common in the context of assisted ventilation or lacrimal stasis.

Herpetic disease may cause a vesicular rash on the eyelids, swollen eyelids, keratitis, and anterior uveitis. Neonatal keratoconjunctivitis can lead to serious systemic comorbidity.

Chemical conjunctivitis develops within 1 or 2 days of topical treatment. Gram stain shows leukocytes but no infiltrates. Symptoms often settle after a couple of days, once the causative treatment is discontinued.

Investigations

Diagnostic certainty may be difficult based on the clinical findings alone. Microbiological investigations are invaluable in confirming the cause and targeting treatment. Discovery of a conjunctival STI mandates referral to genitourinary medicine (GUM) for sexual contract tracing and treatment to prevent further spread of disease and infertility.

In suspected gonococcal disease, a Gram stain on conjunctival scrapings from the palpebral conjunctiva should be performed urgently. Gram-negative diplococci in polymorphonuclear leukocytes suggest gonococcal conjunctivitis. Multinucleated giant cells may be present in HSV. Conjunctival scrapings should be taken for PCR; especially useful in chlamydial and HSV infection. Intracytoplasmic inclusion bodies on a Giemsa stain support chlamydial conjunctivitis but unlike adults are non-specific. PCR and ELISA have superseded other chlamydial tests with the advantage of greater sensitivity and specificity (**Table 59.2**).

Conjunctival cultures are useful in determining a bacterial cause.

Fluid from skin vesicles can be sent for viral culture for HSV. Epithelial cells infected with HSV may show eosinophilic intranuclear inclusions on Papanicolaou smear.

Diagnosis

Clinical syndromes are distinctive and determined by the responsible organism. These are summarised in **Table 59.1** and

Table 59.2 Key points for management of ophthalmia neonatorum according to pathogenic organism

Pathogenic organism	Confirmatory/ supportive tests	Suggested treatment	Further management
Chlamydia	Chlamydial culture or PCR	Oral erythromycin – neonate Adult carriers: azithromycin single dose – mother and sexual partners	GUM referral for contact tracing of sexual partners Repeat swabs to confirm eradication
Gonococcus	Urgent Gram stain and gonococcal culture on Thayer-Martin medium	IM ceftriaxone	GUM referral for contact tracing of sexual partners
Bacterial (non-gonococcal)	Bacterial cultures on blood and chocolate agar	Broad-spectrum topical antibiotics until culture results available	
Herpetic	HSV culture, PCR, enzyme immunoassays/ multinucleated giant cells on Giemsa / deranged liver function	IV acyclovir	Liaison with paediatrician for inpatient care. Management of disseminated disease (encephalitis, pneumonitis, hepatitis). Confirmed disease requires oral acyclovir for 6 months to prevent recurrence
Chemical	None	Consider stopping topical treatment	May continue treatment if the consequences of incomplete treatment outweigh the advantages of resolving the chemical inflammation

inform investigation, where appropriate, to confirm the diagnosis.

Treatment

If gonococcal disease is suspected and urgent Gram stain confirms gram-negative diplococci, treatment should be commenced as an emergency and before confirmatory cultures. The conjunctivitis can threaten globe integrity. *Gonococcus* can penetrate intact epithelium causing corneal neovascularisation and perforation (**Table 59.2**).

In cases which do not suggest gonococcal or herpetic disease, it is reasonable to take microbiological swabs and initiate an empirical topical antibiotic. This is most commonly chloramphenicol (0.5% qds) in the UK. A dangerous mistake, avoided by prior discussion with microbiology, is to take inappropriate samples and fail to exclude or identify chlamydial infections.

Specific treatment regimens are as follows:
- *Chlamydia:*
  - Oral erythromycin: 12.5 mg/kg qds 14 days
  - Mother and sexual partners: single dose of 1 g oral azithromycin
  - Erythromycin is safe in pregnancy, however, due to the side effects and reduced efficacy, the WHO recommends oral azithromycin
- *Gonococcus:*
  - Single dose IV or IM ceftriaxone: 25–50 mg/kg up to 125 mg maximum
  - Also treat asymptomatic infants from mothers confirmed to have *N. gonorrhoeae*
- Neonatal HSV:
  - Asymptomatic infants to mothers with primary genital HSV infection: IV acyclovir, 60 mg/kg three times daily for 2–3 weeks
  - The risk of systemic complications indicates inpatient management
  - Topical antimicrobials, steroids, and cycloplegics as required
  - Confirmed disease mandates > 6 months of oral treatment to prevent recurrence
- Maternal HSV:
  - Oral acyclovir 400 mg tds, 3–5 days. Suppressive treatment may be initiated from 36 weeks onwards at 400 mg twice a day until delivery

Further reading

Fransen L, Klauss V. Neonatal ophthalmia in the developing world: epidemiology, etiology management and control. Int Ophthalmol 1988;189–196.

Gupta N, Bowman C. Managing sexually transmitted infections in pregnant women. WHE 2012; 8:313–321.

Laga M, Meheus A, Piot P. Epidemiology and control of ophthalmia neonatorum. WHO 1989; 67:471–478.

Matejcek A, Goldman R. Treatment and prevention of ophthalmia neonatorum. Can Fam Physician 2013; 59:1187–1190.

Simon J. Povidone-iodine prophylaxis of ophthalmia neonatorum. Br J Ophthalmol 2003; 87:1437.

Related topics of interest

- Conjunctivitis (p. 72)
- Orbital cellulitis (p. 242)

Optic disc imaging

Key points

- Imaging of the optic nerve head (ONH) and retinal nerve fibre layer (RNFL) using photography or optical coherence tomography (OCT) is essential for documenting baseline appearance and monitoring for progression in glaucoma
- OCT can provide objective quantitative measurements, which can be compared to a reference database to measure rates of change using trend-based analysis
- Faster rates of change on OCT are associated with increased risk of worsening visual field loss
- It is essential to check scans for artefacts and to be aware of limitations of a normative database

Imaging options

Detection of ONH and RNFL change is essential for the diagnosis and monitoring of glaucoma. Changes can be observed using fundoscopy, but because of wide variation in normal disc appearance, drawing optic discs alone is not enough.

Photography

Traditionally, photography has been the imaging modality of choice. Photography is useful for documenting baseline disc appearance, disease progression and as a reference standard for diagnosis of glaucoma. Glaucomatous changes include narrowing of the neuroretinal rim, increased cup–disc ratio, and diffuse or localised loss of the RNFL (**Figure 60.1**). However, photographs are subjective and do not provide quantitative measurements. There is often disagreement even among specialists in judging change.

Confocal scanning laser ophthalmoscopy

Confocal scanning laser ophthalmoscopy (CSLO) and OCT have advantages over photography in providing quantitative measurements. CSLO (e.g. Heidelberg retina tomography) takes multiple measures of retinal height to produce a colour-coded topography image. Although quantitative measures such as optic disc and rim areas can be obtained, measurements from CSLO rely on a reference plane. This is a contour line placed along the inner edge of the scleral rim by the technician. Placement of the line varies and, therefore, measurements are not truly objective.

Optical coherence tomography

Optical coherence tomography was first used to image the human eye in 1991 and it has evolved considerably. The original time domain OCT has been superseded by spectral domain OCT (SDOCT), which offers enhanced image quality (**Figure 60.2**). SDOCT devices incorporate real-time eye tracking to compensate for eye movements during scanning. It includes software to automatically centre follow-up scans on previously scanned locations by identifying retinal landmarks. This ensures reproducibility and better ability to detect progression.

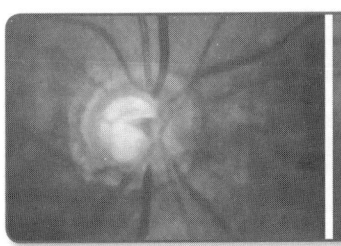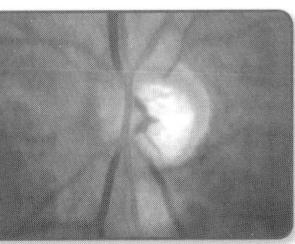

Figure 60.1 Optic disc photographs of patient with glaucoma in both eyes. (*For colour version see plate 4*)

Diagnosis (classification)

Retinal nerve fibre layer

Optical coherence tomography can be used to classify eyes as normal (green), borderline (yellow, < 5% probability of being normal) or outside normal limits (red, < 1% probability of being normal) with RNFL thickness, the most commonly used parameter. An overall classification is provided along with quadrants, sectors or clock hours (**Figure 60.2**). The TSNIT (temporal, superior, nasal, inferior, temporal) plot displays measurements along a calculation circle. A normal TSNIT configuration is a 'double hump' pattern due to thicker RNFL in the superotemporal and inferotemporal regions.

Classification

Before classification, the whole scan should be checked for quality and artefacts, such as decentration and segmentation errors, which may be manually corrected. Several conditions other than glaucoma may cause RNFL thinning (e.g. optic disc drusen, multiple sclerosis); therefore, the results of OCT should be considered in conjunction with information from the history, examination, and other tests. OCT aids diagnosis but cannot make the diagnosis alone.

Normative databases

Optical coherence tomography normative databases are useful for classification but have limitations: limited number of eyes, consist primarily of white subjects, and exclude those with high refractive errors. High myopia (≥6D) especially are associated with a higher risk of glaucoma (odds ratio of 5.8). They often have atypical disc appearances leading to false positives on OCT. The normal peaks in the double hump pattern on the TSNIT plot are displaced temporally due to a narrow angle between their arcuate RNFL bundles.

Several case-control studies have shown OCT to have excellent ability to differentiate glaucomatous and healthy eyes even in early disease. However, these studies used strict inclusion criteria and may overestimate performance. The GATE study examined the ability of an OCT normative database to detect glaucoma among 943 suspected patients referred from community optometrists. A RNFL global classification of outside normal limits had a 76.9% sensitivity for a 78.5% specificity.

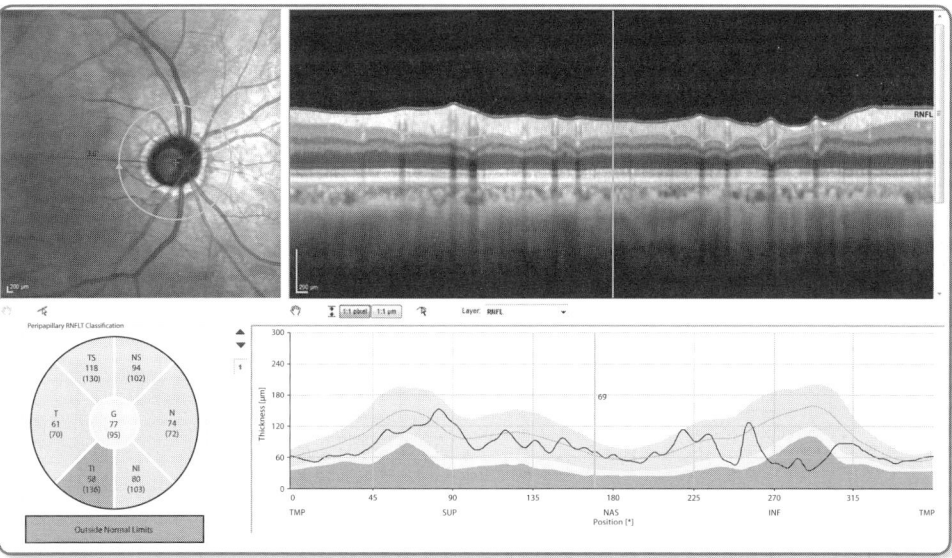

Figure 60.2 Optical coherence tomography (OCT) retinal nerve fibre layer (RNFL) scan for the right eye of the patient in Figure 1 showing segmentation of the RNFL and classification as outside normal limits. (*For colour version see plate 4*)

Other optic nerve head parameters

Optic nerve head parameters are traditionally measured from the disc margin, e.g. cup–disc ratio, but the location of the disc margin is subjective and not identifiable on OCT. Measurements taken relative to Bruch's membrane opening (BMO, termination of Bruch's membrane on OCT) are likely to be more reproducible. BMO-minimum rim width (BMO-MRW), which is defined as the minimum distance between BMO and internal limiting membrane (ILM), is a new parameter now available commercially. However, it is not yet clear whether this is superior to RNFL thickness.

The macula

Imaging of the macula may be useful for glaucoma management, as it is important for central vision and contains a large number of retinal ganglion cells (**Figure 60.3**). However, a systematic review comparing macular (e.g. ganglion cell layer) and RNFL measures for glaucoma detection concluded that RNFL parameters are still preferable although the differences are small. Using multiple measurements would increase sensitivity but increase the number of false positives. Macular measurements may be useful in eyes with unusual disc appearance, e.g. tilted discs.

Detecting progression

Variability in normal optic nerve appearance makes diagnosis of glaucoma challenging, and observing for change over time may be more useful. Imaging is useful for detecting progression in patients with established glaucoma, although it should be used in conjunction with assessment of visual fields.

The OCT devices include software to aid detection of progression, and can calculate rates of change in RNFL over time (measured as μm per year). Eyes with faster rates of change have been shown to be at increased risk of worsening visual field defects.

Reproducibility

Detection of progression depends on the ability to differentiate true change from the noise of test variability. OCT RNFL measurements have excellent short-term reproducibility (intraclass correlation coefficient 97.2%). A short-term change in average RNFL thickness of 4 μm or more has been suggested as suspicious of progression. Due to lower reproducibility of sector measurements, a relatively greater change is

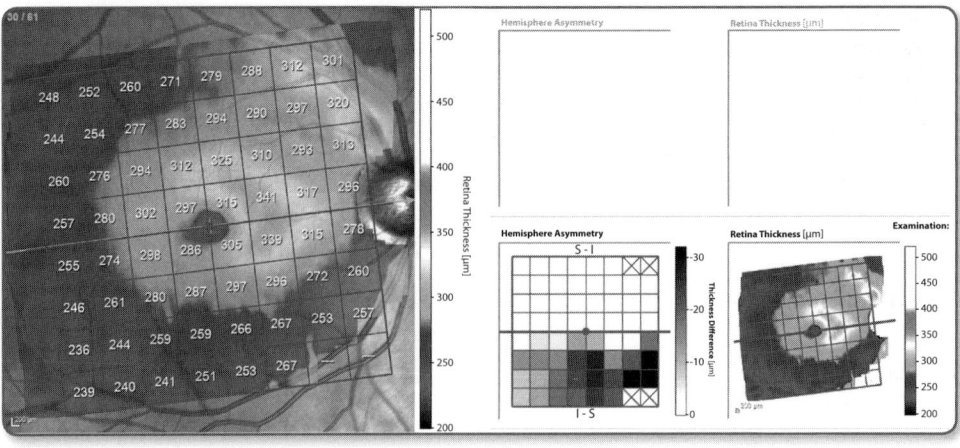

Figure 60.3 Macular retinal thickness analysis for the same patient. (*For colour version see plate 4*)

needed for similar confidence of true change (approximately 7 μm for temporal, superior and inferior quadrants, and 8 μm for the nasal quadrant).

Age-related changes

Glaucoma progression must be differentiated from normal age-related changes. Mean rates of age-related change in average, superior and inferior RNFL thickness have been reported as −0.52, −1.35 and −1.25 μm per year, respectively.

Optic disc imaging in other diseases

Optic nerve head drusen

Drusen are acellular deposits primarily consisting of calcium, buried or at the surface of the optic disc with 75% being bilateral. The frequent associated visual field defects may mimic glaucoma. ONH drusen can be visualised using B-scan ultrasonography (appearing as highly reflective round structures with acoustic shadowing), fundus autofluorescence (inherent autofluorescent properties) or using OCT with enhanced depth imaging (EDI-OCT). Drusen tend to produce a lumpy ONH internal contour on OCT with normal or thinned RNFL.

Papilloedema

Optic disc swelling due to papilloedema tends to cause a dome-shaped elevation of the ONH on OCT radial scans, and increased RNFL thickness especially in the nasal sector. There may be a subretinal hypo reflective space between the photoreceptor layer and RPE at the neural canal opening, and inward angulation of the peripapillary RPE and Bruch's membrane.

Multiple sclerosis

Longitudinal studies have shown patients with multiple sclerosis, including those with no history of optic neuritis, often have progressive RNFL thinning. Thinning is most pronounced in the temporal sector of the ONH (papillomacular bundle), with the arcuate fibres relatively spared.

Congenital defects

Congenital defects such as optic disc pits and colobomas may be associated with peripapillary subretinal fluid or schisis. Both can be visualised on OCT scans through the affected area, with the degree of vitreous condensation and adhesion overlying the optic disc determined.

Further reading

Azuara-Blanco A, Banister K, Boachie C, et al. Automated imaging technologies for the diagnosis of glaucoma: a comparative diagnostic study for the evaluation of the diagnostic accuracy, performance as triage tests and cost-effectiveness (GATE study). Health Technol Assess 2016; 20:1–168.

Oddone F, Lucenteforte E, Michelessi M, et al. Macular versus retinal nerve fiber layer parameters for diagnosing manifest glaucoma: a systemic review of diagnostic accuracy studies. Ophthalmology 2016; 123:939–949

Tatham AJ, Medeiros FA, Zangwill LM, et al. Strategies to improve early diagnosis in glaucoma. Prog Brain Res 2015; 221:103–133.

Related topics of interest

- Glaucoma – inflammatory (p. 159)
- Glaucoma – medical management (p. 162)
- Glaucoma – primary open angle (p. 165)
- Normal tension glaucoma (p. 219)
- Ocular hypertension (p. 226)
- Retinal imaging (p. 277)

61 Optic neuritis

Key points

- Optic neuritis (ON) is a syndrome of inflammatory optic neuropathy
- A working diagnosis of typical or atypical ON is made based on the clinical features and history. The final diagnosis is established retrospectively, based on diagnostic workup and observed clinical course
- Typical ON refers to idiopathic demyelinating ON, often associated with MS
- All other types of ON are considered as atypical which is an umbrella diagnosis for ON with underlying inflammatory autoimmune conditions or infectious and post-infectious aetiology
- Only two main forms of atypical ON associated with specific antibodies (anti- AQP4-Ab and anti- MOG-Ab) are discussed further in this chapter. For other forms of atypical ON see Chapter 60
- If not specified, the term optic neuritis usually implies a typical form of ON

Epidemiology

The typical age of patients with ON is between 20 and 40, with females predominantly affected twice as often as males. The incidence of ON and MS is highest in populations living at higher latitudes, and is lowest in equatorial regions. Around 50% of patients with optic neuritis will develop MS within 15 years from diagnosis, and similarly more than half of patients with MS will have at least one episode of ON during the course of the disease.

Pathophysiology

In typical ON, it is presumed that an autoimmune reaction to the nerve sheath myelin leads to demyelination and axonal loss. Certain human leukocyte antigen (HLA) types are more common and risk is increased if family history is positive. Similarly to most autoimmune diseases, the exact trigger is not known. In atypical ON Anti-aquaporine 4 antibodies (anti-AQP4-Ab) targeting astrocytes, and anti-myelin oligodendrocyte glycoprotein antibodies (anti-MOG-Ab) targeting oligodendrocytes are involved in the pathogenesis of optic neuritis.

Clinical features

Optic neuritis is characterised with subacute visual loss accompanied by pain or eye tenderness which often worsens on eye movements. Symptoms typically develop over hours to days with spontaneous improvement usually in a third week. Positive visual phenomena (i.e. photopsias) can occur spontaneously or on eye movements and loud noises. This symptom was present in 30% of patients in the Optic Neuritis Treatment Trial (ONTT). Some patients may have temporary worsening of vision caused by increased body temperature known as Uhthoff's phenomenon. It is a poor prognostic indicator as it carries a higher risk for MS.

The severity of visual dysfunction can vary from normal visual acuity to no light perception. Visual field defects are almost always present and can be central, diffuse or variable focal patterns. Loss of colour vision is typically disproportionately severe compared with the loss of visual acuity. If the lesion is unilateral or asymmetrical, the relative afferent pupillary defect (RAPD) will be positive. Basic neurological tests should be performed to exclude focal deficits. Presence of limb weakness or paraesthesia is suggestive of CNS involvement.

There are not many clinical intraocular signs; optic disc can be normal (retrobulbar ON) or mild to moderately swollen, mild pars planitis and retinal venous sheathing are rare, but when present, indicate higher risk of developing MS.

Atypical features that suggest alternative diagnosis are:
- Age of onset > 50 years
- Severe optic disc swelling, haemorrhages, hard exudates, cotton-wool spots, vitritis or uveitis

- Symptoms worsening after 2 weeks, or absence of significant recovery within 3–4 weeks of the onset of symptoms
- Severe (no light perception) or bilateral visual loss
- Absence of pain, or severe pain on eye movements
- Recent onset of other cranial neuropathies

In children, the clinical picture tends to be different. Bilateral involvement and disc swelling are more common. They have a lower risk of developing MS than adults, especially if the optic neuritis is preceded by a viral illness or vaccination.

Investigations

- *Visual field:* Static perimetry is helpful in detecting mild to moderate loss of light sensitivity, while kinetic perimetry is more useful in patients with large field defects or VA below 6/24
- Optical coherence tomography (OCT) of the disc and macula are useful for diagnosis and assessment of the extent of axonal damage. Loss of ganglion cells in the macula is present in most patients after the first 2 weeks which precedes peripapillary RNFL thinning by approximately 4 weeks
- Visual-evoked potentials (VEP) is electrodiagnostic test which typically shows delay of signal. However, this investigation is mainly of value in selected cases, and for confirmation of functional visual loss or functional overlay when this is suspected. It may also uncover previous episodes of subclinical optic neuritis of the other eye
- MRI scan of brain and orbits (shows high signal on T2, and intravenous gadolinium enhances active inflammatory lesions within first 6 weeks)
- Lumbar puncture (LP) in atypical cases (e.g. when symptoms suggest infectious aetiology), CSF may show oligoclonal bands (increases the risk of developing MS), lymphocytosis and elevated proteins

Diagnosis

- MRI scan of brain and orbits with contrast typically shows enhancing demyelinating lesion within the affected optic nerve. Another value of an MRI scan is to provide prognosis regarding the risk of developing demyelinating disease. This is based on size, location and number of brain white matter lesions. Every patient with diagnosis of optic neuritis should have this done for a baseline as sometimes lesions on MRI scan can be subclinical (i.e. asymptomatic). However, some patients prefer not to have a scan. Furthermore, the diagnosis of MS can be made on the basis of changes identified on MRI findings over a period of 6–12 months allowing treatment to be initiated. The ON associated with NMO produces much more extensive optic nerve inflammation than the short segments seen in most cases of MS-associated ON
- Anti-MOG-Ab and anti-AQP4-Ab are found in a significant proportion of patients with optic neuritis. Some patients may have both antibodies positive, but there are also a considerable number of seronegative patients (some of whom may develop antibodies later on the course of disease). Generally, AQP4-Ab is associated with NMO, while anti MOG-Ab can be found in acute disseminated encephalomyelitis (ADEM) in children, neuromyelitis optica spectrum disease (NMOSD) in adults and as an isolated recurrent optic neuritis.

Optic neuritis is considered as a clinically isolated syndrome if there are no clinical or MRI findings that suggest an underlying diagnosis of demyelinating disease. Some of these patients may develop a demyelinating condition in their lifetime, but the risk is much lower in comparison with patients with neurological deficits or demyelinating lesions at presentation.

Treatment

Pulse corticosteroid therapy should be considered especially in those cases with moderate to severe visual loss. Commonly used regimes include; intravenous methylprednisolone 1,000 mg daily for 3 days

or oral methylprednisolone 500 mg daily for 5 days. The rationale for steroid use is to:
- Speed up recovery
- Improve visual prognosis in cases of severe visual loss (which implies extensive inflammation commonly seen in NMO and some cases of atypical ON), as a delay in treatment may increase the likelihood of developing permanent optic nerve damage

On the other side of spectrum, mild optic neuritis has good visual prognosis and the vast majority spontaneously recover to almost normal vision. Prior to initiating systemic steroid therapy:
- The patients need to be informed of all potential side effects
- Medical contraindications and malignancies should be excluded
- Blood and urine for analysis – to exclude active infection
- Baseline serum glucose level and blood pressure
- Some patients at significant risk of TB need a chest X-ray

Patients should be referred to a neurologist for further assessment and investigation if there are clinical or MRI signs suggestive of an associated demyelinating condition. Disease-modifying drugs (DMD) are used for reducing the number of relapses and severity of episodes once the diagnosis of relapsing-remitting MS is established. Also, when an MRI scan suggests a higher risk of progression into demyelinating disease, DMD should be considered as there is evidence suggesting that some DMD have the potential for preventing new episodes that would lead to the diagnosis of MS.

Plasma exchange is used in acute NMO/NMO spectrum disease if there is no improvement on steroids. Steroid-sparing agents are introduced when long-term immunosuppression is required.

Further reading

Liu GT, Volpe NJ, Galetta SL. Neuro-ophthalmology Diagnosis and Management, 2nd edition. New York: Elsevier 2010: 131–141.

Miller NR, Subramanian P, Patel V. Walsh & Hoyt's Clinical Neuro-ophthalmology: The Essentials, 3rd edition. Philadelphia: Lippincott Williams & Wilkins 2016: 130–144.

Pane A, Miller N, Burdon M. The Neuro-ophthalmology Survival Guide, 2nd edition. New York: Elsevier 2017:57–67.

Related topics of interest

- Optic neuropathies (p. 239)
- Perimetry (p. 248)
- Imaging in ophthalmology (p. 176)

62 Optic neuropathies

Key points

- Optic neuropathies (ON) are the diverse group of conditions with various underlying aetiologies that eventually lead to ganglion cell loss and visual loss
- Detailed history, clinical presentation, associated ocular and systemic signs are important for guiding further diagnostic workup
- In acute visual loss with normal optic disc appearance and presence of relative afferent pupillary defect (RAPD), urgent diagnostic workup is required as prompt treatment may prevent irreversible axonal loss
- Some conditions can be sight-threatening while others can be life-threatening, hence, timely diagnosis is essential for prevention of permanent visual loss or death

Clinical features

Non-arteritic anterior ischaemic optic neuropathy

Non-arteritic anterior ischaemic optic neuropathy (NAION) is the most common optic neuropathy in the age group above 50. Visual acuity can be anywhere between 6/6 to no perception of light, with variable visual field loss (often inferior altitudinal) and dyschromatopsia. These patients typically have crowded optic disc appearance with small cup to disc ratio. Cardiovascular risk factors like diabetes, hypertension, hypercholesterolaemia and smoking are known to be more common in these patients but exact pathophysiology is unknown.

To minimise the risk for the fellow eye, potential triggers like obstructive sleep apnoea and hypotensive events should be ruled out. In patients younger than 50 years of age, one should think of non-giant cell arteritis (GCA) types of arteritis and hyperhomocysteinaemia.

Posterior ischaemic optic neuropathy

Main risk factors for posterior ischaemic optic neuropathy (PION) are major surgeries complicated with prolonged hypotension with or without significant blood loss.

Hereditary autosomal and mitochondrial optic neuropathy

Dominant optic atrophy (DOA) may present in two different ways; as slowly progressive bilateral visual loss or as an incidental finding on routine eye testing. Vision can be in the range from normal (6/6) to 6/60. DOA typically presents in the first two decades, but if visual loss is mild to moderate, it may be discovered later in life. It is caused by mutation of the *OPA1* gene, which is responsible for intracellular signal processing and mitochondrial function.

Leber's hereditary optic neuropathy (LHON) is classically characterised by sequential or rarely simultaneous bilateral painless visual loss (vision worse than 6/60). It predominately affects males in their 2nd or 3rd decade. In the acute stage of the disease, optic disc is hyperaemic with telangiectatic blood vessels. Interestingly, in the population there are more carriers of the LHON mutation, but not all of them develop the disease. Smoking, alcohol and some medications toxic to mitochondria are considered as potential triggers for the disease conversion, therefore risk factors should be explained to the patient and family members, potential carriers. The three most common mutations m.11778, m.3460, and m.14484 account for about 90% of cases. Several studies have shown the beneficial effect of the antioxidant idebenone for LHON patients with mutation 11778, and gene therapy is showing promising results as well (**Figure 62.1**).

Toxic/metabolic/nutritional deficit optic neuropathy

Nutritional vitamin B12 and folate deficiency, tobacco and alcohol optic neuropathy (usually come together) have a direct effect on mitochondrial metabolism, hence clinical presentation is similar to hereditary ON with bilateral central or caecocentral scotoma.

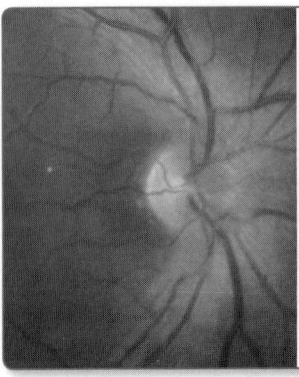
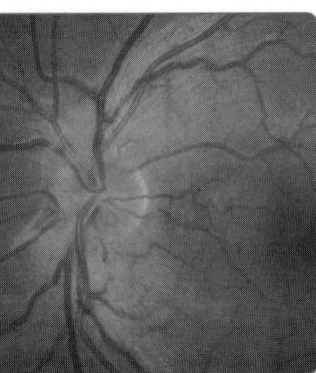

Figure 62.1 Leber's hereditary optic neuropathy. Description: patient presented with worsening vision in the left eye (6/24), and 6 week history of visual loss in the right eye (CF). (*For colour version see plate 5*)

Methanol-related toxic ON presents as acute severe bilateral visual loss accompanied with bilateral disc swelling and other systemic symptoms of poisoning.

Ethambutol-related optic neuropathy is dose and treatment duration dependent. It is potentially reversible, therefore, early detection is paramount for prevention of permanent visual loss.

There have been some reports of NAION-like ON in men after taking sildenafil or other phosphodiesterase 5 inhibitors.

Inflammatory optic neuropathy

Optic neuritis associated with systemic autoimmune disease: Systemic lupus erythematosus, sarcoidosis, Wegener's granulomatosis, Sjögren's syndrome.

Chronic relapsing inflammatory optic neuropathy (CRION) is a recurrent autoimmune optic neuritis without any underlying systemic condition, hence it is a diagnosis of exclusion. Persistence of pain for weeks after visual loss and relapse on steroid withdrawal are two main characteristics in clinical presentation.

Infectious optic neuropathy

Syphilis, tuberculosis and Lyme disease are great mimickers as their ophthalmic and systemic presentation is very variable. One should always look for signs of intraocular inflammation: uveitis, vasculitis and chorioretinal involvement.

These sometimes present as perineuritis with moderate to severe pain on eye movements or neuroretinitis with the development of lipid exudates in a form of a macular star, usually 1–2 weeks following the onset of disc swelling.

Protozoa (e.g. Toxoplasma) and viruses (e.g. VZV) can cause optic neuritis in immunocompetent patients but more often affect those who are immunocompromised (i.e. AIDS).

Infiltrative optic neuropathy

Lymphoma, leukaemia and solid tumour metastasis may cause ON in the clinical course of the disease but sometimes it can be the first sign of systemic disease.

Compressive optic neuropathy

Compression within the optic nerve (glioma or disc drusen), or extrinsic compression alongside the pathway of the optic nerve such as tumours (sphenoid or optic nerve sheath meningioma, craniopharyngioma, pituitary adenoma, and metastatic lesions), carotid-ophthalmic artery aneurysms, dysthyroid optic neuropathy, mucoid cyst and abscess. Gaze-evoked transient visual loss, orbital signs, diplopia and pain are suggestive symptoms. Lesions affecting posterior segment of the optic nerve are less likely to present with disc swelling the more posterior the lesion is and the slower it grows.

Post-radiation optic neuropathy

Typically develops 1–3 years after the optic nerve was exposed to radiation. There can be a diverse range of visual loss and the clinical picture resembles diabetic retinopathy when the retina is involved. It may be treated with systemic steroids.

Post-traumatic optic neuropathy

It can be caused by two mechanisms:
1. *Primary:* By direct injury to the optic nerve (an object penetration through the orbit or bone fragment) and indirect blunt trauma by transmitting force to optic canal and optic nerve.
2. *Secondary:* It is caused by haematoma (e.g. iatrogenic haemorrhage following parabulbar injection) or soft tissue swelling, consider steroids within 24 hours from the onset of injury.

Post-infection and post-vaccination optic neuropathy

Typically presents in children or young adults within few weeks of respiratory or gastrointestinal infection or vaccination. Spontaneous recovery to normal vision is common, however, it is reasonable to consider steroids especially if visual loss is severe and/or concurrent meningeal involvement.

Paraneoplastic optic neuropathy

Usually presents with bilateral disc swelling and accompanying CNS symptoms. Lung carcinoma is the most common associated cancer.

Diabetic papillopathy

It is a diagnosis of exclusion, hence main diagnostic challenge is to rule out other causes of disc swelling. Patients typically present with mild or no visual loss. Apart from standard management of diabetic retinopathy, there is no specific treatment, and swelling usually resolves within 3–4 months.

Diagnosis

Clinical intraocular examination and meticulous history will guide further diagnostic tests: contrast-enhanced MRI scan of brain and orbits (to look for compressive lesions, inflammation), blood tests (to look for infective causes, vitamin deficiencies), genetic tests, electrodiagnostics (in equivocal cases) and lumbar puncture (in selected patients). Sometimes it is difficult to identify the exact cause when a patient presents with signs of already established optic neuropathy.

Treatment

Depending on the underlying cause of ON, treatment can be: replacement of deficient vitamins, cessation of toxin exposure, antibiotics for infective causes, surgery for compressive lesions, neuroradiological intervention for aneurysm, treatment of systemic conditions, steroids or decompressive surgery for dysthyroid orbitopathy. In some cases, there is no proven efficient treatment, like in NAION or DOA.

Further reading

Chan JW. Optic Nerve Disorders. New York: Springer; 2007.

Liu GT, Volpe NJ, Galetta SL. Neuro-ophthalmology Diagnosis and Management, 2nd edition; New York: Elsevier; 2010:103–183.

Miller NR, Subramanian P, Patel V. Walsh & Hoyt's Clinical Neuro-ophthalmology: The Essentials, 3rd edition. Philadelphia: Lippincott Williams & Wilkins; 2016:161–208.

Related topics of interest

- Giant cell arteritis (p. 156)
- Glaucoma – primary open angle (p. 165)
- Normal tension glaucoma (p. 219)
- Ocular hypertension (p. 226)
- Optic neuritis (p. 236)
- Papilloedema (p. 245)

63 Orbital cellulitis

Key points
- Microbial orbital cellulitis is a true defined as an acute infection of orbital tissue posterior to the orbital septum
- *An ophthalmic emergency:* Treatment should be initiated immediately to prevent permanent visual loss and life-threatening spread of infection to intracranial structures
- Management of patients requires a multidisciplinary approach with input from ophthalmologists, physicians/paediatricians and ENT surgeons

Epidemiology
Orbital cellulitis is more common in winter months when predisposing factors, particularly sinusitis, are more common. It occurs more commonly in children than adults. There is no association with race but in children it is twice as common in males.

Anatomy
The orbital septum is a tough sheet of fibrous tissue that marks the anterior boundary of the orbit and separates orbital tissue from preseptal tissue. It attaches to the periosteum of the orbital rim and extends to the upper and lower tarsal plates. The medial wall (lamina papyracea) is the thinnest of the orbital walls and spread of infection from the adjacent ethmoid sinus is the most common cause of orbital cellulitis. Valveless orbital veins allow direct communication between the ethmoids sinuses, orbit, and cavernous sinus.

Pathophysiology
Sources of infection
There are three main routes of infection:
1. Direct inoculation of the orbit from trauma, foreign bodies or surgery (infected orbital implant)
2. Spread from adjacent tissues:
   - *Sinusitis:* the most common cause of orbital cellulitis is a result of direct extension from the paranasal sinuses or haematogenous spread via valveless connections between sinus and orbital veins
   - Preseptal cellulitis: Secondary to eyelid trauma or localised infections, e.g. infected chalazia
   - Dacryocystitis, dacryoadenitis or endophthalmitis
   - Facial cellulitis or dental infections
3. Haematogenous spread from distant sites

Common microbial pathogens in orbital cellulitis secondary to sinusitis *Staphylococcus aureus, Staphylococcus epidermidis,* and *Streptococcus pneumoniae. Haemophilus influenzae* is more common in older children. Older children (>9 years) and adults are more likely to have polymicrobial infections and anaerobic infections. Gram negative organisms are more common in traumatic and dental infections.

Fungal infections, in particular mucormycosis, should be considered in immunocompromised patients, progresses more rapidly than bacterial orbital cellulitis due to a tendency to invade vessel walls and causes more ischaemia and tissue necrosis.

Clinical features
Patients typically present with unilateral upper and lower lid swelling and pain. A careful history and examination will differentiate orbital cellulitis from preseptal cellulitis and other inflammatory conditions.

History
A detailed history can help to establish the diagnosis and source of infection. Record the following:
- *Onset and precipitating factors:* Time of onset, speed of spread, current or recent associated infections, e.g. upper respiratory tract or sinus infections, fever, headache, sinus pressure
- *Associated ocular symptoms:* Visual changes pain, diplopia, proptosis
- *Associated neurological symptoms:* Headache weakness or numbness
- Systemic symptoms of sepsis, e.g. fever, lethargy, confusion

- *Past ocular history:* Periocular surgery, trauma, infections or insect bites
- *Past medical history:* Sinus disease, predisposing conditions, e.g. immunosuppression, diabetes
- *Drug history:* Immunosuppressive medications and current or recent antibiotic regimens
- *Systems review:* To identify a distant source of infection if no local source found

Examination
Record the following:
- Vision and colour vision
- *Pupillary reactions:* Record presence or absence of a relative afferent pupillary defect
- Ocular motility
- *Proptosis:* Exophthalmometry
- *Extent of lid swelling:* Take photographs and mark edge of cellulitis
- Fundus examination including appearance of optic nerve
- Cranial nerve and neurological examination
- *Baseline observations:* Blood pressure, pulse, respiratory rate, temperature

Diagnosis
Orbital cellulitis is primarily a clinical diagnosis. Proptosis and ophthalmoplegia are key features of this condition. Other typical features include:
- Eyelid oedema and erythema; patients often cannot open the affected eye easily
- Raised intraorbital pressure with a tense orbit on retropulsion, often raised intraocular pressure
- Retrobulbar ache and pain on eye movement
- Conjunctival injection and chemosis
- Optic nerve compression in severe cases may cause reduced visual acuity, reduced colour vision, relative afferent pupillary defect and optic disc swelling
- Systemic signs and symptoms of infection; fever, headache, malaise

Preseptal cellulitis may be considerd as stage 1 orbital cellulitis. The differential diagnosis includes carotid cavernous fistula, cavernous sinus thrombosis, herpes zoster ophthalmicus, thyroid eye disease, idiopathic orbital inflammation, neoplasia with inflammation, e.g. rhabdomyosarcoma, histiocytosis X, leukemia, metastatic carcinoma

Investigations
These baseline tests should be performed for all patients at first presentation:
- *Blood tests:* Full blood count, renal function, C-reactive protein, erythrocyte sedimentation rate, serum glucose, urinalysis
- Blood cultures if the patient is febrile (33% positive in children and < 5% in adults)
- Microbial swabs: Swab conjunctiva and collect purulent material from the nose with a cotton or calcium alginate swab, smear for Gram stain, and culture on aerobic and anaerobic media

Computed tomography (CT) imaging, thin axial and coronal cuts, with or without contrast, is essential to review the paranasal sinuses and identify the presence of intraorbital gas, subperiosteal abscess or intracranial extension. If the intraconal space is predominantly involved in the absence of associated sinus disease, an intraorbital foreign body should be suspected. Initiation of intravenous (IV) antibiotics should not be delayed by imaging. In view of the radiation risk posed by CT imaging, it is appropriate to start empirical antibiotic treatment for babies and young children and image only if there is clinical deterioration or no clinical improvement after 48 hours.

Treatment
Management of sepsis, including administration of high-dose broad-spectrum IV antibiotics, according to local antimicrobial guidelines, should be administered without delay. Antibiotics should cover gram-positive and gram-negative pathogens and, in adults and older children, anaerobic cover should also be considered. Patients with orbital cellulitis should be admitted for monitoring and should remain in hospital until afebrile and clinically improving. At least 48 hours of IV antibiotics are usually required and antibiotics should be adjusted depending on the response to treatment and results of

cultures. Patients require hourly monitoring of visual function and neurological condition during the first 24 to 48 hours following admission with a low threshold for repeat imaging in cases of clinical deterioration. Patients should be managed jointly with paediatricians or physicians. Patients with sinus disease require ENT input, as sinus drainage is frequently required. Input from other specialities including infectious disease and neurosurgery may also be required.

If orbital compartment syndrome is suspected, an emergency lateral canthotomy and cantholysis is indicated. Adjuvant treatment includes ocular anti-hypertensives for raised intraocular pressure and nasal decongestants for concomitant sinusitis. Use of steroids in orbital cellulitis is controversial. Chen et al. suggested that concomitant steroid use shortened hospital stays in children with orbital cellulitis but did not affect outcomes.

Ferguson and McNab demonstrated that 62% children and 5% adults developed a subperiosteal abscess and 9% of children and 22% adults developed an orbital abscess. Garcia and Harris suggested that urgent drainage should be considered if the following criteria are met:
- Patient > 9 years old
- Presence of frontal sinusitis
- Non-medial location of subperiosteal abscess
- Large subperiosteal abscess
- Suspicion of anaerobic subperiosteal infection (e.g. presence of gas within the abscess space as visualized on CT scan)
- Recurrence of subperiosteal abscess after previous drainage
- Evidence of chronic sinusitis (e.g. nasal polyps)
- Acute optic nerve or retinal compromise
- Infection of dental origin, as anaerobes infection more likely

The surgical approach to drainage of a subperiosteal abscess depends on its location and the preference of the surgeon and includes a transcutaneous, transconjunctival, retrocaruncular approach combined with an endoscopic sinus drainage technique.

Complications

In the pre-antibiotic era, 20% of patients with orbital cellulitis developed permanent visual loss but this is now rare with appropriate treatment and monitoring. Visual loss is commonly due to ischaemic optic neuropathy secondary to direct infection of the nerve, raised intraorbital pressure leading to central retinal artery occlusion or thrombophlebitis affecting the blood supply to the nerve. Spread to intracranial structures may cause cavernous sinus thrombosis, intracranial abscesses, meningitis and encephalitis. These complications are very rare but have a high mortality and survivors have a high risk of permanent neurological deficit.

Further reading

Chaudhry IA, Al-Rashed W, Arat YO. The Hot Orbit: Orbital Cellulitis. Middle East African J Ophthalmol 2012; 19:34–42.

Duke-Elder S, MacFaul PA. The ocular adnexa: part 2. Lacrimal orbital and paraorbital diseases. In: Duke-Elder S (Ed). System of Ophthalmology. London: Henry Kimpton; 1974:859–889.

EyeRounds. Orbital Cellulitis in a Child (Hong ES, Allen RC). [online] Available from: http://www.EyeRounds.org/cases/103-Pediatric-Orbital-Cellulitis.htm. [Last Accessed October, 2019].

Ferguson MP, McNab AA. Current treatment and outcome in orbital cellulitis. Aust N Z J Ophthalmol 1999; 27:375–379.

Harris GJ. Subperiosteal abscess of the orbit: computed tomography and the clinical course. Ophthal Plast Reconstr Surg 1996; 12:1–8.

Uddin JM, Scawn RL. Preseptal and orbital cellulitis. In: Hoyt CS, Taylor D (Eds). Pediatric Ophthalmology and Strabismus, 4th edition. China: Elsevier Saunders; 2013:89–99.

Related topics of interest

- Chalazion (p. 63)
- Imaging in ophthalmology (p. 176)

64 Papilloedema

Key points

- Papilloedema refers to bilateral optic disc swelling caused by raised intracranial pressure
- When bilateral disc swelling is suspected, two questions need to be answered – are discs truly swollen, and if they are, is it papilloedema or some other cause?
- If one makes working diagnosis of papilloedema, the second step is to find the cause for raised intracranial pressure. In many cases, papilloedema is a presenting sign of life-threatening conditions, therefore appropriate imaging needs to be done urgently

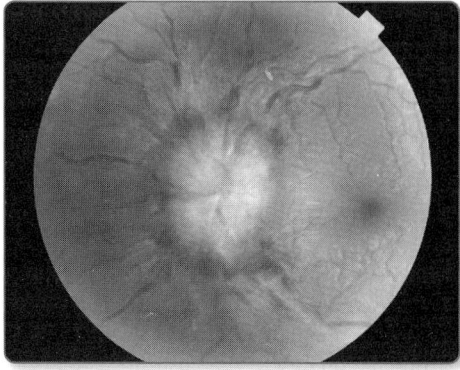

Figure 64.1 Acute papilloedema. (*For colour version see plate 5*)

Pathophysiology

There are three main reasons for raised intracranial pressure (ICP):
1. Increased brain volume (space-occupying lesions and cerebral oedema).
2. Decreased cerebrospinal fluid drainage (hydrocephalus secondary to various intracranial pathology, dural venous sinus thrombosis or fistula, extracranial venous obstruction).
3. Pseudotumour cerebri (PTC) (idiopathic intracranial hypertension as primary PTC, and various types of secondary PTC).

Clinical features

In the early stage of papilloedema, optic discs have subtle signs of indistinct disc margins and mild blurring of blood vessels. As papilloedema evolves, the disc becomes hyperaemic, elevated and the cup obliterates. Haemorrhages, cotton wool spots and retinal striae may be present (**Figure 64.1**). Due to anatomical variations in optic nerve canal, disc swelling can be asymmetrical to the point that clinically it may seem like unilateral swelling, but additional diagnostic tests will reveal some degree of peripapillary retinal nerve fibre layer (RNFL) swelling. Optic discs in chronic papilloedema show signs of gliosis, and hyperaemia is replaced with pallor. Even years after the swelling resolves, discs may remain elevated. Visual function is typically spared in the early course of papilloedema, but prolonged moderate to severe papilloedema leads to loss of nerve fibres and secondary optic neuropathy.

Clinical presentation consists of the combination of different symptoms, but rarely patients can even be completely asymptomatic, some will have no headache while it can be very mild in others. They typically complain of a new type of a headache, occasionally accompanied with nausea and vomiting. It is constant, but tends to fluctuate during the day, worse in the morning (patient tends to wake up with it), when lying down, bending over, coughing or straining (Valsalva manoeuvre). It is important to distinguish this type of headache from coexisting underlying headaches that are triggered by raised ICP. These headaches can have migrainous features and tend to remain for some period of time after the ICP normalises. Whooshing sound synchronous with pulse is often present in one or both ears. Transient visual obscurations (TVO) are episodes of blurring or even complete blackouts lasting for a couple of seconds. Sometimes patients report pressure behind eyes or retrobulbar pain. Flashing lights or zig-zag lines are uncommon but can be present. Double vision (usually horizontal) is secondary to 6th nerve palsy as it is the most susceptible cranial motor nerve to be damaged from raised ICP.

Most important underlying conditions to think of for ophthalmologists:
- Subarachnoid haemorrhage (SAH) and space-occupying lesions (SOL) – different types of tumours and cysts (cystic echinococcosis, arachnoid cyst)
- *Dural sinus thrombosis and fistula:* Detailed history is essential to rule out acquired prothrombotic conditions and disorders such as oral contraceptive pill use, pregnancy, immobility, Behcet disease, obstructive sleep apnoea and antiphospholipid syndrome. Some genetic causes include protein C/protein S deficiency, factor V Leiden mutation and antithrombin deficiency. Apart from headaches, an altered mental status, focal neurological deficits and/or seizures may be present.
- Idiopathic intracranial hypertenion (IIH) is a condition of raised ICP with normal neuroimaging and normal cerebrospinal fluid composition. It predominately affects overweight women of childbearing age.
- *Secondary PC:* Most common medications associated with secondary PC are tetracyclines, exogenous growth hormone, hypervitaminosis A and retinoids.

Various other causes of swollen discs:
- Optic neuropathies will have some signs of impaired visual function while acute papilloedema usually does not affect visual function unless rise of ICP is rapid or severe
- Malignant hypertension presents with swollen discs and plentiful signs of flame-shaped haemorrhages, cotton wool spots and lipid exudates in macula
- Ocular hypotony of 5 mmHg or less (usually after eye surgery or post-traumatic) and intraocular inflammation (uveitis) can cause disc swelling. These causes can be revealed easily with slit lamp examination.

Pseudopapilloedema refers to a suspicious optic disc appearance which resembles swollen discs. These discs are usually congenital anomalies, crowded hyperopic discs or optic disc drusen. Main distinguishing feature from papilloedema is the absence of peripapillary retinal RNFL swelling.

Optic disc drusen represent calcified extruded axoplasmic material. If superficial, they are easy to diagnose, but younger patients tend to have buried drusen which might be challenging to distinguish from true disc swelling. Discs are often elevated with indistinct margins. Peculiar vascular branching with irregular disc contour might be the only giveaway sign. Superficial drusen can be confirmed with autofluorescence while buried with presence of a hyper-reflective material on ultrasound.

Investigations

The best neuroimaging method is MRI with venography (to rule out sinus venous thrombosis). A CT scan should be done if MRI is not available. An LP is performed if the cause for raised ICP was not found on neuroimaging. It acts to therapeutically relieve the pressure and improves patient symptoms immediately. Opening pressure and constituents are analysed.

An ocular coherence tomography (OCT) of the optic disc is useful for measurement of RNFL thickness and assessing various optic disc parameters. This sensitive method is used for detecting early disc swelling, distinguishing from pseudopapilloedema and for monitoring purposes. Fluorescein angiography (showing early disc leakage) is rarely used, in equivocal cases.

Treatment

Treating the underlying cause – surgery for tumours or cysts, blood thinners for thrombophilia, cessation of medication that can cause increased ICP.

The aim of treatment in IIH is to prevent irreversible loss of nerve fibres and permanent visual loss. After LP is performed, the ICP is decreased temporarily as it builds up again in days to weeks. Serial LP can be considered for control of ICP in selected patients, such as in pregnancy.

Second-line treatment is acetazolamide (carbonic anhydrase inhibitor) which reduces cerebrospinal fluid production. The common starting dose is 500 mg BD, which can be increased if tolerated by the patient. An alternative to acetazolamide is another carbonic anhydrase inhibitor, such as topiramate, which is also an anti-epileptic drug. The starting dose is 25 mg BD, and can be gradually increased to a daily dose of 100–150 mg. The topiramate has additional beneficial effects on migrainous headaches and helps with weight loss.

The mainstay treatment of IIH is weight loss. An LP and carbonic anhydrase inhibitors should be considered only as temporary measures. This can be achieved by a change in diet, increased physical activity, and bariatric surgery or gastric balloon for severely obese patients.

For those patients who are deteriorating and severe visual loss is imminent, surgical procedures like optic nerve fenestration, ventriculo-peritoneal or lumbo-peritoneal shunts are available. Dural stents are used for transverse dural sinus stenosis.

Further reading

Liu GT, Volpe NJ, Galetta SL. Neuro-ophthalmology Diagnosis and Management, 2nd edition. New York: Elsevier 2010:199–230.

Miller NR, Subramanian P, Patel V. Walsh & Hoyt's Clinical Neuro-ophthalmology: The Essentials, 3rd edition. Philadelphia: Lippincott Williams & Wilkins 2016:109–129.

Pane A, Miller N, Burdon M. The Neuro-ophthalmology Survival Guide, 2nd edition. New York: Elsevier 2017:125–142.

Related topics of interest

- Cranial nerve palsies – multiple cranial nerves palsies (p. 104)
- Cranial nerve palsy – abducens nerve palsy (p. 98)
- Headache (p. 172)
- Imaging in ophthalmology (p. 176)

65 Perimetry

Key points

- Visual field is a helpful tool in evaluation of the pathology of the optic disc and the visual pathway
- The patterns of defects differ depending on the localising of disease along the afferent visual pathway
- It is a key element in the detection/assessment of disease progression in glaucoma patients
- Accuracy of data entry, patients' understanding of the procedure and the reliability of the visual fields are important parts of the interpretation of the results

Perimetry

Monocular visual field is defined as the ability of a static eye gazing into infinity to discriminate a stimulus from a homogeneous background. Due to differences in sensitivity, a typical 'Island hill of vision' first described by Traquair in the 1930s is seen. Perimetry determines the dimensions of this island, including its height and extension. In a typical visual field, the fovea is the peak of the vision island, point of maximal retinal sensitivity. The regular dimensions of the island are 60° nasal and superior, 70–75° inferior and 100–110° temporal. The physiological blind spot is localised below the horizontal meridian, 15.5° temporal to fixation point and it corresponds to optic nerve head position.

An area of diminished retinal sensitivity embedded in an area of greater sensitivity is called a scotoma.

There are two main types of perimetry:

1. *Manual kinetic perimetry* using a Goldman-type bowl perimeter: It is performed by testing a stimulus from an area with no visual sensitivity to where the stimulus is just seen, along a preselected meridian. A line connecting the points with the same threshold sensibility in a two-dimensional chart is called an isopter.

2. *Static perimetry* using a bowl-type perimeter or video monitor: The size and localisation of the stimulus are fixed. Every point sensibility threshold is determined by changing the brightness of the stimulus and it is expressed in decibels (dB) (0.1 log unit). This is the most widely used current automated method.

Standard automated perimetry

Humphrey (HFAs; Carl Zeiss Meditec, Dublin, CA) and Octopus (Haag-Streit, Mason, OH) are the most common computerised perimeters in Europe.

Examination strategies that employ threshold estimations and full threshold strategy are used to monitor the disease and to detect the glaucoma progression. The threshold estimations strategies like Swedish Interactive Thresholding Algorithm (SITA) of Humphrey and Tendency Oriented Perimeter (TOP) of Octopus can obtain the same information as full threshold strategy in far less time.

The usual algorithms in glaucoma are central 24° (24-2 in Humphrey) and 30° (30-2 in Humphrey and G1 in Octopus) with test points 6° apart. In order to help with the identification of defects that respect vertical and horizontal midline, they examine locations 3° above, below, temporal and nasal to those lines.

The central visual field can also be tested with 10-2 (Humphrey) or C8 (Octopus) algorithms. They focus on the central 10-8° of the field and localisations are tested every 1–2° intervals. They are the choiced programs to detect and follow very focal central scotomas and in cases of advanced visual fields that threaten the fixation.

There are 30–60° algorithms available but they are seldom performed as they are very time consuming and offer little additional information as far as glaucoma management is concerned.

Visual field results interpretation

The results of the visual field can vary between devices but they have certain elements in common (**Figure 65. 1**).
A. Patient information:
- *Age:* correct age ensures an appropriate age match analysis
- *Patient refraction:* It must be accounted for. The corrective lens adequately centred and needs to be closed to the eye in order to avoid lens rim artefact

B. *Size of stimulus:* The sizes of standard stimuli are $0 = 1/16$ mm^2, $I = 1/4$ mm^2, $II = 1$ mm^2, $III = 4$ mm^2, $IV = 16$ mm^2, $V = 64$ mm^2. The usual size stimulus in SAP is III
C. *Reliability indices:* Fixation monitor-fixation losses, false-positives and false-negatives
- *Fixation monitor-fixation losses:* A blind spot map is outlined before the full test. During the test if a patient responds stimuli within the blind spot, the device interprets this as a fixation loss

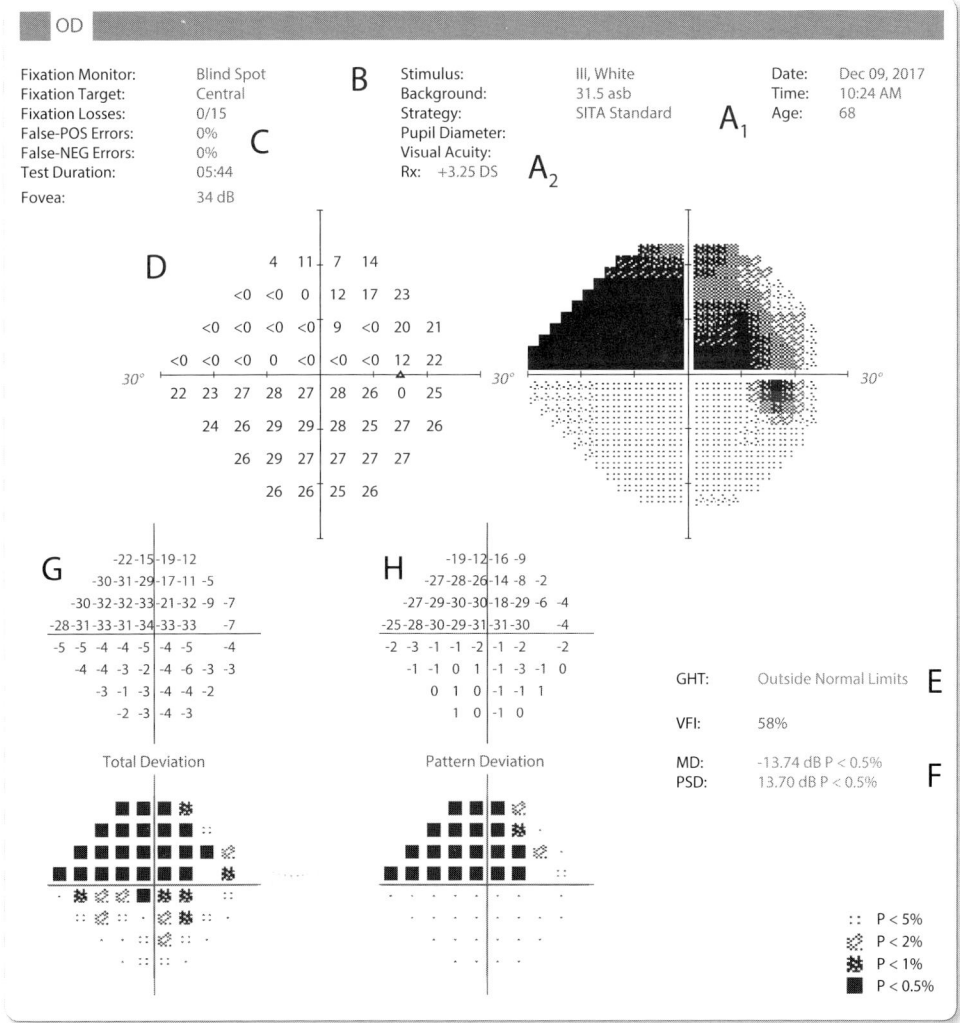

Figure 65.1 Single visual field printout (Humphrey visual field analyser). Glaucoma patient, superior nasal step defect that respects the horizontal meridian combined with arcuate superior defect, the confluence of these defects results in a superior altitudinal defect.

- *False-positives:* The perimeter intermittently reproduces the sound of the shutter without projecting any lighted stimulus. When a patient responds to this sound, a false-positive is registered. False-positive rates that exceeds 20% (happy trigger patients) can camouflage defects and produce fields with inaccurate threshold sensitivities
- *False-negatives:* The perimeter projects a lighted stimulus 9 dB brighter than the quantified threshold of an already examined point. If the patient fails to respond to this stimulus, a false-negative is registered
    - False-negative rates greater than 33% are indicative an unreliable visual field test. However, it is important to be aware that patients with advanced field loss can exhibit high false-negative rates that do not reveal lack of reliability
    - A typical visual field produced as a result of a patient failing to pay attention partway throughout the test is the known as the cloverleaf pattern
D. Threshold value of the test localisation points. Raw values for the points examined in a routine examination, expressed in dB. Alongside is presented a greyscale map that has to be assessed always in conjunction with the raw data
E. *Glaucoma hemifield test (GHT):* This test compares the test localisations above and below the horizontal meridian in order to detect any significant difference between the analysed points. The power of GHT analysis to identify glaucoma damage derives from the segregation of upper and lower retinal ganglion cells axons at the optic disc
F. *Global indexes:*
    - Mean deviation (MD): This quantifies the global impairment. It is age-corrected
    - Pattern standard deviation (PSD): This quantifies the focal defect. It is a global index of the irregularities of the field defects
    - Visual field index (VFI): This is calculated as a percentage of an expected normal visual field. It is based in pattern deviation maps with central field values being more heavily weighted. This is an attempt at improving detection of the central visual field progression by reducing confounding factors (e.g. cataract)
G. *Total deviation map:* This shows the difference between the observed values and the expected normal values for every test localisation
H. *Pattern deviation map:* This is calculated by ranking test points based on the observed values and the expected age-matched values and general sensitivity is measured using the 85th percentile sensitivity. The aim of this calculation is to eliminate the non-glaucomatous diffuse VF loss due to a progressive cataract for example

Patterns of visual field loss

Due to the characteristic distribution of the retinal ganglion cell (RGC) axons in the retina and along the afferent visual pathway, patterns of defect differ according to location. A detailed, comprehensive description of patterns of visual fields loss are beyond the scope of this chapter, however a brief summary is outlined later.

Pre-chiasmal visual field defects

Retinal superior, inferior and nasal RGC fibres travel in a somewhat straight course to the optic nerve, however, because the nasal location of the optic disc, temporal axons must separate to avoid the macula and enter in the optic nerve at either the superior or inferior pole. This also means that some of the nasal fibres access the optic disc through its temporal side.

Thus, depending on the main group of RGC fibres affected, lesions of the optic nerve can be classified into:
1. *Papillomacular fibres:* Central, paracentral and central scotoma
2. *Arcuate fibres:*
    - Nerve fibre bundle defects: Arcuate scotoma (Bjerrum)

- Wide area of arcuate fibres: Altitudinal defect (Seidel)
- Temporal area of arcuate fibres: Nasal step defect that typically respects the horizontal meridian. While bi-nasal defects occur rarely in neurological disease, defects of both nasal field areas are more characteristic of glaucomatous neuropathy, though these do not typically respect the vertical midline

3. *Nasal radial fibres:* Temporal wedge defect blind-spot enlargement results from optic disc edema of any cause or from large areas of peripapillary atrophy or tilting

Chiasmal visual field defects

The typical visual field defect of the chiasmal compression is a bitemporal hemianopia. These defects can be relative or complete. A chiasmal lesion that

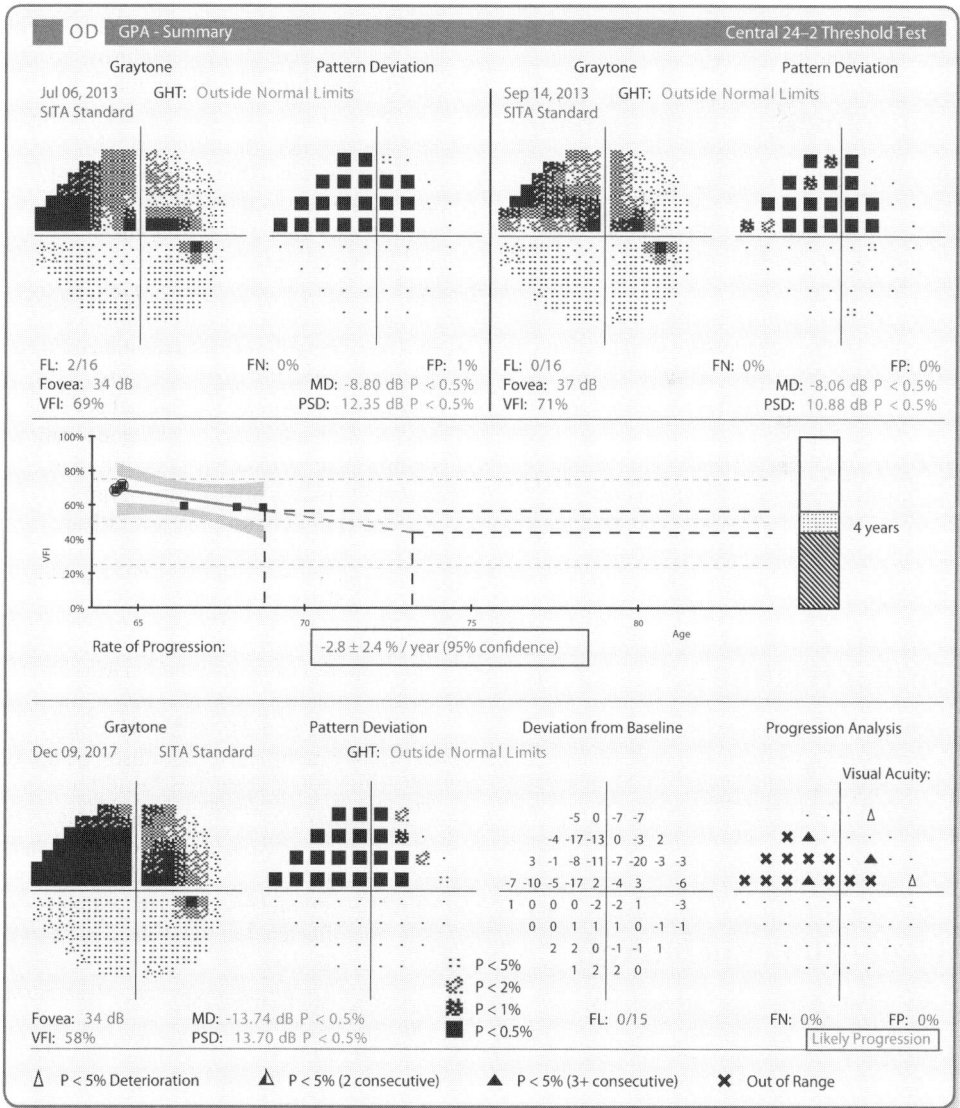

Figure 65.2 Guided progression analysis printout.

compresses only the nasal fibres of one eye can lead a unilateral temporal hemianopia.

Lesions that affect the optic nerve when reaching the chiasm cause junctional scotomas with a central scotoma and decreased visual acuity in the ipsilateral eye and a temporal hemianopia in the contralateral.

Post-chiasmal visual field defects

These lesions produce homonymous visual field defects (depending on location it may be congruous or incongruous) that respect the vertical midline.

Glaucomatous visual field loss

The typical glaucomatous visual field scotomas include: arcuate or Bjerrum, paracentral, nasal step, altitudinal or Seidel, temporal wedge and diffuse depression (**Figure 65.1**).

The most common automated methods for detection of deterioration are usually either 'event based' or 'trend analysis'.

Event analysis identifies changes in a given test localisation compared to this specific point in the initial baseline reference examination, e.g. Guided Progression Analysis software (GPA; Carl Zeiss Meditec, Inc.) included in the Humphrey visual field analyser is the most widely protocol used (**Figure 65.2**). It compares the pattern deviation value of each test localisation with the average value of that specific point in the two baseline visual fields. It highlights the test localisations which show a worsening greater than the expected normal test-retest variability. This is a normal variability that has been previously studied in a group of stable glaucoma patients during a short period of time. The software alerts of possible progression when the same three points (not necessarily contiguous) have met this criterion on two consecutive visual fields. When the criterion is met in three consecutive visual fields, the GPA indicates likely progression on the printout.

Trend analysis: These methods employ regression analysis of the test parameters to determine the quantity and the rate of change in global indices as MD, PSD or VFI or individual test localisations. The main limitation of this method is the requirement for a greater number of visual fields than would be required for event-based methods to detect a significant change.

A final point to bear in mind is that visual fields should not be used in isolation when assessing glaucoma patients and other parameters such as optic disc changes (e.g. using OCT correlation) and clinical examination findings should also be taken into account.

Further reading

Alward WLM. Glaucoma: The Requisites in Ophthalmology. St Louis: Mosby Inc.; 2000.
Aref AA, Budenz DL. Detecting Visual Field Progression. Ophthalmology 2017; 124:S51–S56.
Azarbod P, Mock D, Bitrian E, et al. Validation of point-wise exponential regression to measure the decay rates of glaucomatous visual fields. Invest Ophthalmol Vis Sci 2012; 53:5403–5409.
Chauhan BC, Garway-Heath DF, Goñi FJ, et al. Practical recommendations for measuring rates of visual field change in glaucoma. Br J Ophthalmol 2008; 92:569–573.

Related topics of interest

- Glaucoma – primary open angle (p. 165)
- Normal tension glaucoma (p. 219)
- Ocular hypertension (p. 226)
- Optic neuropathies (p. 239)

66 Peripheral retinal degenerations

Key points
- Peripheral degenerations affecting the inner retina and the vitreoretinal interface are more likely to predispose to formation of retinal breaks
- With the exceptions of horseshoe tears (U-tears) or higher-risk lattice degeneration in fellow eyes of patients with detachments, most peripheral retinal degenerations do not generally require routine prophylactic treatment/ monitoring to prevent retinal detachment

Outer retinal degenerations

Pavingstone degeneration
Discrete, 'punched-out' depigmented yellowish-white areas of chorioretinal atrophy. Large choroidal vessels can be seen beneath the absent RPE and choriocapillaris. These may be solitary or in groups/confluent, most often anterior to the equator in the inferior retina and are found in > 20% of the population. Areas of pavingstone degeneration can limit the spread of subretinal fluid in a detachment.

Reticular degeneration
A fine network of 'honeycomb' pigmentary changes, reticular degeneration is typically found in older patients and is associated with AMD.

Peripheral drusen
Clusters of pale yellow lesions located near the equator, typically found in older patients.

Congenital hypertrophy of the retinal pigment epithelium
These benign, flat, dark grey-black well-defined lesions found just posterior to the ora serrata are present at birth and are hence not a 'true' degeneration, these lesions can depigment over time with a thin rim of residual pigment at the edge of the lesion which may then be mistaken for a hole.

Inner retinal degenerations

Microcystoid
Microcystoid change is the most frequently encountered peripheral retinal degeneration. This appears as small clusters of closely-spaced vacuoles in greyish retina in the OPL/INL near the ora and can be found in all eyes, increasing with age. These vacuoles can coalesce to form retinoschisis cavities.

Retinoschisis
'Senile' retinoschisis develops from the coalescence of microcystoid cavities resulting in asymptomatic splitting within the neurosensory retina. Retinoschisis appears as a smooth, thin, convex, immobile 'dome-shaped' retinal elevation, most often seen bilaterally (80%) in the inferotemporal quadrant. Other features distinguishing these from retinal detachments include the absence of tobacco dust and stable absolute visual field defect. Small round inner leaf breaks or larger rolled-edge outer leaf breaks may also be noted. Retinoschisis is present in 5% of the population and much more prevalent in hypermetropes. Typical retinoschisis involves splitting of the OPL whilst the reticular type shows splitting of the NFL. Retinal detachment risk is < 0.05% and as they are usually non-progressive and asymptomatic, these cases rarely require surgery.

Cystic tufts
Small, discrete elevated whitish equatorial lesion mainly comprising glial tissue with strong vitreoretinal adhesion. Round holes and tears can occur. Present in up to 5% population. RD risk in presence of cystic tufts is < 1%.

White without pressure
Fixed geographic regions of grey-white translucence in the absence of scleral indentation. White without pressure (WWP) is found in 30% of normal eyes (often young, pigmented) just posterior to the ora and

is often bilateral. These areas represent stronger adhesion of condensed vitreous with increased density of collagen fibrils at the vitreoretinal interface. Giant retinal tears may rarely develop along the borders of WWP areas, although the presence of WWP is not specifically associated with increased RD risk.

Lattice degeneration
These are localised circumferential oval patches of retinal thinning with criss-cross networks of sclerosed vessels. Commonly found between the equator and the vitreous base, areas of lattice degeneration may contain small holes and are often bilateral. Radial/paravascular lattice may be associated with Stickler syndrome. Vitreoretinal interface adhesions are particularly strong at the borders of lattice and the overlying vitreous is liquefied, resulting in a higher risk of retinal tears following a PVD. Lattice degeneration is found in 5–8% of eyes, more commonly in young adult moderate myopes. It is found in 30–40% of eyes with retinal detachments, but the chance of developing an RD is only 1% in the presence of lattice degeneration. Natural history studies suggest that only 3% will develop tractional tears over 10 years. Prophylactic treatment of asymptomatic lattice degeneration is not routinely recommended.

Snailtrack degeneration
A frost-like variant/precursor of lattice degeneration known as 'snailtrack' degeneration can sometimes be seen, consisting of glistening bands of tightly-packed 'snowflakes.' Although these lesions do not tend to result in horseshoe tears from vitreous traction, snailtrack degeneration is associated with atrophic holes and asymptomatic detachments in eyes where the vitreous remains attached.

Table 66.1 Retinal detachment risk from peripheral retinal degenerations

Moderate	Lattice degeneration
Low	White without pressure Retinal tufts Microcystoid Retinoschisis
None	Pavingstone degeneration Reticular degeneration CHRPE Peripheral drusen

Atrophic round holes
Chronic atrophy results in a round full-thickness peripheral retinal defect with smooth borders, often associated with myopia or lattice degeneration. Surrounding pigmentation is often a sign of chronicity. Since round holes are typically not associated with PVD/vitreous traction even though some lesions may have a surrounding cuff of subretinal fluid, they therefore do not tend to recruit more fluid through the break and the hole remains typically 'stable' and asymptomatic.

Prophylactic retinopexy
All tractional (PVD-related) u-tears should be treated with laser or cryotherapy retinopexy. **Table 66.1** stratifies the risk of progression to retinal detachment associated with various peripheral degenerations. The risk of retinal detachment from peripheral degenerations is low and the natural history data that underpins most of our current understanding does not provide sufficient evidence to suggest significant benefit from routine prophylactic treatment of peripheral degenerations. Exceptions can be made on a case-by-case basis with higher-risk patients, e.g. lattice degeneration in a high myope with retinal detachment in the fellow eye.

Further reading

AAO. Peripheral Retinal Abnormalities (Section 12: Retina and Vitreous). In: Basic and clinical science course (BCSC) San Francisco: American Academy of Ophthalmology 2011–12:283–291.

Macalister G, Sullivan P. Peripheral retinal degenerations. Optometry Today CET 2011:44–53.

Wilkinson CP. Interventions for asymptomatic retinal breaks and lattice degeneration for preventing retinal detachment. Cochrane Database Syst Rev 2012; 14:CD003170.

Williamson T. Peripheral Retinal Degenerations. In: Vitreoretinal Surgery, 2nd edition. Berlin Heidelberg: Springer 2013:96–98.

Related topics of interest

- Vitreoretinal surgery – retinal breaks and detachment and vitreomacular interface disorders (p. 350)
- Vitreoretinal surgery – management of complications of cataract surgery, post-operative endophthalmitis and vitreoretinal biopsy (p. 360)
- Vitreoretinal surgery – intraocular haemorrhage, complications of vitreoretinal surgery and modern developments (p. 365)
- Retinal detachment (p. 270)

67 Pigmentary glaucoma

Key points

- The typical patient affected by the condition is a young, myopic male
- The risk of glaucoma is about 10% within 5 years and 15% within 15 years
- Laser iridotomy may have a role in reducing the risk of raised intraocular pressure and therefore pigmentary glaucoma in individuals at high risk

Epidemiology

The prevalence of pigment dispersion syndrome (PDS) is approximately 1.9% in the general population. However, in a population of over 6 thousand patients with glaucoma, 1.7% were found to have PDS with or without secondary ocular hypertension and 4.4% had an established diagnosis of pigmentary glaucoma (PG). A number of studies have reported PDS/PG to be more common amongst males and is almost exclusively seen in the Caucasian population. Although there is no definite data on the age of onset of PDS, it is commonly diagnosed between the 3rd and 4th decade. Phenotypic manifestations of the condition are rare under the age of 20 years. The vast majority of patients with PDS have mild-to-moderate myopia with patients developing PG tending to be affected by a greater degree of myopia.

Pathophysiology

Pigment dispersion syndrome is likely to be caused by a combination of mechanical and genetic factors.

Mechanical factor

In 1979, it was proposed that mechanical rubbing between the concave posterior iris surface and the anterior zonules was responsible for the release of pigment from the iris epithelium, which can be exacerbated by mydriasis. With the advent of ultrasound biomicroscopy (UBM), it has been shown that patients with pigment dispersion have a more posterior inserted iris on the ciliary body, a concave iris profile with a deeper anterior chamber, and iridozonular and iridociliary contact. Furthermore, activities such as blinking, accommodation, and exercise can increase posterior bowing of the iris and contact with anterior lens surface/zonules. This later was termed as 'reverse pupil block'.

Genetic factor

Pigment dispersion syndrome and PG have strong hereditary associations; however, to date, consistent data and causative mutations in the genome have not been found.

Clinical features

The diagnosis of PDS is based on the classical clinical triad of slit-like mid-peripheral iris transillumination defects (**Figure 67.1**), diffuse and dense homogenous brownish pigmentation of the angle (**Figure 67.2**), and pigment granules on the corneal endothelium (Krukenberg's spindle) with a normal intraocular pressure (IOP). When the IOP is elevated, this is regarded as secondary ocular hypertension. With the development of glaucoma, the condition is referred to as PG. Pigmentation can also be seen in some

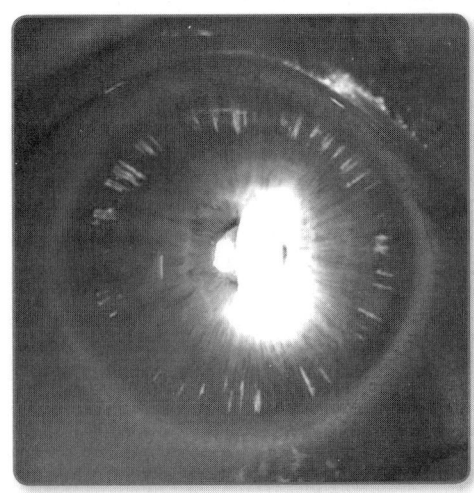

Figure 67.1 Mid-peripheral iris transillumination defects typical of pigment dispersion syndrome.

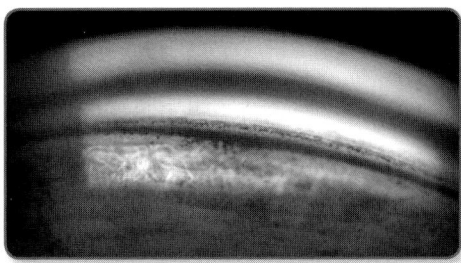

Figure 67.2 Diffuse and homogenous pigmentation of the drainage angle.

patients on the iris surface, zonules, and lens capsule (Zentmayer ring and Scheie stripe). The retina is often abnormal in PDS/PG with lattice degeneration, full thickness retinal breaks, and retinal detachment occurring more frequently compared to patients with other forms of glaucoma.

The course of the disease can be divided into three phases:
- *'Active' pigment dispersion phase:* During this phase, which is largely asymptomatic, pigment is actively liberated into the anterior segment. The release of pigment in some patients can be accelerated by physical exercise, stress, and mydriasis. The IOP is normal during this phase
- *'Conversion' phase:* Based on a retrospective population-based study, 10% of patients with PDS are likely to develop glaucoma within 5 years and 15% after 15 years
- *'Burnt-out' or 'regression' phase:* Where, with age, the pigment starts to clear from the anterior segment such that the Krukenberg's spindle and iris transillumination defects disappear partly or completely, the pigmentation of the trabecular meshwork starts to clear, and the IOP normalises. This can often cause a diagnostic dilemma in the older patient group who may be labelled as 'glaucoma suspect' or 'normal tension glaucoma'. The only sign of PDS remaining may be homogenous pigmentation of the trabecular meshwork predominantly in the superior angle

Investigations

No investigations are required to make the diagnosis of PDS. However, it is important to monitor these patients due to the risk of conversion of PG.

Diagnosis

The diagnosis of PDS and PG is clinical – by identifying the classical triad of the Krukenberg's spindle, mid-peripheral iris transillumination defects, and homogenous pigmentation of the angle on clinical examination with or without raised IOP or glaucoma.

Treatment

Medical treatment

The medical treatment of IOP is indifferent to that of primary open angle glaucoma. Pilocarpine has been shown to reduce both liberation of pigment by reversing iris concavity and 'reverse pupil block' and decreasing the IOP by increasing trabecular outflow. However due to the relative young age of patients and the induced myopia, pilocarpine is often poorly tolerated by patients due to pain/brow ache, poor night vision, and increase in myopia.

Laser treatment

Both argon (ALT) and selective laser trabeculoplasty (SLT) can be used to lower the IOP in patients with PDS/PG. However, due to the greater amount of pigmentation in the angle in PDS, there is a higher risk of a significant IOP rise post-treatment and, therefore, care must be taken to minimise the energy used and treat a maximum of 180 degrees at a time. In a retrospective review of 32 eyes of 32 patients with uncontrolled PG treated with ALT, the success rate (defined by IOP < 21 mmHg without additional treatment or glaucoma surgery) at 1, 3, and 5 years was 80%, 58%, and 45%, respectively. However, two patients (6.2%) had a significant IOP rise within the 1st week requiring a trabeculectomy. Similarly, in a retrospective review of 30 eyes of patients with PG treated with SLT, the success rate (defined as IOP reduction > 20% without additional medication or surgery) was 85%, 44% and 14% at 1, 3, and 4 years, respectively. An IOP spike (defined as an IOP rise > 6 mmHg) was seen in two patients (6.7%) within 2 hours after SLT laser.

Laser iridotomy has been shown to reverse iris concavity in the majority of patients with PDS to a more planer configuration. Furthermore, this reduction is also seen in patients where the iris only becomes concave during accommodation. Although iridotomy reverses the anatomical iris changes seen in PDS, two questions frequently asked are: (1) is this treatment clinically beneficial? and (2) at what stage of the disease process should it be performed (PDS or PG)? To answer question one, a 10-year prospective clinical trial of patients with PDS (with normal IOP) who were randomised to either Nd:YAG laser iridotomy or observation found that laser iridotomy reduced the risk of developing a significant rise in IOP (5 mmHg or more) in the treated 'high risk group' (positive phenylephrine provocation test*) (14.3%) compared to the control group (untreated 'high risk') (61.9%). In the 'low risk' control group (negative phenylephrine provocation test), only 11.4% developed a significant rise in IOP. Overall, in the observation group, there was a 30% risk of a significant IOP rise in 10 years. Furthermore, younger age was an independent risk factor for development of raised IOP in the 'high-risk' group. To answer question two, a 3-year prospective trial of 116 patients with PDS and secondary ocular hypertension randomised to either Nd:YAG laser iridotomy or observation showed no benefit of laser iridotomy in preventing progression to PG. This suggests that once the IOP has become elevated, it is assumed that the trabecular meshwork is already damaged and, therefore, a reduction in pigment liberation by performing laser iridotomy will have no beneficial effect on the IOP. In fact, laser iridotomy liberates significant amount of pigment into the anterior chamber, which could result in a significant rise in the IOP.

Surgery

Surgery is indicated when the IOP is uncontrolled following medical and/or laser treatment or there is evidence of progressive glaucoma. The gold standard procedure used is a trabeculectomy with mitomycin C (MMC) augmentation. Factors to consider when operating in this patient's group are: (1) *intraoperatively* – minimising fluctuation in the anterior chamber during surgery due to the risk of inducing traction on the retina by the vitreous base and (2) *post-operatively* – as these patients are predominantly young myopes, there is a risk of hypotony.

Complications

The principle complication of PDS is PG. Risk factors for development of PG include male gender, black race, and degree of myopia.

---

*Three doses of phenylephrine 10% are instilled 5 minutes apart. The presence of anterior chamber pigment and IOP is checked before and 60 and 120 minutes after instillation of phenylephrine.

Further reading

Gandolfi SA, Ungaro N, Tardini MG, et al. A 10-year follow-up to determine the effect of YAG laser iridotomy on the natural history of pigment dispersion syndrome: a randomized clinical trial. JAMA Ophthalmol 2014; 132:1433–1438.

Potash SD, Tello C, liebmann J, et al. Ultrasound biomicroscopy in pigment dispersion syndrome. Ophthalmology 1994; 101:332–339.

Siddiqui Y, Hulzen Ten RD, Cameron JD, et al. What is the risk of developing pigmentary glaucoma from pigment dispersion syndrome? Am J Ophthalmol 2003; 135:794–799.

Related topics of interest

- Secondary open angle glaucoma (p. 305)

68 Posterior uveitis

Key points
- Intraocular inflammation primarily affecting the retina and choroid but frequently involves the whole eye and is known as *panuveitis*
- It includes a spectrum of diseases from self-limiting white-dot diseases confined to the eye, to severe life-threatening disseminated fungal infections manifesting with choroidal lesions
- Nearly always requires extensive investigation and treatment from uveitis specialists
- Although the rarer form of uveitis, it results in 10% of all severely sight impaired registrations

Epidemiology
Posterior uveitis makes up just 7% of all uveitis cases with a wide spread of ages and equal sex distribution due to the heterogeneity of the many and varied potential causes listed here. Some conditions are usually bilateral but others may be unilateral, particularly infections.

Risk factors
It may be infectious, non-infectious or neoplastic (masquerade). Unlike anterior uveitis, when microbes are infiltrating the retina or choroid it can suggest a systemic infection from either bacteria, viruses or fungi. Non-infectious causes result from immune dysregulation as discussed later and can be localised to the eye as in the white dot syndromes or part of a widespread manifestation like Behçet's disease. Equally, there are idiopathic cases as with all forms of uveitis.

Bird shot chorioretinopathy is one of the few posterior uveitis syndromes with a clear genetic risk factor – the presence of the human leucocyte antigen (HLA) – A29 is arguably required for diagnosis and present in over 99% of cases.

Pathophysiology
Direct infiltration of tissue by microbes in infectious uveitis is a clear pathophysiological cause for inflammation but the aetiology of non-infectious remains largely unknown. Experimental models of posterior and panuveitis exist which can be prompted sensitisation of the immune system to retinal peptides such as S antigen. This suggests the trigger for the immune system attacking the eye is sensitisation to retinal or choroidal antigens possibly by molecular mimicry from an otherwise innocuous viral infection in a predisposed individual. The final pathway of this immune reaction is better characterised with T-lymphocytes and macrophages the inflammatory cells entering the retina and choroid.

Clinical features
There are many different diseases included under the umbrella of posterior/panuveitis and this list of features cannot be conclusive. Individual diseases such as Behçet's disease and sarcoidosis warrant entire textbooks themselves.

Symptoms
Blurred vision, floaters and visual sensations like central scotomas or photopsias (flashing lights) are most common. Pain is rare unless there is panuveitis and therefore secondary anterior uveitis is developing. The onset of symptoms can be sudden, e.g. in infections, or slow and insidious if the underlying lesions occur sporadically. It is also not uncommon for patients to present only when the fovea is involved by the chorioretinal lesions and therefore vision precipitously drops.

Symptoms related to possible causative systemic disease should be sought with specific questioning about respiratory symptoms, skin rashes, orogenital ulceration, arthritis or neurologic symptoms.

Examination

Although described later are conditions primarily of chorioretinitis, all the features of anterior, intermediate and retinal vasculitis may be present alongside these lesions. Look for vitritis, cystoid macula oedema, retinal vasculitis sheathing and cuffing and optic nerve head swelling (much more common in posterior uveitis).

Choroidal inflammation (choroiditis) may present with deep yellowish lesions and granulomas which may be of a distinctive size and distribution (birds hot chorioretinopathy) or solitary large granulomas in tuberculosis. Active lesions are more likely to be white with fluffy edges whereas they will pigment with well-defined borders as they become inactive (**Figure 68.1**). When these lesions extend into the retina as well, they are termed chorioretinitis.

Retinal inflammation (retinitis) presents with white fluffy areas in the retina with an anterior appearance and involving the vasculature often leading to intra-retinal/pre-retinal haemorrhages (**Figure 68.2**).

Other manifestations include serous retinal detachment and swelling such as in sympathetic ophthalmia or Vogt-Koyanagi-Harada (VKH) syndrome.

Investigations

As posterior uveitis could be related to a serious systemic disease all cases should be investigated. See the *Retinal Vasculitis* chapter for details on urgent intravitreal tap if viral infection is suspected. Taking a comprehensive history will allow investigations to be targeted and the appropriate imaging modalities to be selected to aid in diagnosis. Syphilis testing with treponemal serology is required in all due to potential for almost any presentation of uveitis and the need for urgent treatment and potential cure.

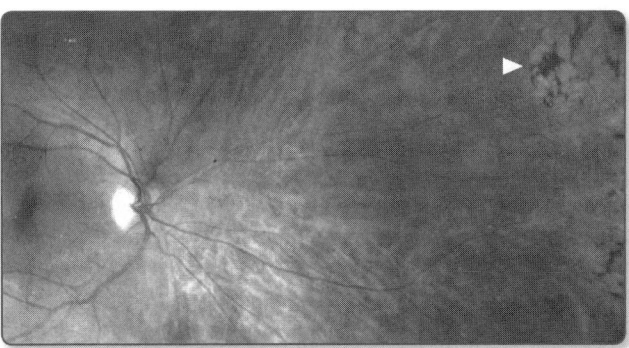

Figure 68.1 Wide field fundus colour photograph of a right eye showing (white arrowhead) pigmented chorioretinal scars as a sign of chronicity.

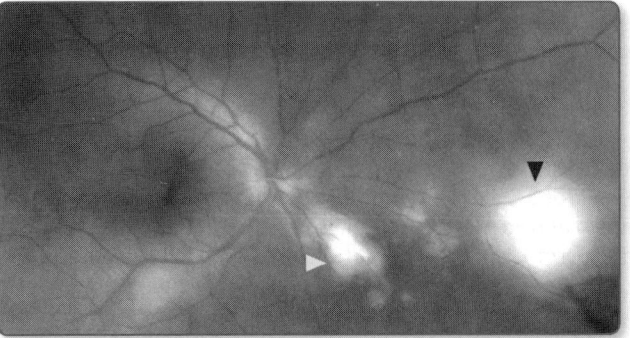

Figure 68.2 Wide field fundus colour photograph of a right eye showing (black arrowhead) an active focus of retinitis secondary to toxoplasmosis, note the fluffy poorly defined edges. In contrast older lesions are well defined with pigmented borders (white arrowhead). The view is hazy due to vitritis. (*For colour version see plate 5*)

Initial investigations

- *Blood testing:* FBC, U&E, ESR, ACE, treponemal (syphilis) serology
- *Chest X-ray:* Sarcoid and TB
- Urinalysis – looking for blood and protein
- Optical coherence tomography (OCT) may show cystoid macula oedema or lesions affecting the inner or outer retina.
- Fundus fluorescein angiogram (FFA) should be considered on all – where not contraindicated – this may show characteristic changes aiding diagnosis, e.g. 'starry sky' of multiple pinpoint leaks in the detached RPE in VKH disease

Further multimodal imaging

- Indocyanine green angiography should be done where possible and may reveal choroidal changes not visible clinically or on FFA which can direct the diagnosis clearly, e.g. choroidal granulomas indicated TB or sarcoidosis likely
- Fundus autofluorescence imaging may show characteristic changes, e.g. bright areas of RPE disturbance indicate new expanding active lesions in APMPPE or serpiginous choroidopathy
- Ultrasonography may show choroidal thickening suggestive of VKH or sympathetic ophthalmia

Targeted investigations

Based on results earlier/suspicions:

- Low threshold for TB testing with Mantoux or interferon gamma release assay tests
- *Blood tests:* Serology for HIV, *Toxoplasma*, Lyme disease, *Bartonella*
- HLA-B51 testing for Behçet's disease, HLA-A29 testing for bird shot
- Further testing under medical physicians including sarcoid specific imaging, etc.

Diagnosis

Infectious causes should be ruled out as quickly as possible with appropriate blood or ocular testing but given the likely complex nature of disease, and need for long-term treatment, onward referral to a specialist uveitis clinic would be advised in most cases.

Clinical examination, imaging and other testing may indicate pathognomonic changes associated with one diagnosis, e.g. bird shot chorioretinopathy or *Toxoplasma* chorioretinitis. But the anatomical location of inflammation may give clues to the underlying cause as follows:

- Choroiditis
  - Isolated ocular disease/white-dot syndromes: Punctate inner choroidopathy, multifocal choroiditis, bird shot chorioretinopathy, multiple evanescent white-dot syndrome (MEWDS), acute posterior multifocal placoid pigment epitheliopathy (APMPPE)
  - Non-infectious systemic disease: Sarcoidosis, VKH
- Retinitis and retinal vasculitis
  - Non-infectious: Behçet's disease, sarcoidosis
  - Infectious: Viruses such as herpes simplex, herpes zoster alongside concurrent HIV infection
- Chorioretinitis
  - Infectious: *Toxoplasma, Toxocara*, Fungi such as *Aspergillus* or histoplasmosis
- Any variation of the above
  - Infectious: Syphilis, tuberculosis, Lyme disease
  - Non-infectious: Sarcoidosis

Treatment

Observation without treatment should only be used in the mildest cases with good visual acuity and no evidence of infection. Treatment is indicated to preserve or improve vision. Treat the underlying cause where possible:

- Antibiotics for posterior uveitis secondary to systemic infection, e.g. doxycycline for Lyme disease or voriconazole for *Aspergillus*

Control the inflammation:

- Immunosuppression starting with corticosteroids delivered either intraocular, e.g. dexamethasone 700 µg implant, oral (prednisolone 1 mg/kg/day and taper) or intravenous (pulsed methylprednisolone 1g OD for 3 days)
- Second-line steroid sparing treatments are more likely to be needed than in other forms of uveitis and include

cyclosporine/tacrolimus, methotrexate and mycophenolate mofetil
- Third-line treatment will be with an anti-TNF biologic, e.g. adalimumab

Complications

Posterior uveitis/panuveitis is a leading cause of blindness in the working age population with irreversible visual loss occurring due to retinal scarring at the macula, macula ischaemia, hypotony with phthisis and due to secondary glaucoma. Other common complications which may respond to immunosuppression or surgery include cataract, cystoid macula oedema, optic nerve swelling or retinal detachment

Further reading

Jabs DA, Rosenbaum JT, Holland GN, et al. Guidelines for the use of immunosuppressive drugs in patients with ocular inflammatory disorders: Recommendations of an expert panel. Am J Ophthalmol 2000; 130:492–513.

Pivetti-Pezzi P, Accorinti M, La Cava M, et al. Endogenous uveitis: an analysis of 1417 cases. Ophthalmol 1996; 210:234–238.

Related topics of interest

- Anterior uveitis (p. 14)
- Intermediate uveitis (p. 185)
- Retinal vasculitis (p. 286)
- Birdshot chorioretinopathy (p. 29)
- White dot syndromes (p. 372)

69 Refractive surgery

Key points

- The most important aspect of preoperative assessment for refractive surgery is understanding of the patient's visual expectations
- Laser refractive surgery is the most common refractive surgery procedure, and is associated with very high patient satisfaction
- There are currently no good surgical methods to perfectly restore accommodation in presbyopia. Surgery in presbyopia aims to achieve spectacle independence at distance and near vision

Correction of refractive error

- *Myopia:* The refractive power of the eye must be reduced
- *Hypermetropia:* The refractive power of the eye must be increased
- *Astigmatism:* Flattening of the cornea at its steepest meridian and/or steepening the cornea at its flattest meridian, or with an astigmatic intraocular lens (IOL)
- *Presbyopia:* Accommodation cannot be restored surgically; however, optical techniques are used to achieve near points of focus using various methods described in this chapter

Refractive error and aberrations

Refractive error is estimated to affect 1 to 2 billion people worldwide. It is estimated that 153 million people globally are visually impaired, and 8 million people are blind, as a result of uncorrected refractive errors (Pascolini D et al. 2012).

The eye is not a perfect optical system and has inherent optical aberrations; however, the emmetropic eye can achieve a high level of resolution when a distant object is focussed onto the retina. Imperfections in an optical system cause optical aberrations because incident light is deviated, preventing the convergence of light to a single point of focus.

Optical aberrations reduce the resolving power of the eye, and therefore visual acuity. Defocus (myopia/hyperopia) and cylindrical refractive errors (astigmatism) are examples of low-order aberrations. These are normally correctable with spectacles. However, the way the human eye handles light is more complex than this and includes higher-order aberrations such as spherical and coma aberration which can cause halo and glare, respectively. They can be detected by wavefront scanning aberrometry, which analyses a wavefront profile as light is transmitted through the eye. An emmetropic eye has good distance vision, however to allow good near vision the refractive power of the eye must increase by accommodation.

Clinical assessment for refractive surgery

Table 69.1 outlines the history, examination and investigations necessary during preoperative evaluation for refractive surgery. The priority is to understand the patient's visual expectations. Any unrealistic expectations must be addressed prior to considering surgery.

Recent contact lens wear can affect subjective refraction, corneal thickness, keratometry and topography. Remove soft contact lenses 1 week prior to investigations, rigid gas permeable lenses 3 weeks prior, and hard lenses 4 weeks prior. In general, two consecutive similar topographies confirm refractive stability.

Laser refractive surgery

Laser refractive surgery is the commonest refractive surgery procedure and has very high rates of patient satisfaction. The anterior corneal surface is reshaped to alter its refractive power. The cornea accounts for two-thirds of the refractive power of the eye, and the anterior surface is the most important refractive interface. Removal of 12–18 μm of corneal stroma by stromal ablation corrects roughly 1.00 D of refractive error.

Wavefront-guided laser is used to treat pre-existing higher-order aberrations in addition to refractive error, while wavefront-optimised laser aims to avoid inducing

Topic 69

Table 69.1 Preoperative clinical assessment for refractive surgery

History	• Vision requirements: consider work, leisure, sports • Past ocular history: amblyopia, keratoconus, previous surgery • Past medical history: including diseases which affect corneal healing • Family history: including keratoconus • Lifestyle risks, e.g. competitive professional contact sport
Examination	• Subjective refraction (before and after cycloplegia) • Slit-light examination: lid margin, tear film, corneal dystrophy or degeneration, lens opacity, macular disease • Intraocular pressure: corneal refractive surgery decreases corneal thickness which can affect post-operative IOP measurement • Anterior chamber depth for phakic intraocular lenses • Mesopic pupil diameter for optimal width of laser treatment zone
Investigations	• Corneal topography: corneal ectasia can occur in early keratoconus following photoablation • Pachymetry: The minimum recommended residual stromal bed thickness by the US FDA is 250 μm; however, many surgeons prefer a 300 μm bed thickness after LASIK • Keratometry • Endothelial cell count for phakic intraocular lenses • Aberrometry

additional aberrations during refractive laser surgery. These methods were developed to reliably optimise and preserve the natural aspheric prolate corneal shape, to improve quality of vision and reduce night vision problems.

Lasers used in refractive surgery

- Excimer laser – photoablation of corneal tissue (UV light, 193 nm)
- Femtosecond laser – photodisruption using extremely short duration pulses which produce cavitation bubbles in the corneal stroma (1040 nm)

General risks include, under/overcorrection, corneal haze, haloes, glare and night-vision problems. Rare complications are recurrent erosions, corneal infiltrates, infectious keratitis, and corneal ectasia.

Laser-assisted stromal *in situ* keratomileusis (LASIK)

This is the most common form of laser refractive surgery. A femtosecond laser precisely cuts a flap of thickness 80μm to 160 μm into the superficial corneal stroma. The flap is reflected back and an excimer laser is used to modify the anterior curvature of the stromal bed (**Figure 69.1**). The flap is then replaced.

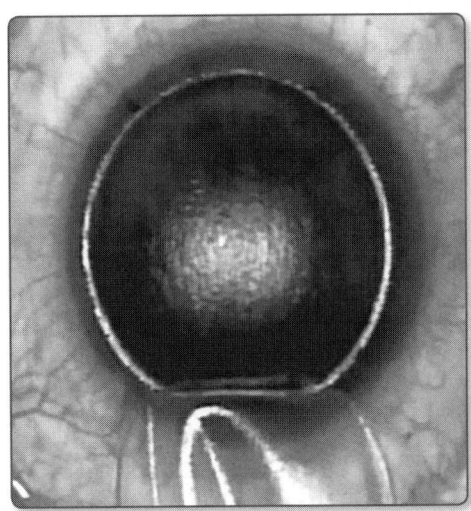

Figure 69.1 LASIK flap reflected back to expose the underlying stromal bed. (*For colour version see plate 6*)

Advantages: Relatively painless, rapid visual recovery, reduced risk of infection and corneal haze compared to surface treatments (such as PRK, LASEK and epi-LASEK).

Disadvantages: Greater risk of ectasia compared to surface treatments, flap-related complications (torn, incomplete or free flaps, buttonholing, postoperative folds, striae, dislocation or epithelial ingrowth), post-operative diffuse lamellar keratitis, and dry eye due to corneal nerve damage.

Photorefractive keratectomy (PRK)

The corneal epithelium is loosened with 20% alcohol, debrided and discarded. An excimer laser is used to reshape the corneal stromal surface. A contact lens is worn for several days postoperatively.

Advantages: Lower risk of ectasia, no flap-related complications, more suitable in patients who need to make a quick return to competitive contact sport.

Disadvantages: Painful, large epithelial defect post-operatively, slower visual recovery, greater risk of infection and postoperative corneal haze.

Laser-assisted subepithelial keratomileusis (LASEK)

Similar to PRK, however the epithelium is not discarded but swept aside and then replaced over the stromal bed following excimer laser treatment.

Epithelial laser-assisted in situ keratomileusis (Epi-LASIK)

Similar to LASEK, however instead of using 20% alcohol, a microkeratome is used to cut an epithelial flap prior to excimer laser treatment.

Refractive lenticule extraction (ReLEx)

Femtosecond laser cuts a disc-shaped lenticule from the corneal stroma which is then extracted manually. No excimer laser is used. The procedure is also called SMILE (small incision lenticule extraction). Disadvantages presently include no pupil tracking for properly centred treatments and no cyclotorsional control for precise astigmatism treatment

Other corneal refractive procedures

Corneal relaxation procedures

These procedures flatten the cornea along the treated meridian. *Limbal relaxing incisions* of varying arc are used during cataract surgery to reduce pre-existing corneal astigmatism using a guarded blade. *Opposite clear corneal incisions* are made opposite to the primary incision during cataract surgery to enhance its astigmatic effect. An *arcuate keratotomy* using a diamond knife or femtosecond laser is performed in the clear cornea, and is often utilised after corneal graft surgery. *Wedge resections* are used to treat high astigmatism. A wedge of corneal tissue is removed from the flat axis and the defect sutured to steepen the cornea in that axis. *Radial keratotomy* is a now obsolete procedure that involves multiple deep stromal incisions in the clear cornea to treat myopia and astigmatism.

Corneal addition procedures

Intracorneal ring segments were originally developed for the treatment of myopia but are now used to treat keratoconus by inserting a semi-circular ring segment into the corneal stroma after a channel is cut manually or with a femtosecond laser. *Compression sutures* can be placed along the flattest meridian to reduce astigmatism. Epikeratophakia, keratophakia and intracorneal implant procedures are other rarely used corneal addition procedures.

Phakic IOL surgery

Phakic IOLs correct refractive error in phakic eyes when laser refractive surgery is unsuitable or when clear lens extraction is not appropriate (e.g. pre-presbyopia). This technique is mainly used in myopia, and anterior chamber depth must be assessed preoperatively due to the risk of endothelial trauma and pupil block glaucoma. The procedure is reversible and accommodation is preserved. New versions available have central holes to prevent pupil block and secondary angle-closure glaucoma.

Refractive lens surgery

Removal of the crystalline lens and implantation of an IOL for correction of refractive error is mostly performed in the context of conventional cataract surgery. Refractive lens exchange may also be used in the absence of cataract when laser surgery and phakic intraocular lenses are unsuitable in patients who are presbyopic.

'Premium' IOLs have additional refractive properties compared to conventional monofocal IOLs. *Aspheric IOLs* have zero or negative spherical aberration. *Multifocal IOLs* (**Figure 69.2**) have optics divided into zones focussing for distance and near and in the case of trifocal lenses also intermediate. This increases spectacle independence; however, patients may report glare, haloes and reduced contrast sensitivity. *Light-adjustable IOLs* allow correction of up to 2.00 D of residual refractive error after implantation using UVA irradiation. *Accommodating IOLs* have so far failed to demonstrate clinically significant accommodation and are associated with posterior capsule opacification, however newer designs are offering encouraging preliminary results. Extended depth of focus lenses work in a variety of different ways and in general offer independence of glasses for distance and intermediate tasks but not close reading.

Piggyback IOLs are used for implantation of more than one IOL following crystalline lens removal (polypseudophakia). This may be planned, for example in high hyperopia when an IOL of sufficient power is unavailable, or it may be carried out as a secondary procedure to correct residual refractive error after cataract surgery. Usually, one IOL is implanted into the capsular bag, and the other into the ciliary sulcus.

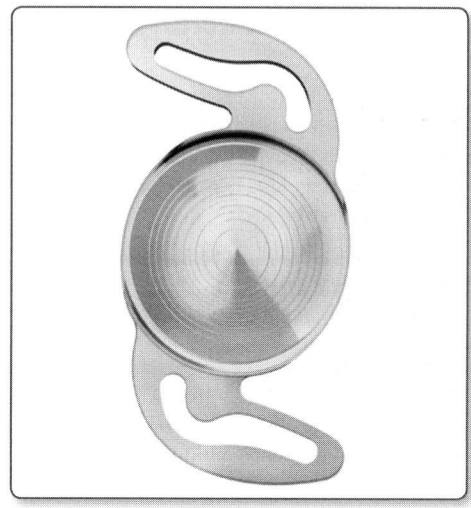

Figure 69.2 Diffractive optical rings of a multifocal intraocular lens.

Refractive surgery in presbyopia

Accommodative function, and therefore near visual ability, reduces with age leading to presbyopia. The aim of surgery is to achieve spectacle independence for distance and near vision. There are currently no methods available to perfectly restore accommodation, however the following paragraph describes optical methods used to achieve good near vision without glasses.

Monovision is a method utilising contact lenses, laser refractive surgery, or IOL implantation, whereby the dominant eye is treated to allow emmetropia for distance, and the other eye is treated to allow myopia for near, with up to 2.50 D of anisometropia. *Multifocality* is a common technique using bilateral multifocal IOLs or contact lenses. *Enhanced depth of focus* is a method which utilises the pinhole effect by inserting small, disc-shaped corneal inlays into the central corneal stroma or small aperture IOLs. *Accommodating IOLs* were discussed earlier in this chapter.

Further reading

Barsam A, Allan BD. Excimer laser refractive surgery versus phakic intraocular lenses for the correction of moderate to high myopia. Cochrane Database Syst Rev 2014:CD007679.

Sundaram V, Barsam A, Barker L, et al. Training in Ophthalmology: the essential clinical curriculum, Refractive Surgery, 2nd edition. New York: Oxford University Press; 2016.

The Royal College of Ophthalmologists. Professional Standards for Refractive Surgery; 2017. [online] Available from https://www.rcophth.ac.uk/wp-content/uploads/2017/04/Refractive-Surgery-Standards-for-Refractive-Surgery-3-April-2017.pdf. [Last Accessed October, 2019].

Related topics of interest

- Cataract – complications of surgery (p. 50)
- Corneal dystrophies (p. 79)
- Corneal topography (p. 94)

70 Retinal arterial occlusion

Key points

- Retinal arterial occlusions are rare but can result in significant permanent visual loss
- They are associated with systemic disease and carry a high mortality rate
- In the absence of any effective treatment for visual loss, prevention is the key

Epidemiology

Central retinal artery occlusion (CRAO) is a rare cause of visual loss with an incidence of 1 per 100,000 people in the USA. In 1–2% of cases, there is a bilateral involvement. Branch retinal artery occlusions (BRAO) are also uncommon. The Blue Mountains Eye Study identified asymptomatic retinal emboli in about 1.4% of the population studied, increasing to a 3% in the 10-year survivors.

The incidence of retinal artery occlusions (RAOs) increases with age (peaking near age 80). A male gender predilection has been found in CRAO but not BRAO. Systemic risk factors for embolic occlusions include cigarette smoking, hypertension, body mass index, hyperlipidaemia, diabetes, and cardiac disease. Retinal arterial occlusions are associated with an increased risk of mortality.

Pathophysiology

Both CRAO and BRAO are usually a result of an embolus. Three main types of emboli recognised are:

- Cholesterol emboli (Hollenhorst plaques) arising in the carotid arteries
- Platelet-fibrin emboli associated with large-vessel arteriosclerosis
- Calcific emboli arising from diseased cardiac valves

Other rare causes of emboli include septic emboli from infective endocarditis, long bone fracture related fat emboli and talc emboli in intravenous drug users.

The inner layers of the retina derive its blood supply entirely from the central retinal artery except in the presence of a cilioretinal artery which arises from the short posterior ciliary artery and provides blood to a variable portion of the nasal macula. Rapid neuronal atrophy from sustained retinal ischaemia (within 90 minutes based on primate studies) remains the limiting factor for visual recovery.

Clinical features

The signs and symptoms of RAO depend on the size and location of the occluded vessel. Visual loss may be transient (up to 20 minutes duration) or persistent. Ophthalmic artery occlusions result in total loss of vision in the affected eye. Non-perfusion of the choroid and retina causes ischaemia of all retinal layers (the resulting vision is typically perception of light to no perception of light). Typical presentations of CRAO are profound monocular vision loss, with vision ranging from count fingers to hand motion in the majority of patients. Central vision may be spared if a cilioretinal artery is present (20–23% of eyes). A relative afferent pupillary defect occurs in ophthalmic and CRAOs. Isolated cilioretinal artery occlusions may result in localised central, paracentral, or centrocecal scotoma. Peripheral BRAO may be asymptomatic. Involvement of a major macular arcade results in sectoral visual field loss.

Within hours of infarction of the inner retina, the retina appears oedematous and opacified. The 'cherry red spot' sign is typically seen in CRAO. This results from the orange reflex arising from the intact choroidal vasculature beneath the foveola, which contrasts with the surrounding opaque neural retina. Inhibition of axoplasmic transport in the nerve fibre layer results in cotton wool spots. Later, the occluded vessel may recanalise, and the retinal colour returns to normal as perfusion returns.

Investigations

History and examination

A careful medical history to identify systemic disease should be taken. Evidence of embolic disease includes transient ischaemic symptoms, lateralizing weakness and paresthesia. Symptoms of giant cell arteritis (GCA) include headaches, scalp tenderness, malaise, temporal tenderness, jaw claudication, fever, proximal stiffness and a history of polymyalgia rheumatica.

Older individuals presenting with a RAO should be evaluated for GCA and embolic disease in a stroke centre, assessing cardiac status, heart valves, and carotid arteries. Younger patients should be assessed for autoimmune, hypercoagulable and inflammatory disorders.

Clinical evaluation should include fundoscopy to identify emboli, carotid and cardiac auscultation and palpation of the scalp for the presence of tenderness and pulse of the temporal arteries.

Giant cell arteritis is estimated to account for 1–2% of cases of CRAO. Isolated cilioretinal artery occlusions should raise suspicions of GCA. Patients over the age of 50 should be investigated for GCA with erythrocyte sedimentation rate (ESR) and C-reactive protein (CRP) levels as markers of inflammation. An elevated platelet count detected on a full blood count may also be suggestive of GCA. A temporal artery biopsy should be performed within 14 days (preferably 1–2 days) of initiating corticosteroid therapy in suspected GCA cases.

Optical coherence tomography
Inner retinal hyperreflectivity is evident in acute RAO. Patchy areas of deep capillary-bed ischaemia can manifest as increased reflectivity on OCT, referred to as paracentral acute middle maculopathy.

Fluorescein angiography
It may demonstrate delays in retinal arteriolar flow and a delayed arteriovenous transit time. Ophthalmic or carotid artery obstruction may cause delayed choroidal filling as well.

Diagnosis
Acute, symptomatic RAO is regarded as an ophthalmic emergency and should be regarded as a clinical indicator of a more severe systemic disorder. Other associations include cardiac arrhythmias, mitral valve prolapse, sickle cell disease, coagulation disorders, pregnancy, oral contraceptive use, occult malignancy and inflammatory and infectious aetiologies such as *Toxoplasma* chorioretinitis and syphilis. Rarely, migraine can cause RAO in patients and should be considered in patients younger than 30–40 years of age. Susac syndrome should be considered in recurrent BRAO (leakage of the vessel wall on fluorescein angiography, Gass plaques in the retinal arterioles on fundoscopy, MRI brain and audiology evaluation).

The Royal College of Physicians (RCP) stroke guidelines include transient ocular ischaemic events in the definition of a transient ischaemic attack (TIA). An ophthalmologist and a stroke physician should jointly manage visual loss due to RAO.

Treatment
Embolic retinal artery occlusion
Several interventions have attempted to dislodge an embolus towards a peripheral location to enable retinal reperfusion. These include lowering the intraocular pressure with a paracentesis or intravenous acetazolamide, carbogen vasodilatory inhalation therapy (a mixture of 95% oxygen and 5% carbon dioxide) and applying intermittent pressure on the globe ('ocular massage'). The effectiveness of these manoeuvres in improving vision outcomes is limited. Hyperbaric oxygen therapy, catheterisation of the ophthalmic artery with a thrombolytic infusion, and transvitreal neodymium–yttrium–aluminium-garnet laser embolysis also lack good evidence of efficacy.

The greatest risk of a vascular event is highest early after a stroke or TIA (25% within 3 months), half of which is within the first 4 days. An acute RAO presentation should be referred to a stroke centre. Commencing secondary prevention promptly can substantially reduce the risk of recurrent ischaemic events. There is no evidence in support of treating asymptomatic patients who have a BRAO with an expedited stroke workup.

Please refer to the latest RCP stroke guidelines for details but in principle it is recommended that patients with a confirmed diagnosis of TIA should receive and oral antiplatelet agent and high intensity statin therapy started immediately.

Giant cell arteritis

High-dose corticosteroids should be initiated in all patients with suspected GCA. Generally, high dose oral prednisone (1 mg/kg body weight) is initiated. A 3-day course of intravenous pulsed methylprednisolone at a dose of 500–1,000 mg daily followed by high-dose oral prednisone is an alternate approach.

Complications

Approximately 18% of eyes develop iris neovascularization after an acute CRAO. This can develop 1–12 weeks after the CRAO, with a mean time interval of approximately 4–5 weeks. Complete panretinal photocoagulation can induce regression of anterior segment neovascularisation in approximately 60% of cases.

Further reading

American Academy of Ophthalmology. Retinal and Ophthalmic Artery Occlusions. Preferred Practice Pattern. San Francisco: AAO; 2016.

Vodopivec I, Cestari DM, Rizzo JF III. Management of transient monocular vision loss and retinal artery occlusions. Semin Ophthalmol 2017; 32:125–133.

Related topics of interest

- Diabetic eye disease (p. 116)
- Giant cell arteritis (p. 156)
- Retinal imaging (p. 277)
- Retinal vein occlusion (p. 290)

71 Retinal detachment

Key points

- For the best visual prognosis, acute rhegmatogenous retinal detachment (RRD) requires urgent surgical repair (within 24 hours if macula-on)
- Tractional retinal detachment is usually associated with advanced diabetic eye disease and carries significant risk to vision, including when surgery is performed
- Exudative retinal detachment is rare and management tends to be targeted at the underlying cause, which is often inflammatory

Retinal detachment is the separation of the neurosensory retina from the retinal pigment epithelium. There are a number of causes, each with significantly different management and urgency of needing repair.

Rhegmatogenous retinal detachment

Rhegmatogenous retinal detachment is the most common type of retinal detachment (incidence 1/10,000/year), and usually associated with evolving posterior vitreous detachment (PVD). Patients usually complain of photopsia and floaters, and may have a visual field defect depending on the severity and extent of the RRD. There are other indicators, such as the presence of pigment in the anterior vitreous, which indicates that a retinal break is highly likely to have occurred. Following a retinal break, there is a 50% chance of progression to a retinal detachment due to subretinal accumulation. RRD can also occur in the absence of PVD, secondary to round holes in myopes. Occasionally, an RRD is chronic and progresses slowly, if at all. In such cases, retinal thinning and demarcation lines may be present as well as reduced intraocular pressure (Schwartz's syndrome).

Clinical examination of acute RRD shows retinal detachment and usually a visible retinal break (although sometimes the break is only fully identified during surgical repair).

RRD is usually described as 'macula on' or 'macula off', depending on the extent of the subretinal fluid and whether the macula is involved. Those with macula-on RRD tend to have preserved visual acuity at the time of diagnosis. The position of the RRD gives information regarding the likely position of the primary retinal break, according to Lincoff's rules (Lincoff and Gieser, 1971).

Lincoff's rules

- In 96% of superior nasal or temporal detachments, the hole is within 1.5 clock hours of the highest border
- In 93% of total or superior detachments crossing the midline, the primary hole is at 12 o'clock or in a triangle; the apex is at the ora serrata, and the sides intersect the equator one hour either side of 12 o'clock
- In 95% of inferior detachments, the higher side indicates to which side of the disc an inferior hole lies
- In bullous inferior detachments, the primary hole lies above the horizontal meridian

Once the diagnosis of acute RRD has been established, the clinician must arrange surgical repair. Acute macula-on RRD is a relative emergency, and should be repaired within 24 hours to reduce the likelihood of subsequent macular involvement and visual loss. There is less consensus on timing of surgery for macula-off detachments, and it must take into account duration of symptoms, although as a rule, retinal reattachment should be arranged as a priority and it is advised that cases are discussed with vitreo-retinal specialists at the time of diagnosis.

The most common technique for retinal reattachment is pars plana vitrectomy, combined with cryo- or laser-retinopexy and intraocular gas tamponade. It is important to note that patients who have intraocular gas must not fly until the gas bubble has fully absorbed, due to the potential problem of IOP fluctuation at high altitude. In certain scenarios, such as lack of PVD, the vitreoretinal surgeon may decide to perform a scleral buckling procedure (i.e. indenting the RPE towards the retina with a scleral sutured silicon explant) combined with cryotherapy of the retinal breaks, although this is clinician dependent. An approximate success rate (retinal reattachment) of 80–90% with one operation is usually quoted. The prognosis of macula-off RRD is highly variable, but in general the resultant visual acuity is worse than predetachment.

Tractional retinal detachment

Tractional retinal detachment (TRD) refers to retinal detachment secondary to abnormal intraocular membranes which exert a pulling effect on the retina. They are most commonly seen in the context of advanced diabetic eye disease (see other chapters), although rarer causes such as familial exudative vitreoretinopathy must be considered in the differential diagnosis. The cause is usually evident from the history and examination findings.

TRD may be asymptomatic until it affects the macula, and due to the surgical complexity in repairing them, treatment is often deferred until the macula becomes involved. Vitrectomy and delamination carry significant risk, and patients must be carefully consented regarding the risk and benefit of surgery.

Exudative retinal detachment

This is a less common condition where fluid accumulates in the subretinal space, causing retinal detachment, secondary to a non-functioning outer blood-retinal barrier. The causes for exudative retinal detachment (ERD) include inflammatory conditions (e.g. posterior scleritis, posterior uveitis), choroidal tumours and vascular conditions (e.g. central serous retinopathy). Rarely, it can be seen following panretinal photocoagulation.

The work-up for patients with ERD is significantly different from RRD or TRD, and should include a full systemic examination to look for underlying aetiology as well as a B-scan ultrasound which is helpful for identifying posterior scleritis. The well described symptom of 'shifting fluid' may be present, this described subretinal fluid which moves dynamically, as the position of the eye moves. Once the cause of the ERD is established, specific treatment of the underlying condition is the main aspect of management, rather than vitrectomy.

Further reading

Williamson TH. Vitreoretinal Surgery, 2nd edition. US: Springer-Verlag Berlin Heidelberg; 2011.

Related topics of interest

- Vitreoretinal surgery – retinal breaks and detachment and vitreomacular interface disorders (p. 350)

72 Retinal dystrophies

Key points
- Inherited retinal diseases represent the commonest cause of visual impairment in England and Wales in the working age population, and the second commonest in children
- Inherited retinal conditions are clinically highly variable and are the most genetically heterogeneous of all diseases in medicine
- Careful history and examination, detailed retinal structural and functional assessments, and genetic testing, is often needed to establish an accurate diagnosis, provide informed genetic counselling and advice on prognosis
- There are no proven cures to date, however, recent advances in genetic testing, retinal imaging, surgical techniques, and along multiple avenues of research including gene therapy, have led to a new era of a rapidly increasing number of ongoing and planned clinical trials, with cautious optimism for the future

Overview
Inherited retinal disorders are a diverse group of retinal conditions, varying both clinically in terms of presentation, severity and progression, and genetically – with over 300 disease-causing genes identified to date. They can be usefully sub-classified on the basis of either natural history: stationary (dysfunction syndromes) versus progressive (dystrophies); or retinal involvement: predominantly isolated to the macula (developmental macular disorders and macular dystrophies) versus generalised retinal involvement (rod-cone, cone, and cone-rod dystrophies, and chorioretinal dystrophies). In addition, they can be classified on the basis of whether they are syndromic or isolated to the eye, with the majority being non-syndromic.

Presentation
Diseases affecting predominantly rod photoreceptors present with peripheral visual field loss and impaired night vision (nyctalopia). Diseases affecting mainly cone photoreceptors, can cause photophobia, central scotomata, and decreased VA, contrast sensitivity and colour vision.

Diagnosis
Detailed clinical history (including family history) and examination, retinal imaging [including SD-OCT and fundus autofluorescence (FAF)], perimetry, electrophysiological testing, and assessments of colour vision help establish a diagnosis. Examination of other family members is also often necessary. Molecular genetic testing is valuable to confirm the clinical diagnosis or establish the specific underlying genetic basis.

Examples of inherited retinal disorders
There are a huge range of inherited retinal disorders (IRD) that are beyond the scope of this chapter, so further reading is provided. Selected conditions are described later.

Retinitis pigmentosa
Retinitis pigmentosa (RP) is the commonest IRD, affecting approximately 1 in 3,000. 50% of patients have no family history of RP. Autosomal dominant RP is often of later onset and slower progression than autosomal recessive and X-linked forms. The majority of cases are non-syndromic. Mutations in over 100 genes have been implicated.

Clinical features
- Progressive nyctalopia and peripheral visual field constriction initially, followed by central visual loss over time

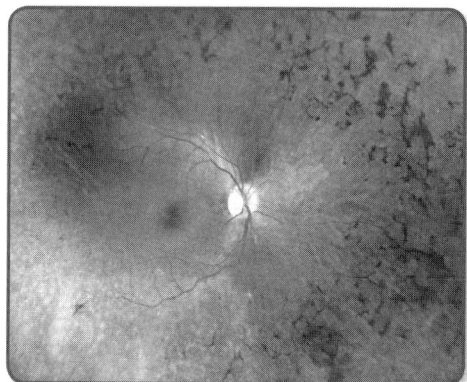

Figure 72.1 Fundus photograph showing the mid-peripheral 'bone-spicule' retinal pigmentation, optic disc pallor and arteriolar attenuation of retinitis pigmentosa. (*For colour version see plate 6*)

- Mid-peripheral 'bone-spicule' retinal pigmentation, optic disc pallor, arteriolar attenuation (**Figure 72.1**)
- Ocular associations: Cataract (especially posterior subcapsular), myopia (particularly in X-linked RP), and cystoid macular oedema (CMO)

Investigations
- *SD-OCT and FAF:* Useful for both diagnosis and monitoring change over time
- *Full-field electroretinogram (ERG):* Greater degree of generalised rod than cone dysfunction in early disease
- *Perimetry:* Recording progressive constriction of visual fields

Treatment
- *Supportive measures:* Genetic and psychological/emotional counselling, visual impairment registration, glasses and low vision aids, support from social services
- *CMO:* Carbonic anhydrase inhibitors are the mainstay currently; topical agents initially for 6 months minimum to determine effect, proceeding to oral if no improvement
- *Cataract surgery:* Reduce operating light levels, slowly taper post-operative topical steroids
- *Disease progression:* Role of nutritional supplements controversial; supplementation with vitamin A palmitate no longer recommended; Omega-3 and lutein may be worth considering, although the current evidence base is limited
- *Future therapies:* Gene and stem cell therapies are promising with various phase I/II clinical trials underway (clinicaltrials.gov); the Argus II epiretinal prosthesis system has been licenced for use in advanced RP

Differential diagnosis
Several conditions may cause a pigmentary retinopathy mimicking advanced RP. These include: retinal inflammatory diseases (e.g. rubella, syphilis, infectious retinitis), advanced autoimmune and paraneoplastic retinopathies, drug toxicity (e.g. chloroquine), traumatic retinopathy and long-standing retinal detachment.

Leber congenital amaurosis (LCA)
- Group of clinically heterogeneous disorders caused by mutations in at least 25 genes
- Characterised by severe visual impairment from birth or early infancy, nystagmus, absent/diminished pupillary light reflexes, and extinguished ERG responses. Also associated with oculodigital syndrome and keratoconus
- Usually normal fundus appearance, or only subtle retinal pigment epithelial (RPE) changes/vessel attenuation in the early stages. Characteristic retinal phenotypes are seen with certain causes, including *RPE65*, *RDH12* and *CRB1*-associated LCA
- Multiple phase I/II and III gene therapy clinical trials are ongoing or planned (clinicaltrials.gov)

Bietti crystalline chorioretinal dystrophy
- Autosomal recessive dystrophy, characterised by multiple small intraretinal crystalline deposits
- Common in East Asia, especially Japan and China
- *CYP4V2* mutations believed to result in disordered lipid metabolism
- Patients present following routine optician retinal evaluation or due to increasing

nyctalopia and peripheral visual field constriction
- Degenerative changes begin in the RPE and choriocapillaris, leading to a 'moth-eaten' appearance on FFA. Perilimbal subepithelial corneal deposits may be seen. With extension of atrophy, ERG responses diminish, visual fields constrict, and VA decreases
- Often leads to legal blindness by the fifth or sixth decade

Congenital stationary night blindness (CSNB)

- Group of disorders associated with early, non-progressive, nyctalopia
- *Other features may include:* Reduced VA, refractive error (commonly myopia but occasionally hyperopia), nystagmus, and strabismus
  - Divided into those with a normal fundus, including myopic fundi (with autosomal dominant, autosomal recessive, and X-linked subtypes); and those with fundus abnormalities (Oguchi's disease and fundus albipunctatus)
  - CSNB with normal fundi
    - Complete CSNB: No detectable rod-specific ERG and a profoundly electronegative bright flash response (reduced b-wave to a-wave ratio). Cone ERGs show subtle abnormalities
    - Incomplete CSNB: detectable rod-specific ERG, and a profoundly negative bright flash response. Cone ERGs are much more abnormal than in complete CSNB
  - CSNB with abnormal fundi
    - Oguchi disease: Fundus has a golden-yellow metallic sheen, but appears normal following prolonged dark adaptation (Mizuo phenomenon)
    - Fundus albipunctatus: Autosomal recessive. Numerous tiny radially distributed white dots/flecks over most of the fundus, but usually absent at the macula

Achromatopsia

- Non-progressive, autosomal recessive disorder affecting 1 in 30,000
- Lack of function of all 3 cone subtypes
- Patients have poor VA (6/36-6/60) and colour vision from birth/early infancy, pendular nystagmus and marked photophobia
- Fundus appearance is usually normal, or with mild RPE changes
- Complete or incomplete forms – residual colour vision and slightly better VA (6/24-6/36) in the incomplete form
- *ERG:* Non-recordable cone responses with normal rod responses. Differentiates from LCA
- *OCT:* Appearances range from normal to a hyporeflective optically empty zone in the outer retina at the fovea, to outer retinal atrophy; foveal hypoplasia may be present

Stargardt disease (STGD)

- Commonest macular dystrophy
- Autosomal recessive, due to *ABCA4* mutations
- *Three presentations:* Childhood-onset (worst prognosis), adult-onset, and late-onset/foveal-sparing STGD (best prognosis). Childhood-onset is commonest, with VA reducing to approximately 6/60 by end of teenage years; second commonest peak is early adulthood
- Diagnosis can be delayed as often initially minimal fundus signs on examination [classical retinal phenotype is macular atrophy with yellow/white retinal flecks (**Figure 72.2**)]; however, clear structural disturbance can be seen on SD-OCT and FAF, and retinal dysfunction on ERG
- ERG is helpful in providing advice on prognosis: Group 1 – isolated macular dysfunction; Group 2 – macular and generalised cone dysfunction; Group 3 – macular and both generalised cone and rod dysfunction. Best prognosis associated with Group 1 and worst with Group 3

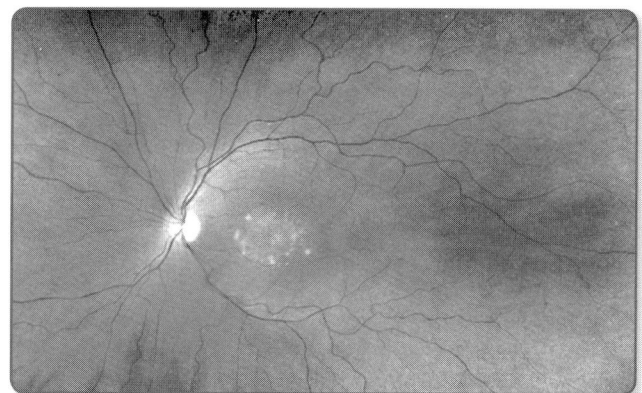

Figure 72.2 Fundus photograph of Stargardt disease showing areas of macular atrophy. (*For colour version see plate 6*)

- *FFA:* Classically 'dark choroid', due to blockage of choroidal fluorescence by accumulation of lipofuscin in the RPE

Best disease

- Second most common macular dystrophy
- Onset usually in childhood, with highly variable expression
- Autosomal dominant, associated with *BEST1* mutations
- Usually asymptomatic initially. Most patients retain reading vision beyond the fifth decade
- Most easily recognised by yolk-like lesion at the posterior pole (**Figure 72.3**); may later be replaced by scarring, atrophy, or choroidal neovascular membrane (CNVM)
- Electrooculogram (EOG): Reduced Arden ratio and ERG; normal
- Anti-vascular endothelial growth factor (VEGF) agents are very effective in both childhood and adulthood CNVM

Adult vitelliform macular dystrophy

- Often confused with Best disease, though has later onset with often less progression
- *EOG:* Often normal
- Bilateral, round or oval, yellow, symmetrical, sub-retinal lesions, typically one-third to one-half optic disc diameter in size. *PRPH2* mutations

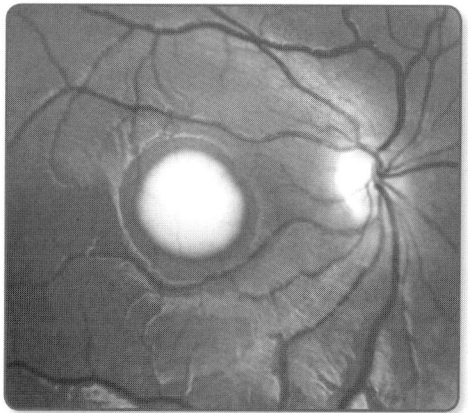

Figure 72.3 Fundus photograph of Best disease showing a yolk-like lesion at the posterior pole.

identified in approximately 20% of affected patients

Autosomal dominant drusen

- Caused by *Fibulin-3* mutation
- Often incidental finding in adults
- Often associated with a good prognosis, with reading difficulties in later life due to macular atrophy
- Yellow–white drusen at the posterior pole; characteristically abutting the optic disc (may be better seen on FAF)
- Infrequently complicated by CNVM for which anti-VEGF agents are very effective

Further reading

Michaelides M, Holder GE, Moore AT. Inherited Retinal Disorders. In: Taylor & Hoyt's Pediatric Ophthalmology and Strabismus, 5th edition. New York: Elsevier 2017. pp. 462–486.

Michaelides M, Moore AT. Inherited Macular Dystrophies. In: Taylor & Hoyt's Pediatric Ophthalmology and Strabismus, 5th edition. New York: Elsevier 2017. pp. 502–515.

Smith J, Ward D, Michaelides M, et al. New and emerging technologies for the treatment of inherited retinal diseases: a horizon scanning review. Eye (Lond) 2015; 29:1131–1140.

Related topic of interest

- Retinal imaging (p. 277)

73 Retinal imaging

Key points

- Retinal imaging is essential in diagnosis, documentation, and monitoring of retinal diseases (**Figure 73.1**)
- Multimodal imaging can aid diagnosis
- Optical coherence tomography has become the essential tool of retinal practice
- Newer imaging modalities combined with functional tests can monitor small changes even before a change of symptoms

Fundus colour photography

Fundus colour photography can be easily performed with a retinal fundus camera. Many cameras can be used without pupillary dilation (non-mydriatic). However, with most of these cameras, a better quality picture is obtained with a dilated pupil. Recently, adapters and attachments have been commercialised to enable smartphones to take fundus pictures. It is a potentially powerful technique with the development of

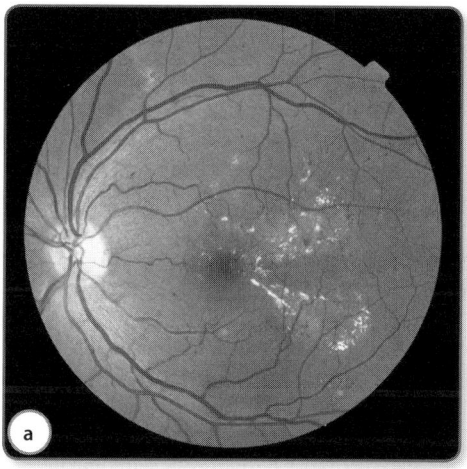

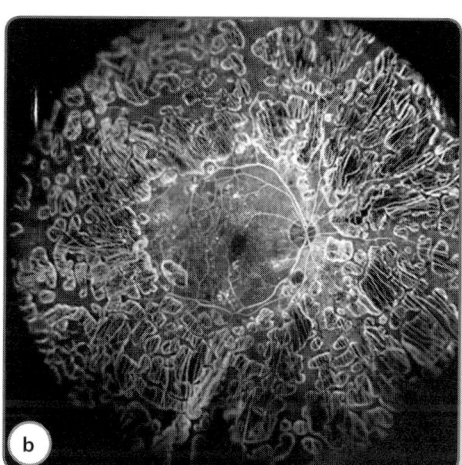

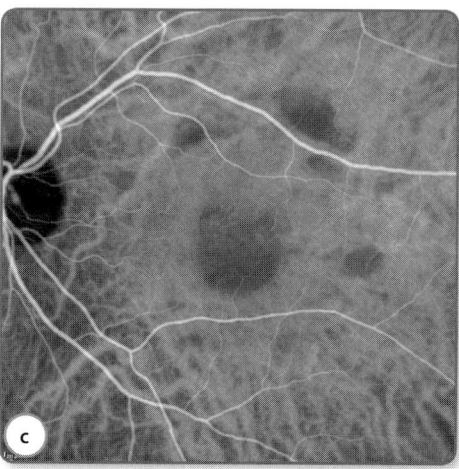

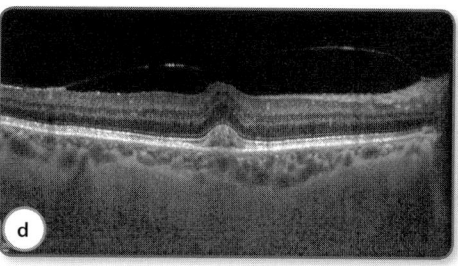

Figures 73.1 Fundus photos to show examples of different imaging modalities. (a) Fundus colour photography (*For colour version see plate 6*); (b) Fundus fluorescein angiogram; (c) Indocyanine green (ICG) angiogram; (d) Optical coherence tomography (OCT); (e) Optical coherence tomography angiogram (OCTA); (f) Auto-fluorescence (AF) imaging; (g) Ultra-widefield imaging (*For colour version see plate 6*); and (h) Ultrasound of the retina. *Continues overleaf...*

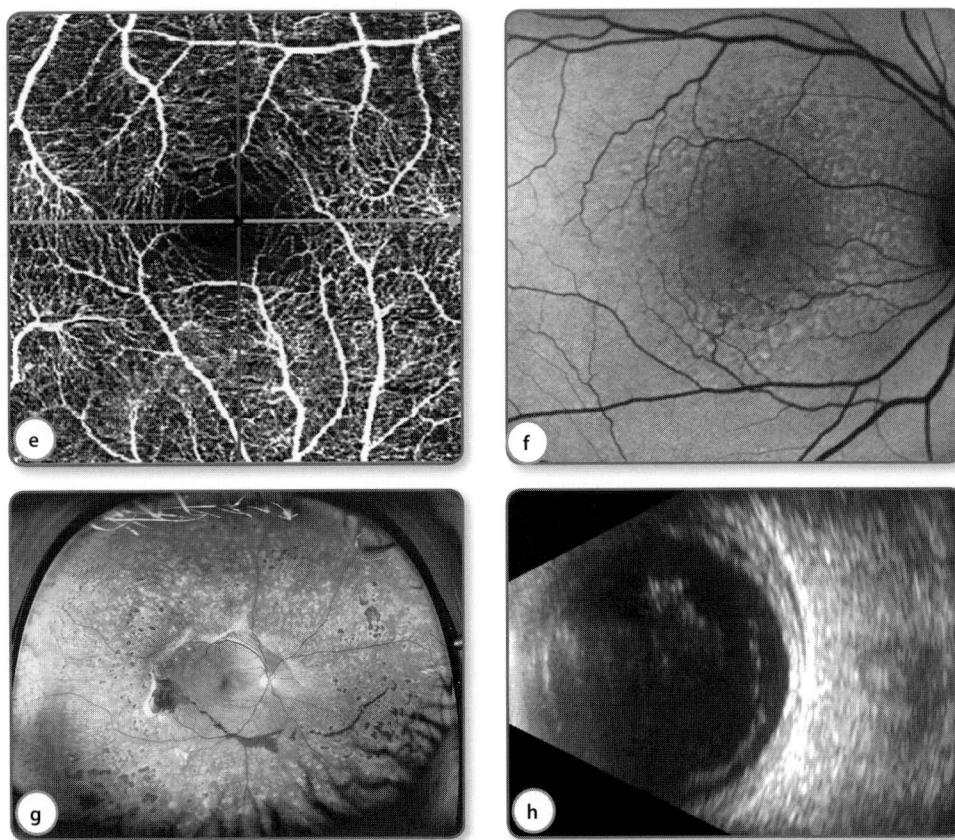

Figures 73.1 *Continued...*

real-time telemedicine. Most of the current adapters are quite difficult to use, as they need the camera to focus on the retinal image, so dilatation is usually needed. Many systems also use a video stream for recording. After the video is recorded, software in the phone is used to identify a good quality picture to be saved, sent, and analysed. The ultimate goal would be to make an adapter that the patient can use to perform a retinal selfie without pupillary dilatation. One would need to use infrared to focus, auto-focus, and auto-shoot.

Fundus colour photography is the original and still most commonly used method to document and monitor diabetic retinopathy. The Food and Drug Administration (FDA) uses the Early Treatment Diabetic Retinopathy Study (ETDRS) trial defined Diabetic Retinopathy Severity Score (DRSS) to assess whether a treatment is beneficial for diabetic retinopathy or not. Similarly, diabetic eye screening programmes use a modified/simplified system to assess the risk of sight-threatening retinopathy for referral to hospital eye service.

The standard picture is 30°, but newer cameras have a wider angle of 45/50°. The ultra-widefield camera can capture up to 200° (see later). ETDRS uses seven fields (of 30°) or four wide field (of 45°) to assess the DRSS. The English diabetic eye screening programme uses two images, one centred on the macula, and one centred on the optic disc.

Fundus fluorescein angiogram

Fundus fluorescein angiogram (FFA) usually uses an intravenous fluorescein dye to examine the retinal circulation. The dye can be visualised by using different filters to allow the retina to be illuminated by the camera light and through a different channel detected by the fundus camera as black and white images. Recently, instead of using the flash light of the camera, a scanning laser is used to pick up the signal. The latter allows better quality images with less illumination, and hence is more comfortable for the patient. In addition, video can be recorded, allowing us to see the retinal vascular dynamic instead of just a snapshot in the traditional fundus camera.

Fundus fluorescein angiogram was indicated for most retinal diseases in the past. Optical coherence tomography (OCT) is enough to make the diagnosis in many typical cases. With the advances of OCT-angiogram (OCT-A), the role of FFA will change further in the coming years (vide infra).

The basic terminology of FFA includes the following:
- *Leakage:* Lesions, such as choroidal neovascularisation are hyper-fluoresce (brighter) initially and become more hyper-fluorescent and extends beyond the lesion border
- *Staining:* Lesions, such as a fibrotic scar, are hyper-fluoresce initially and become more hyper-fluorescent but don't extend beyond the lesion border
- *Window defect:* Lesions hyper-fluoresce all the way through with similar intensity, due to the overlying tissue, usually the retinal pigment epithelium (RPE) is atrophic or gone
- *Blockage:* Hypo-fluorescence areas are due to a superficial lesion, such as blood, which blocks visualisation of the dye

Indocyanine green angiogram

Indocyanine green (ICG) angiogram is similar to FFA, but a different dye is used which is less permeable thereby improving the visualisation of choroidal lesions. It is most commonly used in the diagnosis of polypoidal choroidal vasculopathy (PCV) or central serous chorioretinopathy. It is also useful in inflammatory eye diseases and ocular oncology.

Optical coherence tomography

Optical coherence tomography is based on low-coherence interferometry. The use of relatively long wavelength light allows it to penetrate deeper into the choroid. It allows 'in vivo' cross-sectional 'histology' of the retina and choroid. The origin commercial device is called time-domain OCT. Its use has been expanded dramatically with the advance of anti-vascular endothelial growth factor (anti-VEGF) therapy for macular diseases. The concept that OCT can be used to make the diagnosis and allow personalised dosing frequency in these patients is highly popularised; however, this also lead to significant under treatment, with poor real-life outcomes as compared to clinical trial outcomes of anti-VEGF therapies. The move to spectral-domain OCT (SD-OCT) allows faster scanning and higher resolution. Some machines also have eye-tracking and image averaging ability with combined fundus camera or even FFA/ICG cameras, allowing multi-modal imaging by one machine with same area of the retina examined at the same time. Traditional SD-OCT biased the image quality on the vitreous side of the retina. When examining the choroid is more important (in various retinal diseases), Rick Spaide introduced enhanced depth imaging (EDI) by flipping the image, so the choroid and outer retina can be better visualised. Recently, swept source OCT (SS-OCT) using even faster scanning and even longer wavelengths, beyond 1,000 nm, deep into the infrared range, can visualise the choroid more clearly even when there are overlying retinal pathologies such as pigment epithelial detachment and drusen. The scans can be lined up into a cube, and hence the software can 'optical cut' the section parallel to the retinal surface, this is called en-face OCT. Using the different cut level, the 'slab', the drusen volume, for example, can be measured. Furthermore, the different layers of the retinal can be segmented. Therefore, as well as the overall retinal thickness, the individual layers of the retinal can also be measured. Most of this can be very easily done in a normal retina but segmental errors are common in disease. Manual adjustments are, therefore, required in order to get accurate measurements. These measurements are mostly for research rather than clinical use.

The OCT has not replaced FFA, but it has become the standard screening device in retinal practice. FFA/ICG is only used as confirmatory or if the diagnosis is in doubt.

Optical coherence tomography angiogram

Optical coherence tomography angiogram combines en-face OCT and the understanding that the only moving parts in the retina are blood cells in the retinal and choroidal blood vessels. Analysing the same image taken in the same spot of the retina, any differences are likely to be due to the presence of blood vessels. Using very dense and fast scanning, with software analysis of the differences between scans, blood vessels can be mapped without the use of any dye, and everything can be captured just like the OCT scan. Eye tracking and averaging are also able to enhance the image. However, one needs to understand that a large retinal vessel would cast a shadow on the layers in outer the retina and choroid, this is called projection artefact. Fortunately, commercial machines can now correct for projection and motion artefact. With improved optics and even faster scanning devices, we can now visualise most of the posterior retina. One of the limitations of OCTA is that it cannot see active leakage, and if the blood flow is too slow, then the blood vessel cannot be detected. Hence, it still cannot replace FFA/ICG completely, but it is predicted that the latter will be used less and less.

Auto-fluorescence imaging

It was noted, even before the injection of the fluorescence dye, that the retina auto-fluoresces; however, the signal is very low. With the advance of scanning laser ophthalmoscopy (SLO) imaging and adding averaging, this signal can be recorded.

It was found that the RPE cells provide most of the signal. It has become the gold standard measurement of geographic atrophy of the RPE cells, the advanced dry form of age-related macular degeneration. It is also commonly used to diagnose macular dystrophies.

Ultra-widefield imaging

Traditional fundus cameras can only take a 30° or 45° shot in one go, as mentioned previously. Even taking seven fields for diabetic retinopathy staging, only up to about 100° of the retina can be visualised. Using a curved mirror, ultra-widefield imaging can extend the view to over 200° in one go. As well as taking fundus images, auto-fluorescence (AF)/FFA/ICG can also be performed. The main limitation is that eyelashes can often block the view of the inferior retina. However, peripheral retinal lesions can be documented with ease and it is an essential tool in ocular inflammatory diseases to make diagnoses and document progression or improvement. There is also increasing evidence that patients with predominantly peripheral diabetic retinopathy lesions may be more likely to progress. The slightly distorted peripheral areas make standardised measurements for research slightly difficult and need correction. There are some newer devices with about a 120–150° view without peripheral distortion and with less interference by eyelashes.

Ultrasound of the retina

Like fundus cameras and FFA, ultrasound (US) is one of the earlier tools in the diagnosis of retinal diseases. It is still useful when there is a dense vitreous haemorrhage to see whether there is an underlying retinal detachment and/or retinal tears. It is also used in the diagnosis for choroidal tumours. However, ultra-widefield imaging, OCT, and OCTA will slowly replace US when the media is clear.

Further reading

Cassels NK, Wild JM, Margrain TH, et al. The use of microperimetry in assessing visual function in age-related macular degeneration. Surv Ophthalmol 2018; 63:40–55.

Frampton GK, Kalita N, Payne L, et al. Fundus autofluorescence imaging: systematic review of test accuracy for the diagnosis and monitoring of retinal conditions. Eye (Lond) 2017; 31:995–1007.

Keane PA, Sadda SR. Retinal imaging in the twenty-first century: state of the art and future directions. Ophthalmology 2014; 121:2489–2500.

Rabiolo A, Parravano M, Querques L, et al. Ultra-wide-field fluorescein angiography in diabetic retinopathy: a narrative review. Clin Ophthalmol 2017; 11:803–807.

Sharma A. Emerging Simplified Retinal Imaging. Dev Ophthalmol 2017; 60:56–62.

Spaide RF, Fujimoto JG, Waheed NK, et al. Optical coherence tomography angiography. Prog Retina Eye Res 2018; 64:1–55.

Related topics of interest

- Age-related macular degeneration (p. 1)
- Diabetic eye disease (p. 116)
- Retinal detachment (p. 270)
- Retinal dystrophies (p. 272)
- Retinal vasculitis (p. 286)
- Retinal vein occlusion (p. 290)

74 Retinal lasers

Key points

- Lasers are focused light energy with high spatial and temporal coherence
- Different wavelengths are absorbed by different ocular tissues
- Laser lenses have different properties that need to be considered when delivering treatment

Background

The term *laser* is an acronym for "light amplification by stimulated emission of radiation". The high spatial coherence properties enable laser light to maintain a narrow beam over long distances and concentrate power over small focussed areas. Temporal coherence permits emission of light within a very narrow wavelength spectrum (emit a single colour of light).

Types of retinal lasers

Solid state laser

These lasers use a crystalline or glass rod that is "doped" with ions to provide the required energy states. Examples include the neodymium-yttrium aluminium garnet (Nd-YAG) laser. The standard emission wavelength is about 1064 nm. This is doubled to 532 nm when used as a retinal laser.

Diode laser

These use semiconductors (similar to a light-emitting diode) that are electrically pumped to generate optical gain. The wavelength most commonly used for retinal treatment is 810 nm.

Mechanism of action on tissues

Laser light absorbed by tissues induces photothermal, photochemical and vapourisation effects on the selected tissues. Photothermal reactions occur when laser light is absorbed and is converted into thermal energy (coagulation), producing rise in temperature up to 65°C, which causes denaturation of tissue proteins and coagulative necrosis. Photodynamic therapy utilises photochemical reactions induced by ultraviolet or visible light. This is absorbed by tissue molecules or by molecules of a photosensitizing medication (e.g. verteporfin), producing cytotoxic reactive oxygen species. Vapourisation results from a rise in water temperature above the boiling point within tissues, which causes micro-explosions, as can occur in overly intense burns.

The different pigment compounds found within the retina selectively absorb different wavelengths of laser (**Table 74.1**). As a result of these absorption characteristics, the green and yellow lasers are the most commonly used for treating vascular disorders at the macula.

Laser treatment aims to selectively target the tissue to be treated while sparing adjacent normal tissue.

$$\text{Laser fluence} = \frac{\text{Laser pulse energy (J)}}{\text{Effective focal spot area (cm}^2\text{)}}$$

$$\text{Laser intensity} = \frac{\text{Laser peak power (W)}}{\text{Effective focal spot area (cm}^2\text{)}}$$

The effectiveness of treatment depends on the laser parameters used, the clarity of the ocular media, and the extent of fundus pigmentation. Smaller spot sizes and longer duration exposures require less energy than larger spot sizes to achieve the same intensity effects.

A slit lamp mounted transpupillary approach is the commonest method of treating retinal vascular disorders. Other methods include indirect ophthalmoscopes, endophotocoagulation during vitrectomy, or trans-scleral application with a contact probe when ocular media opacities are significant.

Clinical application of lasers

The advantages of the yellow laser include minimal scatter through nuclear sclerotic lenses, low absorption by macular xanthophyll,

Table 74.1 Absorption spectra of retinal pigment

Pigment	Blue (488 nm)	Green (514 nm)	Yellow (570 nm)	Red (647 nm)
Melanin	Yes	Yes	Yes	Yes
Haemoglobin	Yes	Yes	Yes	Poor
Macular xanthophyll	Yes	Yes	Poor	Poor

and little potential for photochemical damage. As such, it is useful for treating vascular structures while causing minimal damage to adjacent pigmented tissue.

The red and infrared lasers can penetrate through nuclear sclerotic cataracts and moderate vitreous haemorrhages and are also minimally absorbed by xanthophyll. However, they result in deeper burns with inhomogeneous absorption at the level of the choroid so titrating the correct level of energy during treatment is more challenging. Patient discomfort can be more of a problem.

Panretinal photocoagulation (PRP)

This aims to deliver relatively high-intensity burns with large spot sizes (200–500 μm) that are of a creamy pale colour. Treatment is usually applied up to the arcades, sparing 2 disc diameters from the temporal macula and disc. Targeted panretinal photocoagulation (PRP) involves the delivery of laser to ischaemic retina identified on fluorescein angiography. Care should be taken to avoid the long ciliary nerves located in the 3 and 9 o'clock positions if possible.

A complete PRP typically delivers 1,500 burns of 500 μm size. Multi-spot pattern lasers that are in use do not incorporate the 500 μm spot size and most clinicians select the 400 μm spot size. This would require a total of 2,340 burns to give an equivalent treatment area to 1,500 × 500 μm (the treatment *area* with conventional settings is 1.56X bigger than with a 400 μm spot size). If this reduction in treatment area is not accounted for, it could result in under-treatment.

Macular laser

Laser is applied to areas of thickening avoiding the retina 500 μm from the foveal centre and the temporal margin of the disc. The laser spot sizes used are smaller than in PRP (100–200 μm) and the duration of the burn is typically ≤0.1 seconds.

Sub-threshold laser is a modification of conventional macular laser that aims to minimise thermal damage to macular tissues such as photoreceptors and choriocapillaris. Micropulse lasers that administer short pulses of laser (≤ 0.1 ms) have emerged as the main modality to achieve sub-threshold treatment where a visible laser burn is not detectable. Trials in diabetic macular oedema have demonstrated visual outcomes that are either equivalent to or better than conventional laser.

A further evolution in macular laser is navigated laser therapy (NAVILAS; OD-OS, Inc. Germany) that utilises eye-tracking with the ability to overlay infrared, fluorescein angiography, and optical coherence tomography images onto the real-time fundus image for precise mapping and treatment of target areas.

Laser retinopexy

Approximately, 2–3 concentric rings of laser are placed around the retinal break to create chorioretinal adhesion and prevent progression of the subretinal fluid and retinal detachment. The laser burns are usually 200–500 μm in size and are more intense (whiter appearance) than PRP burns.

Other retinal lesions

Photocoagulation can be used to ablate small retinal angiomas and their feeder vessels. Half fluence photodynamic therapy has been used to treat choroidal polyps and central serous retinopathy. Conventional macular laser has also been used to treat retinal pigment epithelial (RPE) disturbances in central serous retinopathy.

Laser lenses

There are two types of lenses that are used to treat retinal disorders:
1. Negative-power planoconcave lenses: These provide an upright image with superior resolution of the macula. The spot size of the laser on the retina is similar to that selected on the slit lamp setting.
2. High-plus power lenses: These lenses provide an inverted image with a wide field of view. Fine resolution at the macula is relatively reduced. These lenses are ideal for panretinal photocoagulation and retinopexy. The spot size of the laser beam is magnified and the image seen is minified.

Table 74.2 details the magnification characteristics of commonly used laser lenses.

Complications

- Macular oedema may develop. Any pre-existing oedema must be treated prior to commencing PRP
- Reduction in visual field and nyctalopia can develop after PRP
- Inadvertent foveal burns with resultant central micro-scotomas
- Bruch's membrane ruptures can develop with high intensity foveal burns of short duration and small spot size (< 100 µm) with secondary choroidal neovascularisation
- Iris burns with iris atrophy and iritis
- Exudative choroidal detachment can result from intense PRP. This reaction peaks 1–3 days after treatment and resolves spontaneously within a few weeks. This can result in forward rotation of the ciliary body, narrowing of the anterior chamber, raised intraocular pressure and aqueous misdirection, which requires urgent treatment

Safety

Careful preparation of the patient including comfortable positioning on the slit lamp and using a fixation target is important successful laser treatment. Subtenon or peribulbar anaesthesia can minimise eye movements in challenging circumstances such as nystagmus.

Ophthalmic lasers are class 4 lasers. The machine should be serviced regularly. The laser treatment room must have safety locks, blackout blinds over windows, warning signs indicative of use and appropriate eye filters for persons within the room not receiving treatment.

Table 74.2 Magnification factors for commonly used retinal laser lenses

	Type of lens	Magnification of image	Magnification of spot size
Panretinal photocoagulation	Ocular Mainster PRP 165	0.51	1.96
	Rodenstock Panfundoscope	0.7	1.43
	Volk Equator Plus	0.44	2.27
	Volk Superquad 160	0.5	2.0
Macular laser lenses	Goldmann 3-mirror central	0.93	1.08
	Ocular Mainster High Magnification	1.25	0.8
	Volk Area Centralis	1.06	0.94
	Volk Fundus Lens	1.25	0.8
	Volk PDT Len	0.66	1.5
	Ocular PDT 1.6	0.63	1.6

Further reading

American Academy of Ophthalmology. 2017–2018 Basic and Clinical Science Course (Section 12: Retina and Vitreous). San Francisco: AAO; 2018.

Public Health England. Ubiquitous Lasers. [online] Available from https://www.gov.uk/government/uploads/system/uploads/attachment_data/file/496266/Ubiquitous_Lasers_StdQ.pdf. [Last Accessed October, 2019].

Sivaprasad S, Sandhu R, Tandon A, et al. Subthreshold micropulse diode laser photocoagulation for clinically significant diabetic macular oedema: a three-year follow-up. Clin Exp Ophthalmol 2007; 35:640–644.

Su D, Hubschman JP. A review of subthreshold micropulse laser and recent advances in retinal laser technology. Ophthalmol Ther 2017; 6:1–6.

Related topics of interest

- Diabetic eye disease (p. 116)
- Retinal vein occlusion (p. 290)
- Retinal arterial occlusion (p. 267)

75 Retinal vasculitis

Key points

- This is potentially sight-threatening intraocular inflammation that primarily involves the retinal vasculature
- Retinal vessel inflammation can be a part of the spectrum of signs in panuveitis but can also be the sole presenting feature of a myriad of diseases
- As with all uveitis, it can be a primary condition or secondary to infections or systemic diseases
- Arterial involvement may represent an infectious viral retinitis where delaying treatment for angiography is not recommended, if in doubt 'tap and inject'

Epidemiology

The prevalence of uveitis has been estimated around 4–5 per 10,000 and within this group retinal vasculitis makes up around 10%, leading to an approximate prevalence of 4 per 100,000. However, most prevalence studies come from Western populations, and in countries with high rates of tuberculosis (TB) and Behçet's disease, the numbers will be much higher.

There is a female to male preponderance in some studies and most patients present in young adulthood. Both eyes are usually affected although it can be asymmetrical.

Pathophysiology

Retinal vasculitis is an immunological condition as evidenced by rare post-mortem samples and animal models of uveitis which stimulate the systemic immune system and lead to marked retinal vasculitis.

In patients with proven systemic vasculitis, it is likely circulating immune complexes are reaching the retina but in patients where only the eye is affected, there may be local organ-specific auto-reactive T cells as the culprit. Either case should respond to broad-spectrum immunosuppression such as corticosteroids.

The inflamed vessel walls can leak fluid leading to oedema or inflammatory cells and proteinaceous material leading to a cuff of exudate around the vessel. This should be distinguished from fibrotic thickening and sheathing of vessel walls which can occur in the chronic stages or from non-inflammatory processes.

This material can build up and vessel walls thicken until there is occlusion. If the occluded vessel is an artery, there will be ischaemia, cotton-wool spots and eventually neovascularisation may occur. If the occluded vessel is a vein, there will be typical signs of venous occlusion with oedema, intraretinal haemorrhages and microaneurysms.

Clinical features

Symptoms

Retinal vasculitis may be asymptomatic if the affected vessels are peripheral. If it is causing a secondary vitritis, then patients may complain of floaters and decreased vision. If affecting the posterior pole, then they may experience positive scotomata. The eye may remain white and painless during these attacks.

Symptoms related to possible causative systemic disease should be sought with specific questioning about respiratory symptoms, skin rashes, orogenital ulceration, arthritis or neurologic symptoms.

Examination

Anterior uveitis and scleritis can occur alongside retinal vasculitis although that starts to suggest more of a panuveitis picture. Vitreous inflammation and cellular activity are common as is cystoid macula oedema. The optic nerve may appear hyperaemic and be swollen.

The hallmark of retinal vasculitis is, of course, the changes to and around the retinal vessels. The vessels will develop a thickening and cuff of inflammatory material which may be widespread or focal and segmental in nature (**Figures 75.1a** and **b**). The most important decision to be made on examination is whether arteries, veins

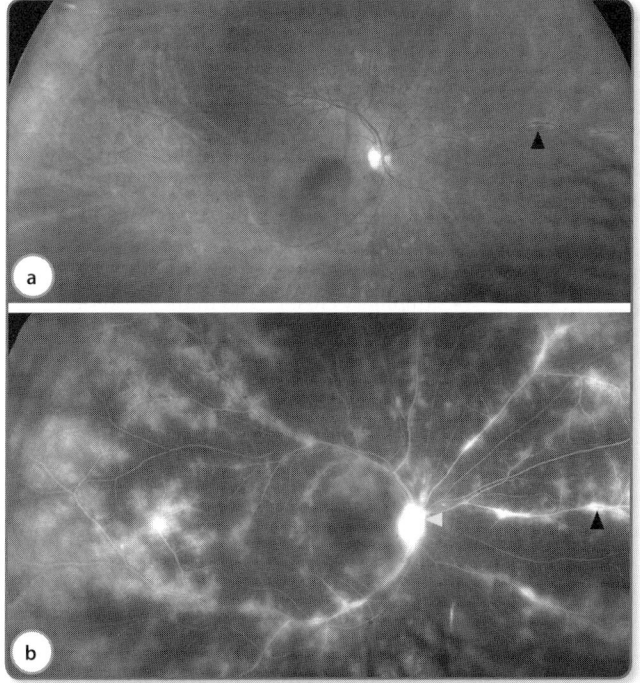

Figures 75.1a and b (a) Wide-field fundus colour photograph of a right eye showing (black arrowhead) cuffing of a retinal vein (*For colour version see plate 7*). (b) Fluorescein angiogram of the same eye showing staining and leak from the same vessel visualised on colour photo (black arrowhead). The optic nerve also leaks in this late phase leading to a 'hot disc' (white arrowhead). There is also widespread small vessel leak leading to 'ferning' temporally.

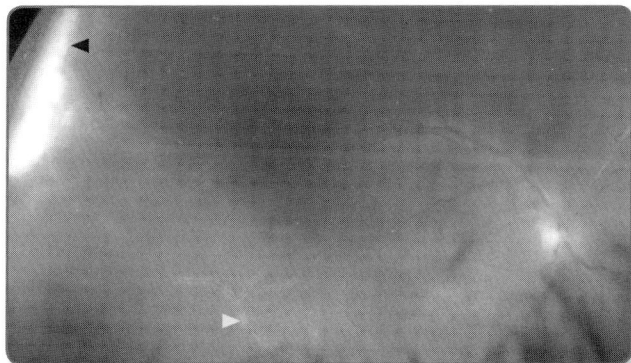

Figure 75.2 Wide-field fundus colour photograph of a right eye showing (black arrowhead) peripheral acute retinal necrosis with opaque whitening of the retina. There is additional vascular cuffing of arteries and veins leading towards the area (white arrowhead). The picture is hazy due to vitritis. (*For colour version see plate 7*)

or both are affected. Capillary involvement may not be visualised until angiography is performed. Retinal haemorrhages are common and may suggest frank vascular obstruction such as a branch retinal vein occlusion (BRVO).

Due to the asymptomatic nature of some early disease the patient can also present with secondary complications like vitreous haemorrhage from neovascularisation, central retinal vein occlusions (CRVO) or even retinal detachment form peripheral traction.

Investigations

As retinal vasculitis could be related to a serious systemic disease, all cases should be investigated. Most importantly, if infectious viral retinitis causing arteritis is suspected, then there should be no delay in further investigation and imaging (**Figure 75.2**). The eye should have a 'tap and inject' with a sample of intraocular fluid sent for viral testing [polymerase chain reaction (PCR)] and intravitreal anti-viral treatment such as Foscarnet (2.4 mg in 0.1 mL).

Initial investigations
- *Blood testing:* FBC, U&E, ESR, treponemal (syphilis) serology, ANA, ANCA
- *Chest X-ray:* Sarcoid and TB
- *Urinalysis:* Looking for blood and protein
- *Optical coherence tomography (OCT):* It may be normal or show cystoid macula oedema

Imaging: Fundus fluorescein angiogram (FFA) (wide-field if possible)
- *Posterior pole features:* 'Hot' disc with leakage, cystoid macula oedema, enlarged foveal avascular zones due to macula ischaemia
- *Vascular features:* Vessel wall staining, vessel leakage, skip lesions, widespread capillary leakage (ferning), ischaemic areas can just show capillary dropout or be dark due to total lack of flow (**Figure 75.1**)

Targeted investigations
Based on results above/suspicions:
- Brain imaging if suspecting multiple sclerosis
- Blood tests: Serology for HIV, toxoplasma, Lyme disease, Bartonella
- HLA-B51 testing for Behçet's Disease
- Further testing under medical physicians including sarcoid-specific imaging, etc.

Diagnosis
Initial ruling out of infectious causes should be done locally, medical physicians can help with systemic diseases but onward referral to a specialist uveitis clinic would be advised in most cases.

Using the clinical examination and FFA imaging, there should be an attempt to classify anatomically which vessel is primarily affected as this will give clues to the underlying cause.
- Arteries (Arteritis)
  - Isolated ocular disease: Viral retinitis, e.g. acute retinal necrosis, IRVAN syndrome (idiopathic retinal vasculitis, aneurysms and neuroretinitis)
  - Systemic disease: Syphilis, Susac syndrome, systemic vasculitides, e.g Churg–Strauss syndrome, systemic lupus erythematosus (SLE), polyarteritis nodosa (PAN), granulomatosis with polyangiitis (GPA)
- Veins (Periphlebitis)
  - Syphilis, sarcoidosis, TB, SLE, Behçet's disease (may present with vein occlusion)
- Capillary bed (leading to ferning on FFA)
  - Behçet's disease, sarcoid, intermediate uveitis
- Capillary closure and frank ischaemia
  - TB, multiple sclerosis, sarcoidosis.

Treatment
Conservative management with close observation may be used in static cases of peripheral vasculitis. Treatment is indicated if there is severe vitritis, cystoid macular oedema, posterior pole involvement or for extensive peripheral ischaemia. If there is systemic vasculitis driving the retinal changes, then treatment is more likely to be needed to prevent eventual visual loss. The use of wide-field digital photos to allow inter-visit comparison is recommended.

Principles of treatment
- Treat the underlying cause
  - Antibiotics for vasculitis secondary to systemic infection, e.g. penicillin for syphilis
- Control the inflammation
  - Immunosuppression starting with corticosteroids delivered periocular, intraocular, e.g. dexamethasone 700 µg implant, oral (prednisolone 1 mg/kg and taper) or intravenous (pulsed methylprednisolone 1 g OD for 3 days)
  - Second-line steroid-sparing treatments include cyclosporine/tacrolimus, methotrexate and mycophenolate mofetil
  - Third-line treatment will be an anti-TNF biologic, e.g. adalimumab or rheumatologists may consider giving interferon alfa for Behçet's disease or cyclophosphamide for granulomatosis with polyangiitis (GPA)
- Treat the complications
  - Peripheral ischaemia may lead to neovascularisation and pan-retinal

photocoagulation is recommended to the ischaemic areas only, guided by the FFA
- Vitrectomy may be required if there is persistent vitreous haemorrhage from peripheral traction bands

Complications

Some complications of retinal vasculitis may be the presenting feature like BRVO/CRVO or vitreous haemorrhage. Neovascularisation occurs in 15% of patients with retinal vasculitis and is usually associated with areas of ischaemia on FFA.

Persistent vitreous haemorrhages can worsen fibrotic vitreoretinal changes and lead to blinding tractional retinal detachments. Involvement of perifoveal capillaries can lead to sudden central visual loss due to ischaemic maculopathy and is an indication for urgent aggressive treatment.

Visual prognosis depends on whether there is a large ischaemic element, being worse if there is, and if there is a systemic disease which can continue to drive the vasculitis for many years. Of note, up to one-third of women presenting with non-ischaemic retinal vasculitis could develop multiple sclerosis over the next 5 years.

Further reading

Abu el-Asrar AM, Herbort CP, Tabbara KF. A clinical approach to the diagnosis of retinal vasculitis. Int Ophthalmol 2010; 30:149–173.

Dick A, Azim M, Forrester J. Immunosuppressive therapy for chronic uveitis: optimizing therapy with steroids and cyclosporin A. Br J Ophthalmol 1997; 81:1107–1112.

Suhler EB, Adan A, Brezin AP, et al. Safety and efficacy of adalimumab in patients with non-infectious uveitis in an ongoing open-label study: VISUAL III. Ophthalmology 2018; 125:1075–1087.

Related topics of interest

- Intermediate uveitis (p. 185)
- Posterior uveitis (p. 259)

76 Retinal vein occlusion

Key points
- Retinal vein occlusions (RVOs) are the second commonest retinal vascular disorders
- Visual loss results from macular oedema, retinal ischaemia and neovascularisation
- Visual outcomes from delayed treatment remain inferior to those from early treatment of macular oedema

Epidemiology
Retinal vein occlusion is the second most common cause of blindness from retinal vascular disease after diabetic retinopathy. It may be subdivided into branch retinal vein occlusions (BRVO), hemiretinal vein occlusions (HRVO) and central retinal vein occlusions (CRVO).

The prevalence of retinal vein occlusion is 5.20 per 1,000 for any RVO, 4.42 per 1,000 for BRVO, and 0.80 per 1,000 for CRVO. It is estimated that 14–19 million adults are affected by RVO worldwide.

Age
Increasing age is associated with a higher prevalence of all types of RVO and most patients affected are over 60.

Gender
There is no gender difference in RVO prevalence.

Race
Some studies found the prevalence of RVO is greater in black, Asian and Hispanic ethnic groups than in Caucasians but this difference may reflect variation in underlying systemic risk factors.

Systemic factors
Arterial hypertension, hyperlipidaemia, diabetes mellitus (DM) and peripheral vascular disease are more prevalent in BRVO but not in CRVO and HRVO.

Hyperhomocysteinaemia and anti-phospholipid antibodies (aPL) have been implicated in meta-analysis studies. Elevation of plasma homocysteine is found in 5–7% of normal people and aPL are a common incidental finding. Hyperviscosity due to high haematocrit has been associated with BRVO. Obstructive sleep apnoea has recently been associated with all types of RVO.

Ocular risk factors
Glaucoma carries the highest risk.

Pathophysiology
The pathogenesis of RVO is multifactorial. Compression of the vein at the arteriovenous (A/V) crossing and degenerative changes of the vessel wall may result in turbulent blood flow in BRVO.

Visual loss results from retinal bleeding, cystoid macular oedema (CMO), retinal ischaemia, primary damage to the neuroretina and secondary complications such as retinal neovascularisation, vitreous haemorrhage and rubeosis iridis.

Inflammatory mediators upregulated in RVO include vascular endothelial growth factor (VEGF), placental growth factor (P1GF), platelet-derived growth factor (PDGF)-AA and interleukin (IL)-6, 8, 12, and 13. These increase vascular permeability and promote the breakdown of the blood-retina barrier with resultant CMO.

Clinical features
Patients typically present with painless visual loss or disturbance in their visual field that is more commonly noticed on waking. Extra-macular BRVOs may be asymptomatic.

In the early stages of RVO, superficial and deep retinal haemorrhages, macular oedema, cotton-wool spots and optic disc hyperaemia and oedema predominate. In later stages, sheathing of retinal veins and venous-venous collaterals may develop on the retina or optic disc.

Poor prognostic markers for the development of rubeosis are poor vision at presentation, retinal ischaemia, deep retinal haemorrhages, optic disc swelling and the presence of a relative afferent pupillary defect.

Diagnosis

Slit lamp biomicroscopy is sufficient to make the diagnosis of an RVO. Evaluation of the angle for rubeosis is mandatory at initial presentation. Four weekly gonioscopy for the first 4 months was recommended in CRVO and HRVO, regardless of perfusion status, given the incidence ischaemic conversion. However, the risk of ischaemic conversion is low in the absence of significant ischaemia at baseline (**Table 76.1**).

The differential diagnosis of CRVO includes ocular ischaemic syndrome, and hypertensive retinopathy and diabetic retinopathy (when bilateral).

Investigations

Fluorescein angiography (FA) has limited use in the early stage of RVO as retinal blood may mask angiographic findings. It can differentiate between ischaemic and non-ischaemic RVO. Angiographic findings include dilatation of retinal veins and capillaries, a "petaloid pattern" of leakage around the macular and delayed dye transit time. It is also useful in differentiating collateral vessels from neovascular vessels (collateral vessels do not leak).

Ultra-widefield angiography using Optos imaging (Optos Plc, Dunfermline, Scotland) has allowed visualization of up to 3 times the area captured with a standard 7-field Early Treatment of Diabetic Retinopathy Study (ETDRS) imaging protocol in a single capture. However, artefacts that magnify the peripheral image more than the centre need to be corrected for.

Spectral domain optical coherence tomography (OCT) is the most widely used method of evaluating the retina in RVO. It gives information about structural changes within the retina and quantitative information about retinal thickness that can be used to monitor response to treatment.

Features on OCT that are significantly correlated with worse baseline vision include the presence of disorganization of retinal inner layers (DRIL), disruption of the external limiting membrane and the ellipsoid layer.

OCT angiography can be used to visualise the central retinal circulation without the use of intravenous fluorescent compounds. It detects vessels based on blood flow.

Systemic investigations can be limited to assessing arterial hypertension, hyperlipidaemia and blood glucose, FBC and ESR. Treatment should be directed at improving or preventing visual loss and underlying atherosclerosis risk factors should also be addressed.

Treatment

Laser was the standard treatment for macular oedema for patients with a vision of 20/40 or worse in BRVO (Branch Vein Occlusion Study) and was not beneficial in CRVO (CVOS). Retinal blood usually prevented treatment for 3 months.

Intravitreal injections of corticosteroid or anti-VEGF agents have replaced laser as the standard of care for treating macular oedema in RVO. The major trial outcomes are detailed in **Table 76.2**. A direct comparison between the trials cannot be made as the treatment protocols and selection criteria varied between trials, namely in the proportion of ischaemic RVO, duration of disease and in the number of injections given.

The cumulative proportion of patients who had ever gained 15 letters or more over the 12-month study period was 71% (ranibizumab 0.5 mg) in the BRAVO study and 66.4% (0.5 mg ranibizumab) in CRUISE and 58.5% (aflibercept 2 mg), in COPERNICUS.

Table 76.1 Risk of anterior and posterior neovascularisation in CRVO based on ultra-widefield imaging of ischaemia

Area of non-perfusion (disc areas)	Neovascularisation development at 12 months (%)
< 10	0
10–30	14.3
30–75	20
75–150	80

Table 76.2 Summary of major trial outcome data

Trial	Disease type		Follow-up period (months)	Mean change in BCVA from baseline (ETDRS)	Comments
BRAVO	BRVO	Ranibizumab 0.5 mg	12	+18.3	
		Sham (+ rescue Ranibizumab after 6 months)	12	+12.1	
		Sham before rescue	6	+6.9	
		Laser before rescue	6	+7.3	
COMRADE-B	BRVO	Ranibizumab (3+ PRN)	6	+14.2	Dexamethasone duration of action is less than 6 months. BCVA endpoints in both trials did not measure peak vision
		Dexamethasone 0.7 mg implant	6	+9.66	
GENEVA	Mixed	Sham	12	+4.9	
		Dexamethasone 0.7 mg implant	12	+7.4	
CRUISE	CRVO	Ranibizumab 0.5 mg	12	+13.9	Duration of oedema < 3 months at baseline and 1.5% had posterior non-perfusion
		Sham (+ rescue Ranibizumab 0.5 mg	12	+7.3	
COPERNICUS	CRVO	Aflibercept 2 mg	6	+17.3	Duration of oedema at baseline < 9 months and 15.5% of patients had posterior non-perfusion
		Sham before rescue	6	-4	
		Aflibercept 2 mg	12	+16.2	
		Sham + rescue Aflibercept after 6 months	12	+3.8	Actual gain of +7.8 letters as vision fell from baseline to -4 prior to rescue injections

The key distinctions from these trials are:
- Treatment with anti-VEGF agents alters the natural history of RVO. Retinal blood appears to clear faster and macular oedema resolves faster
- Oedema was found to resolve within the first 3 years in 43.8% of CRVO patients compared with 26% spontaneous resolution in the Central Vein Occlusion Study (CVOS). The remaining 56% with unresolved oedema required a mean of 5.9 injections in year 4 and had lower visual acuity gains
- Median time to first 15-letter or more gain from baseline was about 12.0 months in sham-treated eyes and 4.0 months in BRVO and 5.2 months in CRVO (ranibizumab 0.5 mg)
- Patients initially given sham treatment and then treated with ranibizumab had persistently poorer gains in vision compared with early treatment group
- The efficacy of laser alone was similar to sham intervention
- Less frequent injections were associated with poorer visual outcomes

Complications

Visual loss

Although visual loss from macular oedema may be largely reversed by current treatment, macular ischaemia and neuroretinal damage cannot. Epiretinal membranes, lamellar macular holes and retinal gliosis are common secondary complications that contribute to visual loss.

Neovascularisation

The risk of anterior segment neovascularisation in untreated eyes with CRVO with more than 10 disc areas (DA) of retinal capillary non-perfusion is 35% over 3 years and 10% in perfused eyes (CVOS). Ultra-widefield imaging studies have identified posterior pole non-perfusion as a more significant driver of retinal and anterior neovascularisation than peripheral non-perfusion (**Table 76.2**). Treatment with anti-VEGF agents can delay the onset of neovascularisation by 6.2 ± 7.3 months during the treatment-free period but does not ameliorate the risk.

Complications of treatment

Major complications include exogenous endophthalmitis, and retinal detachments. Perforation of the crystalline lens and intraocular hypersensitivity inflammation occur with all intravitreal agents. Ocular hypertension and cataract progression are more common with corticosteroid injections.

Further reading

Jonas J, Paquesb M, Monésd J, et al. Retinal vein occlusions. Dev Ophthalmology 2010; 47:111–135.

Mimouni M, Segev OR, Dori D, et al. Disorganization of the retinal inner layers as a predictor of visual acuity in eyes with macular edema secondary to vein occlusion. Am J Ophthalmol 2017; 182:160–167.

Nicholson L, Vazquez-Alfageme C, Patrao NV, et al. Retinal nonperfusion in the posterior pole is associated with increased risk of neovascularization in central retinal vein occlusion. Am J Ophthalmol 2017; 182:118–125.

Regnier SA, Larsen M, Bezlyak V, et al. Comparative efficacy and safety of approved treatments for macular oedema secondary to branch retinal vein occlusion: a network meta-analysis. BMJ 2015; 5:9–12.

Royal College of Ophthalmology. Retinal Vein Occlusion Guidelines. London: RCO; 2015.

Related topics of interest

- Diabetic eye disease (p. 116)
- Retinal arterial occlusion (p. 267)
- Retinal imaging (p. 277)
- Retinal laser (p. 282)

77 Retinoblastoma

Key points
- Retinoblastoma is the most common ocular tumour in childhood
- Individuals with a history of retinoblastoma can be at a lifetime risk of other malignancies
- Timely detection and appropriate treatment can be successful in preventing extraocular spread and death

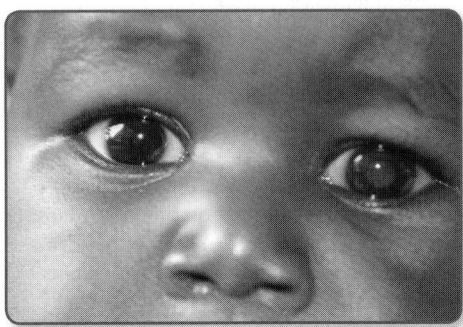

Figure 77.1 A child with leucocoria +/− squint.
(*For colour version see plate 7*)

Epidemiology

Retinoblastoma is the most common malignant ocular tumour in childhood, usually occurring before the age of 5 years. The incidence of retinoblastoma is estimated at between 1:15,000 and 1:20,000 live births. Untreated retinoblastoma is fatal, the greatest predictor of which is extraocular extension directly through the sclera or through invasion of the optic nerve at diagnosis. Timely detection and appropriate treatment, however, can be successful (up to 95%) in preventing spread out of the eye.

About 60% of those affected have unilateral retinoblastoma and tend to present at a later average age of 24 months. The remaining 40% are bilateral and present at 13 months of age. In the presence of a family history, diagnosis is often made earlier.

Pathophysiology

Retinoblastomas are neuroblastic tumours in origin, affecting photoreceptor precursors. Histologically, the cells contain little cytoplasm and the finding of fleurettes and Flexner–Wintersteiner and Homer Wright rosettes is classic. As the cells rapidly outgrow their blood supply, necrosis, haemorrhage, and calcification are often seen within the retinoblastoma.

Clinical features

Leucocoria is the most common presentation (60%) (**Figure 77.1**). This is usually accompanied by or followed by strabismus (20%). Other features include reduced vision, nystagmus, and more unusually glaucoma, orbital cellulitis, uveitis, hyphaema, retinal exudates, and vitreous haemorrhage.

Retinoblastomas can exhibit endophytic or exophytic growth. Rarely, they can present as a diffuse infiltrate.

In endophytic growth, a white or cream-coloured mass with no surface vessels or small irregular vessels breaks through the internal limiting membrane. Endophytic retinoblastoma is occasionally associated with vitreous seeding where the broken tumour fragments are visible in the anterior chamber and vitreous, thus mimicking endophthalmitis or uveitis, which can confound the diagnosis. Deposits or seeding of tumour in the retina can be mistaken for multicentric tumours.

Exophytic tumours appear yellow-white and occur in the subretinal space. The overlying vessels are commonly increased in calibre and tortuosity. The accumulation of subretinal fluid can obscure the tumour and resemble an exudative retinal detachment. Tumour cells can infiltrate through Bruch's membrane into the choroid and blood vessels or ciliary nerves. Large tumours can exhibit both endophytic and exophytic growth.

Diffuse infiltrating growths comprise 1.5% of all retinoblastomas. In the absence of a discrete tumour mass, there is a relatively flat infiltration of the retina by tumour cells.

The growth is slower than that of typical retinoblastoma.

Retinoblastomas might also regress spontaneously. They can result in benign retinocytomas when asymptomatic, or can cause inflammation leading to phthisis bulbi. The genetic implications for these individuals are the same as those with active retinoblastoma.

Differentials include:
- Congenital disorders such as persistent hyperplastic primary vitreous and Coats disease
- Hereditary disorders including tuberous sclerosis, Norrie disease, incontinentia pigmenti, familial exudative vitreoretinopathy, and von Hippel–Lindau disease
- Ocular infestation by *Toxocara canis*

Genetics

Two different genes have been identified in retinoblastoma: *RB1* and *MYCN*.

RB1 is present on the long arm of chromosome 13 (13q14) and codes for the tumour suppressor gene *pRB*. 90% of *RB1* mutations are heterozygous de novo mutations. The remaining 10% have the inherited pathogenic variant of *RB1*. Individuals with a germline *RB1* mutation have a 50% risk of passing the mutation on to their offspring; autosomal dominant inheritance pattern. Prenatal testing for those at increased risk (with an affected family member) is possible.

Though it is inherited in an autosomal dominant pattern, only 90% of those with germline mutations will exhibit the retinoblastoma phenotype through reduced penetrance, i.e. 45% risk of tumour in children born to an individual with the mutation. 10% develop no tumour and remain an unaffected carrier of heritable retinoblastoma. The risk to their offspring is, however, the same as in those with the mutation.

In germline mutations, every cell in the body is missing one copy of the *RB1* tumour suppressor gene. Every photoreceptor can therefore produce a tumour; multiple or bilateral tumours are a feature. Most of the de novo mutations are somatic, where only one retinal cell loses a copy of the *RB1* gene and so there is a need for a random event to provide a second hit for a tumour to develop; usually unilateral and unifocal tumours (**Figures 77.2** and **77.3**). An alternative possibility for non-hereditary retinoblastoma is for a single small mutation such as a chromosomal aberration to be capable of producing a tumour, particularly where there is more than one primary tumour.

Overall, 60% of tumours are unilateral and unifocal; 40% are bilateral or trilateral. Trilateral retinoblastoma is where bilateral ocular disease occurs with a pinealoblastoma (retina-like tissue in the pineal gland) which is rare but fatal. In unilateral cases, the

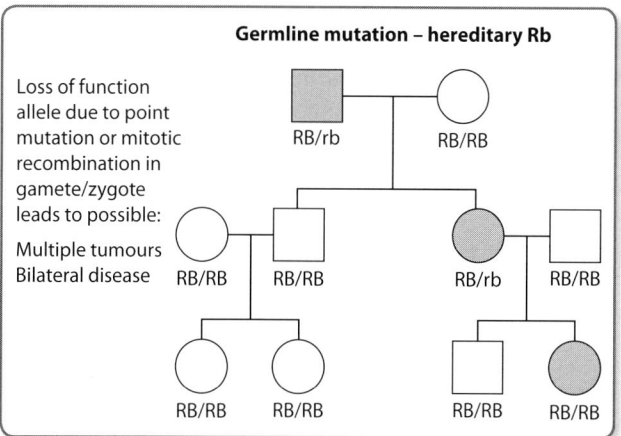

Figure 77.2 Germline mutation – hereditary retinoblastoma.

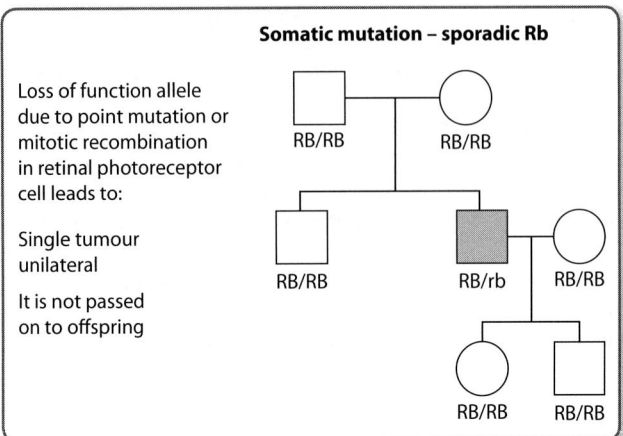

Figure 77.3 Somatic mutation – spontaneous retinoblastoma.

majority are somatic mutations; however a small proportion (10–15%) are germline mutations, which has implications for heritability.

The *MYCN* oncogene is on chromosome 2p. Multiple copies of this gene in a single retinal cell lead to retinoblastoma.

Genetic counselling of retinoblastoma families is complex, and must rely on accurate interpretation of clinical and molecular data in order to provide individuals and families with information on the nature, inheritance, and implications of the genetic disorder to help them make informed medical and personal decisions. When a child has unilateral disease and no family history, precise molecular genetic testing is required to determine their risk of heritable retinoblastoma. Where the mutation is proven to be confined to the tumour alone through molecular analysis, the risk to the siblings is that of the general population and so regular monitoring is not required. Otherwise, in the absence of genetic testing, first-degree relatives are at a significant risk of retinoblastoma and require regular clinic follow-up or examinations under anaesthesia. They will also have a lifetime risk of secondary non-retinoblastoma cancers.

Investigations

The diagnosis can be supported with imaging to evaluate any extraocular extension (tumour-optic nerve relationship) and any potential intracranial changes in trilateral disease.

Computed tomography scans may demonstrate intraocular calcification, but non-radiation modes of imaging are preferred due to the higher risk of secondary tumours in these patients. B-scan ultrasonography and magnetic resonance imaging (MRI) are used more commonly for this reason. Aspiration of ocular fluids should be avoided in most circumstances due to the risk of seeding malignant cells from the tumour.

Diagnosis

Retinoblastoma is usually diagnosed on dilated fundal examination of the affected child. This may be due to the common presentation of a white pupil or due to a masquerade symptom. In difficult cases, this might require examination under anaesthesia.

Bone marrow aspiration and examination of cerebrospinal fluid (CSF) may also be performed when pathologic examination of the enucleated eye reveals optic nerve invasion or significant risks for extraocular extension.

Treatment

Molecular and clinical genetic input is important in the management of these patients, and joint care with ophthalmology, paediatric oncology, pathology, and radiation oncology in a tertiary centre is essential. Supportive treatment is fundamental.

Focal therapy with laser or cryotherapy can destroy dividing and non-dividing tumour cells and surrounding tissues. This makes it effective in destroying small retinoblastoma tumours and residual intraocular tumours after chemotherapy. Laser is best delivered at repeated regular intervals to reduce complications. Cryotherapy is primarily used for small peripheral lesions. For superior lesions, a laser barrier is useful in preventing serous retinal detachments. Fluorescein angiography is a useful tool in showing recurrence in the form of tumour blood vessel reactivation.

Chemotherapy can be delivered locally or as an adjunct to systemic treatment for chemoreduction and in extraocular extension. It reduces tumour size and retinal detachment, and promotes regression of vitreous seeds. Focal therapy can then be used for final tumour control. Direct intra-arterial (ophthalmic artery) melphalan is the newest modality.

External beam radiation therapy is less commonly used due to the high risk of secondary tumours and cosmetic side effects (midface hypoplasia due to cessation of bone growth). Plaque brachytherapy is useful in localised disease in non-critical areas.

Enucleations are used in advanced disease or where any other treatment has failed, in order to preserve the life of the child.

Indicators of poor prognosis include large size of tumour, optic nerve involvement, extraocular spread, and older age at presentation.

Complications

Children with heritable retinoblastoma are at an increased risk of bone (osteosarcoma) and soft tissue tumours (e.g. leiomyosarcoma and rhabdomyosarcoma), malignant melanoma, and epithelial cancers (e.g. lung, bladder, oesophagus, and breast).

This risk increases in those who have received external beam radiation therapy. Their exposure to ionising radiation, e.g. X-rays should be limited. Metastases occur in the bone marrow, liver, and lungs.

Further reading

AE Singh, BE Damato. Clinical Ophthalmic Oncology: Retinal Tumors, Springer, 3;2019.

Community Eye Health Journal vol. 31:101;2018; 11–16

NCBI. (2018). Retinoblastoma. (online) Available from https://www.ncbi.nlm.nih.gov/books/NBK1452/ [Last accessed November, 2019].

The Royal College of Ophthalmologists. (2008). Retinoblastoma for Life. (online) Available from https://www.rcophth.ac.uk/wp-content/uploads/2014/08/Focus-Summer-2008.pdf [Last accessed November, 2019].

Related topics of interest

- Cataract – Congenital (p. 55)

78 Retinopathy of prematurity

Key points

- Screening protocols identify those cases, which require treatment
- Timely, adequate treatment significantly reduces the chance of blindness
- Premature babies have a high incidence of cortical visual impairment (CVI), nystagmus, refractive error and strabismus

Epidemiology

Retinopathy of prematurity (ROP) in the UK affects babies with the following risk factors:
- Low birth weight
- Prematurity
- Multiple gestation births and assisted reproductive techniques

Babies requiring treatment are born at mean corrected gestational age (CGA) of < 26/40 and mean birth weight of 800 g.

There have been three ROP epidemics:
1. Associated with supplementary oxygen in the 1950s in the UK.
2. Improved neonatal care increasing the survival of extremely premature babies.
3. Lower income countries without access to titrated oxygen therapy like the first epidemic in the UK.

Variability in ROP rates and severity depend upon standards of neonatal care, hence one country's screening programme cannot apply necessarily to another.

High-income countries with good access to ROP treatment have rates of severe sight impairment (SSI) due to ROP of < 10% of blind individuals. In lower income countries, this is over 40%.

Pathophysiology

In utero, the retina and associated vasculature develop in tandem in relative hypoxia and physiological vascular endothelial-derived growth factor (VEGF) levels. Insulin-derived growth factor (IGF-1) transfers from mother to baby in the last trimester stimulating weight gain.

Following premature birth, two phases of ROP may occur:
1. Weeks 22–30 CGA: *Vasculogenesis*. A consequence of premature birth is cessation of neonatal hypoxia (even in room air), VEGF drops from physiological levels, avascular retinal growth proceeds exceeding its blood supply.
2. Weeks 31–45 CGA: *Angiogenesis*. Hypoxic retina releases VEGF causing pathological extraretinal vessel growth.

Earlier birth and higher supplemental oxygen exacerbates phase 1, giving a higher ROP risk. Sicker babies often require higher oxygen concentrations, for longer periods to prevent death, adversely affecting retinal development.

Additional risk factors for ROP include:
- Low birth weight, low IGF1 levels and slow weight gain
- Brain-derived neurotrophic factor (BDNF) gene mutations are associated with severe ROP

Transfusion of adult haemoglobin with a lower affinity for oxygen than the foetal form releases oxygen to the retina more easily resulting in hyper-oxygenation of the retina. Donor twins in twin-twin transfusion syndrome are more likely to receive blood transfusions and this is an independent risk factor.

Other factors influencing retinal vascularisation include placental growth factor, erythropoietin, and alpha-B crystalline.

Clinical features

- International Classification of ROP (1984) standardised the description of retinal vasculature: disc vessel calibre and tortuosity (termed *plus* or *pre-plus*), area of vascularisation (zone) and the delineation between vascularised and avascularised retina (stage) (**Table 78.1**)

Retinopathy of prematurity

Table 78.1 International classification of ROP (ICROP): ROP staging

Vessels	Zone	Stage
Plus: Increased tortuosity and dilation of retinal arterioles and veins at the optic nerve in two or more quadrants as compared with standard photographs	I: Area with a radius of twice the distance between the optic nerve and the fovea, centred on the optic disc	0: No demarcation between vascularised and avascularised retina
		1: White demarcation line
	II: Area with a radius of the optic nerve to the nasal ora serrata	2: Line thickens and elevates into a salmon pink ridge
Pre-plus: Increased tortuosity and dilation that does not meet criteria for plus disease		3: Extra-retinal neovascularisation on the ridge (**Figure 78.1**)
	III: Remaining temporal crescent of retina	4: Subtotal retinal detachment, not involving the macula (4a), or macula involving (4b) (**Figure 78.3**)
		5: Total retinal detachment: open (5a), closed funnel (5b)

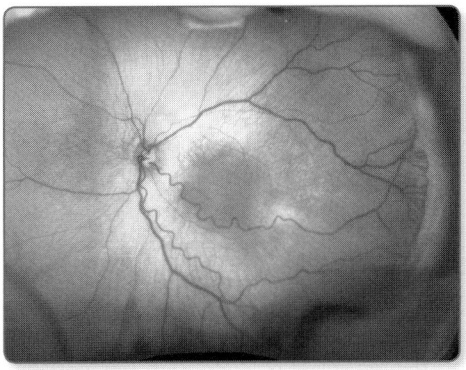

Figure 78.1 AP-ROP with extensive arteriolar and venular dilatation and tortuosity in zone I. (*For colour version see plate 7*)

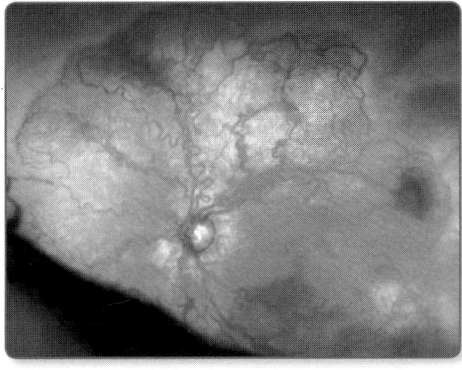

Figure 78.2 Temporal zone II, stage 3 ROP with plus disease in superotemporal and inferotemporal quadrants. This is type 1 ROP and should be treated as per ET-ROP criteria. (*For colour version see plate 7*)

- Poorly dilating pupils can indicate more severe disease because of a stiffer vascularised iris.
- Severity may increase steadily during development, but in the majority of cases will stabilise and regress
- Persistent tunica vasculosa can obscure the retinal view
- AP-ROP (aggressive posterior ROP) is vascularisation limited to zone I or posterior zone II with prominent plus disease and flat neovascularisation occurring usually at 33–35 weeks CGA. It can rapidly progress to stage 4 (**Figure 78.2**)

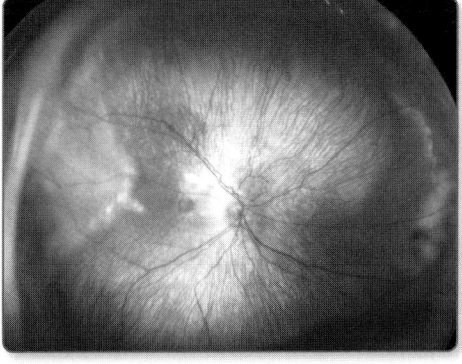

Figure 78.3 Temporal zone II, stage 4a ROP with a localised area of retina under traction extending towards the fovea. (*For colour version see plate 8*)

Investigations

- Fundal examination with indirect ophthalmoscopy and 28D lens. A speculum and indentation may be required to visualise anterior retina. Topical anaesthetic, oral sucrose and swaddling improves comfort
- Retinal imaging can be useful to document, monitor and remotely manage
- Fluorescein angiography can guide the treatment

Diagnosis

- UK screening criteria: Babies weighing < 1,501 g and/or born at less than 32 weeks' gestation should be screened, whilst all babies weighing < 1,251 g or born less than 31 weeks' gestation must be screened. Babies born at less than 27 weeks have their first retinal examination between 30 weeks and 31 weeks. Babies born after 27 weeks have their first examination at between 4 weeks and 5 weeks after birth
- Minimum of fortnightly examinations until the retina is fully vascularised or characteristics of regression are seen on two successive examinations

Treatment

- Treatment aims to reduce circulating VEGF, by ablation of avascular retina with laser, or anti-VEGF intravitreal injections. Treatments can be stressful for inants; sedation or general anaesthetic may be required
- Two major studies guide the treatment:
  - Cryotherapy for retinopathy of prematurity (CRYO-ROP) study defined *threshold disease* as the severity at which 50% of babies would have a retinal detachment (**Table 78.2**)
  - Early treatment for retinopathy of prematurity (ET-ROP) study defined type 1 disease for earlier treatment (**Table 78.2**). Type 2 ROP should be considered for treatment if there is progression to type 1 disease
- Anti-VEGF agents are unlicensed therapies. Advantages are quick treatment time, less physiological stress, and relatively better efficacy if there is no view to deliver laser. Regression is faster than laser
- Retinal surgery in cases of stage 4a or 4b, rarely 5. Endoscopic lens-sparing vitrectomy has superseded conventional vitrectomy augmented with encirclement because it allows release of tractional bands in all vectors thereby improving likelihood of anatomical retinal architecture post-procedure. Encircling bands can be considered as a secondary procedure

Complications

- Prematurity:
  - Intraventricular haemorrhage, post-haemorrhagic ventricular dilatation, periventricular leucomalacia and hydrocephalus can lead to CVI
- Retinal ablation:
  - Reduced peripheral field, reduced night vision, reduced acuity though in CRYO-ROP study, visual field was constricted by 5–10° whether treated or not
  - > 8D of myopia; 52% for zone I disease versus 36% zone II. ET-ROP 6-year outcomes: SSI 25%; unfavourable structural outcome 9%, glaucoma 9%, strabismus 42%
- Anti-VEGF:
  - > 8D myopia; 4% zone I disease, 2% zone II
  - ~8% require re-treatment, sometimes more than 65 weeks CGA

Table 78.2 Classification of disease for treatment decisions

Type I ROP	Type II ROP	Threshold
Zone I, any stage with plus* (*in 2 quadrants or more)	Zone I, stage 1 and 2 without plus disease	5 contiguous, or 8 non-contiguous clock hours of stage 3 ROP in zone I or II in the presence of plus disease
Zone I, stage 3, without plus	Zone II, stage 3 without plus disease	
Zone II, stage 2 or 3 with plus*		

Further reading

Good WV1, Early treatment for retinopathy of prematurity cooperative group. (2004). Final results of the Early Treatment for Retinopathy of Prematurity (ETROP) randomized trial. Trans Am Ophthalmol Soc 2004; 102:233–250.

Hartnett ME. Advances in understanding and management of retinopathy of prematurity. Surv Ophthalmol 2017; 62:257–276.

Mills MD. Evaluating the Cryotherapy for Retinopathy of Prematurity Study (CRYO-ROP). Arch Ophthalmol 2007; 125:1276–1281.

Royal College Ophthalmologists. Guideline for the Screening and Treatment of Retinopathy of Prematurity. London: Royal College Ophthalmologists; 2008.

Related topics of interest

- Esotropia (p. 137)
- Glaucoma in children (p. 169)
- Leucocoria (p. 205)
- Nystagmus (p. 222)
- Retinal lasers (p. 282)

79 Scleritis

Key points

- Scleritis is a sight-threatening inflammation of the outer scleral coat of the eye which may be anterior or posterior, necrotising or non-necrotising
- Scleritis is commonly misdiagnosed as episcleritis, an entirely avoidable mistake if the vasoconstrictor test is used in clinic with instillation of a drop of 2.5% phenylephrine into the affected eye(s)
- Half of all affected individuals also have an associated systemic condition such as granulomatosis with polyangiitis or rheumatoid arthritis
- Aggressive treatment with oral nonsteroidal agents, steroids, steroid-sparing agents or even biologics may be needed

Epidemiology

Scleritis has an annual incidence of 3.4 cases per 100,000 people per year, with a prevalence rate of 5.2 cases per 100,000 people per year. Scleritis is the most common amongst females and older individuals with both of these trends being more pronounced than with those suffering from episcleritis. It is essential to know the difference between these two very similar conditions as the treatment is very different and there are very real risks present if scleritis is misdiagnosed as the more benign episcleritis.

Pathophysiology

The sclera is the protective dense collagenous coat of the eye which overlies the highly vascular uveal tract and sits underneath the two layers of connective tissue that form the episclera. It has a vascular plexus associated with the most superficial layers which results in an area of injection overlying any portion of inflamed sclera, which may also involve the episclera. A systemic association is present in almost 50% of cases of scleritis so certain tests are mandatory in order to pick up any other potentially life-threatening conditions which might also be present. Initially, the area of inflammation results in thickened patches of sclera though if timely diagnosis is not made, local vasculitis can result in ischaemic patches of sclera which then becomes necrotic and melts away, so-called "necrotic" disease. Trauma to the eye caused by accidents or surgery can also set up an inflammatory cascade.

Clinical features

The presentation of scleritis is entirely dependent on the location and severity of the inflammation. The condition is termed "anterior scleritis" if any patch of redness can be seen, and this is further divided into anterior non-necrotising and anterior necrotising scleritis if the blue tinge of the underlying uveal tract is hidden or now visible due to thinning dying overlying sclera respectively. Anterior non-necrotising scleritis can be isolated to one area of thickened sclera, in which case it is termed "nodular", or it can be widespread throughout the whole visible anterior sclera in which case it is termed "diffuse". Should the telltale bluish tinge of choroid that indicates anterior necrotising scleritis (**Figure 79.1**) be present, this can be associated with a lot of injection and inflammation, though a rare variant affecting less than 5% of scleritis sufferers called scleromalacia perforans may be present in which there is no sign of inflammation whatsoever and the eye is white. If scleritis is present but no injection or necrosis can be seen, then this indicates posterior involvement only, so-called "posterior scleritis".

Half of all cases are bilateral, though the figure is lower for posterior scleritis. The typical presentation of anterior scleritis is with an acute history of a red, deeply injected eye and a deep seated boring pain in the eye which wakes the sufferer at night. Whilst episcleritis tends to build over a week, scleritis may gradually worsen over 4 or more weeks. It is very common for scleritis to be initially diagnosed as the much more benign and

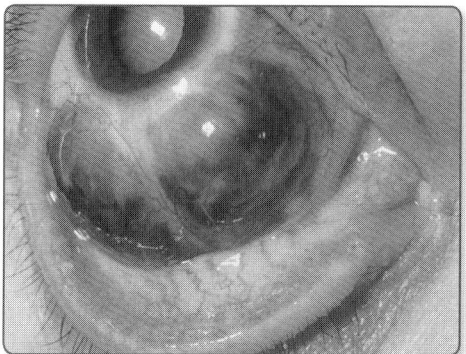

Figure 79.1 Necrotising scleritis.

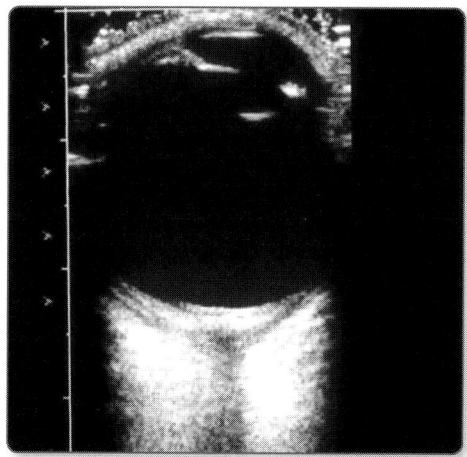

Figure 79.2 B-scan showing "T sign".

usually self-limiting superficial episcleritis and a patient who complains of an episcleritis that simply does not go away should be considered at risk of suffering from scleritis.

Posterior scleritis, affecting around 10% of scleritis patients, presents with no history of injection or redness whatsoever, but rather pain out of all proportion to what can be seen with fundal examination revealing choroidal folds and possibly even a swollen optic disc.

Investigations

Investigations are divided into those needed to diagnose scleritis in clinic and those needed to investigate for systemic disease associations. As with episcleritis in clinic the vasoconstrictor test in which a drop of 2.5% phenylephrine is instilled into the conjunctival sac is highly useful. If the injection does not disappear, scleritis is present. If posterior scleritis is suspected then a B-scan ultrasound can be performed which can indicate thickening of the posterior coats (>2 mm) and fluid under Tenon's capsule which shows up the pathognomonic "T-sign" (**Figure 79.2**) where the stem of the letter T seen is represented by the optic nerve and the arms the subtenon inflammatory fluid.

Systemic conditions associated with scleritis include granulomatosis with polyangiitis (Wegener's disease), rheumatoid arthritis, polyarteritis nodosa, relapsing polychondritis, and other vasculitides, as well as infectious cases such as varicella zoster virus, syphilis, and tuberculosis. Ask about the presence of other vasculitic conditions and if absent, specific symptoms such as joint issues, respiratory tract or sinus problems as well as nasal symptoms. Investigations can include full blood count (FBC), urea and electrolytes (U and E), erythrocyte sedimentation rate (ESR), C-reactive protein (CRP), rheumatoid factor (RF), cyclic citrullinated peptide (CCP), syphilis serology, and cytoplasmic antineutrophil cytoplasmic antibodies (c-ANCA), with other investigations being tailored to that discovered during history taking.

Diagnosis

The diagnosis of scleritis is made on clinical features, with the vasoconstrictor test and B-scan ultrasound used as adjuncts to help diagnose anterior and posterior scleritis, respectively. Associated systemic diseases, present in 50% of patients, can either be asked about in the history or, if not present, the above investigations carried out. It is important to do this as granulomatosis with polyangiitis, as well as many other vasculitic conditions, can be lethal if not diagnosed in time through damage to the respiratory tract and other organs.

Treatment

Unlike with episcleritis, treatment must always be commenced here. Provided there are no contraindications, the lowest ring on the ladder consists of an oral nonsteroidal agent such as flurbiprofen 100 mg tds for 2 weeks. This can be augmented with topical maxidex (0.1% dexamethasone) six times a day in cases of anterior scleritis. If the scleritis responds well, then the flurbiprofen can be tapered down over a 6-week period before being stopped altogether. If a patient cannot take a classic nonsteroidal agent, then a cyclooxygenase-2 (COX-2) inhibitor such as oral meloxicam 15 mg can be used instead in mild cases. If despite this treatment the disease continues unabated, then the next course of action consists of oral steroids in the form of prednisolone 60 mg a day for a week, tapering by 10 mg per week over a 6-week period. This is particularly good if bilateral disease is present though systemic steroids do have myriad side effects and so if the disease is unilateral and anterior, then local steroid in the form of subconjunctival triamcinolone (kenalog) 40 mg, in divided doses over the affected areas, can be useful. If any local steroid is used, it is important to monitor the intraocular pressure at each visit.

It must always be remembered; however, that if there is any hint whatsoever of an infectious element, steroids should be avoided. In addition, if necrosis is present, then local steroids should be avoided. In such cases, rapid escalation to immunosuppressives and biologicals is advised.

If the scleritis flares up after treatment is tapered or stopped, then a steroid-sparing agent should be considered, of which, methotrexate is a preferred option as it is more effective against scleritis compared with other agents. In resistant cases biologic agents need to be considered, most commonly the anti-tumour necrosis factor (TNF) drugs, or rituximab.

Where the sclera has become thinned in cases of anterior necrotising scleritis, special measures are indicated. Copious amounts of ocular lubrication are needed as well as some form of eye protection in the form of a shield to avoid accidental perforation of the eye. Early involvement of an anterior segment surgeon is needed if there is a large area of necrotic sclera present or the disease is rapidly progressive as patch grafting of donor sclera may be needed to save the eye.

Complications

By far the most common complication is misdiagnosis of scleritis as episcleritis, with consequent delayed diagnosis and missed opportunity to bring the disease under early control. Similarly, posterior scleritis is often missed entirely and the patient is dismissed as a malingering dramatist. Complications also arise from the side effects of steroids, namely cataract formation and raised intraocular pressure.

Further reading

Akpek EK, Uy H, Christen W, et al. Severity of episcleritis and systemic disease association. Ophthalmology 1999; 106:729–731.

Honik G, Wong IG, Gritz DC. Incidence and prevalence of episcleritis and scleritis in Northern California. Cornea 2013; 32:1562–1566.

Williams GS, Westcott M. Practical Uveitis: Understanding the Grape. London, United Kingdom: Taylor & Francis; 2017.

Related topic of interest

- Episcleritis (p. 134)

80 Secondary open angle glaucoma

Key points
- Secondary open angle glaucoma refers to the wide range of open angle glaucomas where there is an identifiable primary underlying mechanism
- A helpful but arbitrary classification is based on the level of insult in relation to the trabecular meshwork
- An important part of treatment involves the identification and management of the underlying primary condition

Epidemiology

Given the diversity of conditions in this category, it is difficult to give a precise incidence report on 'secondary glaucoma', however, a mention of the epidemiology of the individual conditions is included in **Table 80.1**, as well as elsewhere in related chapters within this book.

Pathophysiology

To provide a comprehensive account of secondary open angle glaucoma, it is beyond the scope of this chapter. However, we feel that a very helpful way to conceptualise this heterogeneous group is to categorise the individual underlying primary conditions using three levels of primary insult based on the trabecular meshwork (TM). These are pre-trabecular, trabecular, and post-trabecular. The end result of all of which is raised intraocular pressure and glaucoma.

Pre-trabecular meshwork level

The two main conditions in this category are:
1. Ischaemic/neovascular glaucoma (NVG)
2. Iridocorneal endothelial syndrome (ICE)

Neovascular glaucoma leading to the abnormal growth of fibrovascular membrane over TM is often secondary to significant ischaemia at posterior segment. Proliferative diabetic retinopathy and central retinal artery occlusion are the two main pathologies in which significant ischemia, if left untreated, results in raised vascular endothelial growth factor (VEGF) in anterior chamber (AC), leading to the growth of abnormal fibrovascular membrane over trabecular meshwork.

Iridocorneal endothelial syndrome which has three variants, namely, Chandler syndrome (most common), essential/progressive iris atrophy, and iris naevus/Cogan–Reese syndrome causes a secondary rise in intraocular pressure (IOP) due to abnormal activity and growth of endothelial cells (the cause of which is not entirely clear), forming a membrane over the trabecular meshwork.

At the trabecular meshwork level

Damage to or obstruction of the trabecular meshwork is responsible for the mechanism of the majority of secondary open angle glaucoma. One way to review this group of conditions is to classify them according to the type of cellular material/insult causing disruption to the TM. The following list is by no means comprehensive but covers the most common causes:
- *Pigment:* Pigment dispersion syndrome (covered elsewhere), pigment release following procedures such as cataract surgery, uveitis–glaucoma–hyphaema (UGH) syndrome
- *Exfoliative:* Pseudo exfoliation syndrome/glaucoma
- *Lens material/altered macrophages:* Phacolytic glaucoma
- *Iatrogenic:* Ophthalmic viscosurgical devices (e.g. high-molecular weight hyaluronic acid, which swells by binding to water molecules) following cataract surgery, emulsified silicone oil following vitreoretinal surgery, and steroid induced (complex mechanism of reduced aqueous outflow)
- *Photoreceptor outer segment/retinal pigment epithelial cells:* Schwartz–Matsuo syndrome in retinal detachment

Table 80.1 Summary of ocular and systemic findings in a sample group of conditions leading to secondary glaucoma. Continues opposite...

Conditions	Incidence	Systemic findings	Ocular findings	
			Anterior segment [apart from raised intraocular pressure (IOP)]	Posterior segment (apart from signs of glaucoma)
Carotid cavernous fistula (direct or indirect)	Rare Traumatic type is the most common (accounts for > 70% of cases)	Audible bruit	Depends on direct/indirect or high flow/low flow: Asymptomatic, reduced vision, conjunctival chemosis and episcleral venous engorgement, proptosis, diplopia, and ophthalmoparesis	Retinal vein engorgement, disc swelling
Cavernous sinus thrombosis	Rare Any age Typically young adults	Fever, sepsis, headache and signs of meningism	Reduced vision, ptosis, dilated pupil, reduced corneal reflex, and altered sensation in the distribution of ophthalmic and maxillary nerves	Retinal vein engorgement and disc swelling
Fuchs' heterochromic cyclitis	Typically young adults	–	Usually unilateral, asymptomatic or blurred vision and discomfort Iris heterochromia (lighter), mild chronic anterior uveitis, diffuse stellate KPs, cataract, and fine iris vessels crossing the TM	Anterior vitreous cells (from anterior chamber spill over), normal or glaucoma
Ghost cell glaucoma	Occurs in the context of recent vitreous haemorrhage	–	Blurred vision, corneal oedema, and ghost cells (red blood cells that have lost their haemoglobin) in AC	Vitreous haemorrhage
Iridocorneal endothelial syndrome (ICE)	More common in females, age 20–50 years typically	–	Unilateral discomfort, reduced vision, and corneal oedema/endothelial cell changes (beaten bronze, hammered silver) Peripheral anterior synechiae, iris atrophy, and corectopia (Chandlers syndrome) Full-thickness iris holes and polycoria (progressive iris atrophy) Iris nodules and atrophy (Cogan-Reese syndrome)	Normal or glaucoma
Neovascular glaucoma	See Chapter on Neovascular Glaucoma			
Phacolytic glaucoma	Elderly	–	Reduced vision, pain, hypermature cataract, AC flare, and pseudo-hypopyon with no KPs and deep AC	No fundal view due to cataract but expected to be normal
Pigment dispersion syndrome	See Chapter on Pigmentary Glaucoma			
Posner-Schlossman syndrome	Typically young males but also occurs in middle age	–	Reduced vision, haloes, minimal AC flare/cells with no conjunctival hyperaemia ('white eye') with very high IOP (40–50 mmHg)	Normal or glaucoma
Pseudo-exfoliation (PXF) syndrome/glaucoma	More prevalent in Scandinavian countries and some Mediterranean regions Up to 25% risk of glaucoma	–	PXF on pupil border and anterior lens capsule (described as dandruff-like material) Sampaolesi's line–irregular pigment in TM and anterior to Schwalbe's line, narrow angles and phacodonesis	Normal or glaucoma

Secondary open angle glaucoma

Table 80.1 Continued...				
Schwartz-Matsuo syndrome	Occurs in the context of retinal detachment	–	Normal or blurred vision. Aqueous cells (typically larger than inflammatory cells seen in anterior uveitis)	Rhegmatogenous retinal detachment and retinal tears
Sturge-Weber syndrome	1 in 20,000–50,000 live births	Port-wine stain, developmental delays, cognitive impairment, seizures, and paralysis	–	–
Superior vena cava syndrome	15,000/year cases in the USA >65% due to malignancy	Systemic symptoms of malignancy (e.g. weight loss, anorexia, etc.), headache, haemoptysis, dyspnoea, distended neck and chest vein, hoarseness, oedema and plethora of face	Depends on the degree of obstruction: Blurred vision, engorged episcleral/conjunctival vessels, and peri-orbital oedema	May be normal
Thyroid eye disease	See Chapter on Thyroid Eye Disease			
Uveitis-glaucoma-hyphaema syndrome	Associated with a malpositioned IOP	–	Intermittent reduction in vision, discomfort, photophobia, and AC cells/hypopyon/hyphaema. Localised iris changes with iris lens contact. Malpositioned IOL/haptic	Possible vitreous haemorrhage or macula oedema

AC, anterior chamber; IOL, intraocular lens; KPs, keratic precipitates; TM, trabecular meshwork

- *Inflammatory cells/trabeculitis:* Uveitis, episcleritis/scleritis, alkali burns, Posner-Schlossman syndrome (possibly as a result of viruses including cytomegalovirus, herpes simplex and herpes zoster causing low-grade inflammation), and Fuchs' heterochromic cyclitis
- *Blood/altered macrophages:* Hyphaema, ghost cells (red blood cells that have lost their haemoglobin), and UGH syndrome
- *Neoplastic cells:* Tumours of the anterior segment can lead to direct invasion of TM, direct compression or cause iris neovascularisation
- *Trauma:* Due to hyphaema and red blood cells, uveitis, TM damage with recession, and iatrogenic from topical steroids

Post-trabecular meshwork level

Aqueous humour traverses through the trabecular meshwork to Schlemm's canal and then follows to approximately 30 collector canals and eventually to episcleral and conjunctival veins. The pressure within orbital venous system is normally maintained at low levels as due to lack of valves, flow establishes through pressure gradients, and conditions that disrupt this process can lead to secondary raised IOP. There are several levels of the primary venous outflow disruption, namely:

- *Conjunctival level*: For example, damage from alkali burns

- *Episcleral vessels*: For example, Sturge-Weber syndrome
- *Orbital level*: For example, thyroid eye disease, orbital tumour, orbital varix, and iatrogenic post-orbital surgery
- *Intra-cranial level*: For example, cavernous sinus thrombosis, carotid cavernous fistula
- *Extra-cranial level*: For example, superior vena cava syndrome

Clinical features

By definition, all patients will have raised IOPs (incidental finding or symptomatic) and possible signs of glaucoma. Other clinical and systemic features will be disease specific and would need to be actively identified. **Table 80.1** summarises the findings in a sample group of these conditions.

Investigations

These can be categorised into ocular and systemic investigations. Apart from the routine glaucoma staging test in all cases [anterior segment optical coherence tomography (OCT), visual fields, disc and macular imaging OCT], further ocular investigations may include confocal microscopy, ultrasound biomicroscopy (UBM), aqueous humour analysis, fluorescein angiography, posterior segment OCT and ocular ultrasound. Systemic investigation may include blood work up as well as cultures, cardiovascular work up, carotid Dopplers, neuroimaging, tumour staging scans, and lumbar puncture and cerebrospinal fluid (CSF) analysis.

Treatment

This involves control of the IOP, either medically, with laser (iridotomy, selective iridoplasty, and cyclodestructive, as appropriate depending on the circumstances) or surgically. Treatment of the primary underlying condition can involve control of inflammation, ocular surgery [e.g. AC washout, cataract extraction, intraocular lens (IOL) repositioning, vitrectomy, and retinal detachment repair], orbital surgery, retinal laser, and intravitreal injection therapies. Systemic treatment varies from immunosuppression, possible tumour management to neurosurgery.

Prognosis

It varies depending on the underlying primary conditions and ranges from excellent to sight/ocular and even life-threatening.

Further reading

Camp DA, Yadav P, Dalvin LA, et al. Glaucoma secondary to intraocular tumors: mechanisms and management. Curr Opin Ophthalmol 2019; 30:71–81.

European Glaucoma Society (EUGS). (2014). Terminology and Guidelines for Glaucoma, 4th edition. [online] Available from https://bjo.bmj.com/content/bjophthalmol/101/4/1.full.pdf. [Last accessed October, 2019].

Nassr MA, Morris CL, Netland PA, et al. Intraocular pressure change in orbital disease. Surv Ophthalmol 2009; 54:519–544.

Related topics of interest

- Glaucoma – medical management (p. 162)
- Neovascular glaucoma (p. 216)
- Pigmentary glaucoma (p. 256)
- Retinal lasers (p. 282)
- Thyroid eye disease (p. 316)

81 Sickle cell retinopathy

Key points

- Sickle cell disease is a group of autosomal recessive disorders which cause sickling of red blood cells when oxygen levels are low
- The SC genotype is more likely than the SS genotype to be associated with retinopathy, but less likely to cause severe systemic problems
- Rates of permanent visual loss from sickle cell retinopathy are low
- One-third of cases of proliferative sickle retinopathy (PSR) regress spontaneously
- Current management of proliferative sickle cell retinopathy includes the observation of cases which are asymptomatic and sector laser photocoagulation in cases with higher risk of sight-threatening complications

Introduction

Sickle cell disease results from a mutation in the beta-globin gene (see pathophysiology). The homozygous haemoglobin SS (HbSS) causes the most common form of systemic problems. *Sickle cell retinopathy* is the most prominent manifestation of sickle cell disease in the eye.

Epidemiology

Sickle cell disease is one of the most prevalent inherited diseases in England affecting more births than cystic fibrosis. 1:2,000 babies in the UK are screen-positive for sickle cell disease.

The SS genotype of the disease causes the most common and severe form of systemic problems. Patients experience recurrent episodes of vascular occlusion affecting the lungs, liver, kidneys, bone, and skin. The SC and sickle β-thalassaemia genotypes cause milder systemic disease, but have a higher prevalence of proliferative sickle cell retinopathy.

A longitudinal cohort study of over 20 years in Jamaica confirmed that proliferative sickle cell retinopathy was most frequently seen in the SC genotype group (43% of these patients had developed proliferative sickle cell retinopathy by age 26 years compared with 14% in the SS genotype group). The youngest reported case of proliferative sickle cell retinopathy is at 8 years of age, with peak prevalence at 15–39 years.

The study also showed that there was spontaneous regression of proliferative sickle cell retinopathy in approximately a third of the patients.

Pathophysiology

Haemoglobin is composed of two β-globin proteins, two α-globin proteins, and a haem molecule. A point mutation in the beta-globin gene results in the substitution of a valine for glutamic acid on the β-globin protein chain leading to formation of defective HbS.

An individual with sickle cell anaemia inherits two copies of the defective gene (SS genotype). Sickle cell disease also results from a combination of the HbS allele and other beta-globin variants such as the HbC allele (SC genotype) or Hb β-thalassaemia allele (sickle β-thalassaemia). HbD and HbE are also other significant ethnic variants.

Haemoglobin S abnormally polymerizes with other Hb molecules under conditions of low oxygen tension leading to reduced red blood cell deformability, increased blood viscosity, and sickling of the red blood cell.

Although the genotypes are distinct, sickle cell disease has a heterogeneous phenotype and its pathophysiology is complex and multifactorial. Genetic and environmental modifiers are likely to play a role and molecular interactions such as inflammation, vasculopathy, and coagulation responses may explain why the same genotype can display varying clinical manifestations.

Clinical features

In the eye, any tissue can be affected by vascular occlusion in sickle cell disease.

Sickle cell retinopathy is the most prominent manifestation of sickle cell disease in the eye. Clinical features can broadly be divided into nonproliferative and proliferative retinal changes. These are due to vaso-occlusive complications in the retinal and rarely the choroidal circulation.

Nonproliferative sickle retinal signs include salmon patch haemorrhages, black starbursts, venous tortuosity and schisis cavity.

"Salmon-patch" haemorrhages are preretinal or in the subinternal limiting membrane space. Intraretinal haemorrhages also occur and may leave schitic spaces and iridescent deposits on resolution.

Vascular occlusions are more commonly seen in the retinal periphery with signs of blind-ended vessels and hairpin loops. Submacular choroidal infarction may also occur. Clinical features of peripheral ischaemia are more prominent than macular ischaemia in sickle cell retinopathy and account for the difference in sites of neovascularisation as compared with diabetic retinopathy.

Angioid streaks are recognised as a generally benign association with sickle cell disease (1–7% of patients).

Proliferative sickle cell retinopathy

Retinal vascular occlusions at the retinal periphery cause increasing features of demarcation between avascular and vascularised retina over time. Vascular remodelling is seen at the borders of these areas. When neovascularisation occurs at these borders, sea fan configurations are typically seen.

Proliferative sickle cell retinopathy progresses at variable rates between individuals, being more likely to show an increase in proliferative lesions in the under-25 age group. Despite this, the rates of visual loss from proliferative sickle cell retinopathy are low. Spontaneous regression and autoinfarction of neovascular lesions are more common in SS disease.

Investigation

Fundus fluorescein angiography findings

A Jamaican cohort study describes a classification system for angiographic findings:
- Type I vascular/avascular borders have preserved arteriolar and venular loops, but loss of the capillary bed tending to the retinal periphery
- Type II borders show an abrupt demarcation with evidence of blind-ended small and medium calibre retinal vessels as well as loss of the capillary bed

In addition, type IIa borders have capillary buds or stumps which may leak angiographically and have been found by this study to be a strong risk factor for development of proliferative sickle cell retinopathy.

Ocular coherence tomography findings

Recent studies using enhanced depth imaging optical coherence tomography (EDI-OCT) and optical coherence tomography angiography (OCTA) indicates the presence of temporal macular thinning and choroidal thinning in proliferative sickle cell retinopathy.

Diagnosis

Risk factors for proliferative sickle cell retinopathy include genotype (worse in SC), sex, and age (peak prevalence at an earlier age in men with SC).

Other risk factors from a study by Fox et al. in Jamaica show an increased risk of proliferative sickle cell retinopathy in the SS genotype when associated with high Hb levels in men and low foetal Hb in both sexes.

In the SC genotype, risk factors reported are a high mean cell volume and low foetal Hb in both sexes and high Hb and high mean red cell Hb in men.

Treatment

A Cochrane review of laser treatment in proliferative sickle cell retinopathy indicates a paucity of recent robust studies. The review states that laser treatment can be considered an option for treatment of proliferative sickle cell retinopathy; however, patient-related and functional outcomes are unclear. Sectoral retinal argon laser and xenon arc feeder vessel ablation treatments showed an effect in lowering the risk of loss of vision and vitreous haemorrhage. Paradoxically, laser treatment did not show a significant effect in achieving complete regression of neovascular lesions when compared with no treatment.

Medical treatment targeting the pathophysiology of the disease shows promise but requires further clinical research to determine its effect on ocular disease.

Case reports describe the use of intravitreal bevacizumab and associate treatment with regression of neovascularisation and resolution of vitreous haemorrhage; however, it is not possible to determine the clinical efficacy of treatment from these reports.

Importantly, population studies remind us that observation must be considered in the management of sickle cell retinopathy, especially when there is no macular involvement and the patient is asymptomatic. Spontaneous regression of neovascular fronds occurs in a third of those with the SC genotype and there is a low risk of permanent visual loss in those who were observed up to the age of 26 years.

Complications

Vitreous haemorrhages were rare in the Jamaican cohort and tended to last less than 3 months. Even more uncommon was permanent visual loss from retinal detachment which occurred in two patients (from a total of 59 patients with PSR) observed up to the age of 26 years.

Further reading

Barbosa de Melo. An Eye on Sickle Cell Retinopathy. Rev Bras Hematol Hemater 2014; 36:39–321.

Downes et al. Incidence and Natural History of Proliferative Sickle Retinopathy. Observations from a Cohort Study. Ophthalmology 2005; 112:1869–1875.

Elagouz et al. Sickle Cell Disease and the Eye: Old and New Concepts. Survey of Ophthalmology 2010; 4:359–377.

Han et al. Evaluation of Macular Vascular Abnormalities Identified by Optical Coherence Tomography Angiography in Sickle Cell Disease. Am J Ophthalmol 2017; 177:90–99.

Herman, Chaudhry. Sickle Cell Disease. McMaster Pathophysiology Review 2012-2016. http://www.pathophys.org/scd/

Mathew R, et al. Spectral Domain OCT in patients with Sickle Cell Disease. Br J Ophthalmol 2015; 99:967–972.

Myint et al. Laser Therapy for Retinopathy in Sickle Cell Disease. Cochrane Database of Systematic Reviews 2015.

Streetly et al. Positive screening and carrier results for the England-wide universal newborn sickle cell screening programme by ethnicity and area for 2005-07. J Clin Path 2010; 63:626–629.

Related topics of interest

- Retinal imaging (p. 277)
- Retinal lasers (p. 282)

82 Strabismus surgery

Key points

- Most strabismus surgery is performed under general anaesthesia, to relieve diplopia, improve or retain binocular vision, or to reduce disfigurement from a squint
- Most strabismus surgery involves recession, resection/plication, or transposition of the extraocular muscles
- Repeatable measurements are desirable prior to surgery to maximise success

Indications

All patients with strabismus must have a full ocular examination, refraction, and dilated fundus examination. Any underlying secondary cause of strabismus must be addressed. Nonsurgical treatment of strabismus including occlusion, glasses, prism, and botulinum toxin injection may be considered prior to surgery. In children, associated strabismic amblyopia must be managed prior to strabismus surgery.

Strabismus surgery to restore appropriate ocular alignment may be indicated for:
- Binocular function
  - Improve or restore binocular function in infants and young children
  - Increase field of binocular vision or relieve diplopia
- Correction of disfigurement
- Correct abnormal head posture

Preoperative assessment

The diagnosis and surgical plan are confirmed in the clinic. At least two measurements on separate visits are required to ensure the angle is stable and reproducible. Surgical dose is calculated based on the deviation in prism dioptres. **Table 82.1** gives one example of a surgical table and should only be used as a guide. Surgical results depend on the operative technique, the underlying strabismus, and desired endpoint.

General principles in surgical planning are:
- Weaken overacting muscle and/or strengthen antagonist muscle
- Minimise induced incomitance
- Treat pre-existing incomitance by matching duction deficits

The patient's fitness for general anaesthesia and suitability for adjustable sutures is assessed. The consent process includes risks of general anaesthesia, infection, bleeding, loss of vision, new-onset double vision, and need for further surgery if there is under- or overcorrection.

Techniques

Anaesthesia

Strabismus surgery is almost always performed under general anaesthesia in both children and adults. In cases where general anaesthesia is not possible, a peribulbar or retrobulbar orbital block can be used.

Table 82.1 Surgical dose for rectus muscle operations

	Recession	Resection
Medial rectus	1 mm surgery = 3.0 Δ effect	1 mm surgery = 2.5 Δ effect
Lateral rectus	1 mm surgery = 2.5 Δ effect	1 mm surgery = 2.0 Δ effect
Superior rectus	1 mm surgery = 2.5 Δ effect	
Inferior rectus	1 mm surgery = 3.0 Δ effect	

Notes:
- Fibrotic and enlarged muscles (e.g. thyroid): more effect per mm.
- More effect from unilateral recess/resect than bilateral recession.
- More effect advancement previously recessed muscle than virgin resection.

Preparation and forced duction tests

The surgical plan is clearly recorded on the theatre board. Following sterile preparation and drape, forced duction testing is performed, if required, using toothed forceps to move the eye in a direction opposite the muscles to be tested. An episcleral traction suture is used to rotate the eye and maximise the exposure.

Conjunctival incision

The conjunctival incision can be limbal, forniceal or over the muscle. The conjunctiva is handled with nontoothed forceps (e.g. Moorfield forceps) and blunt-tipped spring scissors are used for cutting. Subtenon pockets are created on either side of the muscle using blunt dissection. Tenon capsule is very thick in infants and becomes progressively thinner with age.

Identify and expose the muscle

The borders of the rectus muscle are identified. The muscle is hooked with a curved strabismus hook under direct visualisation. Care should be taken to minimise tissue trauma during this process. When the muscle is hooked or manipulated, bradycardia induced by the oculocardiac reflex can occur. The surgeon and anaesthetist need to be mindful and intravenous atropine may need to be administered. Tenon capsule attachments are dissected from the edges of muscle and directly overlying the muscle until the muscle is clearly visualised. The curved strabismus hook is replaced with one that spreads the muscle. Intraoperative phenylephrine and bipolar diathermy are used for haemostasis.

There are various methods of suturing the muscle. 6-0 polyglactin suture on double-armed quarter-circle spatulated needles are preferred by the authors.

Weakening

Several approaches can be used to weaken an extraocular muscle, i.e. recession, myectomy, tenotomy, myotomy or tendon spacer. Recession is the most commonly performed weakening procedure and involves securing and detaching the muscle from its insertion and moving the muscle edge posteriorly towards its origin, reducing the mechanical advantage, with resultant weakening of action.

Two locking bites are placed through the outer thirds of the muscle. The tendon is disinserted from the sclera using scissors, taking care not to cut the suture. The desired amount of recession is marked on the sclera using callipers. The recessed muscle can be fixed to the sclera directly at the new insertion (fixed recession) or to the original insertion with the muscle allowed to "hang back" by the desired amount. The latter technique can be combined with a small anchoring bite through the sclera and is useful in cases where exposure is difficult (e.g. medial rectus), for large recessions and if postoperative adjustment might be necessary.

Strengthening

Extraocular muscles can be strengthened through resection, advancement, plication or tucking. Resection is the most commonly performed strengthening procedure and involves excision of a length of muscle to shorten and therefore strengthen its action.

A second strabismus hook is placed under the muscle and moved away from the insertion. The desired amount of resection is marked directly on the muscle using gentle diathermy. Two locking bites of suture are placed through the outer thirds of the muscle, just posterior to intended resection. The muscle is resected and then sutured to the original insertion (**Figure 82.1**).

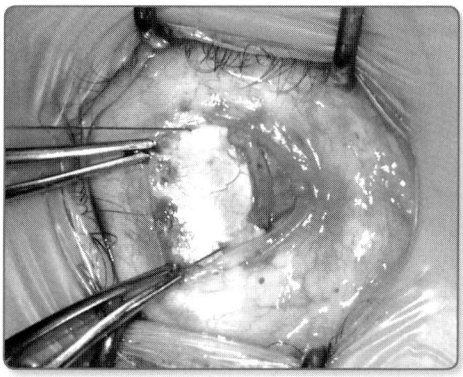

Figure 82.1 Recession of medial rectus (intraoperative).

Special situations

- *Posterior fixation suture (faden operation)*: A nonabsorbable suture is used to secure the muscle belly to the sclera just posterior to the equator. The effect is to selectively weaken the muscle in its direction of action, without altering the primary position alignment
- *Transposition*: When a muscle has no function (e.g. complete lateral rectus palsy), transposition of other muscles, e.g. superior rectus can improve the range of movement as well as primary position alignment
- *Advancement of previously recessed muscle*: Preferred option for consecutive deviation, e.g. medial rectus advancement for consecutive exotropia. The muscle insertion is moved to the original insertion, combined with a small resection if a pseudotendon is present. This is usually combined with recession of antagonist muscle on an adjustable suture to optimise the postoperative outcome
- *Inferior oblique weakening*: The insertion is moved lateral to the temporal border of the inferior rectus muscle. Care is taken during exposure to avoid bleeding and engaging the orbital fat. The surgeon must ensure all of the muscle is hooked as the inferior oblique muscle has a large belly
- *Superior oblique surgery*: Harada–Ito procedure to correct excyclotorsion, tenotomy for weakening (e.g. Brown syndrome), and tucking for congenital palsy with a lax tendon

Conjunctival closure

Local anaesthesia is injected into the subtenon space for cases where postoperative adjustment is not planned. 8-0 polyglactin suture is used to close conjunctival incisions with buried knots.

Adjustable sutures

Surgical results may be improved by the use of adjustable sutures, particularly for reoperations and in patients at risk of postoperative diplopia. They can be performed in conjunction with recessions, resections, and advancements.

Postoperative care

Patients are advised not to drive for at least 3 days postoperatively. It is normal for the eye to be red for 2 weeks and slightly pink for 2 months postoperative. A combination steroid/antibiotic drop is prescribed three times a day for 3 weeks in the operative eye(s). A postoperative review is recommended at 2–3 weeks postoperative to assess alignment and healing.

Complications

- *Under -or overcorrection*: Minimised by accurate preoperative assessment and use of adjustable sutures where possible
- Surgical confusion, i.e. wrong muscle or wrong procedure. Prevented through clear documentation on theatre board and surgical time out
- Scleral perforation, which may result in retinal detachment. Prevented by good surgical technique
- *Anterior segment ischaemia*: If operating on more than 3 muscles simultaneously, higher risk in patients with pre-existing vascular risk factors
- *Infection*: Orbital cellulitis (1:2,000), endophthalmitis with scleral perforation (1:30,000)
- *Double vision*: Usually transient but may require further procedures to resolve
- *Bleeding*: Avoided through use of topical vasoconstrictors and meticulous diathermy
- Slipped muscle due to broken or weak suture. This can be recovered with further surgery
- Suture granuloma
- Amblyopia in children
- Change in eyelid position
- Fat adherence syndrome

Further reading

Edelman PM. Functional benefits of adult strabismus surgery. Am Orthopt J 2010; 60:43–47.

Ferris JD, Davies PEJ. Surgical Techniques in Ophthalmology Series: Strabismus Surgery. China: Saunders Elsevier; 2007.

Wang T, Wang LH. Surgical treatment for residual or recurrent strabismus. Int J Ophthalmol 2014; 7:1056–1063.

Related topics of interest

- Esotropia (p. 137)
- Exotropia (p. 142)

83 Thyroid eye disease

Key points

- Thyroid eye disease (TED) is likely to be an autoimmune process
- Smoking cessation must be recommended to all smokers as it is both a major trigger and drive
- Oral selenium supplements can improve the course of mild disease
- Orbital soft tissue changes include eyelid retraction, proptosis, oedema, and fat hypertrophy
- Myopathic changes cause extraocular muscle swelling and double vision
- The cornea may become involved through impaired blink and exposure keratopathy
- Sight loss can occur through optic nerve compression [dysthyroid optic neuropathy (DON)]

Epidemiology

Thyroid disorders will affect up to 10% of the population during their lifetime, with a higher incidence in females. TED occurs in up to half of patients with Graves' disease and even mild change can have long-lasting residual consequences. The incidence of thyroid orbitopathy is approximately 16/100,000 in women and 2.9/100,000 in men. It is most prevalent in women aged 40–50 years. Smoking tobacco has been shown to increase the risk that patients suffering from hyperthyroidism develop TED, whilst also increasing the severity if it does so.

Pathophysiology

The thyrotropin receptor is uniquely targeted in Graves' disease by pathogenic autoantibodies known as thyroid-stimulating immunoglobulins. These autoantibodies can be detected in most persons who have Graves' disease; however the fact that they are not detectable in some, means that additional autoantigens are likely to be involved. The activation of orbital fibroblasts to secrete glycosaminoglycans, then collagen, is controlled by cytokine release from tissue macrophages and migrating lymphocytes. Many have been implicated, including insulin-like growth factor-1 (IGF-1), platelet-derived growth factor (PDGF), tumour necrosis factor-α (TNF-α), and transforming growth factor-β (TGF-β).

At the onset of TED, a lymphocytic infiltrate sweeps through the affected orbital muscles. Inflammation of affected muscles causes them to fail to contract and move freely during eye movements, resulting in pain and diplopia. Glycosaminoglycans lead to water retention, which causes further muscle swelling. As the volume of the orbital contents increases, orbital tension rises. Patients vary according to the ease with which this is relieved by proptosis.

Antigen release after thyroid destruction by iodine-131 may trigger or exacerbate TED, presumably as a consequence of massive antigen release. It should be avoided in patients with orbital myopathy and covered by systemic steroids.

Clinical features

The clinical course of TED is classically described as somewhat sinusoidal, often reaching a peak in disease activity and severity within 12–24 months of onset. Even though TED is commonly treated medically and surgically, nontreated disease can improve spontaneously in up to 50% of patients.

When considering TED, assess both soft tissue and myopathic involvement. Changes can be mild, moderate or severe and the clinical findings can hint toward whether the disease is active or inactive. At first attendance, it is impossible to tell in whom the condition will progress. One aim of assessment is to formulate a plan for the functional and cosmetic rehabilitation of the patient.

Clinical activity is based on features of inflammation. The clinical activity score (CAS) is the sum of items present below, a score of $\geq 3/7$ indicating active disease:

- Spontaneous retrobulbar pain
- Pain on attempted up-or downgaze

- Redness of the eyelids
- Redness of the conjunctiva
- Swelling of the eyelids
- Inflammation of the caruncle and/or plica
- Conjunctival oedema

Thyroid eye disease has many manifestations including eyelid retraction, exposure keratopathy, proptosis, extraocular motility restriction causing diplopia, and compressive optic neuropathy in its most severe instances. Sight-threatening TED occurs in up to 5% of patients and can occur before, during or after the onset of hyperthyroidism. Impairment of optic nerve function, termed DON occurs through compression of the optic nerve. Corneal breakdown can also occur in patients suffering from proptosis, eyelid retraction, and corneal exposure.

Corticosteroids, radiotherapy, and other immunomodulatory drugs can often be effective in the management of the inflammatory phase of the disease. Surgery, in the form of orbital decompression remains the mainstay of treatment in the presence of optic neuropathy, significant exposure keratopathy, or significant proptosis and disfigurement refractory to medical management.

Investigations

Blood workup includes thyroid status as well as baseline testing of a full blood count, inflammatory markers, renal and liver function as preparation for possible immunosuppressive treatment. Thiopurine S-methyltransferase (TPMT) should be checked if azathioprine is likely to be used as a second-line agent.

Orbital imaging is useful at baseline. This can help to assess the severity and degree of myopathic and soft tissue changes; surgical planning, and to ensure another (less common) diagnosis is not being missed. A computed tomography (CT) of the orbits (request axial and coronal sections, with a soft tissue and bone window) would be adequate for the above, although should be avoided in children. Some clinicians prefer magnetic resonance imaging (MRI) as this can help to pick up active myopathic disease during a short tau inversion recovery (STIR)

sequence. Traditionally, it is thought that the inferior and medial rectus muscles are the most frequently targeted in TED, although the levator palpebrae superioris will also commonly be enlarged.

Diagnosis

With a history of thyroid disorder and typical clinical signs and symptoms, a diagnosis can be established. It is, however, important to ensure that another disease process is not being missed and therefore TED should (almost) be considered a diagnosis of exclusion.

Some patients will present with the clinical features of TED and no history of a thyroid disorder. For example, the most common clinical feature of TED is upper eyelid retraction (**Figure 83.1**). If this is the only sign present, then TED should be considered and investigated as such, along with other causes of eyelid retraction.

Numerous grading systems and questionnaires have sought to measure signs and symptoms, but no consensus regarding their use exists. One way of classifying the severity of TED based on symptoms is shown in **Table 83.1**.

Treatment

Immediate aims should include establishing an euthyroid state, smoking cessation,

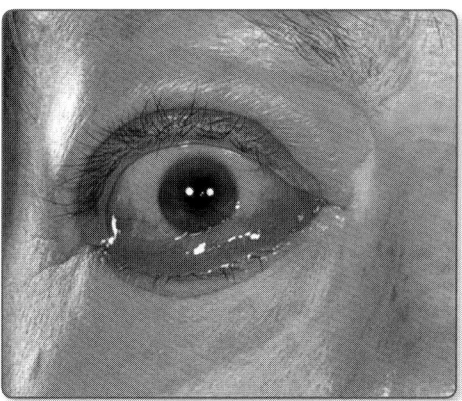

Figure 83.1 Patient demonstrating signs of thyroid eye disease. (*For colour version see plate 8*)

Table 83.1 Severity classification in thyroid eye disease	
Sight-threatening	Dysthyroid optic neuropathy (DON) Corneal breakdown
Moderate-to-severe	Lid retraction ≥2 mm Moderate or severe soft tissue involvement Exophthalmos ≥3 mm above normal Inconstant or constant diplopia
Mild	Minor lid retraction (< 2 mm) Mild soft tissue involvement Exophthalmos < 3 mm above normal Transient or no diplopia Corneal exposure responsive to lubricants

and oral selenium in mild disease. Immunosuppression (oral or intravenous corticosteroid, steroid-sparing agents, and biologics) is likely to be required for moderate soft tissue or myopathic disease. Adjunctive low-dose external beam orbital radiotherapy can be helpful for myopathic disease with impaired motility. These treatments usually have little effect on degree of proptosis.

To minimise the systemic side effects of these drugs, orbital steroid injections (usually triamcinolone) are sometimes used for milder disease. There is encouraging anecdotal evidence that this treatment can be of benefit in select cases.

Orbital decompression surgery is usually delayed until TED is quiescent, unless vision is compromised despite medical treatment (i.e. where there is optic neuropathy, significant orbital congestion or uncontrolled intraocular pressure). There is now a growing acceptance and use of fat removal combined with bone removal during decompression surgery. "Fat only" decompression can also be performed, although less commonly in isolation for the subgroup of patients with DON.

Complications

Since techniques for orbital decompression surgery have evolved, the focus has shifted to reducing complication rates, particularly the incidence of postoperative diplopia. In earlier reported series of orbital decompression, new onset or worsening of pre-existent diplopia has been reported to occur in 15–45% of patients. Removal of the medial and lateral wall preserving the orbital strut (balanced decompression) with or without fat removal has been advocated to decrease the risk of postoperative diplopia. Removal of the deep lateral wall is currently thought to be the safest decompressive procedure, associated with minimal complications. It has no significant effect on horizontal or vertical deviations with a low rate (2–3%) of new onset diplopia.

Further reading

Bartalena L, Baldeschi L, Dickinson A, et al. Consensus statement of the European group on Graves' orbitopathy (EUGOGO) on management of GO. Eur J Endocrinol 2008; 158:273–285.

Dolman PJ, Rootman J. VISA classification for Graves orbitopathy. Ophthal Plast Reconstr Surg 2006; 22:319–324.

Marcocci C, Kahaly GJ, Krassas GE, et al. Selenium and the course of mild Graves' orbitopathy. N Engl J Med 2011; 364:1920–1931.

Related topic of interest

- Imaging in Ophthalmology (p. 176)

84 Trauma – globe rupture

Key points

- Globe rupture is a specific type of open globe injury arising from blunt trauma
- The diagnosis of globe rupture can be difficult and an examination under anaesthetic may be the only way of making the diagnosis
- Prompt, full closure of scleral wounds is recommended; however, very posterior scleral wounds are best left unsutured

Epidemiology

Eye injury is an important cause of vision loss worldwide. There are approximately 1.6 million people blind from injuries. There are estimated to be 200,000 injuries per year that result in an open globe.

Pathophysiology

Ocular trauma has been formally classified by the Ocular Trauma Classification Group as shown in **Figure 84. 1**. A formal classification system allows more accurate communication between healthcare personnel and allows more reproducibility of research studies into ocular trauma. As can be seen in the flowchart (**Figure 84.1**), globe rupture is a specific type of ocular trauma that arises after blunt injury that leads to a full-thickness eyewall wound. It comes about secondary to an inside-out mechanism with the intraocular pressure momentarily increasing and leading to rupture of the eyewall normally at specific weak points such as posterior to muscle insertions or around pre-existing surgical wounds.

Clinical features

Following globe rupture, patients normally present with reduced visual acuity and pain. Examination findings vary and indeed may be subtle. It might be that a full-thickness defect in the eyewall is observed on clinical examination, but often this is not the case and the diagnosis has to be made based on the history and other clinical features. Additional clinical features that may be noted include low intraocular pressure, relative afferent pupillary defect, hyphaema, deep anterior chamber, and haemorrhagic chemosis (**Figure 84.2**). 24 hours after injury, rather than low intraocular pressure, high

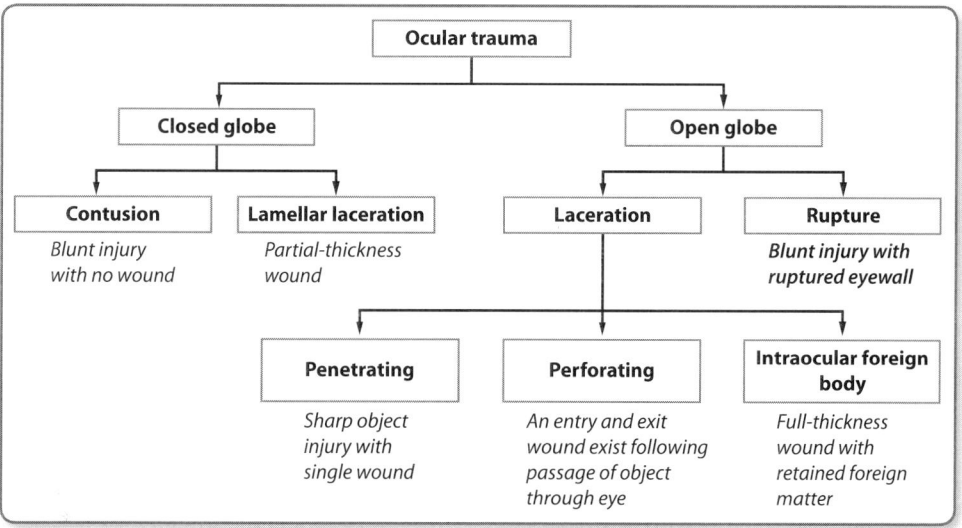

Figure 84.1 Ocular trauma classification group classification of ocular trauma.

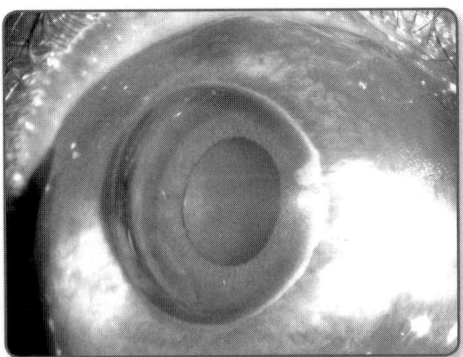

Figure 84.2 Haemorrhagic chemosis and deep anterior chamber following globe rupture. (*For colour version see plate 8*)

intraocular pressure may be seen as fibrinous adhesions form securing the wound.

A thorough examination and good documentation of findings are important not only because they allow further management planning but also because cases of globe rupture can end up with surrounding legal proceedings. Clinical features at presentation are important at predicting final visual acuity. The ocular trauma score (OTS) was developed as a means of predicting final visual acuity following trauma. In its development it was found that the important factors for predicting final visual acuity are initial visual acuity, presence of rupture, endophthalmitis, globe perforation, retinal detachment, and afferent pupillary defect.

Investigations

When the diagnosis of globe rupture is in doubt because of a non-conclusive clinical examination, further investigations are helpful.

Computed tomography (CT) scanning is normally the first investigation performed in patients with suspected globe rupture. It is readily available in most emergency departments, it is non-invasive, and it is not operator dependent. Alteration in globe volume and contour together with scleral discontinuity are seen on CT. CT is also good at identifying both radiolucent and radiopaque intraocular foreign bodies.

Magnetic resonance imaging (MRI) is better than CT at imaging soft tissues and it is thought to be more sensitive at identifying scleral ruptures and organic foreign bodies. The magnetic fields and heat generated during MRI mean that it is contraindicated when a metallic intraocular foreign body is suspected. Ferromagnetic foreign bodies implanted into the vitreous of animal eyes experimentally have been shown to move up to 10 mm when subjected to MRI scanning.

Ultrasonography can be a helpful adjunct in the diagnosis of globe rupture. Ultrasonography is operator dependent and great care must be taken not to exert significant pressure on the globe as this may exacerbate the injury. Posterior scleral wounds may be manifest as echolucent discontinuities in the sclera representing vitreous incarceration. Direct imaging of globe ruptures in the more typical pre- and periequatorial location is difficult but their presence can often be inferred from the presence of massive suprachoroidal haemorrhage.

Diagnosis

The diagnosis of globe rupture is normally made based on the results of the clinical examination and investigations. Sometimes, however, the results of these can be inconclusive and if this is the case, the patient will need to be taken to the operating theatre for examination under anaesthesia together with repair of the rupture if one is identified.

Treatment

Initial treatment of globe rupture is to place a rigid plastic shield over the eye and initiate systemic antibiotic therapy. Tetanus prophylaxis should be administered, if required. Appropriate analgesia and antiemetics should be prescribed. The patient should be prepared to go to the operating theatre for repair of the wound under general anaesthetic as soon as possible.

At surgery, a thorough exploration of the globe is required to identify any wounds. A 360-degree conjunctival peritomy is carefully made and if no anterior wound is visualised, the sub-Tenon's space is opened in all four quadrants to allow exploration of the posterior sclera. Often a small gush of blood or serosanguinous fluid is observed when opening up the quadrant that involves the scleral laceration. Once the wound has been identified, bridle sutures are placed around the recti.

It is extremely important that all episcleral tissue and clotted blood are carefully cleaned away from the wound so that the edges can be clearly defined prior to suturing. If the wound is circumferential, the whole wound can be cleaned before suturing. If it is radial, then the wound is cleaned and sutured progressively from front to back.

Horizontal wound alignment is important and for circumferential wounds the "50% rule" can be used. This relies on the fact that the human brain is good at gauging symmetry. The first suture is placed half way along the wound and then the rest of the wound is treated as two separate wounds and sutures placed half way along these and this is repeated until the wound is closed. Scleral wounds are best closed using the "pull don't push" principle where the tissue is grasped and impaled on the needle. The whole wound needs to be closed unless it extends very posteriorly. Very posterior wounds are best left unsutured because of the high risk of expulsion of globe contents from the manipulation involved in closing them. Temporarily detaching a rectus muscle may be required to aid wound exposure and to allow rotation of the globe without undue elevation of intraocular pressure.

Non-absorbable sutures such as 9/0 nylon are used in the relatively avascular posterior sclera. Absorbable sutures such as 9/0 polyglactin can be used more anteriorly where the sclera is more vascular so heals more quickly. Using an absorbable suture anteriorly prevents the late complication of suture extrusion. The knots associated with scleral sutures should not be buried unless they are very anterior. Inappropriate rotation of knots can cause retinal damage.

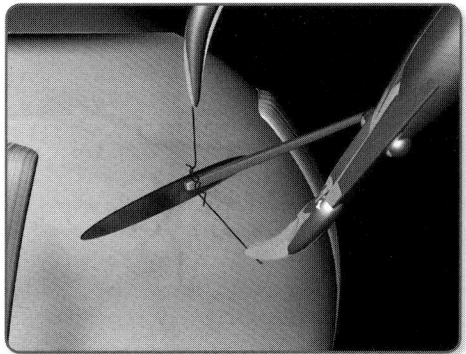

Figure 84.3 An assistant gently presses on prolapsed choroid with an iris repositor whilst the suture is tied.

Choroid can sometimes be seen prolapsing out of scleral wounds. No attempt should be made to excise this given its vascularity. An assistant can gently reposit the choroid whilst the suture is tied over it as shown in **Figure 84.3**. Prolapsed vitreous should be excised and this is best performed with a vitreous cutter. This is preferable to using a sponge and scissors, which pulls more vitreous into the wound and can exacerbate incarceration.

Complications

The two most devastating complications following globe rupture repair are endophthalmitis and sympathetic ophthalmia.

Open-globe injury is a risk factor for the development of endophthalmitis. Recent studies have shown an incidence ranging from 7% to 12%. Delay in primary repair increases the risk of endophthalmitis development.

A retrospective Chinese study of 9,103 patients with globe injury demonstrated a 0.37% risk of sympathetic ophthalmia following open-globe injury. The evidence that enucleation or evisceration is effective at preventing sympathetic ophthalmia is only weak.

Further reading

Gunenc U, Maden A, Kayak S, et al. Magnetic resonance imaging and computed tomography in the detection and location of intraocular foreign bodies. Doc Ophthalmol 1992; 81:369–378.

Kuhn F, Morris R, Witherspoon CD, et al. A standardized classification of ocular trauma. Ophthalmology 1996; 103:240–243.

Sullivan PM. The Open Globe 2013. [online] Available from https://www.eyelearning.co.uk/the-open-globe/ [Last accessed November, 2019].

Zhang Y, Zhang MN, Jiang CH, et al. Development of sympathetic ophthalmia following globe injury. Chin Med J 2009; 122:2961–2966.

Related topics of interest

- Imaging in ophthalmology (p. 176)
- Vitreoretinal surgery – retinal breaks and detachment and vitreomacular interface disorders (p. 350)

85 Tumours – eyelid

Key points

- Basal cell carcinoma (BCC) is the most common eyelid tumour accounting for over 85% of eyelid tumours
- Malignant lesions can result in localised tissue destruction with loss of eyelashes and destruction of meibomian gland orifices
- Management is typically histological margin controlled excision and reconstruction

There are a multitude of tumours arising in the eyelids, and these may be defined according to their cell of origin as epidermal, adnexal, and stromal (**Table 85.1**). The tumours may also be classified according to their invasiveness as benign, premalignant or malignant. This chapter will focus on BCC, squamous cell carcinoma (SCC), sebaceous gland carcinoma (SGC), and melanoma, which together account for 95% of malignant eyelid tumours.

Epidemiology

The eyelids are one of the most common sites for non-melanoma skin cancers, accounting for 5–10% of all skin cancers. BCC is the most common eyelid tumour, accounting for over 85% of eyelid tumours. The incidence of BCC is estimated to be rising by 3–10% globally, in part due to increased longevity. The risk of BCC, SCC, and malignant melanoma is greatest in adult Caucasians with a history of prolonged exposure to ultraviolet light. SCC is the second most common eyelid tumour in this population, comprising 5–10% of all eyelid malignancies. SGC occurs in 1–5.5% of eyelid malignancies, although in Asian countries, it is the second most common, accounting for over 29% of eyelid tumours. Melanoma is much rarer, representing less than 1% of eyelid tumours.

Pathophysiology

The aetiology of eyelid tumours is multifactorial, with significant contributions from the environment, genetics, and the immune system. Immunosuppressed patients have a higher risk of developing SCC, melanoma, and to a lesser extent, BCC. Exposure to ultraviolet radiation inducing cumulative deoxyribonucleic acid (DNA) damage is thought to contribute to most eyelid tumours and patients with fair skin phenotypes show greater susceptibility. There are genetic predispositions to BCC, such as Gorlin–Goltz or naevoid basal cell carcinoma syndrome (NBCCS). This is an autosomal dominant (AD) condition characterised by the early onset of BCCs from puberty onwards, and characteristic abnormalities include odontogenic jaw keratocysts, skeletal abnormalities, and palmar or plantar pits. The causative gene is the *PTCH1* gene, which is activated by the hedgehog pathway, and this has also been implicated in cases of sporadic BCC. Patients with xeroderma pigmentosum (XP) have germline mutations in their nucleotide excision repair genes, and they too have elevated risk of BCC, SCC, and melanoma.

Basal cell carcinomas (BCCs) arise from non-keratinising cells in the basal layer of the epidermis. Histologically, there are different subtypes, with nodular being the most frequent, followed by superficial and infiltrative. There is also the basosquamous carcinoma variant which shows morphologic features of both BCC and SCC. Local invasion to adjacent tissue is particularly a risk with the infiltrating type, and especially high risks are those lesions located in the medial canthus. Although metastasis has been reported, it is extremely rare.

Squamous cell carcinoma is the second most common eyelid tumour, arising in the squamous layer of the epithelium, and comprises 5–10% of all eyelid malignancies. SCC may arise de novo from relatively normal skin or from precursor actinic keratosis (AK), and then develops to in situ Bowen's disease with full thickness involvement of the epidermis, before progressing to invasive and then metastatic disease. Regional lymph node metastasis rates of up to 24% are reported.

Table 85.1 Types of premalignant and malignant eyelid tumours according to their origin. Continue opposite...

Types	Subtypes	Invasiveness	Tumour	Histopathology	Presentation
Epidermal tumours	Non-melanocytic	Premalignant	Actinic keratosis	Squamous dysplasia of epithelium with loss of cell polarity, hyperkeratosis and parakeratosis, may transform to SCC	Small erythematous scaly lesions, in sun-exposed areas
		Malignant	Basal cell carcinoma	Nodular type: Epithelial lobules of cells with oval nuclei and prominent peripheral palisading of the nuclei. Morphoea type: Elongated strands of basaloid cells embedded in a dense fibrous stroma	Most common nodular type is a raised firm, pearly white nodule with surface telangiectasia and central ulceration. Morphoea appears as a pale plaque with poorly defined borders
			Squamous cell carcinoma	Arises from squamous cell layer of epithelium. May be poorly or well-differentiated. Well-differentiated: Polygonal cells, dyskeratotic cells, intercellular bridges. Poorly-differentiated: Pleomorphism with anaplastic cells, abnormal mitotic figures and loss of intercellular bridges. May metastasise to lymph nodes	5% of all eyelid malignancies. Often arises from actinic keratosis or following radiotherapy. Elevated indurated plaque with central ulceration and irregular rolled borders
	Melanocytic	Premalignant	Lentigo maligna	Atypical melanocytes in the basal layers of the epidermis	Precursor to malignant melanoma
		Malignant	Melanoma	Breach of the epidermal basement membrane	< 1% of all eyelid malignancy
Adnexal tumours		Premalignant	Pilomatrixoma	Arise from hair matrix cells. Basophilic basaloid cells peripherally with pale ghost cells centrally. Calcification may be present	Slow-growing solitary solid or cystic pink subcutaneous lesion, usually in the upper lid or eyebrow. Can rarely show malignant transformation

Table 85.1 Continued...

Types	Subtypes	Invasiveness	Tumour	Histopathology	Presentation
		Malignant	Sebaceous gland carcinoma	Well-differentiated: Neoplastic cells with sebaceous differentiation and vacuolated cytoplasm. Poorly-differentiated: Hyperchromatic atypical cells, pleomorphism and high mitotic activity. Oil Red-O staining for lipids is helpful for diagnosis. Shows "pagetoid spread" intraepithelialy into epidermis of lid and conjunctival epithelium	Higher prevalence in Asian countries. Highly malignant, capable of metastasis as well as local invasion. More common in the upper eyelid and in women. Firm, painless subcutaneous lesion, may mimic a chalazion but causes loss of eyelashes
Stromal tumours	Fibrous tissue tumours	Malignant	Fibrosarcoma	Closely packed cells with a woven herringbone interlacing pattern	Rapidly progressive solitary eyelid nodule or second malignancy in patients with retinoblastoma (postradiotherapy)
	Vascular tumours	Malignant	Kaposi's sarcoma	Spongy network of endothelial cells that form slit-like vascular spaces surrounded by spindle-shaped mesenchymal cells and collagen	Caused by human herpesvirus 8. Commonly in AIDS patients. Presents as a blue subcutaneous lesion which may be solitary, multifocal, circumscribed or diffuse
	Neurogenic tumours	Malignant	Merkel cell tumour (cutaneous neuroendocrine carcinoma)	Arises from Merkel cells, neuroendocrine receptors. Lobules of poorly differentiated round cells with abundant mitotic figures. Immunohistochemical staining is helpful in diagnosis	Solitary violaceous nodule commonly in the upper lid. Rapidly progressive, over weeks, frequently metastasises and recurs locally

(AIDS: acquired immunodeficiency syndrome)

Sebaceous gland carcinoma can arise from meibomian glands, glands of Zeis or glands associated with the caruncle, and typically affect the upper lid due to the higher density of meibomian glands there. There is often aggressive local extension and pagetoid (intraepithelial) spread, which can result in skip lesions and also affects the conjunctiva. Metastasis can occur both via lymphatic and haematogenous routes, with reported regional lymph node involvement in up to 18% after surgical excision. Muir–Torre syndrome, a rare AD condition, carrying a higher risk of visceral malignancies, should be suspected if there are multiple sebaceous neoplasms.

Melanoma usually arises de novo, although it can arise from premalignant lesions like congenital naevi, dysplastic naevi or lentigo maligna (LM). 1–5% of congenital naevi transform to melanoma, and up to 30% of dysplastic naevi. LM is considered to be melanoma in situ until it has invaded the dermis, when it becomes malignant melanoma. Sunlight is the greatest risk factor for transformation of melanocytes to melanoma, as is the frequent use of tanning beds. The presence of increased mitotic figures on histology, as for all eyelid tumours, is associated with more aggressive tumours.

Clinical features

Both BCCs and SCCs are most common in the lower lid, followed next in frequency by the medial canthus and then the upper lid. There are several clinical variants of BCC: nodular, noduloulcerative, pigmented, infiltrating (morphoea or sclerosing). Nodular is the most common subtype and these lesions have pearly raised edges, surface telangiectasia, and central ulceration. Morphoea is a rare subtype which can present as a flat and pale or skin-coloured ill-defined lesion, and is often located in the medial canthus. This subtype is associated with a higher rate of deep infiltration. All BCCs are slow-growing lesions which can distort the normal architecture and can result in madarosis.

Whereas the clinical diagnosis of BCC is more straightforward, that of SCC maybe more variable. SCCs can arise de novo or from AK. They typically present as a raised plaque or nodule with keratinisation, scaling or ulceration, but can have a wide spectrum of clinical appearances. SCC can be locally aggressive and results in perineural invasion with cranial neuropathies, causing paraesthesia, pain, ptosis, and diplopia.

Sebaceous gland carcinoma may present as a solid solitary nodule or as diffuse erythematous lid disease with thickening of the lid. The solitary lesion arises deep to the epidermis, from the tarsus, and is associated with madarosis. Diagnosis may be delayed due to initial labelling as recurrent chalazion or blepharoconjunctivitis.

About 25% of patients with melanoma are under 40 years old. The lower lid is also more commonly affected. Superficial spreading is the most common subtype of melanoma on the eyelid, followed by nodular. The lesions are not always pigmented, which can make diagnosis challenging. The ABCDE guidelines for diagnosis of melanoma are widely used. "A" refers to lesion asymmetry, "B", border irregularity, "C" to colour variation, "D" to diameter > 6 mm, and "E" to evolving lesion with time. These should be used to guide assessment of suspicious lesions.

Diagnosis

The gold standard of diagnosis remains histological. BCC is slow growing and rarely metastasise, however, SCC is potentially fatal and early detection and treatment can greatly improve the prognosis. Incisional biopsies may be performed in cases of diagnostic uncertainty, to help with subsequent management. Biopsy of suspected melanoma helps determine the depth of invasion (Breslow thickness). Prognosis is affected by presence of ulceration, mitosis, and lymphatic invasion. Permanent section is required before reconstruction for melanoma, as frozen section is inaccurate. Frozen section is however often sufficiently accurate to allow reconstruction for BCC or SCC. In cases of suspected SGC, a full-thickness biopsy may be preferred and mapping biopsies are often advocated due to the possibility of skip lesions. Traditionally, fresh specimens for SCG were advocated to facilitate confirmatory lipid stains like Oil Red-O and Sudan Black to be used, although newer immunohistochemical stains which allow confirmation of SGC in formalin-fixed specimens. Good communication with the reporting histopathologist is recommended.

Treatment

The gold standard treatment of eyelid malignancies remains surgical excision, with histological margin control to ensure tumour-free margins. Mohs micrographic surgery (MMS) has been reported to achieve high cure rates of 98.1% and if available maybe favoured for the management of BCC and SCC. MMS involves layered excision of the tumour, with further removal where tumour is present until there is clearance. It offers the benefits of determining margin control during excision and maximal preservation of normal tissue. This is valuable in optimising functional and aesthetic outcomes. There have also been comparable cure results with intraoperative frozen section (IFS), where the margins are examined on the day of surgery to enable same day repair. Typical clinical surgical margins for BCC are 3–4 mm, whereas more aggressive tumours such as SGC and melanoma require greater margins, up to 5 mm when feasible. Reconstruction options depend on defect size and may include a combination of direct closure, local flaps, grafts or "laissez-faire" (where the defect is allowed to heal naturally).

Other available treatment modalities for eyelid tumours include topical chemotherapy and immunomodulatory agents, cryotherapy, radiotherapy, and systemic chemoprophylaxis. Topical immunomodulatory treatments like imiquimod 5% cream, a synthetic toll-like receptor agonist can be used for AK and superficial BCC. Topical imiquimod has also been reported as a successful treatment for LM. Typical treatment duration is 6 weeks, although this has been extended for longer, until the lesions become undetectable on slit lamp examination. Adverse events include conjunctivitis, keratitis, and ectropion. Topical chemotherapy agents like 5-fluorouracil, a pyrimidine analogue that preferentially affects DNA synthesis in neoplastic cells, have also been used successfully for AK and superficial BCC.

The double freeze-thaw cryotherapy technique can be useful when margins are not cleared or when patients are not good surgical candidates. Radiotherapy can likewise be used for the same indications. Without adjuvant radiotherapy, perineural involvement in SCC carries a high risk of recurrence, up to 36.9% at 5 years.

The hedgehog pathway inhibitor vismodegib has been used in patients with locally advanced BCC inappropriate for surgery or radiotherapy or symptomatic metastatic BCC; however, looking at current evidence, the National Institute for Health and Care Excellence (NICE) has found that it currently has uncertain clinical benefit in terms of overall survival, in addition to not being cost-effective. It also has significant adverse events, and tumour regrowth occurs upon discontinuation of treatment.

Squamous cell carcinoma and AK have epidermal growth factor receptor (EGFR) overexpression, and EGFR inhibitors have been used for locally advanced SCC, but larger trials are needed.

A history of eyelid tumours increases the risk for subsequent lesions, so advice on ultraviolet protection and self-monitoring for new lesions should be given to all patients. Higher risk lesions such as recurrent and morphoeic BCC, SCC, SGC, and melanoma, as well as lesions with perineural invasion and those located in the medial canthus, may have longer follow-up periods.

Complications

Removal of eyelid tissue can make reconstruction challenging and also result in suboptimal outcomes like ptosis, lid retraction, lagophthalmos, lid malposition, and exposure keratopathy. Delay in diagnosis and treatment can result in disease progression and orbital invasion, which may require exenteration. If there is local or perineural invasion or metastasis, adjuvant therapies like radiotherapy and chemotherapy may be considered. Adverse effects of radiotherapy can include the development of cataract, keratopathy, optic neuropathy, and retinopathy. If surgery becomes necessary in a previously irradiated area that may complicate healing any reconstruction. Complications of cryotherapy include chemosis and skin depigmentation, particularly in more pigmented skin types.

Further reading

Kanski JJ, Bowling B. Kanski's Clinical Ophthalmology E-Book: A Systematic Approach, 8th edition. Amsterdam, Netherlands: Elsevier Health Sciences; 2015.

Pe'er J, Singh AD, Damato BE. Clinical Ophthalmic Oncology: Eyelid and Conjunctival Tumors, 2nd edition. Berlin, Germany: Springer; 2013.

Shields JA, Shields CL. Eyelid, Conjunctival, and Orbital Tumors: An Atlas and Text, 2nd edition. Philadelphia: Lippincott Williams & Wilkins; 2008.

Related topics of interest

- Tumours of the choroid (p. 329)
- Tumours of the retina (p. 345)
- Tumours of the uvea (p. 340)

86 Tumours of the choroid

Key points
- Choroidal naevi require careful monitoring – there are set criteria to determine suspicion for growth
- Choroidal melanomas have a favourable prognosis if diagnosed and treated early
- Choroidal haemangioma or osteoma, though benign, bears features that could compromise vision and in case of diffuse haemangiomas have a devastating effect

Epidemiology

Choroidal naevi are the most common fundus tumours – they have been reported to correspond to 10% of the white population without a particular predilection for age or sex.

Choroidal melanoma is the most common primary intraocular malignancy which can be fatal in adults. In the general population it has an incidence of 5.3–10.9 cases per million population per year. Diagnosis is usually in the sixth to seventh decades of life. Overall incidence is lower in populations of Afro-Caribbean or Asian descent. Risk factors include oculodermal melanocytosis, a lightly coloured iris and fair skinned individuals.

Choroidal metastases are the most common intraocular tumours in the adult. They are diagnosed in 10–40% of cancer patients.

Circumscribed choroidal haemangiomas are acquired vascular tumours of the choroid that develop in the 2nd to 4th decades of life. They have no systemic associations. *Diffuse choroidal haemangiomas* are usually diagnosed in children (with a median age of 8 years). Incidence is higher in Sturge–Weber syndrome patients who have both facial naevus flammeus and leptomeningeal angiomatosis.

Choroidal osteoma is an idiopathic osseous tumour of the posterior choroid. It is most often diagnosed in young adult women. Mean age of diagnosis is 25 years though it has been diagnosed in young children with no predilection for race.

Pathophysiology

Choroidal naevi and melanomas arise from melanocytes of the choroidal stroma. The development of choroidal melanoma has been associated with early oncogenic mutations in pathways involved with the regulation of the cell cycle or the control of cell apoptosis (see Prognosis).

Choroidal metastases more commonly develop as a result of haematogenous spread and commonly develop in the posterior pole (90% vs. 10% for a more anterior location). More commonly they develop secondary breast cancer and lung cancer in female patients and lung cancer in male patients. The primary tumour remains unknown in 12–30% of cases possibly because the diagnosis is made at later stages of the disease and at the setting of generalised metastatic disease.

Pathogenesis of circumscribed choroidal haemangiomas and diffuse choroidal haemangiomas is not entirely clear. It has been theorised that both conditions are related but this has not been substantiated. Diffuse choroidal haemangioma is a manifestation of Sturge–Weber syndrome. The latter relates to the disturbance of neural crest precursors with subsequent effect on the central nervous system, skin, and eyes.

Pathogenesis of choroidal osteoma is unknown. They do not seem to be associated with heterotopic intraocular calcification developing in cases of prolonged inflammation and there are no proven associations with hormonal factors (despite high preponderance in females) or disturbances with calcium metabolism.

Clinical features

Table 86.1 presents a list of differential diagnoses of choroidal melanotic and amelanotic lesions.

Choroidal naevi present with varying elevation and extent, fundus location and pigmentation. Most naevi develop over time secondary degenerative changes of the overlying retinal tissue. Customarily

Table 86.1 The main differential diagnoses of choroidal melanotic and amelanotic lesions. The list is by no means exhaustive but it does cover the common or characteristic entities in the differential

Choroidal melanotic lesions	Choroidal amelanotic lesions
Choroidal naevus	Choroidal amelanotic naevus
Choroidal melanoma	Choroidal metastases
Subretinal haemorrhage	Choroidal haemangioma
Neurofibroma (in selected cases)	Choroidal melanoma
CHRPE	Choroidal osteoma
Retinal detachment	Sclerochoroidal calcification
Choroidal detachment	Choroidal granuloma
Choroidal haemangioma	Posterior scleritis
Eccentric disciform scar	Eccentric disciform scar

(CHRPE, Congenital hypertrophy of the retinal pigment epithelium)

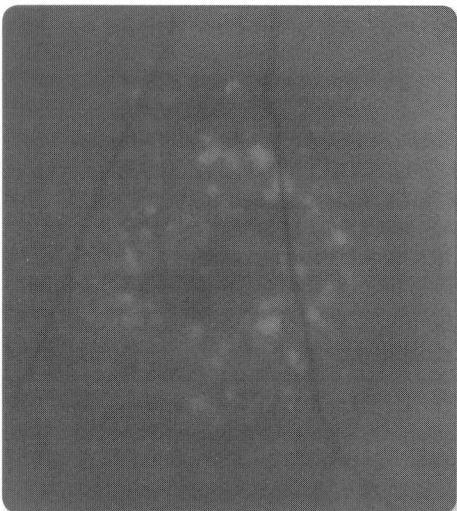

Figure 86.1 Choroidal naevus – note the presence of well defined drusen on the surface. (*For colour version see plate 8*)

these are in the form of drusen (**Figure 86.1**) or disruption of the retinal pigment epithelium (RPE) with formation of pigment clumps, secondary fibrous metaplasia, subretinal or intraretinal fluid or choroidal neovascularisation.

Choroidal melanoma is not always symptomatic and the generation of visual problems is highly dependent on its location.

Melanomas are progressively growing and have varying pigmentation. This growth could be minimal hence the need for careful serial monitoring of suspicious lesions. Alternatively, endophytic extension through Bruch's membrane (attaining a mushroom-shaped configuration) or extrascleral extension could occur. Vitreous seeding has also been documented. Accompanying features also involve actively increasing subretinal fluid and increasing lipofuscin deposits (**Figures 86.2** and **86.3**).

Choroidal metastases present as single or multiple, unilateral or bilateral yellow choroidal lesions that exhibit rapid growth and increased leakage (**Figure 86.4**).

Choroidal haemangiomas are sometimes difficult to detect if too small and could have associated fluid, lipofuscin deposits (rarely) or overlying fibrous or osseous metaplasia (**Figure 86.5**). Circumscribed choroidal haemangiomas are pale orange red lesions commonly encountered in the posterior pole. They are almost always unifocal and unilateral and usually not thicker than 6 mm. They are often asymptomatic, though symptoms can occur as a direct function of the tumour location or behaviour. Subfoveal tumours can induce unilateral hypermetropic shift as a result of anterior displacement of the retina. Juxta- or parafoveal tumours cause vision loss if associated with exudative subretinal fluid or retinoschisis. Diffuse choroidal haemangioma causes diffuse bright red thickening of the posterior choroid (strawberry-coloured fundus). There is usually an associated retinal detachment, which could be much more pronounced causing leukocoria, cataract, and secondary glaucoma (**Figure 86.6**).

Choroidal osteomas are chalk-white or yellow in colour and are located in the juxtapapillary or macular area. They are mostly unilateral but could be bilateral. Typical features include peripheral circumferential growth, gradual decalcification with retinal pigment epithelial disturbance, intraretinal fluid (**Figure 86.7**) or the development of choroidal neovascularisation that is predominantly classic in nature. Vision loss has been reported in up to 60% of cases.

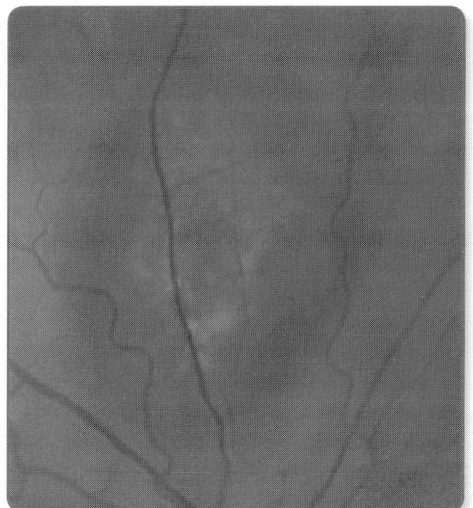

Figure 86.2 Small choroidal melanoma – note the presence of confluent lipofuscin on the surface. (*For colour version see plate 8*)

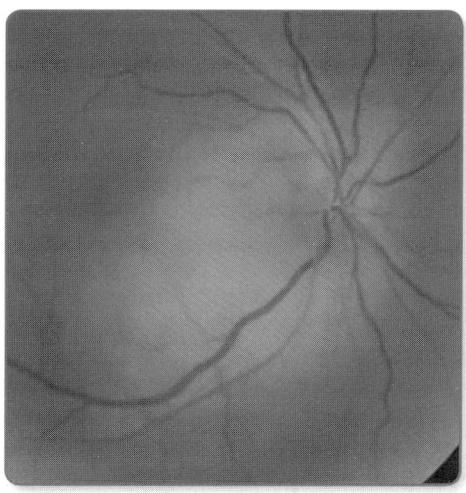

Figure 86.4 Choroidal metastasis – yellowish lesion with feathery margins. (*For colour version see plate 9*)

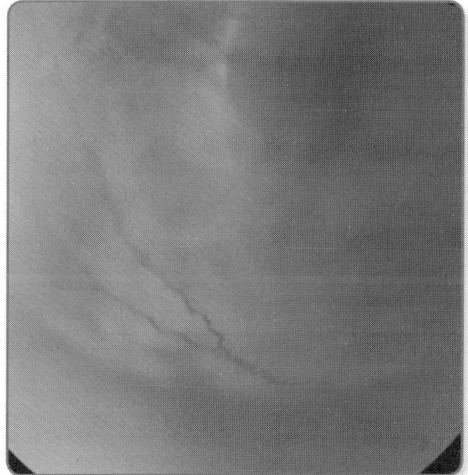

Figure 86.3 Large choroidal melanoma – protruding choroidal mass with associated detachment and disturbance of the overlying retina. (*For colour version see plate 9*)

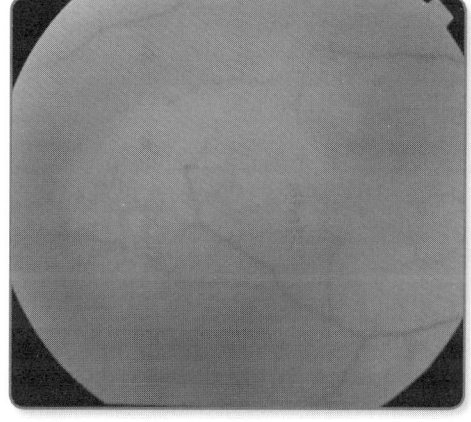

Figure 86.5 Circumscribed choroidal hemangioma – organe mass less distinct with superficial metaplastic features and associated fluid. (*For colour version see plate 9*)

Investigations

Choroidal tumours are typically diagnosed with slit lamp or indirect ophthalmoscopy. Ancillary studies are invaluable in the differential diagnosis.

Fluorescein angiography delineates secondary degenerative overlying retinal changes in choroidal naevi including choroidal neovascularisation. Choroidal melanomas present with increasing mottled hyperfluorescence and late leakage of the lesion and if amelanotic or expanding through Bruch's membrane, they present with the double circulation sign (simultaneous visualisation of the choroidal and retinal circulation). Indocyanine angiography is very useful in diagnosing

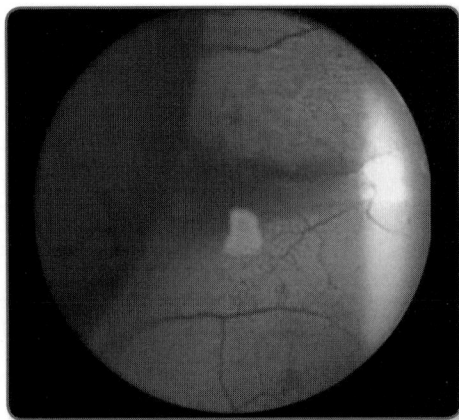

Figure 86.6 Diffuse choroidal hemangioma with extensive exudative detachment visible through the pupil. (*For colour version see plate 9*)

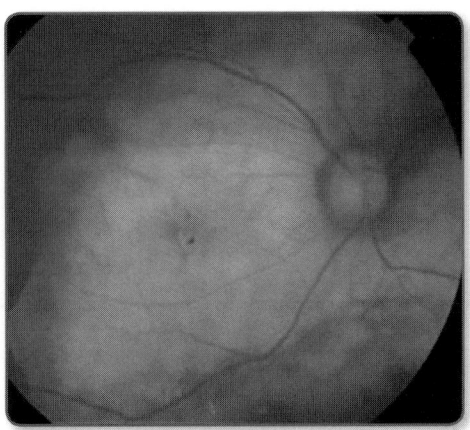

Figure 86.7 Choroidal osteoma white yellow mass with circumferential peripapillary extension, decalcification and macular RPE changes. (*For colour version see plate 9*)

circumscribed choroidal haemangiomas because of their typical presentation of early uptake and late washout (at really late phases of the test – around 25 minutes). Diffuse haemangiomas present with similar features without the late washout stage.

B-mode ultrasonography is not only useful for the estimate of the dimensions of examined tumours but is essential for the differential diagnosis. Choroidal naevi and melanomas are hypoechoic with the latter demonstrating choroidal excavation. In addition, the presence of associated detachment, extraocular extension, and configuration can be assessed. Choroidal metastases and choroidal haemangiomas are hyperechoic and their internal blood flow, as estimated by a Doppler B-scan is customarily higher in comparison with choroidal melanoma. Diffuse choroidal haemangiomas demonstrate diffuse thickening of the choroid and bear similar features as their circumscribed counterpart. Choroidal osteomas or areas of calcification are very hyper-reflective with shadowing.

Autofluorescence is important is accentuating the presence of lipofuscin deposits and delineating the extent of fluid leakage of suspicious lesions. It is helpful in detecting suspicious naevi or small choroidal melanomas or demonstrating the extent of leakage of circumscribed choroidal haemangiomas.

Conventional spectral domain optical coherence tomography (OCT) allows the identification of subretinal fluid associated with a suspicious choroidal lesion of melanoma and importantly the presence or not of chronic anatomic disruption of the neurosensory retina. Newest modules of OCT such as enhanced-depth imaging or swept source have allowed an assessment of the choroidal aspects of lesions and have demonstrated a plethora of new signs such as delineation of the sclerochoroidal interface and posterior scleral bowing, distension of marginal choroidal vessels in naevi and melanomas, presence of vascular channels within small choroidal haemangiomas, bone-like structure with tubules, and channels in choroidal osteoma.

Treatment

Management options

Observation

Monitoring of lesions without any invasive treatment involves choroidal naevi, inactive choroidal haemangiomas or choroidal osteomas without secondary choroidal neovascularisation. Follow-up schedule is customisable based on the individual features of the lesion in question.

Enucleation
Enucleation has been the traditional method of treating large tumours (namely choroidal melanomas) occupying most of the intraocular space or invading the optic nerve or affected eyes with severe secondary glaucoma (as in cases of choroidal metastases with extensive exudative retinal detachment). Secondary enucleation could be done in cases of tumour recurrence following treatment with alternative modalities (see below).

Plaque brachytherapy
This modality involves the placement of a radioactive plaque against the sclera in close proximity to a tumour. All structures close to that source are irradiated resulting in the formation of free radicals, deoxyribonucleic acid (DNA) damage and, eventually, inhibition of cell division and cell death. Radioactive isotopes in use include ruthenium-106, iodine-125 or palladium-103. Plaques are round or curvilinear and of varying diameters. Proper size selection would allow a 2 mm safety margin around the base of the tumour. The radioactive plaque is removed 2–7 days after insertion when the calculated dose of radiation has been locally administered.

Radiation-induced complications occur on average 18–24 months after plaque treatment and include cataract, proliferative radiation retinopathy, and papillopathy, neovascular glaucoma or an exudative tumour response.

Plaque brachytherapy is being used for small or medium choroidal melanomas, circumscribed choroidal haemangiomas or rarely for retinal vascular tumours.

Proton-beam radiotherapy
This modality involves exposure of the tumours to a charged proton beam causing energy deposition to the target tissue. It involves the placement of multiple radio-opaque markers (tantalum rings) to the sclera at the border of the lesion to aid with tumour localisation. A three-dimensional model of the tumour is superimposed on the eye and a face mask and collimator is custom designed for the patient. Administration of treatment is fractionated.

Proton beam radiotherapy has been used for melanomas of up to 14 mm in height and of unusual locations and choroidal haemangiomas (diffuse and circumscribed). Radiation-related complications can occur as cataract, glaucoma, and radiation retinopathy.

Most tumours regress for up to 2 years after treatment. Regression is complete in 15% of patients.

Transpupillary thermotherapy
Transpupillary thermotherapy (TTT) uses modified diode laser delivery system to induce hyperthermia to the tumour with reduced secondary damage to surrounding healthy tissues. Currently it is used as adjuvant treatment for choroidal melanomas or edge recurrence. It has also been used in the past for the treatment of circumscribed choroidal haemangiomas. Complications include scotoma, haemorrhage or retinal vascular occlusion.

Additional treatment options
External beam radiation therapy has been used for the treatment of diffuse or circumscribed choroidal haemangiomas, but not customarily used for choroidal melanomas. Photodynamic therapy has been used for leaking choroidal naevi producing symptoms, active circumscribed choroidal haemangiomas, and individual foci of choroidal metastasis producing symptoms. Anti-vascular endothelial growth factor (VEGF) treatments are reserved for lesions developing secondary choroidal neovascularisation (naevi and osteomas) but also in cases of proliferative radiation retinopathy or maculopathy. The latter have also been treated with dexamethasone implants.

Prognosis
Prognosis for choroidal naevus
The clinical risk factors for growth of a choroidal naevus have been described and include:
- Tumour size over 2 mm
- Fluid (originally described for clinically visible fluid, now refers to clear subretinal fluid on OCT)

- Symptoms (generated from the lesion – vision loss or photopsia or visual field loss)
- Orange pigment (referring to lipofuscin clinically evident or evident with autofluorescence – note it can appear green on amelanotic lesions)
- Margin (distance of 2 disc diameters from the optic disc margin)
- Ultrasonographic hollowness (hypoechoic lesion on B-scan)
- Halo absent (no presence of depigmented halo around the naevus – clear sign of chronicity)
- Drusen absent (no presence of druse over the lesion – clear sign of chronicity)

These factors constitute the mnemonic To Find Small Ocular Melanoma Using Helpful Hints Daily.

Prognosis for choroidal melanoma

Survival rates for choroidal melanoma

Despite the availability of alternative treatment modalities, the survival rates of patients with uveal tract melanoma have not changed in the last decades. Collaborative Ocular Melanoma Study (COMS) reported these to be at 25% and 34% at 5 and 10 years, respectively. Common sites of metastases include the liver (90%), lung (24%), and bone (16%). Patients with metastases confined to extrahepatic locations have longer survival (19–28 months). Median survival in patients with metastasis is 6 months with an estimate of 10% at 2 years.

Metastatic potential

Tumour size for metastatic potential: Tumour size is one of the best parameters used to predict metastatic disease. Increased tumour thickness increases the risk of metastasis. Reported 5-year survival rates after enucleation were 84% for small, 68% for medium-sized, and 47% for large tumours.

Genetic and cytogenetic aspects

Chromosomal and gene alterations: The major chromosome alterations described in choroidal melanoma are chromosomes 3, 6, 8, and 11. The most important of these is monosomy 3 being strongly linked to patient survival. Monosomy 3 is associated with a 5-year survival of approximately 50%, whereas disomy 3 has been reported to predict 100% survival. Chromosomal abnormalities are significantly correlated with the clinical (tumour size) and histopathological (epithelioid cell type) high risk factors for metastasis.

Using gene expression, profiling melanomas have been categorised into two groups, class I and class II. Class I denotes tumours with two copies of chromosome 3 (disomy 3) and other beneficial chromosome changes including gain in chromosome 6p. Class II denoted tumours with only one copy of chromosome 3 (monosomy 3) and other deleterious chromosome changes including gain of chromosome 8p and/or isochromosome 8p.

Mutations in genes *GNAQ* and *GNA11* have been associated with the development of uveal melanoma. No association has been found with chromosome status indicating that these constitute an early pathogenetic event.

Metastatic screening

Currently, here is no universally accepted algorithm for metastatic screening in patients with choroidal melanoma. Customarily, it includes:

- Liver function tests were done every 6 months to annually despite reported low sensitivity, annual abdominal ultrasonography, abdominal CT and preoperatively or on occasion F-18-fluoro-2-deoxyglucose positron emission tomography/computed tomography imaging. MRI of the liver has also been advocated.

Prognosis for choroidal metastases

Patients with uveal metastases usually have coexisting diffuse metastatic disease. Despite the satisfactory response to local treatment, systemic prognosis is poor. Breast cancer and carcinoid tumours have longer survival whereas cutaneous melanoma and lung carcinoma are associated with a worse prognosis.

Visual prognosis depends on size and location of tumour. Vision loss is more common for subfoveal tumours or tumours with retinal detachment involving the fovea.

Prognosis for choroidal haemangioma

Visual prognosis for patients with choroidal haemangioma is only favourable if the choroidal tumour is small and not located at the fovea. However, as most diffuse choroidal haemangiomas are large and associated with a secondary retinal detachment, prognosis is poor, especially in cases of late diagnosis with irreversible amblyopia. An additional confounding factor is the presence of congenital or juvenile glaucoma in the affected eye occasionally leading to enucleation.

Prognosis for choroidal osteoma

Choroidal osteomas can affect visual acuity depending on location, size, decalcification or the development of a choroidal neovascular membrane. The probability of developing choroidal neovascularisation has been shown to be as high as 47% by 10 years and 56% by 20 years. In addition, if osteomas are subfoveal or are decalcified, visual prognosis is worse (34% vs. 10% for subfoveal vs. extrafoveal, and 48% vs. 11% for decalcified vs. noncalcified tumours).

Further reading

Papastefanou VP, Cohen VM. Uveal melanoma. J Skin Cancer 2011; 2011:573974.

Papastefanou VP, Plowman N, Ehud Reich, et al. Analysis of long-term outcomes of radiotherapy and verteporfin photodynamic therapy for circumscribed choroidal hemangioma. Ophthalmol Retina 2018; 2:842–857.

Shields JA, Shields CL, Intraocular tumours: An atlas and textbook, 3rd edition. Philadelphia: Wolters-Kluwer/Lippincott Williams & Wilkins; 2016.

Related topics of interest

- Tumours of the uvea (p. 340)
- Tumours of the retina (p. 345)

87 Tumours – conjunctival neoplasia

Key points

- Conjunctival tumours include a broad array of neoplasms, and can be benign, premalignant or malignant
- Demographic features such as age, race, systemic immune status, chronic exposures (sunlight, smoking), and medical history (xeroderma pigmentosum or Muir-Torre syndrome) are important factors
- Clinical features alone are usually insufficient to make a diagnosis so the 'no touch' surgical technique is used to remove the tumour with minimal handling of abnormal tissue under a dry surgical field

Introduction

Conjunctival tumours include a broad array of neoplasms, some of which are benign, and others that demonstrate premalignant or malignant features. The types and frequency of conjunctival tumours differ with demographic features such as age and race, systemic immune status, and chronic exposures, along with specific location within the conjunctiva. Surgical management is commonly required with 'no touch' excision; double or triple freeze thaw cryotherapy to prevent recurrence; alcohol keratoepitheliectomy, lamellar keratectomy or sclerectomy may be needed for deeper invasion. Ocular surface reconstruction is necessary with amniotic membrane or conjunctival allograft. Intraocular invasion by the cancer may require enucleation and orbital invasion requires orbital exenteration.

Squamous cell papilloma (Figure 87.1)

This is a benign common epithelial tumour associated with human papillomavirus

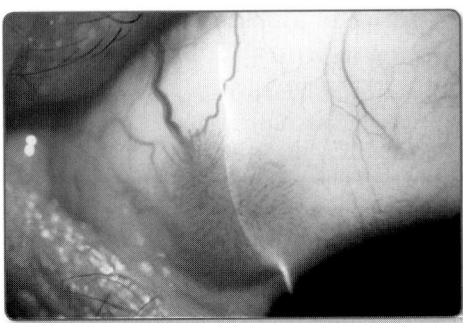

Figure 87.1 Squamous cell papilloma.

(subtypes 6, 11, 16, and 18) and can be found in any age, occurring more commonly in young adults and in males. *Clinical features* include a pink fibrovascular frond of tissue, sessile or pedunculated, with fine stromal vascular channels. In children, they can be multiple, located often in the inferior fornix. In adults, a solitary lesion can extend to cover the entire corneal surface, simulating malignant squamous cell carcinoma. *Management* includes observation (slow spontaneous resolution), no-touch surgical excision with cryotherapy to reduce spread of papillomavirus particles, oral cimetidine, interferon-alpha or mitomycin C drops or systemic interferon-alpha. Recurrences can occur.

Ocular surface squamous neoplasia

Conjunctival squamous carcinoma is included in the general clinical term of Ocular surface squamous neoplasia (OSSN) OSSN, along with the more specific histopathologic terms of conjunctival or corneal intraepithelial neoplasia (CIN) or both (CCIN) and squamous cell carcinoma (SCC). Differentiating these clinically can be challenging. Risk factors include sunlight exposure, HPV (subtype 16), HIV, allergy, immunodeficiency, including iatrogenic and xeroderma pigmentosum.

Clinical features

Usually located at the limbus/bulbar conjunctiva, gelatinous, papillary or leukoplakic; nodular, especially when SCC. Diffuse lesion can masquerade as conjunctivitis. In dark-skinned individuals can pigment mimicking melanoma. SCC can invade the anterior chamber or orbit.

Corneal intraepithelial neoplasia is confined to the surface epithelium without breaching the basement membrane. There can be mild, moderate or severe degrees of cellular atypia and it may involve various thicknesses of the epithelium involved from basal layer outwards (CIN 1-3) as well as modification of cell organisation and loss of polarity. *Carcinoma in situ* may have all the features of SCC but confined to the full-thickness epithelium without breaching the basement membrane.

In SCC, (**Figure 87.2**) the features are similar to carcinoma in situ but the basement membrane is breached and subepithelial layers are involved. Aggressive variants are spindle cell SCC, mucoepidermoid SCC, and adenoid SCC.

Treatment of OSSN

No-touch surgical excision and cryotherapy are commonly used but topical immunotherapy (Interferon) or chemotherapy (Mitomycin or 5-fluorouracil) can be used if diagnosis is known. Neoadjuvant topical immunotherapy can be used to shrink the lesion before surgery. Brachytherapy is also useful in selected SCC cases.

Melanocytic lesions

Racial melanosis is a benign bilateral conjunctival pigmentation usually in the bulbar conjunctiva/limbus in dark-skinned individuals. Avoid surgical excision.

Primary acquired melanosis (PAM) (**Figure 87.3**) is unilateral, flat, benign brown mobile pigmentation of the conjunctiva that usually develops in middle-aged adults with pale skin. It is histopathologically divided into two groups: PAM with atypia which carries 50% lifetime risk of developing melanoma (must be monitored) and PAM without atypia (population risk of melanoma). Management of PAM with atypia is controversial (includes observation, excisional biopsy, map biopsies if extensive, cryotherapy or topical chemotherapy). If an area shows thickening, nodularity or vascularity, then treat it as conjunctival melanoma.

Conjunctival naevus (**Figure 87.4**) is benign and the most common conjunctival tumour, occurring in all races. Onset is in first or second decade of life with a discrete, variably pigmented, slightly elevated sessile lesion, often containing clear cysts. A conjunctival naevus can progress

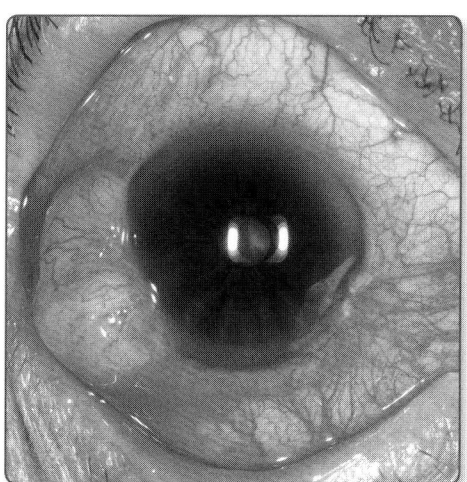

Figure 87.2 Conjunctival squamous carcinoma. (*For colour version see plate 10*)

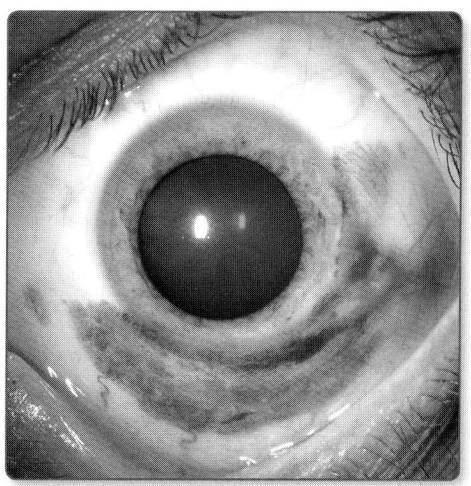

Figure 87.3 Primary acquired melanosis (PAM). (*For colour version see plate 10*)

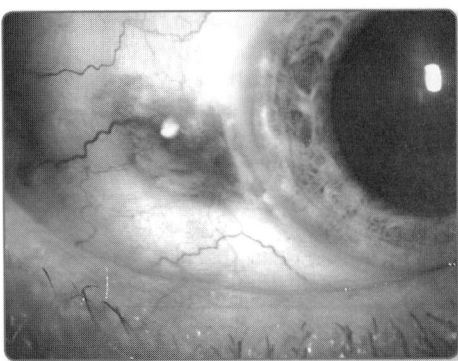

Figure 87.4 Conjunctival naevus. (*For colour version see plate 10*)

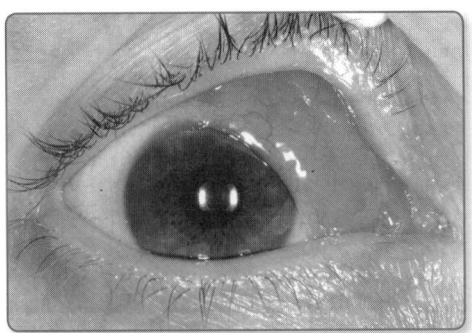

Figure 87.6 Conjunctival lymphoma. (*For colour version see plate 10*)

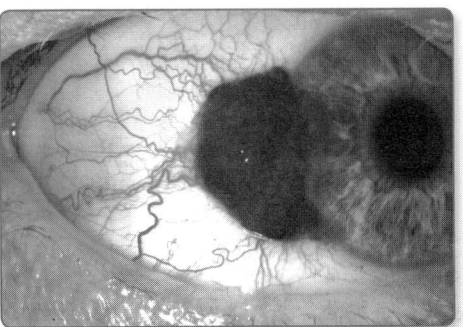

Figure 87.5 Conjunctival melanoma. (*For colour version see plate 10*)

during puberty, but growth in adulthood is highly suspicious of melanoma until proven otherwise (1% chance of malignant transformation). Most are observed periodically but occasionally naevus is excised for comfort or cosmetic reasons.

Conjunctival melanoma (MM) (**Figure 87.5**) onset is in older individuals (median age 62 years old) and can arise from PAM (75%), naevus (20%) or de novo (5%). Located anywhere on the ocular surface or tarsal conjunctiva, they can be pigmented, tan or amelanotic tumours with prominent feeder vessels, corneal or scleral fixity, and surrounding areas of flat PAM. MM can recur locally and develop distant metastasis. If orbital involvement is suspected, imaging with CT or MRI is indicated. Uveal melanoma with extraocular extension mimicking a conjunctival melanoma can be excluded by dilated fundoscopy and ultrasonography. *Management* includes 'no touch' technique wide local excision with cryotherapy. Adjuvant treatments comprise brachytherapy or topical chemotherapy. Orbital involvement usually merits exenteration. Regional lymphadenopathy should be assessed with palpation, head and neck ultrasound, MRI or sentinel lymph node biopsy. Whole body PET/CT scan is useful in disseminated disease. 5-year rates are – recurrence 26%, exenteration 8%, metastasis 16%, and death 7%.

Lymphoid tumours

These are diffuse slightly pink 'salmon patches' usually deep to the conjunctiva or Tenon's fascia, located in fornix or bulbar surface. Clinically, it is hard to differentiate between benign and malignant lymphoproliferative disease. Therefore, a biopsy is necessary.

Benign lymphoid hyperplasia is the benign variant, treated only if symptomatic by excisional biopsy or external beam radiotherapy.

Conjunctival lymphoma (**Figure 87.6**) is a non-Hodgkin's B cell low-grade mucosa-associated lymphoid tissue (MALT) lymphoma, usually isolated in conjunctiva but one-third may have systemic lymphoma. Hence staging is necessary. *Management* of conjunctival lymphoma depends on the extent of periocular and systemic involvement, and general health of the patient. In patients with only conjunctival lymphoma, eradication is achieved by surgery (if unilateral), oral doxycycline (unilateral or bilateral), systemic rituximab (anti-CD20 monoclonal antibody) or external beam radiotherapy (if bilateral).

If ocular and systemic lymphoma is found, then systemic rituximab, chemotherapy or immunotherapy are typically considered. Prognosis is related to lymphoma subtype.

Sebaceous cell carcinoma

This is a rare invasive eyelid skin malignancy that can exhibit pagetoid spread into the conjunctiva to masquerade as a unilateral blepharoconjunctivitis. It occurs in the 6–8th decade of life and is associated with Muir–Torre syndrome. It is capable of metastasis to regional lymph nodes and is potentially lethal. Management involves biopsy for tissue diagnosis followed by exenteration, chemotherapy or radiotherapy.

Further reading

Shields CL, Chien JL, Surakiatchanukul T, et al. Conjunctival tumors: review of clinical features, risks, biomarkers, and outcomes--The 2017 J. Donald M. Gass Lecture. Asia Pac J Ophthalmol (Phila) 2017; 6:109–120.

Shields CL, Shields JA. Tumors of the conjunctiva and cornea. Surv Ophthalmol 2004; 49:3–24.

Shields CL, Sioufi K, Alset AE, et al. Clinical features differentiating benign from malignant conjunctival tumors in children. JAMA Ophthalmol 2017; 135:215–224.

Related topics of interest

- Eyelid trauma (p. 146)
- Tumours of the choroid (p. 329)
- Tumours of the uvea (p. 340)

88 Tumours of the uvea

Key points

- Tumours of the iris and ciliary body could be stationary in development, but special attention is required for ciliary body lesions as they have a late diagnosis due to late generation of symptoms
- Ciliary body melanomas have an unfavourable prognosis and are more aggressive
- Close clinical monitoring is important along with the use of gonioscopy, anterior segment-optical coherence tomography (AS-OCT) or ultrasound biomicroscopy (UBM)

Epidemiology

Melanocytic tumours of the iris include freckles, naevi, and melanomas. Incidence of iris freckles or naevi is unknown as many patients who do bear them do not seek medical or ophthalmological attention. Iris and ciliary body melanomas on the other hand have been reported to correspond to 13–25% of all malignant melanomas of the uvea. These lesions are most common in whites with light-coloured irides and are mostly diagnosed in young adult patients. *Iris and ciliary body metastases* from other primary cancers are very rare.

Vascular tumours of the iris can be classified into iris racemose, cavernous and capillary. Iris racemose haemangioma is an abnormal arteriovenous (AV) communication in the iris stroma with no clear predisposing factors or systemic associations. The other types have systemic associations namely congenital haemangiomatosis for iris cavernous haemangiomas and cutaneous periocular haemangiomas for iris capillary haemangiomas. Congenital tumours of the non-pigmented epithelium as iris and ciliary body medulloepitheliomas usually become symptomatic in early childhood though there are sporadic cases diagnosed and becoming symptomatic during early adulthood or even, more rarely, late adulthood. There is no predilection for sex or race. Acquired tumours of the non-pigmented epithelium as ciliary body adenomas or adenocarcinomas are very rare.

Pathogenesis

Melanocytic tumours of the iris and the ciliary body arise either from uveal melanocytes of the stroma (naevi and melanomas) or the iris pigment epithelium (adenomas and adenocarcinomas). Iris melanomas develop from pre-existing naevi and there has been an association with ultraviolet B (UVB) radiation exposure. Genetic abnormalities have been associated with the development of iris and ciliary body melanoma (loss of chromosomes 3 and 9).

Metastases develop through haematogenous spread and involve the iris and ciliary body in < 10% of cases. *Iris metastases* most commonly originate from breast and lung carcinoma though commonly no primary tumour is identified. *Ciliary body metastases* have been associated with similar primary cancers in individual case reports.

Iris and ciliary body medulloepitheliomas arise from undifferentiated cells of the primitive medullary epithelium. They are comprised of different tissues. Adenomas or adenocarcinomas of the ciliary body arise from fully differentiated ciliary epithelium.

Clinical features

Iris melanocytic tumours appear as discrete masses located in the iris. The degree of pigmentation, location, and dimensions could be variable. An important difference between an iris freckle and an iris naevus is the evident disruption of the anatomy of the stroma upon clinical examination (**Figure 88.1**). This disruption could be associated with ectropion uveae or corectopia when the lesions are located close to the pupillary margin. These lesions can present with intrinsic vasculature when amelanotic (**Figure 88.2**). Shedding of pigment is an additional feature – pigment deposits can also be visualised at the corresponding clock hour

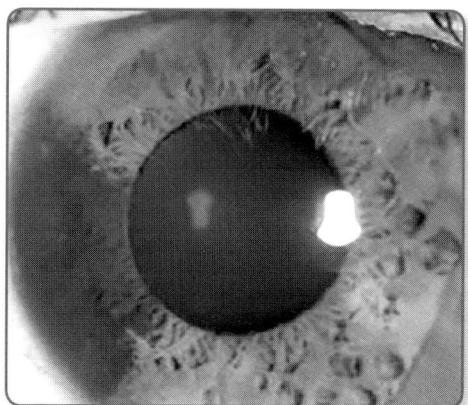

Figure 88.1 Melanocytic iris freckle – note there is no disturbance of the iris stroma. (*For colour version see plate 10*)

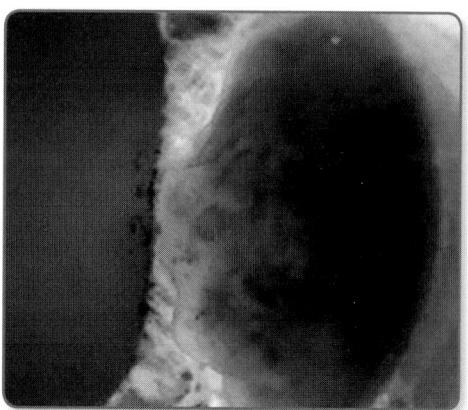

Figure 88.3 Iris melanoma – expansion of the tumour in the anterior chamber with displacement of the iris and shedding of pigment. (*For colour version see plate 11*)

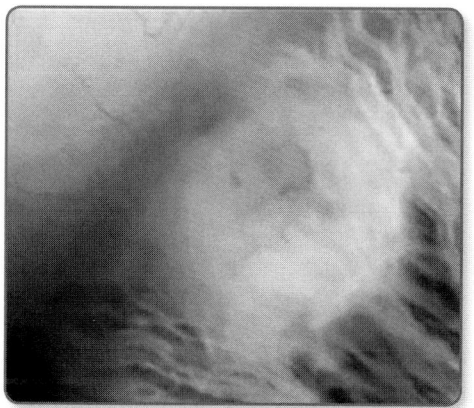

Figure 88.2 Amelanotic iris naevus – note the intrinsic vasculature being discernible. (*For colour version see plate 11*)

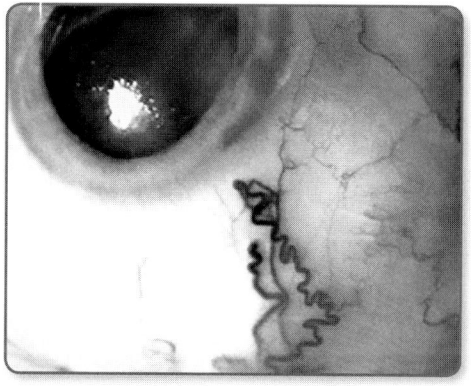

Figure 88.4 Ciliary body melanoma with sentinel episcleral vessels.

of the angle. All these satellite changes are not indicative of malignancy.

A feature indicative of malignancy would be growth of the lesion with or without concurrent haemorrhage in the anterior chamber or compression of neighbouring structures (**Figure 88.3**). Shedding of melanoma cells could lead to multiple foci. Glaucoma in the involved eye could develop in the case of a diffusely expanding iris melanoma. Expansion of the melanoma could be either diffuse or circumferential (ring melanoma). Both these variants are very rare.

Iris and ciliary body metastases are mostly amelanotic, exhibit rapid growth, could be multifocal, and shed cells more commonly.

Ciliary body melanoma can attain a larger size, either dome-shaped or rarely circumferential, before it is recognised clinically. The patient is often asymptomatic. However, a ciliary body mass can cause displacement of the lens resulting in astigmatic error. Signs include dilated episcleral vessels (sentinel vessels) (**Figure 88.4**), focal cataract, and in the case of ring melanoma, raised intraocular pressure. Rarely extrascleral extension is seen at presentation (**Figure 88.5**). Ciliary body melanomas can also extend posteriorly into the choroid (ciliochoroidal melanoma).

Vascular tumours of the iris are commonly unilateral. Iris racemose haemangiomas

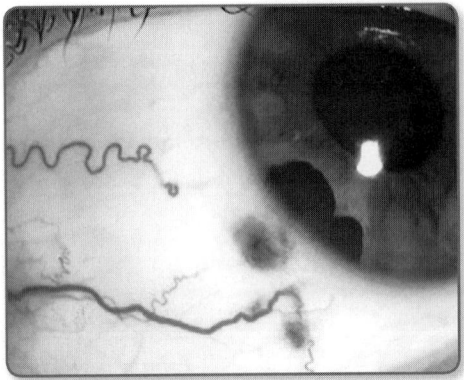

Figure 88.5 Ciliary body melanoma expanding in the iris with sentinel episcleral vessels and two foci of extrascleral extension.

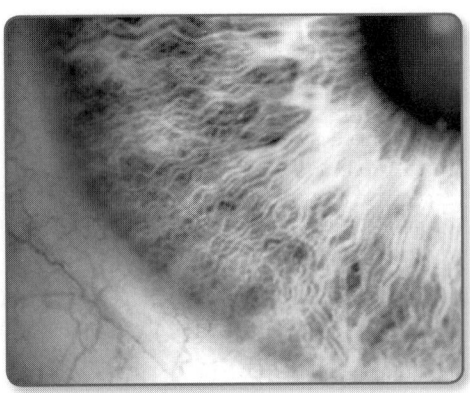

Figure 88.6 Iris haemangioma as discrete vessels discernible in the stroma.

Table 88.1 Main differential diagnoses of iris and ciliary body lesions

Iris melanocytic lesions	Iris vascular tumours	Ciliary body lesions
Iris naevus	Iris metastases	Ciliary body melanoma
Iris melanoma	Iris melanoma	Ciliary body medulloepithelioma
Iris melanocytoma	Iris stromal cyst	Ciliary body adenoma
Iris cyst		Ciliary body adenocarcinoma
Foreign body		Retinoblastoma
Iris haemangioma		
Congenital heterochromia		
Pigmentary glaucoma		
Iris abscess		
Sarcoidosis		
Tuberculosis		

Note: The list is by no means exhaustive, but it does cover the common or characteristic entities in the differential.

are mostly asymptomatic though rarely they might cause hyphaema. They appear in the form of a solitary (simple) or multiple (complex) tortuous vessels located within the iris stroma coursing from the iris root to the pupillary border and back to the iris root in a triangular fashion (**Figure 88.6**). Iris capillary appears as a single red iris lesion that can regress spontaneously. Iris cavernous haemangioma can present either as a small lesion close to the pupillary border producing hyphaema or as a multiloculated mass in the iris stroma.

Medulloepithelioma of the ciliary body commonly presents with poor vision and pain once symptomatic. Displacement of the zonular fibres of the lens in this area produces a characteristic lenticular notch. Eventually, some of these lesions might extend extrasclerally or endophytically and replace intraocular contents. Appearance of the lesion is light-coloured and cystic in appearance. Commonly, the angiogenetic properties of these lesions can produce locally rubeosis. Rarely medulloepithelioma of the iris can produce freely floating cysts.

Adenoma or adenocarcinoma of the ciliary body appears as solid light-coloured masses with differential size and extension. Similarly, to medulloepitheliomas, they might produce secondary glaucoma or subluxation of the lens.

The main differential diagnosis of iris and ciliary body lesions is presented in **Table 88.1**.

Investigations

Iris melanocytic lesions are diagnosed primarily with slit lamp biomicroscopy.

However, additional features of the iris lesion can be determined by gonioscopy, revealing the presence of an expansion towards the angle or the corneal surface or pigment shedding. Sometimes a gonioscopy with a dilated iris might reveal additional features such as an associated cortical cataract in a corresponding location or involvement of the ciliary body.

Transillumination is helpful in differentiating between a posterior expansion of an iris melanotic lesion towards the ciliary body or a ciliary body melanotic lesion. This technique is performed by placing a fibre-optic point light source on the ocular surface and observing the reflection margins of the lesion in the glowing eye. Amelanotic lesions might not be discerned with this method.

The determination of the iris stroma infiltration can be determined by additional imaging such as UBM, high frequency ultrasound or anterior segment OCT. The exact extent of iris vasculature and precise features of an AV iris communication or an iris haemangioma can be revealed more clearly with an indocyanine green (ICG) (**Figure 88.7**). Indirect ophthalmology with scleral indentation might assist in the diagnosis and detection of ciliary body lesions.

In case of uncertainty, a fine needle aspiration (FNA) biopsy might yield the diagnosis. Open biopsy has also been advocated, especially if the FNA tissue yield is insufficient.

Ancillary tests are not helpful in the diagnosis of medulloepithelioma – primarily the diagnosis is set after enucleation.

Similarly, diagnosis for adenomas or adenocarcinomas of the ciliary body can be set histopathologically.

Treatment

Iris freckles or naevi do not require treatment. However, they are monitored for change in their behaviour (especially naevi with considerable or full-thickness stromal infiltration). Iris melanomas can be treated with brachytherapy if well circumscribed and of moderate extent or excision (iridocyclectomy). Enucleation of the eye would be performed for diffuse or ring melanoma of the iris.

Iris or ciliary body metastases as part of generalised cancer have been shown to respond to systemic treatment.

Iris/ciliary body medulloepitheliomas, adenomas or adenocarcinomas have no established treatment – customarily patients with small diagnosed lesions and no sequelae remain under observation or undergo excision. On the contrary, large masses diagnosed in the past led to enucleation as either differential with retinoblastoma was not clinically feasible or because of secondary complications. The role for radiotherapy has not been clearly established for these rare lesions.

Prognosis

Visual prognosis for iris melanomas is good; however, extensive surgical excision or radiation-induced cataract might lead to unfavourable results. Metastases rarely develop with overall mortality rate in the vicinity of 3% from sizeable case series. Transformation of iris naevi to melanomas has been reported to be 4% in 10 years and 11% by 20 years.

For medulloepitheliomas, prognosis is related to their localised extent. Though no distant metastases develop, the lesion does demonstrate local invasiveness. Death can ensue in rare circumstances of orbital and subsequent intracranial extension. Therefore, the important prognostic factor in these lesions would be the presence of extrascleral extension.

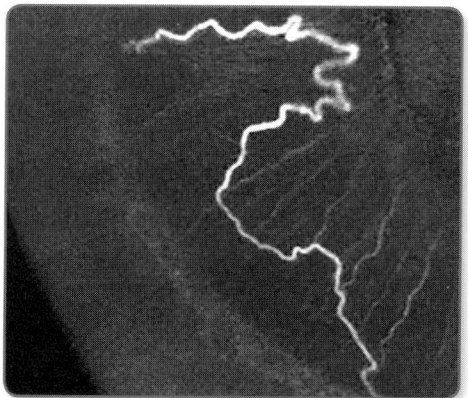

Figure 88.7 Indocyanine green (ICG) of the same patient delineating the course of the haemangioma vasculature.

Further reading

Hau SC, Papastefanou V, Shah S, et al. Evaluation of iris and iridociliary body lesions with anterior segment optical coherence tomography versus ultrasound B-scan. Br J Ophthalmol 2015; 99:81–86.

Shields CL, Shields PW, Manalac J, et al. Review of cystic and solid tumors of the iris. Oman J Ophthalmol 2013; 6:159–164.

Shields JA, Shields CL. Intraocular tumours: An atlas and textbook, 3rd edition. Philadelphia: Lippincott Williams & Wilkins; 2016.

Related topics of interest

- Tumours of the retina (p. 345)
- Tumours of the choroid (p. 329)

89 Tumours of the retina

Key points

- Common retina tumours have systemic associations
- Capillary haemangiomas, especially in cases of von Hippel–Lindau require very attentive monitoring and prompt treatment of new lesions
- Most other lesions require treatment for secondary sequelae they cause despite their overall stationary behaviour

Introduction

The chapter involving tumours of the retina will be dealing with vascular tumours of the retina, glial tumours of the retina and tumours of the retinal pigmented epithelium. Retinoblastomas are covered in a separate chapter.

Vascular tumours of the retina include different types of haemangiomas as capillary, cavernous, and racemose haemangiomas. Glial tumours are primary astrocytic tumours. Tumours of the retinal pigment epithelium (RPE) include the congenital hypertrophy of the retinal pigment epithelium (CHRPE) solitary or multifocal and hamartoma of the retina and the RPE.

Epidemiology

Capillary haemangiomas of the retina are on average diagnosed between the ages of 10 years and 30 years. There does not appear to be any predilection for race or sex. There is a direct association of capillary haemangiomas, especially if they are bilateral and multiple, with von Hippel–Lindau syndrome a hereditary syndrome with concurrent haemangiomas developing in the spine and in the cerebellum along with other tumours as pheochromocytoma. Solitary haemangiomas located either in the retinal periphery or in the juxtapapillary area have no hereditary background and are sporadic.

The incidence of cavernous haemangiomas is unknown and manifestation is associated with concurrent skin and central nervous system lesions. Racemose haemangiomas [a misnomer for a cluster of arteriovenous (AV) retinal communications] have been observed in association with Wyburn–Mason syndrome, a syndrome with coexistent racemose haemangioma of the midbrain.

Glial tumours of the retina are associated with syndromes as tuberous sclerosis or neurofibromatosis. Astrocytic hamartoma is benign and has a high incidence in patients with tuberous sclerosis a syndrome bearing concurrent intracranial astrocytomas and other hamartomatous lesions in the heart and kidney and other locations. Astrocytic hamartomas can also be encountered in patients with neurofibromatosis I.

Tumours of the RPE include CHRPE, solitary or multifocal. Multiple hamartomas of the RPE are associated with familial adenomatous polyposis (FAP). Described incidence has been to 67–100% in these patients. Mean age of diagnosis is at 45 years of age for solitary lesions.

Congenital hamartoma of the retina and RPE is a congenital non-hereditary lesion. Systemic associations have been done with neurofibromatosis and branchio-oculo-facial syndrome.

Pathophysiology

A capillary haemangioma consists of proliferating retinal capillaries that occupy most of the neurosensory retina. The proliferation involves endothelial cells, pericytes, and glia. A cavernous haemangioma consists of clusters of venules located in the inner retina. These are interconnected with a thin endothelial lining. A racemose haemangioma is associated with a thinned and degenerated neurosensory retina but as specified early on, it is a misnomer as it is in essence an AV communication.

Glial tumours are primarily composed of astrocytes. Astrocytic hamartomas bear a variance in the type of astrocytes that they bear namely pleomorphic astrocytes in some of the more common benign tumours and poorly differentiated subependymal astrocytes in the invasive variant.

Congenital hypertrophy of the RPE is characterised by taller and densely packed cells of the RPE with increased pigment and hypertrophy. In multifocal CHRPE the pigmentation of these cells is retained, but hypertrophy is not significant. Similar configurations with variants of pigment cells location are noted in the RPE hamartomas associated with FAP. Hamartoma of the retina and the RPE is composed of a mixture of proliferating blood vessels, glial tissue, and proliferating RPE cells.

Clinical features

Peripheral capillary haemangiomas can be very subtle and difficult to identify. Close inspection will reveal direct feeder vessels in a red or whitish peripheral retinal area. Feeder vessels are more distinct upon growth of the lesion. The growth can be toward the vitreous (endophytic) or towards the choroid (exophytic). Clinically the arterial and the venous feeder vessels might be indistinguishable (**Figure 89.1**). Juxtapapillary capillary haemangiomas present as a sessile mass and feeders are difficult to distinguish.

These lesions do have increasing exudative activity analogous to growth. The extent of oedema can extend from the periphery to the macula. Tractional vitreous bands might be present with coexisting exudative or tractional retinal detachment.

Cavernous haemangiomas appear as clusters of dark-coloured intraretinal microaneurysms. They are associated with overlying fibroglial tissue with minimal progression and exudation. Their main complication is vitreous haemorrhage. They are located in the periphery or in the juxtapapillary area.

Racemose haemangiomas are of three principal types depending on the anatomical level and extent of the AV communication – Type I consists of AV communications in the capillary level, Type II, looks like a capillary haemangioma with our progression or exudation, and Type III consists of large tortuous vessels emanating from the disc and expanding in variable levels in the retina only to return to their point of origin. There is no exudation or growth, though blood redistribution might change over time.

Glial tumours have a different clinical presentation. Astrocytic hamartomas have the appearance of either a translucent thickening of the nerve fibre layer (noncalcified type) or a larger-sized lesion with nodules of calcification (calcified type) (**Figure 89.2**). Growth is a rare event in these tumours and rarely associated with retinal traction, detachment or extraocular extension.

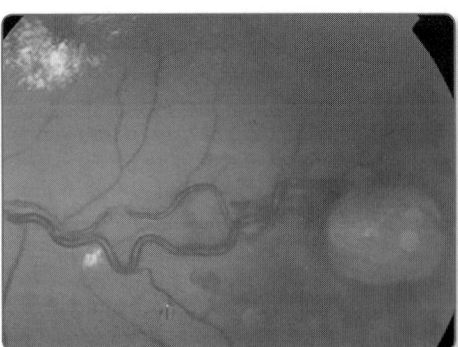

Figure 89.1 Peripheral capillary hemangioma – note the distended feeder vessels and the extent of edema to the macula creating a macular star. (*For colour version see plate 11*)

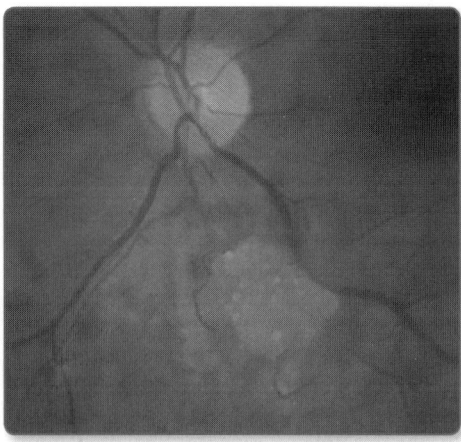

Figure 89.2 Calcified astrocytic hamartoma with discrete nodules on its surface. (*For colour version see plate 11*)

Tumours of the RPE are well-demarcated lesions of varying pigmentations. The most commonly encountered – CHRPE – is located in the mid or far periphery of the fundus and has varying pigmentations. It commonly bears depigmented areas called lacunae that tend to extend (**Figure 89.3**). Nodular growth and rare conversion to adenocarcinoma of the RPE has been reported. Multifocal CHRPE lesions are smaller, ovoid-like, bilateral, and multiple lesions (**Figure 89.4**). These are of varying sizes though more posterior lesions tend to be smaller.

Congenital hamartoma of the retina and the RPE is a light-coloured grey retinal lesion with excessive contractile glial tissue on its surface (**Figure 89.5**). It is the tissue that invariably causes superficial retinal vascular traction with subsequent metamorphopsia to amblyopia due to foveal ectopia. The lesion per se is more stationary. Associations have been made with ischaemia and subsequent neovascularization, exudation or haemorrhage in the vitreous.

As these lesions are located in the juxtapapillary area, they are detected early.

Differential diagnosis

The main differential diagnosis of retinal lesions is presented in **Table 89.1**. The list is by no means exhaustive but it does cover the common or characteristic entities in the differential.

Investigations

Capillary haemangiomas have a rather typical appearance and on most of the occasions diagnosis with fundus examination is nonproblematic; however, additional imaging tests in these lesions would be useful. A wide-field fluorescein angiogram is useful: (1) For identifying the arterial and venous component of the lesion which is important for the treatment plan and (2) For identifying

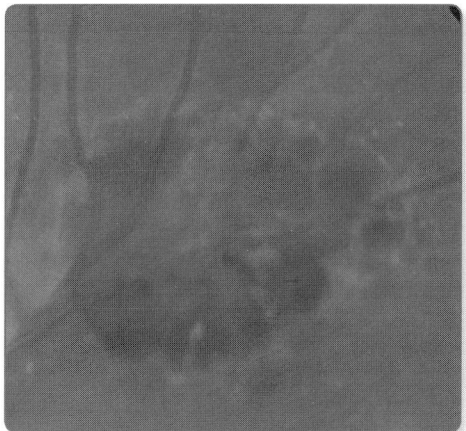

Figure 89.3 Solitary CHRPE with amelanotic lacunae on its surface. (*For colour version see plate 11*)

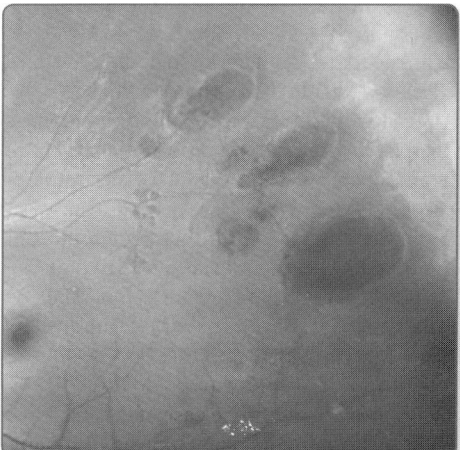

Figure 89.4 Multifocal CHRPE with avoid and spotted configuration. (*For colour version see plate 12*)

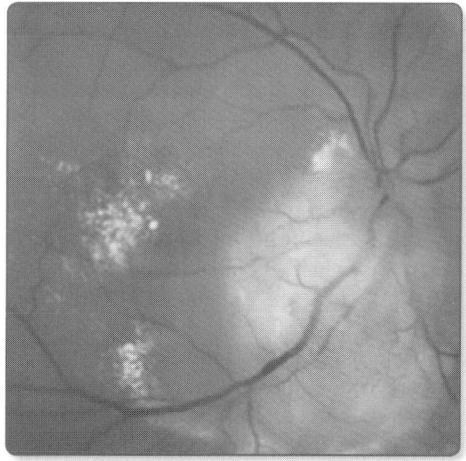

Figure 89.5 Combined hamartoma of the retina and the RPE with evidence of superficial gliosis and associated retinal traction and exudation. (*For colour version see plate 12*)

Table 89.1 Differential diagnosis of retinal lesions

Capillary haemangioma	Glial tumours	Tumours of the pigmented epithelium
Peripheral location: • Retinoblastoma • Vasoproliferative tumours • Coats disease • Eccentric disciform scar • FEVR • Sickle cell retinopathy Juxtapapillary location: • Papilloedema • Optic neuritis	Retinoblastoma Granuloma Myelination of nerve fibre layer	Solitary CHRPE with nodular extension: • Choroidal melanoma • Choroidal naevus Multifocal CHRPE: • Metastases from cutaneous melanoma • Bear track peripheral degeneration Combined hamartoma of the retina and the RPE: • Retinoblastoma • Choroidal melanoma

CHRPE, congenital hypertrophy of the retinal pigment epithelium; FEVR, familial exudative vitreoretinopathy; RPE, retinal pigment epithelium

subtle peripheral coexisting lesions not detected with fundus examination. In this modality, haemangiomas manifest considerable uptake and later leakage.

B-scan ultrasonography indicates the presence of a hyperechoic lesion with increased blood flow on Doppler scan. Optical coherence tomography (OCT) might be useful in determining the extent of retinal oedema.

Cavernous haemangiomas are hypofluorescent at the early stages on fluorescein angiogram with slow filling or pooling at the venous phase. Usually a clinical assessment would suffice for the diagnosis.

Glial tumours of the retina rarely require ancillary studies as their superficial location is rather diagnostic; however, astrocytomas do present with early considerable hyperfluorescence and delineation of vascularity in the late venous phase. The calcified version of the astrocytic hamartoma demonstrated update on autofluorescence (AF) and hyper-reflectivity on B-scan ultrasonography. In case of doubt, fine needle aspiration (FNA) biopsy and immunohistochemical reaction to glial fibrillary acidic protein (GFAP) are diagnostic.

Tumours of the RPE block any signal and they are hypoautofluorescent in AF and hypofluorescent on FFA and indocyanine green (ICG). The hypertrophy of the RPE can be readily depicted on OCT scans with overlying loss/thinning of the neurosensory retina.

Fine needle aspiration of *combined hamartoma of the retina and the RPE* highlights the associated vascular abnormalities with hyperfluorescence and leakage. OCT has a characteristic folded pattern of the retina with replacement of the neurosensory retina structure at the location of the lesion.

Treatment

Treatment of *capillary haemangioma* is done with argon laser or cryotherapy for peripherally located lesions. Argon laser is administered with a particular sequence namely arterial component of tumour, tumour and venous component at the end. If this sequence is not followed, rupture of the haemangioma might develop with associated vitreous haemorrhage. Alternatively, 3× freeze-thaw cryotherapy has been advocated though retina detachment or haemorrhage has been reported as common complications.

Photodynamic therapy has been proposed as adjuvant treatment to laser for sizeable lesions. It is important for the lesion to be fully visualised. Results have been ambivalent due to the rarity of these cases.

Cavernous haemangiomas do not require treatment. In the case of vitreous haemorrhage photocoagulation, cryotherapy or plaque has unproven value.

Glial tumours of the retina do not require treatment though they are periodically observed, especially in case of growth in the invasive variant of astrocytic hamartomas.

Congenital hypertrophy of the retinal pigment epithelium lesions does not require treatment but monitoring in case a nodular growth develops. Prognosis is excellent overall for both solitary and multifocal lesions. RPE hamartomas associated with FAP require close systemic scrutiny due to the high incidence of development of colon cancer.

There is effectively no treatment for combined hamartoma of the retina and the RPE. Though vitrectomy for vitreous haemorrhage or peeling for the superficial gliosis have been attempted.

Further reading

Font RL, Moura RA, Shetlar DJ, et al. Combined hamartoma of sensory retina and retinal pigment epithelium. Retina 1989; 9:302–311.

Papastefanou VP, Pilli S, Stinghe A, et al. Photodynamic therapy for retinal capillary hemangioma. Eye (Lond) 2013; 27:438–442.

Shields JA, Shields CL. Intraocular tumours: An atlas and textbook, 3rd edition. Philadelphia: Lippincott Williams & Wilkins; 2016.

Related topics of interest

- Retinoblastoma (p. 294)
- Tumours of the choroid (p. 329)

90 Vitreoretinal surgery – retinal breaks and detachment and vitreomacular interface disorders

Key points

- Asymptomatic atrophic holes may be observed without treatment
- Prompt diagnosis and treatment of tractional tears lead to a significant reduction in the risk of retinal detachment
- Making the correct diagnosis of the subtype of retinal detachment (RD) (retinoschisis, rhegmatogenous, traction, exudative) is paramount as treatment and prognosis will vary in each case
- Vitreomacular interface disorders are a group of inter-related condition that may affect vision and can successfully be treated surgically to improve the vision

Retinal breaks

Retinal breaks exist in approximately 6% of the population. Any such break may cause RD. The incidence of RD, however, is 1:10,000. Therefore, not all breaks cause detachment.

Pathogenesis and types

Retinal breaks (**Figures 90.1a to e**) can be either: (1) atrophic (idiopathic) breaks 'round holes', that are commonly seen in young, often myopic patients, (2) tractional breaks that develop in upto 30% of patients with symptomatic posterior vitreous detachment (PVD); those include: (i) 'U-shaped' (horse-shoe) tears, (ii) 'operculated' tears, and (iii) giant tears: extending for ≥ 3 hours, and (3) trauma-induced retinal dialysis – disinsertion of the retina at the ora serrata.

Clinical features

Atrophic breaks are typically asymptomatic and are often associated with lattice degeneration. PVD-associated tractional tears often give rise to flashing lights and floaters.

Treatment (Figures 90.2a and b)

Treatment is indicated in patients with tractional tears, i.e. horseshoe and operculated tears and dialysis. Atrophic and asymptomatic tears rarely need treatment. The latter may be treated in fellow eyes of patients that had RD in one eye. Also, the presence of lattice degeneration per se is rarely an indication for treatment.

Laser photocoagulation or cryotherapy may be used. Both work by creating chorioretinal adhesions around the tears. Laser retinopexy is the most commonly used form of treatment and cryotherapy is typically used for anterior peripheral tears, especially in the presence of media opacity, e.g. vitreous haemorrhage. Giant retinal tears and retinal dialysis are almost always associated with RD and need surgery.

Complications

Retinopexy of traction tears reduces the risk of RD by about 10-fold. Epiretinal membrane may develop in 4% of the patients who have retinopexy

Rhegmatogenous retinal detachment

The incidence of rhegmatogenous RD is 1:10,000.

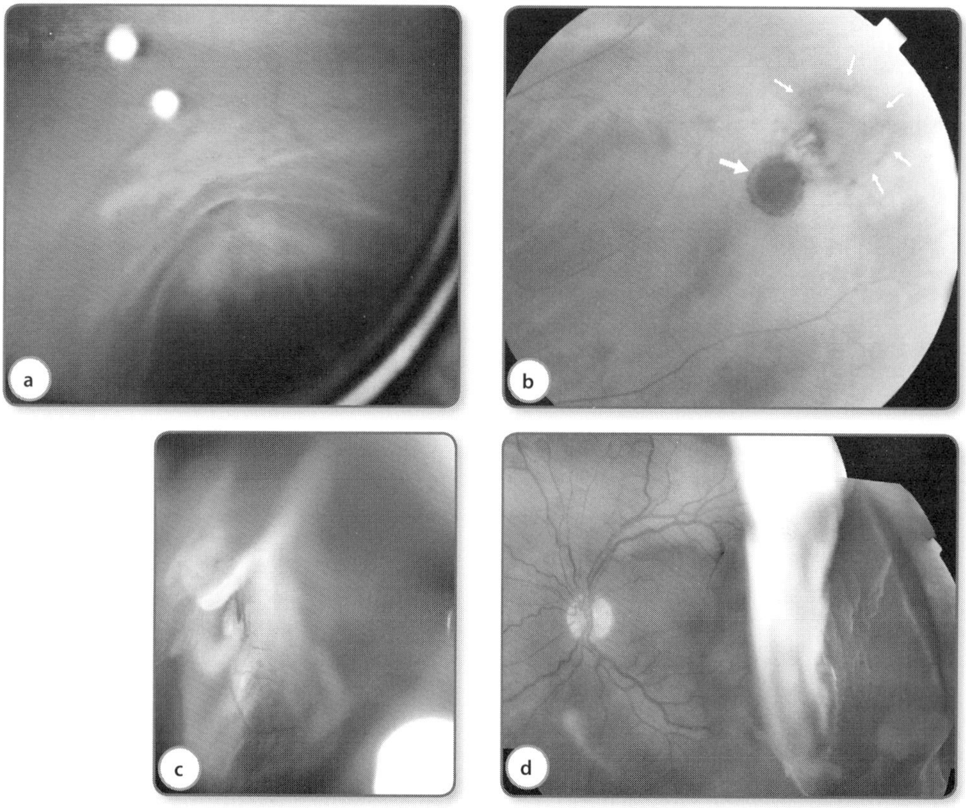

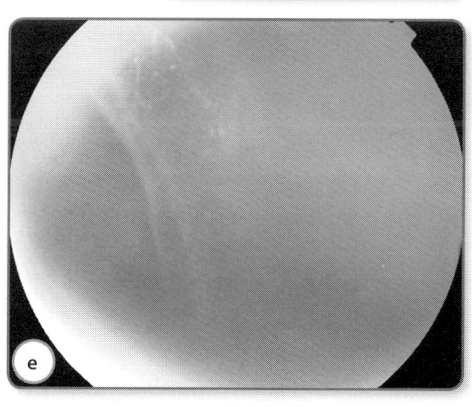

Figure 90.1 Retinal breaks. (a) An atrophic round hole; (b) An operculated tear (the edge-thin arrows and a pigmented operculum-thick arrow); (c) A 'horse-shoe' or U-shaped tear and retinal detachment; (d) A giant retinal tear (≥ 3 hours) with retinal detachment; and (e) Traumatic retinal dialysis. (*For colour version see plate 12 and 13*)

Pathogenesis of retinal detachment

The retina detaches typically as a result of the combination of three factors:
1. A retinal defect (break).
2. Localised traction, on or around break edges.
3. Fluid current within the degenerated vitreous, generated by saccadic eye movements.

Clinical features

Common risk factors are myopia, pseudophakia, and family history of RD.

Retinal detachment typically causes visual field loss, although if it is located anterior to the equator, and extends for no more than 2 hours it may be asymptomatic (subclinical RD).

Visual acuity remains unaffected if the fovea remains attached 'macula-on RD'

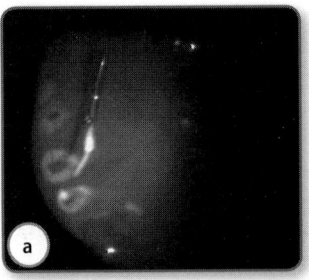 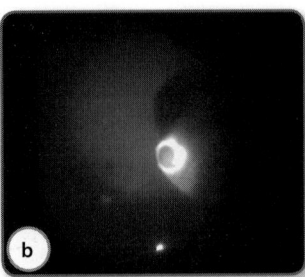

Figure 90.2 Treatment of retinal breaks. (a) Endolaser retinopexy to multiple retinal breaks (during pars plana vitrectomy); and (b) Cryotherapy. (*For colour version see plate 13*)

Table 90.1 Differential diagnoses of rhegmatogenous retinal detachment

	Retinoschisis	Rhegmatogenous RD	Tractional RD	Exudative RD
Symptoms	Asymptomatic	Acute; flashing, falters, fields loss	Gradual; loss of vision	Acute or gradual; loss of vision, floaters, +/- pain, e.g. in posterior scleritis
Field loss	Absolute scotoma	Relative scotoma	Relative scotoma	Relative scotoma
Refraction	Normal or hyperopic	Normal or myopic	Normal	Normal
Anterior chamber	Normal	Normal or faint flare or some cells	Normal or rubeosis irides	Flare or cells
Vitreous	No PVD	PVD + Pigments +/- blood 'tobacco dust'	Blood e.g. in diabetic retinopathy or vitreoretinal adhesions or fibrovascular bands	Inflammatory cells
Retinal break	May be (small inner leaf or large outer leaf breaks)	Yes (atropic or tractional tears)	May be (in combined case)	No
Location of RD	Inferotemporally, occasionally superiorly	Superotemporally, sometimes inferiorly (without atrophic holes)	Mid-peripheral and around the arcades	Inferior and varies with head position
Shape of RD	Smooth, convex	Corrugated, convex, bullies especially in superior RD	Irregular, concave	Convex, smooth, may change position due to shifting of SRF
Laterality of RD	Bilateral	Unilateral	Unilateral or bilateral	Unilateral or bilateral
Chronic changes	No demarcation line	Demarcation pigmented line centrally	No demarcation line	Diffuse mottling of the RPE 'leopard spots'
Treatment	Nil	Surgery (see text)	Surgery, e.g. in proliferative diabetic or sickle cell retinopathy (see text)	Medical (anti-inflammatory), e.g. corticosteroids in posterior scleritis or VKH syndrome

PVD, posterior vitreous detachment; RD, retinal detachment; RPE, retinal pigment epithelium; SRF, subretinal fluid; VKH, Vogt-Kayoing-Harada syndrome

but invariably decreases if it has detached 'macula-off RD'.

Differential diagnosis includes retinoschisis, tractional retinal detachment, and exudative retinal detachment. The management varies with each one of these conditions (**Table 90.1**).

Surgery for retinal detachment (Figures 90.3a to c)

Surgery should be performed within 24 hours in 'macula-on RD' to preserve the foveal vision and within a few days in patients with 'macula-off RD'.

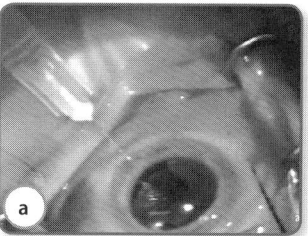 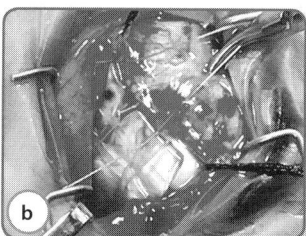 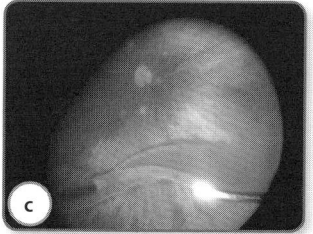

Figure 90.3 Techniques of RD repair. (a) Pneumatic retinopexy (gas injection after cryotherapy); (b) Scleral buckling; and (c) Pars plana vitrectomy.

Successful repair of RD relies on addressing the three pathogenic factors described above, i.e. removing traction on the breaks, closing the breaks and minimising the fluid current until the breaks are sealed.

There are four standard procedures for repairing RD:

1. *Laser photocoagulation:* This may be used in small subclinical RD, i.e. retinal tear with subretinal fluid (SRF) extending no more than 2 hours poterior to the equator.
   Three or four rows of laser burns are applied to create a barrier around the RD.
2. *Pneumatic retinopexy (Figure 90.3a):* This is used in patients with a localised superior with one or more breaks within 1 quadrant and no evidence of proliferative vitreoretinopathy (PVR). 'Rescue' procedure may also be performed in patients with failed primary vitrectomy or scleral buckling due to missed breaks.
   An expansile gas bubble (0.4–0.5 mL of 100% SF6 or C3F8) is injected into the vitreous cavity. The tears are treated with cryotherapy before the gas is injected or with laser retinopexy a few days later, i.e. once the SRF has absorbed.
3. *Scleral buckling (Figure 90.3b):* This procedure is commonly used in young patients with round hole RD, i.e. no PVD, or in cases with localised RD or retinal dialysis.
   Cryotherapy is applied to the area of the breaks followed by suturing of a silicone explant 'buckle' to the sclera. This may be a segment 'segmental buckle' or an encircling band. This helps to create an indent in the sclera, choroid, and retinal pigment epithelium (RPE) towards the retina in the area of the retinal break, which reduces traction and helps to seal on the breaks. High SRF may be drained through the sclera prior to cryotherapy. Laser photocoagulation may be used instead of cryotherapy but a few days later, i.e. once the SRF has absorbed.
4. *Pars plana vitrectomy (PPV) (Figure 90.3c):* Pars plana vitrectomy is the most commonly performed surgical procedure for RD and other vitreoretinal abnormalities. PPV is performed through three ports, each is about 1 mm (depending on the gauge: 20, 23, 25 or 27G). Both the core and cortical vitreous are removed. The posterior hyaloid, if not already detached, must be peeled off the posterior pole.
   In rhegmatogenous RD, PPV is indicated in pseudophakic patients and in patients with multiple breaks, vitreous haemorrhage, giant retinal tears or evidence of PVR.
   Removing the vitreous ensures that traction on breaks is removed. The SRF is then drained through one of the breaks (or a retinotomy) and fluid is exchanged for air. All breaks (and retinotomy sites) are then treated with laser or cryotherapy, followed by replacing the air with a gas (sulphur hexafluoride 20%, perfluoroethane 14%, perfluoropropane 12%) bubble (**Table 90.2**). The gas spontaneously absorbs within 3–6 weeks.

In complex cases of RD, e.g. recurrent RD associated with PVR, a combination of scleral buckling and vitrectomy may be required and other techniques e.g. retinectomy to relieve traction and heavy liquid fluid or silicone oil tamponade (**Table 90.3**) may be used.

Table 90.2 Characteristics of different intraocular gas tamponades

Gas tamponade	Chemical composition	Maximal expansion	Tamponade duration	Non-expansile concentration	100% expansivity
Air	Nitrogen, oxygen, argon and CO_2	None	5–7 days	NA	0
Sulphur hexafluoride	SF_6	24–48 hours	2 weeks	20%	2
Perfluoroethane	C_2F_6	36–60 hours	4–5 weeks	16%	3.3
Perfluoropropane	C_3F_8	72–96 hours	6–8 weeks	12%	4

Table 90.3 Characteristics of other intraocular tamponading agents

Silicone oil and heavy liquid fluids	Chemical composition	Viscosity (centistoke)	Specific gravity (g/cm³)	Refractive index
Conventional SO				
1,000 cSt SO	100% PDMS	1,000	0.97	1.4
5,000 cSt SO	100% PDMS	5,000	0.97	1.4
Heavy SO				
Oxane HD	88.1% 5,700 cSt Oxane/11.9% RMN-3	3,300	1.02	1.4
Densiron 68	69.5% 5,000 cSt PDMS/30.5% F_6H_8	1,400	1.06	1.4
Perfluorocarbon (heavy liquid: heavier than water)				
Perfluoro-n-octane	C_8F_{18}	1.20	1.76	1.3
Perfluorodecalin	$C_{10}F_{18}$	5.68	1.33	1.3

cSt, centistoke; PDMS, polydimethylsiloxane; SO, silicone oil

Outcome of retinal detachment surgery

Anatomical success is achievable in 70–90% of patients with one surgery. Recurrence rate after pneumatic retinopexy is higher than after scleral buckling and vitrectomy (30–40% vs. 20–30% vs. 5–10%).

Visual outcome depends largely on whether the fovea had detached. Visual acuity improvement to ≥20/50 occurs in 60% of patient with mac-off RD.

Complications include cataract especially after gas injection. Other complications of vitrectomy are included in a separate subsection. Transient diplopia and change in refraction is common after scleral buckling.

Tractional retinal detachment

Causes

- Proliferative diabetic retinopathy (PDR)
- Proliferative sickle cell retinopathy
- Proliferative vitreoretinopathy (PVR) (associated with recurrent RD)
- Stage 4 and 5 of retinopathy of prematurity (ROP)
- Familial exudative vitreoretinopathy (FEVR)

Clinical features

The detached retina assumes a concave configuration (unlike the convex configuration in rhegmatogenous RD). Severe traction may lead to the development of a retinal tear, resulting in a combined traction-rhegmatogenous RD (**Figure 90.4** and **Table 90.1**).

Surgery

Indications for surgery include:
- Non-clearing (or recurrent) vitreous or pre-macular haemorrhage (**Figures 90.5a** and **b**), e.g. in PDR
- Traction RD threatening or involving the macula (**Figures 90.6a** and **b**)
- Combined traction-and-rhegmatogenous RD
- Epimacular membrane or vitreomacular traction (taught posterior hyaloid) in cases of persistent diabetic macular oedema (DMO)

Surgery involves core vitrectomy to remove vitreous haemorrhage, followed by complete vitrectomy combined with dissection of the fibrovascular membranes and vitreoretinal adhesions. This may proceed from the periphery towards the macula 'en-bloc dissection' or from the macula towards the periphery 'inside-out dissection'. In children and infants, the posterior hyaloid may be tightly adherent and can be left alone once the visual axis is clear and retinal traction has been relieved. Laser photocoagulation is then performed to areas of retinal ischaemia to reduce the risk of neovascularisation, recurrent bleeding or retinal detachment.

Preoperative injection of anti-vascular endothelial growth factors, e.g. bevacizumab, reduces the risk of intraoperative and postoperative bleeding, e.g. in PDR. This, however, may result in worsening of traction and increased adherence between tissue planes 'crunch syndrome'.

Outcome

Visual outcome depends on the extent and severity of the macular ischaemia and the presence of rhegmatogenous RD.

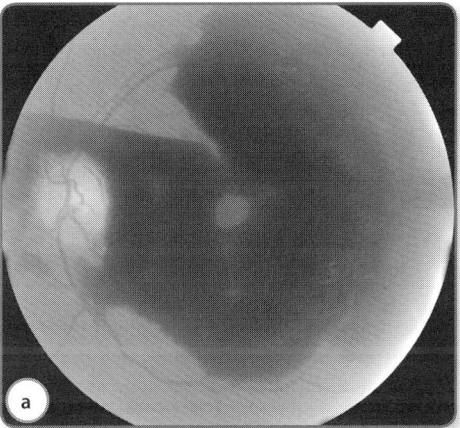

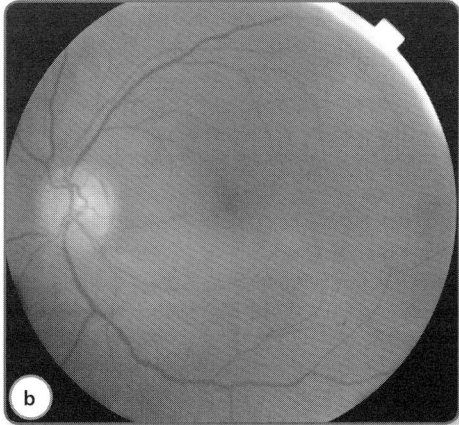

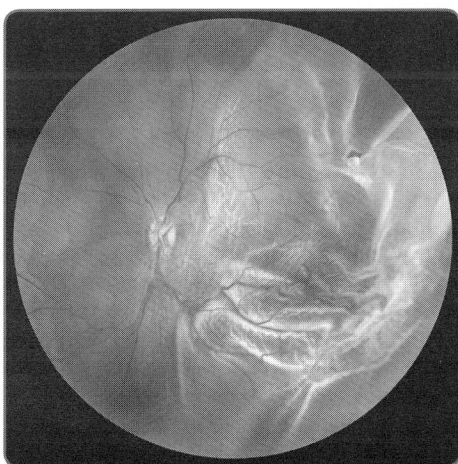

Figure 90.4 Combined tractional and rhegmatogenous retinal detachment in a patient with proliferative sickle cell retinopathy. Note the concave configuration of the area of tractional detachment. There is also a tear with surrounding rhegmatogenous RD that assumes a convex configuration. (*For colour version see plate 13*)
Courtesy: Paul Sullivan, Moorfields Eye Hospital.

Figure 90.5 A case of diabetic premacular haemorrhage: (a) Treated with pars plana vitrectomy and (b) internal limiting membrane peeling.

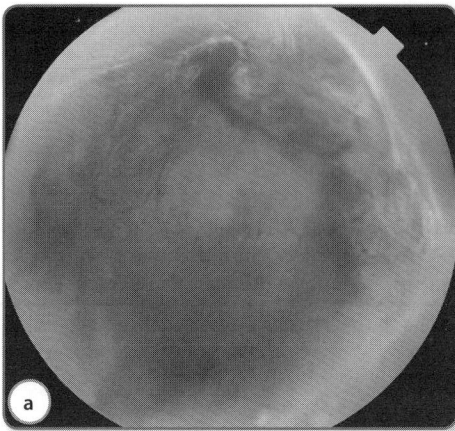 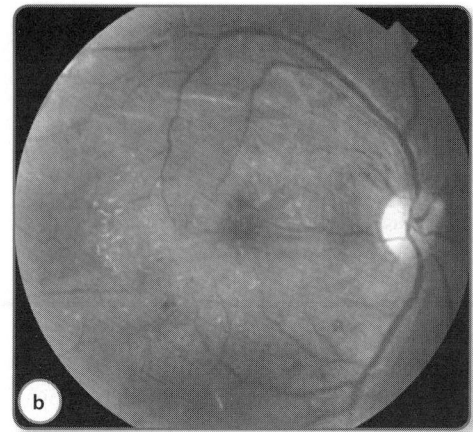

Figure 90.6 A case of proliferative diabetic retinopathy with fibrovascular membrane associated with macular traction along the arcades (a) before and (b) after surgery. (*For colour version see plate 13*)

The most common complication after surgery is vitreous (cavity) haemorrhage (VCH) (up to 40%), cataract (nuclear or posterior sub capsular cataract) (less commonly than in non-diabetics) and epimacular membrane. Rhegmatogenous retinal detachment may occur rarely.

Vitreomacular interface disorders

These are a group of pathologically inter-related conditions (**Figure 90.7**) that include vitreomacular traction (VMT) syndrome, full-thickness macular hole (FTMH), and epiretinal membrane (ERM). The latter may lead to pseudomacular hole (PMH) and lamellar (partial-thickness) macular hole (LMH) formation.

The prevalence of any vitreomacular disorder is 22%, with VMT 0.87% and macular hole (MH) 0.1–0.2% and ERM 9%. The annual incidence of vitreomacular disorders are:
- VMT: 0.6/100,000
- MH: 8.6/100,000
- ERM: 1,000/100,000

Pathogenesis

The three conditions are characterised by two main features:
1. The presence of an abnormal adhesion between the posterior hyaloid face and the internal limiting membrane (ILM) at the macula, and
2. The presence of fibroglial proliferation on the macular surface.

The resulting anteroposterior and tangential (centrifugal) traction forces on the macula lead to the development of either VMT or FTMH. Excessive tangential centrifugal traction forces may cause a lamellar split within the retina, i.e. LMH in the presence of an ERM.

Clinical features (Figures 90.7a to d and Table 90.4)

Patients may be completely asymptomatic or complain of distorted or blurred vision or diplopia. Clinically, VMT may appear as a yellow dot in the fovea and MH shows as a full-thickness defect. Increased reflections from macular surface (celluphane maculopathy), macular wrinkles (puckering) are the main feature of ERM. Defect in ERM may lead to the appearance of a PMH.

Optical coherence tomography (OCT) scan is currently the mainstay for the diagnosis and staging of vitreo macular interface disorders.

Management

Early asymptomatic cases of VMT stages 0 and 1 and even small MHs (< 250 μm) **Table 90.4** may be observed.

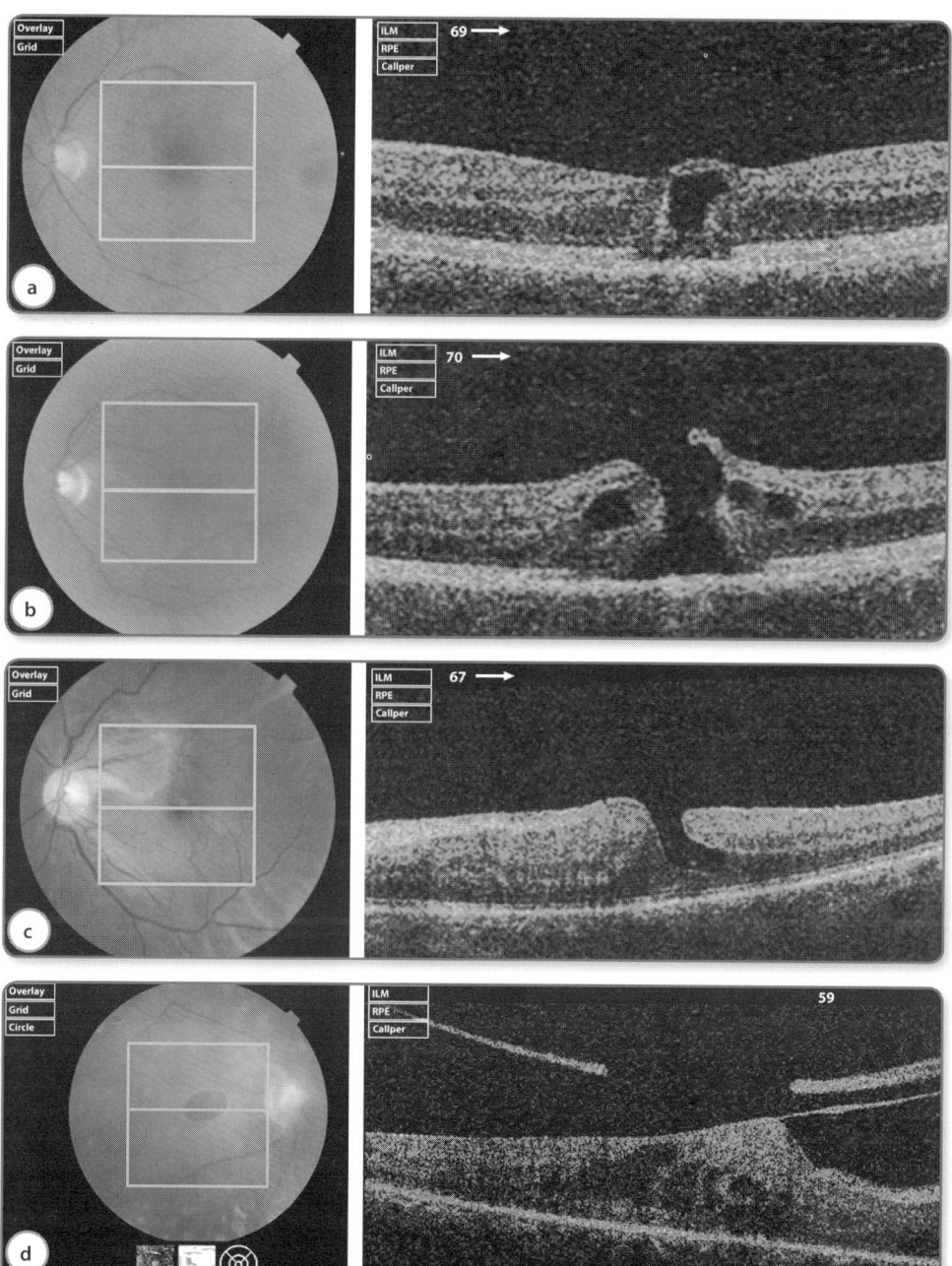

Figure 90.7 Vitreoretinal interface disorders. (a) Vitreomacular traction; (b) Evolution of a full-thickness macular hole from vitreomacular traction; (c) An epiretinal membrane and lamellar hole; (d) An epiretinal membrane and pseudomacular hole.

Table 90.4 Correlation between commonly used clinical macular hole stages and the International Vitreomacular Traction Study Classification System Of Vitreomacular Adhesion, Traction and Macular Hole

Anatomic state	Definition	Gass classification	IVTS classification
VMA	No detectable change in foveal contour	• Stage 0	Size of attachment area: • Focal (≤1,500 μm) • Broad (>1,500 μm) Presence of associated macular abnormalities: • Isolated • Concurrent
VMT	Absence of full-thickness interruption of all retinal layers and vitreous attachment associated with: • Distortion of foveal surface • Intraretinal structural changes • Elevation of the fovea above the RPE	• Stage 1	Size of attachment area: • Focal (≤1,500 μm) • Focal (≤1,500 μm) Presence of associated macular abnormalities: • Isolated • Concurrent
FTMH	Full-thickness foveal lesion from the ILM to the RPE	• Stage 2: Small or medium hole with VMT • Stage 3: Medium or large hole with VMT • Stage 4: Any size hole without VMT	Size – horizontal diameter at narrowest point: • Small (≤250 μm) • Medium (250–400 μm) • Large (>400 μm) Cause: • Primary • Secondary* Presence or absence of VMT
Lamellar macular hole	Irregular foveal contour with defect in the inner fovea and an intact photoreceptor layer	–	–
Macular pseudohole	Concomitant ERM with central opening and invaginated or heaped foveal edges without loss of retinal tissue	–	–

ERM, epiretinal membrane; FTMH, full-thickness macular hole; μm; microns; ILM, internal limiting membrane; IVTS: International Vitreomacular Traction Study; RPE: retinal pigment epithelium; VMA: vitreomacular adhesion; VMT: vitreomacular traction
*Secondary MH may develop in about 3% of the patients with RD or after surgery
Source: Duker JS, Kaiser PK, Binder S, et al. The International Vitreomacular Traction Study Group Classification of Vitreomacular Adhesion, Traction, and Macular Hole. Ophthalmology 2013; 120:2611–2619.

Surgery aims to reduce the distortion and improve visual acuity by restoring the anatomical integrity of the macula. The techniques include:

- *Pharmacologic vitreolysis:* Intravitreal injection of a proteolytic enzyme and ocriplasmin (Jetrea; Alcon) helps to separate vitreomacular adhesion. This is used in symptomatic patients with VMT with "focal" adhesion, i.e. ≤1,500 μm or FTMH ≤400 μm and no evidence of ERM
- *Vitrectomy and macular peeling (Figures 90.8a and b):* This is the standard treatment modality and is indicated in cases of ERM and persistent or progressive VMT with a "broad" VMA, i.e. >1,500 μm or with FTMH that is >400 μm or in patients that failed to respond to ocriplasmin injection or is keen for surgery because of higher success rate

Surgery involves inducing posterior vitreous detachment (PVD) (**Figure 90.8a**) and peeling of ERM (and the ILM in patients with FTMH) (**Figure 90.8b**). The peeling is assisted with the use of a blue dye (trypan blue) to help visualisation of different membranes. In patients with FTMH, a gas bubble is injected and forward head posturing is advised for 5–7 days, especially in large FTMH (i.e. ≥400 μm).

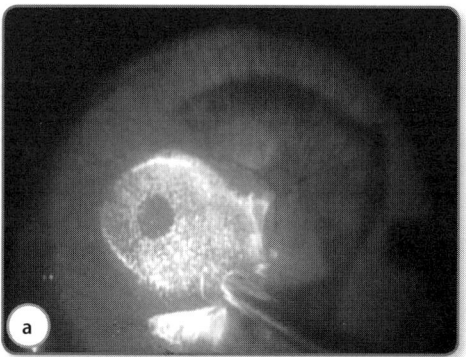 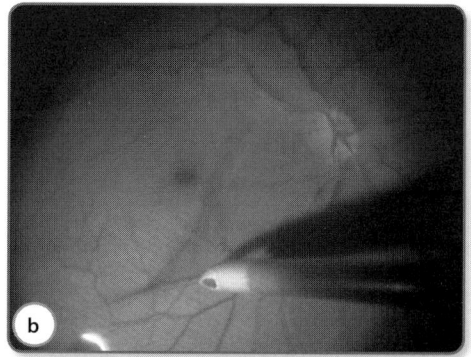

Figure 90.8 Treatment of vitreomacular interface disorders. (a) Posterior vitreous detachment inducement (triamcinolone is used to assist visualisation); (b) Internal limiting membrane peeling during vitrectomy for full-thickness macular hole (trypan blue dye is used to assist visualisation). (*For colour version see plate 14*)

Outcome

Ocriplasmin injection succeeds in releasing VMT and in closure of MHs in about 30–40% of cases. Surgery, on the other hand, results in closure of FTMH in over 90% of cases.

The release of VMT and closure of the hole leads to improvement in visual acuity by two or more lines in 70–80% of patients, with significant reduction in distortion.

Complications of ocriplasmin injection include blurring or worsening of vision (for up to 6 weeks), retinal tears or detachment. After surgery, persistence or recurrence of MH occurs in about 5% of patients.

Further reading

Bainbridge J, Herbert E, Gregor Z. Macular holes: vitreoretinal relationships and surgical approaches. Eye 2008; 22:1301–1309.

Frings A, Markau N, Katz T, et al. Visual recovery after retinal detachment with macula-off: is surgery within the first 72h better than after? Br J Ophthalmol 2016; 100:1466–1469.

Nemet A, Moshiri A, Yiu G, et al. A review of innovations in rhegmatogenous retinal detachment surgical techniques. J Ophthalmol 2017; 2017:4310643.

Oellers P, Mahmoud TH. Surgery for proliferative diabetic retinopathy: New tips and tricks. J Ophthalmic Vis Res 2016; 11:93–99.

Preferred Practice Patterns Committee, Retina Panel. Management of Posterior Vitreous Detachment, Retinal Breaks and Lattice Degeneration. San Francisco: American Academy of Ophthalmology 1998;13.

Sullivan Paul. Vitreoretinal Surgery: An interactive multimedia atlas for ophthalmology trainees, Eyelearning Ltd. 2014.

Williamson TH. Vitreoretinal Surgery, 2nd edition. US: Springer-Verlag Berlin Heidelberg; 2011.

Related topic of interest

- Retinal detachment (p. 270)

91 Vitreoretinal surgery – management of complications of cataract surgery, post-operative endophthalmitis and vitreoretinal biopsy

Key points

- Dropped nucleus has an excellent outcome if vitrectomy and fragmentation are performed promptly
- Vitrectomy plays an important role in managing select cases of postoperative endophthalmitis
- Management of dislocated crystalline lens or lens implants involves vitrectomy and, in the absence of capsular support, alternative lens fixation methods are required
- Vitreous and retinochoroidal biopsy helps in the diagnosis of some intraocular inflammatory and proliferative conditions

Dropped nucleus or nuclear fragments

The crystalline lens nucleus (or fragments) may drop into the vitreous in approximately 0.3% of patients having cataract surgery, especially those that have pre-existing or develop capsular or zonular damage during cataract surgery.

Risk factors for capsular or zonular damage

- Old age
- Dense nuclear cataract
- Zonular weakness, e.g. pseudoexfoliation syndrome
- Trauma
- Surgical inexperience

Clinical features

Left untreated nuclear fragments within the vitreous cavity commonly present with recurrent uveal inflammation, increased intraocular pressure (IOP) or recurrent or persistent cystoid macular oedema.

Surgery (Figures 91.1a to c)

Surgery is indicated in the presence of a large nuclear fragments, more than or equal to

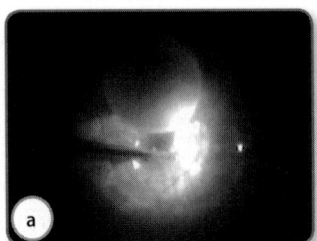
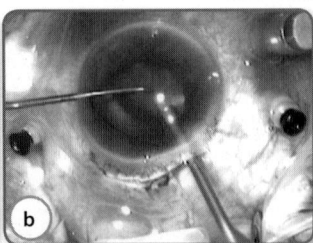
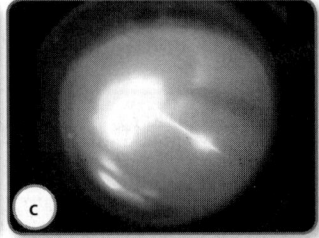

Figure 91.1 (a) Nucleus and nuclear fragments removal by either floating the nucleus to the retropupillary plane using heavy liquid (perfluorocarbon); and (b) Phacoemulsification in the retropupillary plane or (c) Fragmentation using an ultrasound fragmatome or the vitreous cutter on a low cut rate (100–300/min).

one-fourth or smaller fragments associated with any of the above clinical features.

Pars plana vitrectomy (PPV) and fragmentation is performed using either the vitreous cutter or an ultrasound fragmatome or even the phaco tip once the vitrectomy is completed. Heavy liquid may be used to float the nucleus or its fragments away from the macula to enable its safe fragmentation or phacoemulsification in the retropupillary plane.

Outcome

The majority of patients tend to have excellent visual outcome, especially if surgery is performed promptly or within 1 week. Complications include chronic uveitis, cystoid macular oedema, and retinal tears or detachment.

Subluxated and dislocated lens implants

This is a rare but visually disabling complication.

Pathogenesis and risk factors

- *Preoperative*: Traumatic cataract and pseudoexfoliation syndrome
- *Intraoperative*: Posterior capsular tear or zonular dehiscence
- *Postoperative*: Trauma and anterior capsular phimosis in patients with compromised zonules

Clinical features

Patients often present with blurred vision, oscillopsia, double vision, and rarely with pigment dispersion, iris trans-illumination and uveitis-hyphaema-glaucoma syndrome.

Surgery

Before surgery, it is key to establish if reposition or fixation in situ of the subluxed (or dislocated) intraocular lens (IOL) is possible or if IOL exchange will be necessary.
- Pars plana vitrectomy is performed and the subluxed or dislocated IOL is retrieved and fixed in a closed chamber or removed, commonly with the capsular bag, which is often compromised and replaced
- Implantation of IOL in the absence of capsular support:
  - Single-piece IOLs may be sutured to the sclera using 10/0 or 9/0 polypropylene or more favourably 8/0 Gore-Tex sutures. An ab externo (sutures introduced from outside the eye) (**Figures 91.2a** to **f**) or ab interno (sutures brought out from inside the eye) techniques may be used
  - The haptics of three-piece IOLs may be externalised and threaded into the sclera (trans-scleral fixation) (**Figures 91.3a** to **d**)
  - An anterior chamber, angle-fixated or iris-clipped (Artisan-Ophtec) IOLs, may also be used to replace the dislocated or damaged IOLs (**Figures 91.4a** and **b**)

Outcome

Similar visual outcome is achievable with different types of IOL fixation. Notably, however, unlike anterior chamber implantation, mastering the techniques of IOL suturing and trans-scleral fixation fixation involves a long learning curve. A myopic outcome (-1.5 to -2.5) and a higher complication rates are observed with sutured IOLs.

Complications may include corneal oedema, due to endothelial cell decompensation, tilting of IOL, suture erosion or breakage and dislocation. Cystoid macular oedema may occur in up to 30% of patients with angle-supported ACIOL.

Postoperative endophthalmitis

Infectious endophthalmitis may occur rarely, in $\leq 0.1\%$, after any intraocular surgery in patients predisposed to infections, e.g. diabetics.

Pathogenesis

Posterior capsular tear is one of the most common risk factors for acute postoperative endophthalmitis, i.e. occurring within the first 2–6 weeks. The most common causative organisms are coagulase-negative

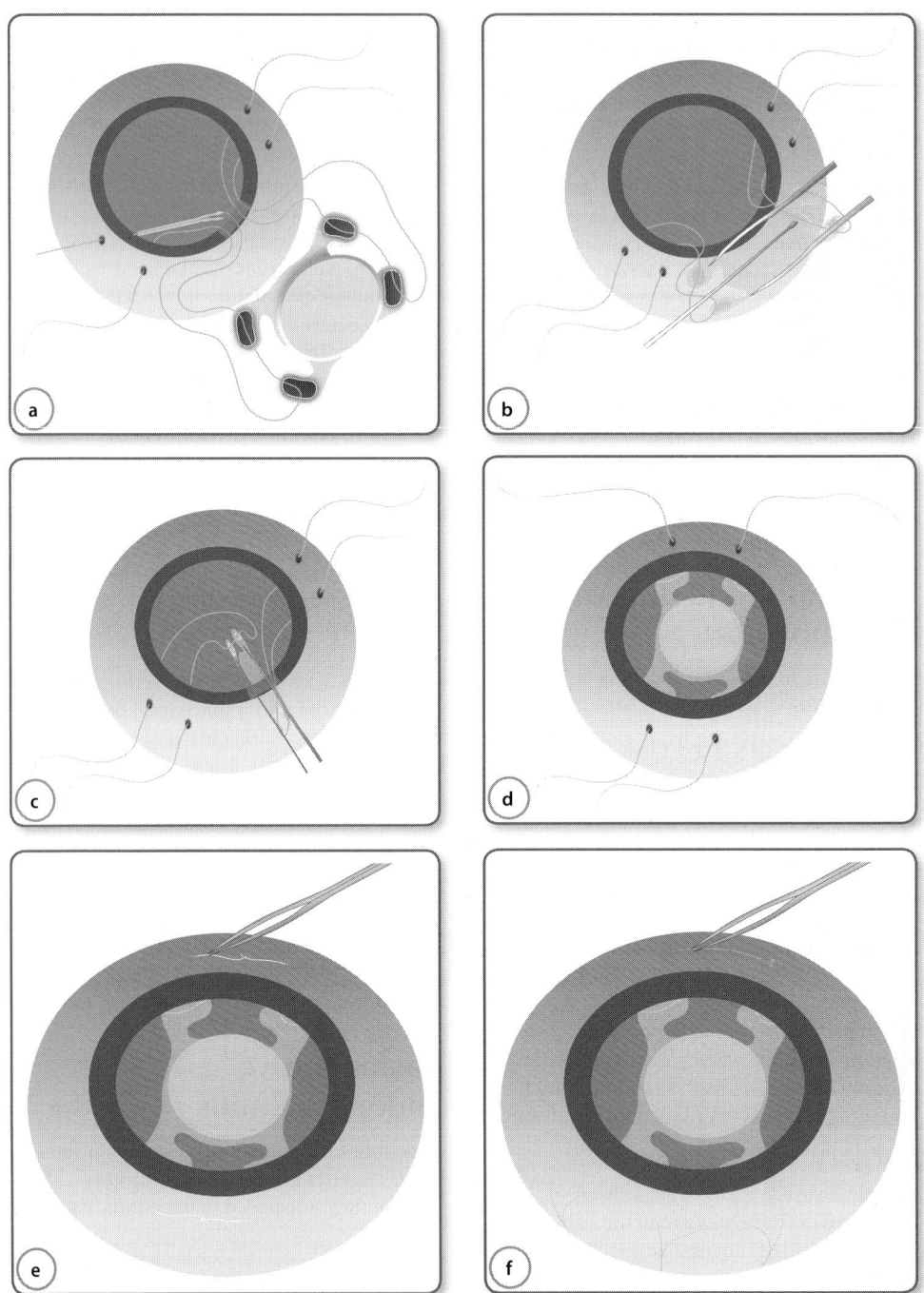

Figure 91.2 Ab externo suturing of a single-piece Intraocular lens (IOL) to the wall of the eye. Two nonabsorbable sutures (e.g. 8-0 Gore-Tex) are attached to the haptics of the lens implant and both are introduced through a corneal incision and pulled out through four 25- or 27-gauge scleral ports (a to c). The sutures are then trimmed and tied off (d and e) and the knots are buried into the sclera (f).

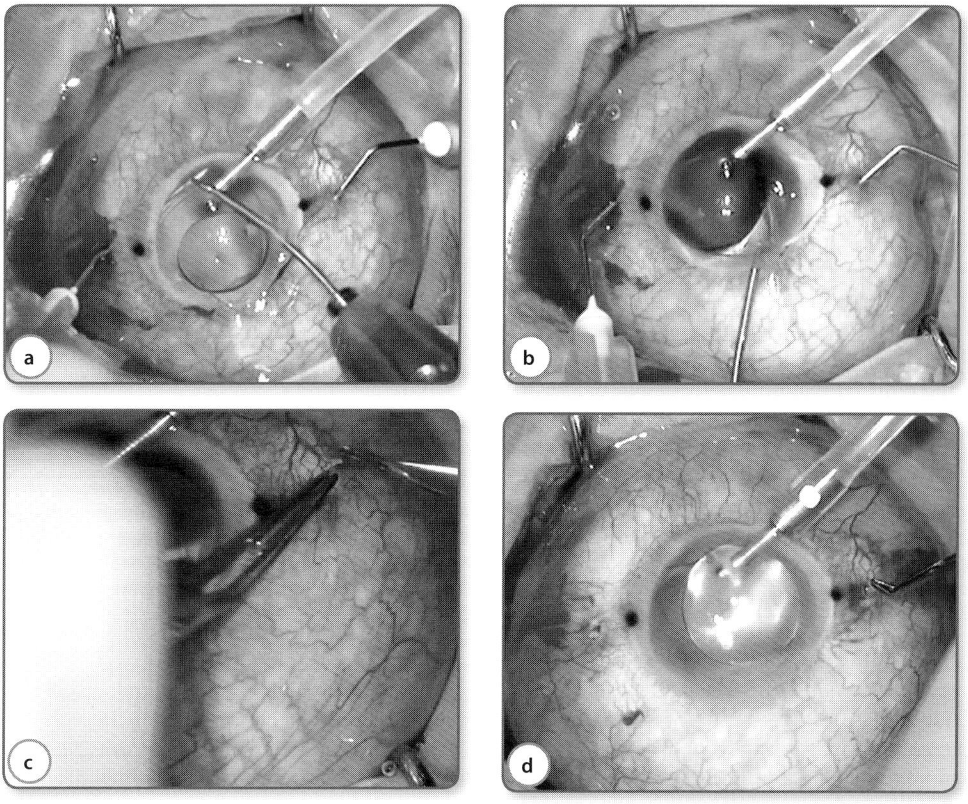

Figure 91.3 Yamane's technique of trans-scleral fixation of intraocular lens. Trans-scleral insertion of two bent needles (25G or 30G) at 2 mm from the limbus (in opposite directions) (a), followed by insertion of three-piece intraocular lens and threading of the leading haptic followed by the trailing haptic through the bore and into the shaft of the needles (a and b), pulling the needles together with haptics through the sclera, followed by using hand-held cautery to create a near-conical bulb at the end of each one of the haptics to reduce the risk of the haptics pulling through the sclera and dislocating (c) and finally allowing the haptic tips to slide back into the sclera and covering it with the conjunctiva (d).

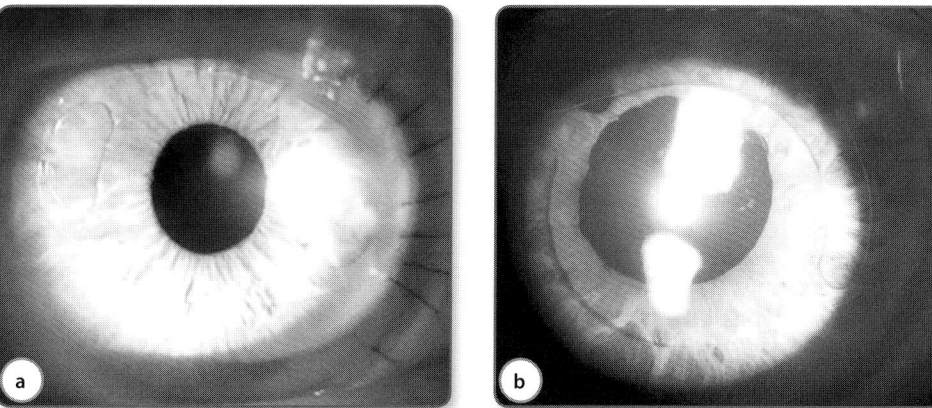

Figure 91.4 Different types of anterior chamber intraocular lens (IOL) implanted in the absence of capsular support. (a) Iris clip (Artisan; Ophtec) IOL; (b) Angle fixation of anterior chamber IOL.

staphylococci, *Staphylococcus aureus*, *Streptococcus* species, and gram-negative organism. *Streptococcus pneumoniae* and *Haemophilus influenzae* are the most common organisms after trabeculectomy. Chronic endophthalmitis is often caused by low-grade organisms, e.g. *Propionibacterium acnes* or fungi and presents much later, i.e. several months after surgery.

Clinical features

In its acute form, patients typically present with pain, lid swelling, conjunctival chemosis, and reduced vision. Hypopyon may be present as well as vitreous cells and exudation. In chronic endophthalmitis, the manifestations are often subtle and may include blurring of vision, anterior chamber and vitreous cells and hypopyon in an otherwise quiescent eye.

Outcome

The Endophthalmitis Vitrectomy Study (EVS) group has shown that vitrectomy and vitreous tap and intravitreal injection of antibiotics resulted in similar visual outcome in patients presenting with visual acuity of more than or equal to hand motion (HM). In patients with perception of light (PL) vision, PPV resulted in improved outcome, i.e. achieving visual acuity of ≥20/40 and 20/100.

Currently, the indications of vitrectomy in patients with endophthalmitis include:
- Patients presenting with PL vision
- No clinical improvement or worsening after intravitreal injection of antibiotics
- Chronic endophthalmitis (e.g. due to *Propionibacterium acnes*)
- Fungal endophthalmitis
- Presence of retinal detachment

Vitreous and retinochoroidal biopsy

Indications and surgery

This is indicated in patients with vitritis or posterior uveitis if the clinical features indicate the possibility of infection, e.g. viral retinitis or neoplasia, e.g. intraocular lymphoma.

Pars plana vitrectomy is used and a dry sample is taken from the vitreous for the purpose of microbial viral polymerase chain reaction (PCR) and microbial culture and antibiotic sensitivity and for cytological examination.

For retinochoroidal lesions, those are reached after vitrectomy is completed and infrared (diode) endolaser is applied around the lesions. Retinal scissors are then used to excise the lesion or a specimen thereof. The specimen is then taken out through an enlarged sclerotomy for histopathological examination.

Outcome

Cultural yield is improved by obtaining vitreous biopsy and retinochoroidal biopsy helps to confirm or establish the diagnosis in up to 50% of infectious and over 30% of masquerade uveitis.

Further reading

Results of the Endophthalmitis Vitrectomy Study: a randomized trial of immediate vitrectomy and of intravenous antibiotics for the treatment of postoperative bacterial endophthalmitis. Endophthalmitis Vitrectomy Study Group. Arch Ophthalmol 1995; 113:1479–1496.

Salehi A, Razmju H, Beni AN, et al. Visual outcome of early and late pars plana vitrectomy in patients with dropped nucleus during phacoemulsification. J Res Med Sci 2011; 16:1422–1429.

Smith JM, Steel DH. Anti-vascular endothelial growth factor for prevention of postoperative vitreous cavity haemorrhage after vitrectomy for proliferative diabetic retinopathy. Cochrane Database Syst Rev 2015, 7:CD008214.

Stem MS, Todorich B, Woodward MA, et al. Scleral-fixated intraocular lenses: Past and present. J Vitreoretin Dis 2017; 1:144–152.

Sullivan Paul. Vitreoretinal Surgery: An interactive multimedia atlas for ophthalmology trainees, Eyelearning Ltd. 2014.

Related topics of interest

- Cataract – complications of surgery (p. 50)
- Intermediate uveitis (p. 185)

92 Vitreoretinal surgery – intraocular haemorrhage, complications of vitreoretinal surgery and modern developments

Key points

- Management of intraocular haemorrhage depends on the duration and the primary cause
- Extensive suprachoroidal haemorrhage (SCH) is rare, but has a poor visual prognosis
- Vitreoretinal surgery is largely safe and both intraoperative and postoperative complications are rare
- Future developments promise better outcome and will enable treatment of currently untreatable conditions

Intraocular haemorrhage

Vitreous haemorrhage

Causes

- Posterior vitreous detachment
- Proliferative retinopathy, e.g. diabetic, sickle cell, and retinal vein occlusions (RVO)
- Age-related macular degeneration (AMD) and choroidal polyps
- Retinal macroaneurysms
- Retinal vasculitis, e.g. Behcet's and Eales disease
- Trauma, e.g. choroidal rupture

Treatment

This often depends on the cause. In the presence of PVD, the likelihood of a retinal tear present is 50–70%. Ultrasound scan will help establish the location of the haemorrhage, e.g. intragel or retrohyaloid, and associated pathological features, e.g. the presence of a retinal tear or tractional retinal detachment. Ultrasound, however, would not be enough to rule out the presence of retinal tears.

Indications for surgery include:
- The presence of tractional retinal tears or detachment
- Recurrent or non-clearing vitreous haemorrhage, e.g. after 2–6 weeks
- Increased intraocular pressure, e.g. due to haemolytic or ghost cell glaucoma or rubeosis iridis
- The presence of visually disabling floaters and vitreous debris after the haemorrhage absorbs

Surgery will include vitrectomy, search, cryotherapy or laser and gas for retinal tears or detachment. It also may include delimitation and endolaser in proliferative retinopathy.

Adjuvant therapy may be needed in the form of intravitreal injection of anti-vascular endothelial growth factors (anti-VEGFs), e.g. bevacizumab, ranibizumab or aflibercept in patients with proliferative retinopathy or macular oedema, be it in diabetic on secondary to RVO.

Patients with retinal vasculitis may need to be started on anti-inflammatory medications to control the inflammation before listing for surgery.

Submacular haemorrhage

Submacular haemorrhage (SMH) is fortunately a rare but sight-threatening condition. The incidence has been estimated to be 1:300 per year in patients with wet AMD and 2.4% in patients with choroidal polyps.

Causes

- Choroidal neovascular membrane (CNVM) or polyps in AMD
- Retinal macroaneurysms
- Ocular trauma, and

- Other causes of CNVM, e.g. high myopia, presumed ocular histoplasmosis syndrome (POHS), etc.

Pathogenesis of visual loss

Although often no apparent risk factors are identified, these may include hypertension and the use of antiplatelets or anticoagulation medications. The main mechanisms of visual loss includes the presence of mechanical barrier to nutrients by the blood clot, dislocation of the photoreceptors by the contracting blood clot, and iron-induced toxic damage to the retinal pigment epithelium (RPEs) photoreceptors and outer retina.

Clinical features (Figures 92.1a to d)

Clinical and OCT scan examination will help establish the cause, size, and location of the haemorrhage, i.e. pre-retinal, sub-hyaloid or sub-ILM, sub-retinal or sub-retinal pigment epithelium.

Treatment

Damage to the retina is time-dependent and therefore treatment should be implemented as soon as possible. Treatment is indicated in patients with large haemorrhage ≥2DD with sub-retinal components.

Clinical trials are underway to establish the most effective treatment method. The two most commonly used, and it seems most effective, treatment methods are:

1. *Pneumatic displacement (Figures 92.2a to d):* An expansile gas bubble [100% sulphur hexafluoride (SF_6) or perfluoropropane (C_3F_8)] or air is injected

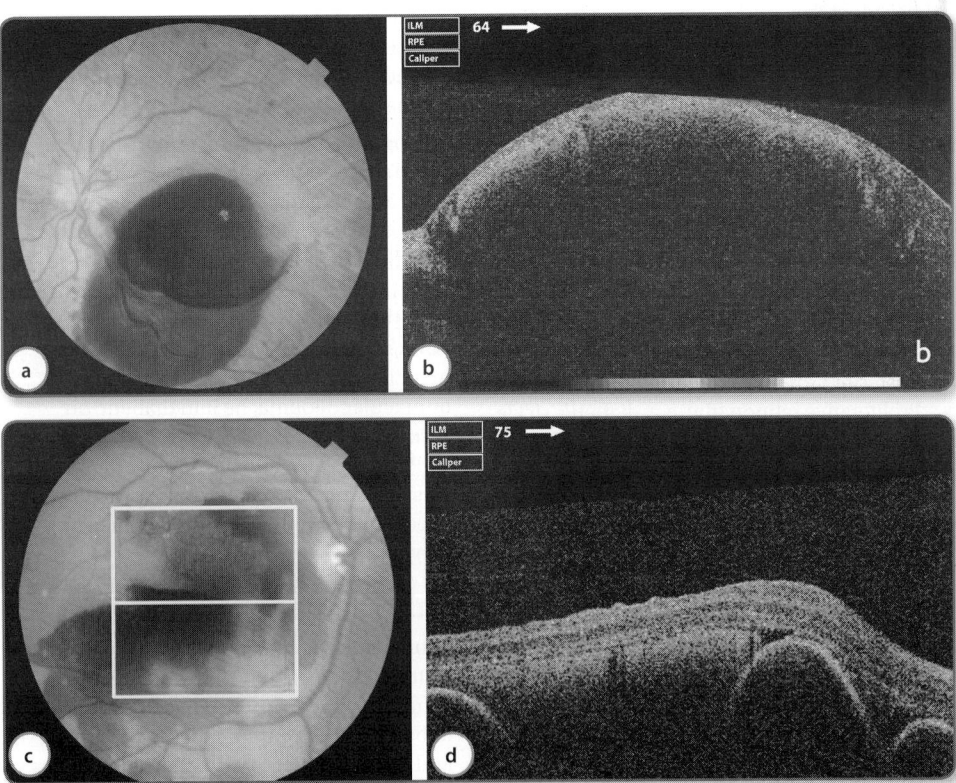

Figure 92.1 Bright sub-internal limiting membrane (ILM) and slightly darker sub-retinal haemorrhage (notice that it masks all the underlying structures) and dark sub-retinal pigment epithelium (RPE) haemorrhage (a and b). Both sub-retinal and sub-RPE haemorrhages have the retinal structures clearly visible over the area of the blood. The cause of submacular haemorrhage in the bottom frames (c and d) is due to choroidal polyps, which appear as saccular protrusions underneath the retina on the optical coherence tomography (OCT) scan. *(For colour version see plate 14)*

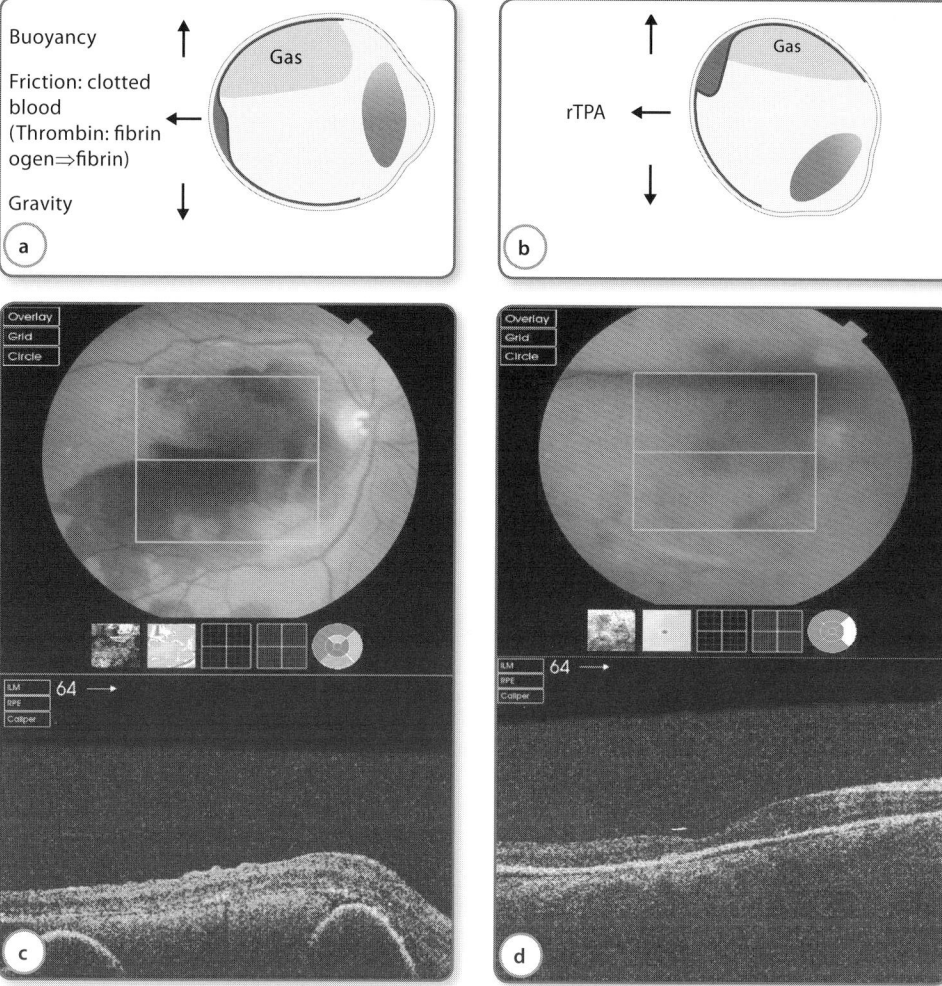

Figure 92.2 Treatment of submacular haemorrhage. (a, b) The forces acting on submacular haemorrhage and modification using rTPA, a bubble of expansile gas and forward head positioning; (c, d) showing displacement and reduced submacular haemorrhage and disappearance of the pigment epithelial detachment. [(a, b) Modified from Stopa and Lincoff, 2007 and 2008]

into the vitreous cavity. This is often combined with or preceded by injection of recombinant tissue plasminogen activator (rTPA), a proteolytic enzyme, to help break down the fibrin and liquefy the blood clot to facilitate its absorption.

2. *Vitrectomy and drainage (Figures 92.3a and b):* In the absence of evidence of SMH displacement, vitrectomy and drainage of blood through one or more retinotomy may be performed.

Outcome

The most common complications are recurrence of SMH, development of FTMH retinal detachment, and rarely rTPA-induced RPE toxicity.

The vast majority of patients have the blood clot displaced or completely absorbed. In a series that was presented at Euretina in 2016, we had 25 patients (mostly of AMD patients) who were treated with either anti-VEGF and rTPA followed by pneumatic

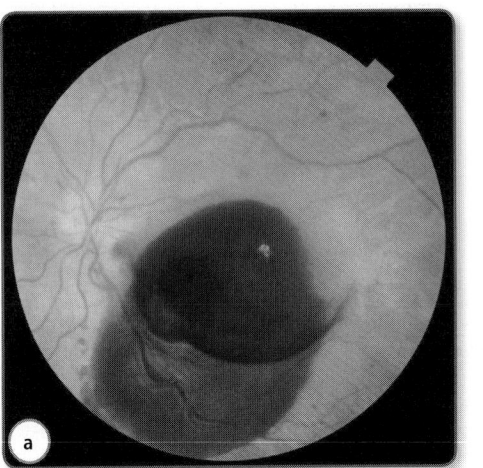
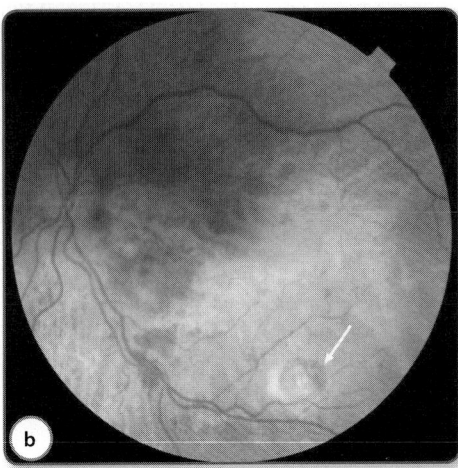

Figures 92.3a and b Treatment of submacular haemorrhage with intravitreal tissue plasminogen activator (TPA) injection followed by vitrectomy and drainage through a retinotomy (arrow).

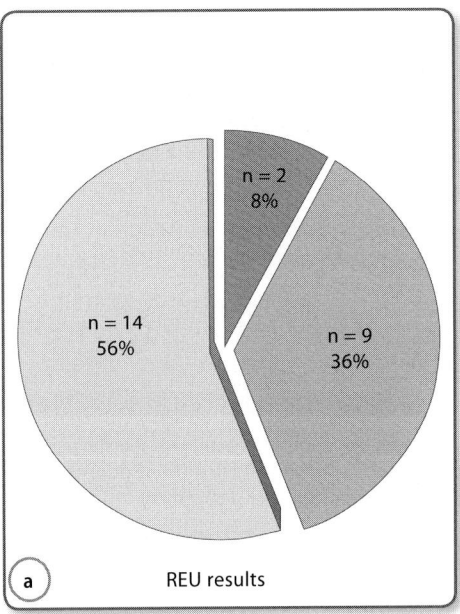
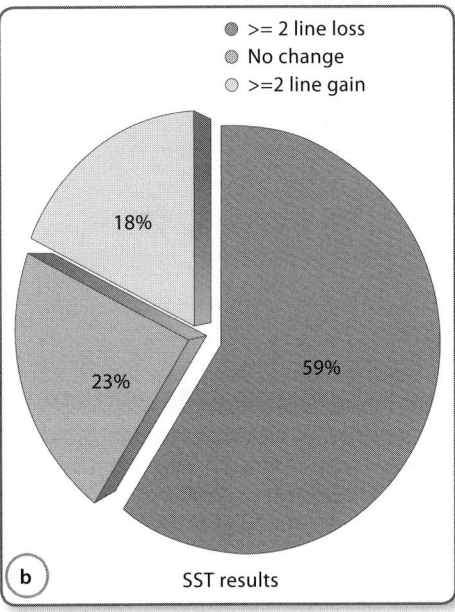

Figures 92.4a and b Outcome of a series of submacular haemorrhage (SMH) mostly due to AMD treated with intravitreal injection of rTPA combined with pneumatic displacement or surgical drainage compared to the natureal history reported by the study of surgery for submacular haemorrhage trial (SST).
Courtesy: Royal eye unit, Kingston Hospital.

displacement or by surgical drainage, the visual outcome improved by 2 or more lines in 56% of patients within 6 to 12 months. This represented nearly a reversal of the natural history reported by the SSM study (**Figure 92.4a** and **b**).

Suprachoroidal haemorrhage

Suprachoroidal haemorrhage, i.e. that occurs within the choroid and suprachoroidal space is another rare but potentially sight-threatening condition.

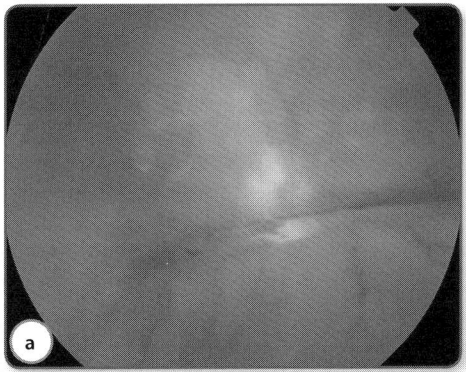 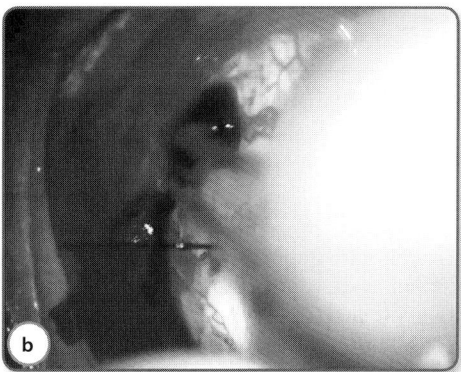

Figure 92.5 (a) Acute (intraoperative) suprachoroidal haemorrhage; (b) Drainage through a sclerotomy incision 2 weeks after the onset of the haemorrhage. (*For colour version see plate 15*)

Acute (intraoperative) (**Figure 92.5a**) and delayed (postoperative) are two common forms of SCH that are related to intraocular surgery.

Causes

- *Iatrogenic*: Intraoperative sudden or prolonged hypotony during phacoemulsification, trabeculectomy, vitrectomy, penetrating keratoplasty or secondary lens implantation
- *Trauma*: Blunt or sharp trauma
- *Spontaneously*: In patients on blood thinners and neovascular AMD or choroidal polyps

Pathogenesis

Acute (intraoperative) and delayed (postoperative) hypotony leads to suprachoroidal effusion which, in turn, leads to excessive stretching, distortion, and ultimately rupture of the long ciliary or vortex vessels.

Risk factors include old age, previous intraocular surgery, cardiovascular medications, glaucoma, elevated intraocular pressure (IOP), extracapsular cataract surgery and posterior capsular tear, long axial length, aphakia, hypertension, and anticoagulation.

The mechanisms of visual loss are similar to those associated with SCH.

Clinical features

Clinical and ultrasound examination will help establish the location and extent of SCH. Ultrasound will also help identify the presence and extent of liquefaction within the blood clot to decide on the best time for drainage surgery.

Management

Increasing IOP intraoperatively as soon SCH is identified is key to limiting its size and reducing the likelihood of visual loss. Surgery should be abandoned and completed at a later date once the haemorrhage has absorbed. Small SCH may be observed with excellent outcome.

Drainage of SCH (**Figure 92.5b**) is indicated in massive SCH "kissing choroidals" and if the haemorrhage extends to the submacular area or is associated with retinal detachment.

Drainage is commonly performed around the 10th day after the onset of haemorrhage, when the blood clot has sufficiently liquefied. Intravitreal injection of rTPA either intraoperatively or preoperatively may help liquefy the blood clot and facilitate early drainage.

Trans-scleral stab incisions are made in the quadrants where the haemorrhage is highermost. The locations of these incisions may be chosen after careful ultrasound examination of extent of SCH. An anterior chamber or pars plana infusion line is inserted to maintain or increase the IOP to facilitate spontaneous drainage of the liquefied blood.

Outcome

Visual outcome depends on the extent of the haemorrhage and underlying disease process. Up to 60% of patients with mild-to-moderate

SCH may achieve 6/12 or better. Extensive SCH, involving the macula or associated with haemorrhagic retinal detachment, carries poor visual prognosis.

Complications of vitreoretinal surgery

Overall, vitreoretinal surgery is safe and both intraoperative and postoperative
sight threatening complications are rare. The following is a list of possible complications that are commonly associated with PPV:
- *Intraoperative*:
  - Lens touch or damage (**Figure 92.6a**)
  - Focal retinal or choroidal damage
  - Retinal incarceration in patients with RD (2–5%)
  - Entry site or iatrogenic retinal breaks (2–10%)
  - Entrapment of heavy liquid fluid underneath the retina (**Figure 92.6b**)
  - Suprachoroidal haemorrhage
- *Postoperative*:
  - Nuclear sclerotic cataract (within 2 years in 80–90% in patients above 50 years)
  - Increased risk of secondary open-angle glaucoma (10–20%)
  - Retinal detachment (<1%) or recurrence (5–10%)
  - Vitreous cavity haemorrhage especially in diabetic patients (20–40% of diabetic patients)
  - Secondary epiretinal membrane or macular hole, especially in patients with macula-off RD (**Figure 92.6c**)
  - Macular fold especially in patients with superior bullous RD
  - Emulsification of silicone oil, secondary glaucoma or band keratopathy

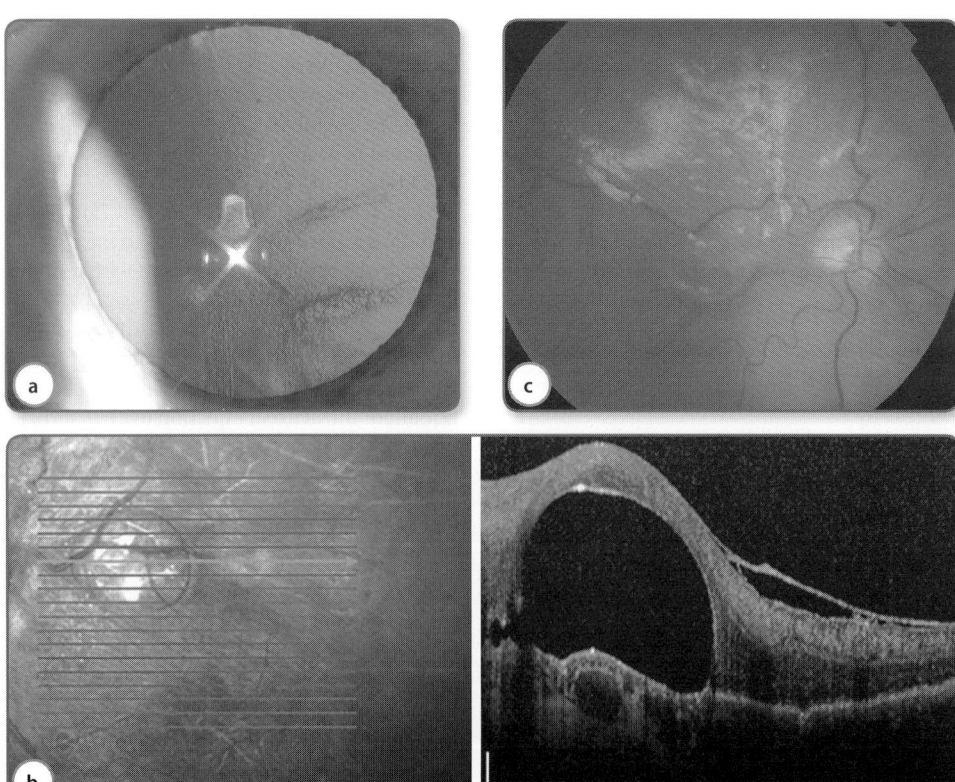

Figure 92.6 Examples of vitreoretinal complications. (a) Intraoperative lens touch with light pipe; (b) Sub-retinal heavy liquid; (c) Secondary epiretinal membrane.
Courtesy: Paul Sullivan, Moorfields Eye Hospital.

- Rare complications are suprachoroidal haemorrhage, endophthalmitis, and sympathetic ophthalmia

Modern and future developments in vitreoretinal surgery

Technical advances in vitreoretinal surgery will help improve surgical performance and outcome and will enable treatments of new conditions. Here are some of the modern and future developments in vitreoretinal surgery and its techniques:

- Increasing use of small gauge trans-conjunctival sclerotomy (25- and 27-gauge) to reduce postoperative pain and intraoperative complications
- Using high cut rare to minimise the risk of traction on the retina, especially in patients with retinal detachment
- Use of chandelier lights to significantly improve visualisation and allow bimanual dissection, e.g. in diabetic delamination
- Use of digital video viewing systems, utilising, ultra-high-definition monitors, and three-dimensional technology, may eventually replace the optical microscope (**Figure 92.7**) in vitrectomy and other intraocular surgery, with clear advantages for improved visualisation and for training
- Improved imaging technology, and using intraoperative OCT scanning to enhance the visualisation and therefore surgical performance

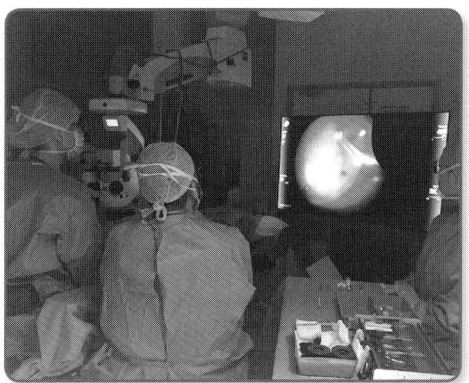

Figure 92.7 Use of 'heads up' video viewing system instead of optical microscope in vitrectomy surgery.

- Use of robots to perform complex surgical procedures, e.g. subretinal injection and macular peeling, may supersede the manual dexterity of surgeons potentially improving the accuracy and precision of those techniques
- Use of gene transfer therapy (via adenovirus or other vectors) for the treatment of inherited macular and retinal dystrophy and use of stem cell transplantation in the treatment of some degenerative conditions, e.g. age-related macular degeneration
- Use of artificial retinal implants (epiretinal and subretinal) in patients with end-stage retinal dystrophy or degeneration

Further reading

Chandra A, Xing W, Kadhim MR, et al. Suprachoroidal hemorrhage in pars plana vitrectomy: risk factors and outcomes over 10 years. Ophthalmology 2014; 121:311–317.

Cole CJ, Kwan AS, Laidlaw DA, Aylward GW. A new technique of combined retinal and choroidal biopsy. Br J Ophthalmol. 2008; 92:1357–1360.

Duker JS, Kaiser PK, Binder S, et al. The International Vitreomacular Traction Study Group Classification of Vitreomacular Adhesion, Traction, and Macular Hole. Ophthalmology 2013; 120:2611–2619.

Khan MA, Haller JA. Ocriplasmin for treatment of vitreomacular traction: an update. Ophthalmol Ther 2016; 5:147–159.

Stanescu-Segall D, Balta F, Jackson TL. Submacular hemorrhage in neovascular age-related macular degeneration: A synthesis of the literature. Surv Ophthalmol 2016; 61:18–32.

Sullivan Paul. Vitreoretinal Surgery: An interactive multimedia atlas for ophthalmology trainees, Eyelearning Ltd. 2014.

Related topics of interest

- Age-related macular degeneration (p. 1)
- Diabetic eye disease (p. 116)
- Full-thickness macular holes (p. 152)

93 White dot syndromes

Key points

- The white dot syndromes are not one entity but many, the aetiologies of which are poorly understood
- It is important to exclude with appropriate investigations, infective and non-infective conditions such as syphilis, tuberculosis (TB), or sarcoidosis, as these may mimic white dot syndromes
- Some variants commonly need no treatment while others need long-term immunosuppression
- Acute posterior multifocal placoid pigment epitheliopathy (APMPPE) can be associated with cerebral vasculitis, a potentially lethal complication that needs immediate inpatient treatment

Epidemiology

The so-called "white dot syndromes" are not one entity. The term encompasses a rather unhelpful phenotypic description of conditions characterised by the appearance of white dots in the fundus. They are poorly understood conditions, some of which may overlap and are idiopathic. They are classified together under this flag of convenience until such time when a more definitive method of determining their aetiology and characteristics has been discovered. For the purposes of this review, we will cover multiple evanescent white dot syndrome (MEWDS), APMPPE, punctate inner choroidopathy (PIC), and multifocal choroiditis with panuveitis (MCP). Restricting our definition to these four conditions listed here gives a combined incidence of 0.45 per 100,000 people per year. MEWDS and PIC are more common in young, predominantly female patients, with PIC common in myopes. Distinct entities such as birdshot and serpiginous choroiditis will be dealt with elsewhere.

Pathophysiology

The main reason these conditions are grouped together is that the exact pathophysiology remains a mystery. PIC and MCP are often treated as being different phenotypes of the same condition, with PIC primarily affecting the macular region and posterior pole and MCP affecting both macula and extramacular retina.

Clinical features

Multiple evanescent white dot syndrome is a name descriptive of the condition as there are indeed multiple white dots present around the posterior pole and mid-periphery of one eye around a tenth of a disc diameter in size, and these dots are indeed "evanescent", in that they quickly disappear. There is also some foveal granularity present and intriguingly a striking relative afferent papillary defect (RAPD) despite good vision. The dots are difficult to see and as such this diagnosis is often missed. A flu-like illness sometimes predates the eye symptoms, which commonly consist of blur and paracentral scotoma.

The APMPPE is another descriptive name as there are multiple areas of posterior lesions seen in both eyes that are "plate-like" in being large, at around a disc diameter in size, and centrally raised. They are initially creamy white but become pigmented over time. In about 30% of patients, there are significant constitutional symptoms such as respiratory difficulties and lymphadenopathy though a portion will also have headache. This is a very serious sign indicative of cerebral vasculitis and prompt action should be taken in this instance. Significant vitritis as well as anterior uveitis may also be present.

Punctate inner choroidopathy and MCP are two sides of the same coin. Patients with PIC have pigmented lesions less than half a disc diameter across in the central macular region of one or both eyes, classically in young myopic females. There is blur and distortion in the affected eye which may be due to either a flare-up of the inflammatory process itself or the development of an associated choroidal neovascular (CNV) membrane. MCP is associated with larger lesions up to a disc diameter across that develop in the extramacular fundus in both eyes. Older dots are pigmented, whereas brand new dots are white with fluffy borders. There can be marked vitritis present, unlike with PIC, with this discrepancy being hypothesised to be down to the number and extent of the lesions present. Patients with MCP present with bilateral blurred vision and floaters, with occasional photophobia.

Investigations

Investigations are primarily aimed at excluding other diagnoses as well as assessing for complications such as the development of a CNV membrane. MEWDS typically is an entirely clinical diagnosis, though fundus fluorescein angiography (FFA) and indocyanine green angiography (ICG) is often undertaken, the appearances of which can be very distinctive (**Figure 93.1**). APMPPE, on the other hand, can vary from mild to severe, and can be sight-threatening (**Figure 93.2**).

In such cases syphilis serology, quantiferon gold, serum angiotension converting enzyme (ACE), inflammatory markers, and even neuroimaging may be needed in order to assess and exclude the differential diagnoses. Certain PIC lesions may be confused with toxoplasmosis scars in which case toxoplasmosis serology may be needed. Optical coherence tomography (OCT) scans are highly useful at differentiating scars from active disease, particularly if serial scans are compared. MCP may present similarly to sarcoidosis, in which case appropriate investigations need to be undertaken. If a patient with PIC has a sudden deterioration in acuity or distortion, OCT combined with OCT angiography, or FFA is vital in determining if this is due to a flare-up in the condition or the development of a CNV membrane.

Diagnosis

If the above investigations, if needed, have excluded other conditions, then a diagnosis of one of the white dot syndromes can be made. Never make a diagnosis of "white dot syndrome" itself as the treatment is very different depending on the exact disease present and such a diagnosis helps nobody.

Treatment

Patients with MEWDS typically need no treatment other than simple reassurance that no other potentially blinding condition is present. The vast majority of patients recover normal vision and typically a patient can be reviewed at 2 months to see that all is well.

The APMPPE is an entirely different entity. If the disease is mild then again no treatment is needed though if the inflammation is severe then a course of steroids in the

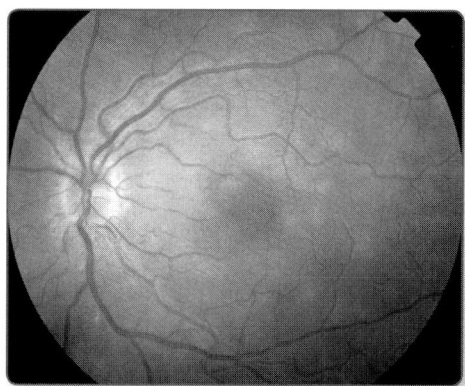

Figure 93.1 Multiple evanescent white dot syndrome (MEWDS).

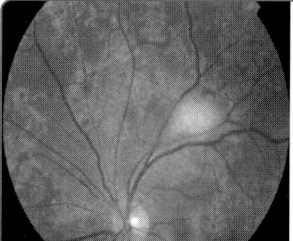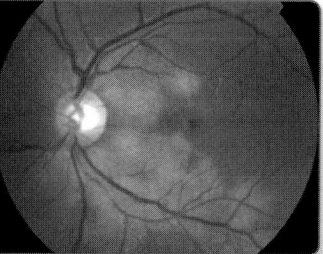

Figure 93.2 Acute posterior multifocal placoid pigment epitheliopathy (APMPPE). (*For colour version see plate 15*)

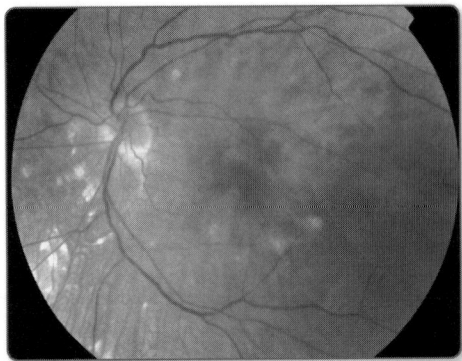

Figure 93.3 Punctate inner choroidopathy (PIC). *(For colour version see plate 15)*

form of a rapidly tapering course of oral prednisolone, starting at 60 mg a day, is the order of the day. Obviously, if this is the case, further investigations would have been needed for conditions that can mimic such as syphilis and TB and should these be positive appropriate treatment instituted. If the patient has a headache, then cerebral vasculitis, a potentially life-threatening condition, should be assumed to be present and arrangements made for immediate admission for treatment with pulsed methylprednisolone infusions under the care of the medical team, with appropriate imaging organised. Whilst most cases of APMPPE settle eventually with the lesions forming scars some unfortunate individuals have chronic disease in which case long-term immunosuppression may be needed.

If patients with PIC have new onset blur and distortion, then investigations should be instituted to find out if this is due to a flare-up of inflammation or a CNV membrane. If the former, then treatment consists of a rapidly tapering course of oral prednisolone starting at 60 mg per day, with appropriate gastric cover, until the condition settles. Long-term immunosuppression may rarely be required in severe cases. If a CNV membrane is the cause, then treatment is typically with an intravitreal injection of anti-vascular endothelial growth factor (VEGF) agent such as bevacizumab (avastin) or ranibizumab. Serial OCT scans are helpful in determining the response to treatment and whether repeat treatment is needed or not.

Immunosuppression, in the form of oral steroids initially, is the treatment of choice for MCP. Progress can be monitored via serial wide-field fundus photographs, OCT, and autofluorescence, and immunosuppression increased or decreased depending on evidence of progression. A steroid-sparing agent may be needed. Patients with MCP cannot be discharged from the uveitis service due to patients usually being unable to report low-grade progression of their disease.

Complications

The main complication to watch out for is the potential for cerebral vasculitis in an APMPPE patient, as this complication can prove fatal. It is, therefore, vital that any APMPPE patient with neurological symptoms and headache is referred immediately. Remember that infective conditions such as syphilis of TB should be investigated for, and excluded, as they may mimic these conditions. Failure to do this may lead to disaster if systemic immunosuppression is instituted in these mimickers.

Further reading

Abu-Yaghi NE, Hartono SP, Hodge DO, et al. White dot syndromes: a 20-year study of incidence, clinical features and outcomes. Ocul Immunol Inflamm 2011; 19:426–430.

Williams GS, Westcott M. Practical Uveitis: Understanding the Grape. United Kingdom: Taylor & Francis; 2017.

Related topics of interest

- Birdshot chorioretinopathy (p. 29)
- Posterior uveitis (p. 259)

Index

Note: Page numbers in **bold** or *italic* refer to tables or figures, respectively.

A

Ab interno canaloplasty 209
Abducens nerve palsy 98, 109
Aberrant regeneration 11
Aberrations 263
Abscess 111
ACAID see Anterior chamber-associated immune deviation (ACAID)
Acanthamoeba 76, 183
    infection 181, 183
    keratitis 76, 77, 182
Accommodative esotropia 137, 139
Acephalgic migraine 173
Acetazolamide 7, 8, 51, 163 see also Diamox
Acetylcholine receptors 212
    antibodies 213
Achromatopsia 274
Acid burn 67
Acne rosacea 63
Acoustic neuroma 107
Acquired cataract
    clinical evaluation of 46
    risk factors for **43**
Acquired immunodeficiency syndrome 325
Acquired myogenic ptosis, causes of 36
Acquired nystagmus 223
    etiological classification of 222
Acrochordon 19
Acrylic intraocular lenses (IOLs) 188
Actinomyces israelii 198
Acute disseminated encephalomyelitis (ADEM) 237
Acute hydrops, treatment of 87
Acute posterior multifocal placoid pigment epitheliopathy (APMPPE) 261, 372, *373*
ADEM see Acute disseminated encephalomyelitis (ADEM)
Adequate immunosuppression treatment 129
Adie's pupil 11, 13
Aflibercept 4, 5, 119, 193, 194, *see also* Eylea
Age-Related Eye Disease Study **4**
Age-related macular degeneration (AMD) 1–5, 59, 193, 195, 365
Agranulocytosis 163
AION see Anterior ischaemic optic neuropathy (AION)
Alcohol 223
Alió-Shabayek classification 86
Alkali burn 67
Alkali burns 307

Allergic eye disease 134
Allergic keratitis 78
Allogeneic haemopoietic stem cell transplant surgery 122
Alpha agonists 163
Alphagan 163
Amblyopia 46, *139*, 145, 314
    risk of 18
Amelanotic iris naevus *341*
Amelanotic lacunae *347*
American Academy of Ophthalmology 117
Amikacin 52, 195
Amitriptyline 174
Amniotic membrane transplant 70
Amphetamines 6
Amphotericin B 195
Amsler sign 159
Amsler-Krumeich classification 86
Amsler-Krumeich keratoconus grading **86**
Anaemia 219
Anaesthesia 312
Ancillary tests 106
Aneurysms 101
Angiotensin-converting enzyme (ACE) 186, 373
Angle closure glaucoma 6–9, 58
    acute 8, 10, 11, 43
    angle imaging 7
    medical treatment 8
Angle grading, shaffer system of **8**
Aniridia 10
Anisocoria 10–13
Anisometropia 205
Anterior capsular
    contraction 53
Anterior cerebellar vermis, lesions of 223
Anterior chamber cells, sun classification for grading **15**
Anterior chamber intraocular lens *188, 363*
Anterior chamber-associated immune deviation (ACAID) 91
Anterior ischaemic optic neuropathy (AION) 156
Anterior subcapsular cataracts, causes of 45
Anterior synechiae 91
    peripheral 161
Anterior uveitis 14–16, 52, 135, 286 *see also* Anterior vitritis
Anticonvulsants 174, 223
Antihistamines 6

Index

Antihypertensives 8
Antimicrobial therapies 196
Anti-myelin oligodendrocyte glycoprotein antibodies 236
Anti-tumour necrosis factor 304
Anti-vascular endothelial growth factor (ANTI-VEGF) 1, 193, 216, 333
Anti-VEGF see Anti-vascular endothelial growth factor (Anti-VEGF)
Anxiety 163
Aphakia 169
Aphakic eyes 160
Aphakic glaucoma, postoperative 57
Aplastic anaemia 163
Apocrine glands 63 see also Moll glands
Apocrine hidrocystoma 19
Aponeurotic ptosis 35
Apraclonidine 13, 163
Aqueous shunt surgery 160
Aqueous-deficient dry eye 123
Arcuate fibres 251
Arcuate keratotomy 265
Arcuate superior defect 249
Argyll Robertson pupil 11
Arterial hypertension 290
Arteries 14, 288 see also Arthritis
Arthritis 14, 288
Artificial tear drops 123
A-scan technique 23, 24
Asthenopia 142 see also Reported diplopia symptoms 138
Astigmatism 97, 190, 263
Atherosclerosis 109
Atopic dermatitis 43, 45
Atrophic round hole 254, *351*
Autoantibodies 213
Autofluorescence 332
   imaging 280
Autologous serum drops 123
Autosomal dominant
   drusen 275
   dystrophy 81
Avastin 4, 119, 194
Avellino dystrophy 81
Axenfeld-Rieger syndrome **10**
Azathioprine 157

B

Background diabetic retinopathy (BDR) 117
Background retinopathy 118
Bacterial conjunctivitis 73
   chronic 73
   pathogens **73**
Bacterial endophthalmitis 195
Bacterial infection, chronic low-grade 32
Bacterial keratitis *181, 182,* 183

Barbiturate intoxication 223
Basal cell carcinoma (BCC) 323
Basal epithelial cells 79
BDR see Background diabetic retinopathy (BDR)
Bear track peripheral degeneration 348
Behçet's disease 14, 261, 286, 288, 365
Bell's palsy 102
Bell's phenomenon 37, 111
Benedikt's syndrome 109
Benign episodic unilateral mydriasis (BEUM) 10, 11
Benign lid lesions 17–21, **19**
Benign tumours 17
Benzalkonium chloride 162
Berry aneurysms 11
Best disease 275, *275*
Beta-blockers 160, 162, 174 see also Propranolol
Betaxolol 163
Bevacizumab 4, 19, 194 see also Avastin
Bietti crystalline chorioretinal dystrophy 273
Bilateral congenital cataract 55
Bilateral orbital venous drainage 40
Bilateral sticky eyelids 73
Bimatoprost 162
Binocular indirect ophthalmoscopy score **185**
Binocular vision 140
   loss of 137
Biometry
   advance of 22
   and lens implant power calculation 22–28
Birdshot chorioretinopathy 29–31, 261
Birdshot, indocyanine green of *30*
Blepharitis 17, 32–34, **33**, 63, 128, 131 see also Rosacea
Blepharophimosis-ptosis-epicanthus-inversus syndrome 36
Blepharoptosis 35–38
Blood dyscrasia 163
Blood testing 186, 243
Blowout fracture 108
B-mode
   technique 24
   ultrasonography 332
Bony facial canal 102
Botulinum toxin 139, 174
   injection 35, 103, 139
Bowman's layer 80, 82
   corneal dystrophies of 80
Bradycardia 163
Brain, computed tomography of 174
Brain-derived neurotrophic factor 298
Branch retinal artery occlusions (BRAO) 267
Branch retinal vein 193
   occlusion (BRVO) 195, 287, 290
Branch vein occlusion study 291
BRAO see Branch retinal artery occlusions (BRAO)
Brimonidine 170
   tartrate 163 see also Alphagan

Brinzolamide 163
British Society of Rheumatology (BSR) 157
Bronchospasm 163
Bruch's membrane 234, 331
Bruckner test 206
Brun's nystagmus 223
Brunescent cataract 45
BRVO see Branch retinal vein occlusion (BRVO)
B-scan ultrasound 217
Bulbar conjunctiva 128
   superior 77
Buphthalmos 169
Busacca's nodules 15
B-wave amplitude 30

C

Calcitonin gene-related peptide (CGRP) 172
Calcium channel blockers 174 see also Flunarizine
Canalicular excision 201
Canaliculitis 198, 199, *199*
Candesartan 174
Capillary bed 288
Capillary haemangioma 17, 19, 36, 345, 347, 348, see also Strawberry naevus
   peripheral 346, *346*
   superficial 18, *18*
Capsulorhexis 149
Capsulotomy 151
Carbachol 164
Carbonic anhydrase inhibitors 160, 163
Carcinoma in situ 337
Cardiac arrhythmias 219
Cardiovascular dysregulation 219
Caroticocavernous fistula (CCF) 179
   endovascular treatment of *179*
Carotid arteries 39
Carotid cavernous fistulas
   barrow classification of **39**
   incidence of 39
Carotid Doppler ultrasound 217
Carotid occlusion 41
Carotid stenosis 218
Carotid-cavernous fistula (CCF) 39–42, 107, 306
   high-flow 40
   low-flow 40
   trauma 39
Cataract 45, 46, 155, 158, 195, 205
   acquired 43–49
   congenital 55–58
   early detection of 56
   early postoperative complications 51
   late postoperative complications 52
   treatment 48
Cataract surgery 43, 57, 58, 90, 145, 169, 188, 273
   management of complications of 360
Cataractous lens, large 46

Cavernous haemangiomas 346, 348
Cavernous portion 110, 113
Cavernous sinus 39, *106*, 110, *177*
   meningioma *177*
   thrombosis 306
CCFs see Carotid cavernous fistulas (CCFs)
Ceftazidime 52, 195
Central anterior chamber depth measurement 7
Central corneal thickness (CCT) 166, 226, 227
Central keratin horn 17 see also Plaque
Central linear B-scans *25*
Central nervous system (CNS) 163, 219
Central retinal artery occlusion (CRAO) 195, 216, 267, 287
Central retinal vein occlusion (CRVO) 193, 195, 290
Central serous chorioretinopathy (CSCR) 59–62, *60*, 279
   chronic 59
Central vein occlusion study 292
Central vestibular nystagmus 223
Cerebellopontine angle syndrome **107**
Cerebral ptosis 35
Cerebrospinal fluid 245, 308
Cervical artery dissection 172
Cervicogenic headache 172
CGRP see Calcitonin gene-related peptide (CGRP)
Chalazion 19, 63–66
   chronic *65*
Chemical burns 91
Chemical conjunctivitis 230
Chemical injuries 67–71
   medical treatment 70
   surgical treatment 70
Chemical ocular injury, clinical course of 69
Chemotherapy 297
Chiasmal visual field defects 251
Childhood glaucoma 170
Childhood onset cataracts 56
Chin depression 114
Chlamydia 73
   disease, prevalence of 229
   infection 229
   trachomatis 73
Chloramphenicol ointment 146
Chorioretinal coloboma 205
Chorioretinitis 261
Choroidal amelanotic
   lesions 330
   naevus 330
Choroidal detachment 330
Choroidal granuloma 330
Choroidal haemangioma 329, 330, *331* see also Osteoma
   circumscribed 329
   prognosis for 335
Choroidal inflammation 260, 261 see also Choroiditis
Choroidal mass lesions 52, 53, 195, 205, 217, 270, 330, 350, *351*, 352 see also Retinal detachment

Index

Choroidal melanoma 216, 329, 330, 348
    large *331*
    prognosis for 334
    survival rates for 334
Choroidal melanotic lesions 330
Choroidal metastases 329, 330, *331*
    prognosis for 334
Choroidal naevus 329, 330, *330*, 348
    prognosis for 333
Choroidal neovascular (CNV) membrane 1, 2, *2*, 59, 193, 365
Choroidal osteoma 329, 330
    pathogenesis of 329
    prognosis for 335
    white yellow mass *332*
Choroidal polyps 365
Choroidal rupture 365
Choroidal tumours 331
Choroiditis 260, 261
Chronic inflammation 69
Chronic relapsing inflammatory optic neuropathy (CRION) 240
CHRPE *see* Congenital hypertrophy of retinal pigment epithelium (CHRPE)
Churg-Strauss syndrome 288
Cicatricial ectropion 125, 126
Ciliary body 216, 340
    adenocarcinoma of 342
    adenoma 342
    lesions 342, **342**
    medulloepithelioma of 340, 342
    melanoma 341, *341*, 342, *342*
    metastases 341
Ciliary muscles 109
Citalopram 6
Citric acid 70
Classical diabetic cataract 45
Clindamycin 195
Clinically significant macular oedema (CSMO) 117, 120
Clomipramine 6
Cluster headache 172, 174
CMO *see* Cystoid macular oedema (CMO)
CNV *see* Choroidal neovascular membrane (CNV)
CO *see* Corneal opacity (CO)
Coats' disease 205–207, 348
Cogan's microcystic epithelial dystrophy 79
Cogan's twitch 37
Collaborative Normal Tension Glaucoma Study 219
Collaborative Ocular Melanoma Study 334
Collamer 189
Coloboma 10
Colour Doppler ultrasonography, role of 157
Colour vision, abnormal 220
Common eyelid lumps 63
Common visual symptoms 156
Complete ophthalmic assessment 37
Computed tomography scanning 320

Confocal microscopy 183
Confocal scanning laser ophthalmoscopy 232
Congenital cranial disinnervation disorders 113, 137
    see also Duane syndrome
Congenital defects 235
Congenital ectropion 125, 128
Congenital entropion require surgery 129
Congenital hypertrophy of retinal pigment epithelium (CHRPE) 253, 330, 345, 348, 349
Conjunctiva 33, 47, 76
    redness of 317
Conjunctival burns 67
Conjunctival chemosis 73
Conjunctival closure 314
Conjunctival goblet cells 122
Conjunctival incision 313
Conjunctival injection 40, 77, 105, 173
Conjunctival level 307
Conjunctival lymphoma 338, *338*
Conjunctival melanoma 338, *338*
Conjunctival naevus 337, *338*
Conjunctival oedema 317
Conjunctival scarring 129, 160
Conjunctival squamous carcinoma 336, *337*
Conjunctival tumours 336
Conjunctivitis 15, 72–74
    acute 72
    bacterial 73
    bilateral 73
    ocular signs in **73**
Conjunctivochalasis 131
Connective tissue pulleys 138
Consecutive exotropia 142
    correction of 145
Contact lens 75, 77, 78, 86
    mechanical complications 76
    wear 75, 122
Contralateral fourth nerve palsy 115
Contralateral hemiplegia 109
Conventional phacoemulsification 151
Convergence insufficiency 143
Cornea 33, 47, 75, 81, 95, 149, 170
    anterior 94
    cross-linking of 87
    reaction of 76
    superior 77, 122
    tear film 94
Corneal abrasion 195
Corneal addition procedures 265
Corneal anaesthesia 22
Corneal crystals 81
Corneal cysts 77
Corneal damage, severe 70
Corneal decompensation 51
Corneal distortion 85
Corneal dystrophies 79–83
    gelatinous drop-like 80
    honeycomb-shaped 80

Corneal ectasia 84–89
Corneal elevation 95
Corneal epithelium 75, 77, 122
Corneal erosion, recurrent 131
Corneal exposure 5
Corneal gluing 70
Corneal graft 22, 90–93
　　surgery 92
　　survival of 91
　　thickness 91
　　type of 91, 92
Corneal hydration 51
Corneal hypoxia, acute 76
Corneal infections 75
Corneal infiltration 76
Corneal intraepithelial neoplasia 336, 337
Corneal metabolic changes 77
Corneal oedema 76, 217
Corneal opacification 90
Corneal opacity (CO) 73
Corneal pannus 128
Corneal pathologies 46
Corneal power 22
Corneal punctate lesions, superficial 91
Corneal refractive
　　procedures 265
Corneal scrape 93, 183
Corneal sutures entail 92
Corneal thickness 167
Corneal tissue 90, 181
　　photoablation of 264
Corneal topography 26, 94–97
Corneal transplantation 70, 87, *191*
Corneal ulceration 42, 70
Corneal vertex 24
Cortical cataracts 45
Cortical venous drainage 40, 41
Cortical visual impairment 298
Corticosteroids 33, 187, 194, 196
Corynebacterium 72
Cover test 48
Cranial nerve palsy 98, 101, 104, 109, 113, 178
　　abducens nerve palsy 98–100
　　facial nerve palsy 101–103
　　multiple 104, 106, **107**
　　multiple cranial nerves palsies 104–108
　　oculomotor (third) nerve palsy 109–112
　　third 11, 12
　　trochlear nerve palsy 113–115
Cranial neuropathies, painful 172
Craniopharyngioma 110
CRAO *see* Central retinal artery occlusion (CRAO)
C-reactive protein (CRP) 157, 186, 268
Creating subconjunctival filtration pathway 210
CRION *see* Chronic relapsing inflammatory optic
　　neuropathy (CRION)
CRVO *see* Central retinal vein occlusion (CRVO)

Cryotherapy 297, *352*
Crystalline lens surface, anterior 22
Crystallins 44
CSCR *see* Central serous chorioretinopathy (CSCR)
CSMO *see* Clinically significant macular oedema (CSMO)
Cyclodiode laser 8, 218
Cycloplegia 16, 78
Cycloplegic agents 16
Cycloplegic refraction 144
Cyclosporine 33
Cyst of Moll glands **19**
Cystoid macular oedema (CMO) 30, 52, 185, 187, 290

D

Dacrocystography 176, 198, 199
Dacryoadenitis 131, 242
Dacryocystitis 132, 198, 201, 242
　　acute *198*, 198, 199
　　chronic 198, 199
Dacryocystorhinostomy (DCR) 201
　　external 203
DALK *see* Deep anterior lamellar keratoplasty (DALK)
Dark sub-retinal pigment epithelium haemorrhage
　　366
DCR *see* Dacryocystorhinostomy (DCR)
Deep anterior chamber following globe rupture *320*
Deep anterior lamellar keratoplasty (DALK) 82, 87,
　　90, *90*
Demodex infestation 32
Dendritic ulcer 159
Deoxyribonucleic acid 323
Depression 163
Dermoid cyst 36
Descemet's membrane 51, 81, 169
　　endothelial keratoplasty (DMEK) 82, 90
Descemet's stripping automated endothelial
　　keratoplasty (DSAEK) 82, 90
Dexamethasone 16, 120, 160
　　implant 194, 196 *see also* Ozurdex
Diabetes 109, 114, 158
　　mellitus 43, 45, 290
　　retinopathy 45
　　type 2 118
　　uncontrolled 45
Diabetic eye disease 116–121
　　classification 116
　　management 118
Diabetic macular oedema (DMO) 116, 119, 193, 195
Diabetic maculopathy 193, 196, 241
　　classification of **117**
Diabetic premacular haemorrhage *355*
Diamox 7, 8, 51, 163
Diffuse choroidal haemangioma 329, *332*
Digital subtraction
　　angiogram *179*
　　angiography 111

Dilated pupil 11, 13 *see also* Tonic pupil
Diode laser 282
Diplopia 10, 14, 40, 115, 143
Disc angle, gonioscopy of 167
Discharging eye 125
Disease-modifying drugs 238
Dissociated optic nerve fibre layer (DONFL) 155
DMEK *see* Descemet membrane endothelial keratoplasty (DMEK)
DMO *see* Diabetic macular oedema (DMO)
Dominant optic atrophy (DOA) 239
DONFL *see* Dissociated optic nerve fibre layer (DONFL)
Donor tissue 91
Dorzolamide 163
Down syndrome 169
Doxycycline 70
Dresden protocol 87
Dropped nucleus 360 *see also* Nuclear fragments
DRSS *see* Diabetic retinopathy severity score (DRSS)
Drusen, peripheral 253, 254
Dry eye syndrome 122–124
DSAEK *see* Descemet stripping automated endothelial keratoplasty (DSAEK)
Duane syndrome 137, 140
Dural sinus thrombosis 246
Dysgenesis, anterior segment 57
Dysphasia 173
Dysthyroid optic neuropathy 316
Dystrophies 272

E

Eales disease 365
Early manifest glaucoma trial (EMGT) 167, 221
Early treatment diabetic retinopathy study (ETDRS) 116, 117, 278, 291
ECCE *see* Extracapsular cataract extraction (ECCE)
Eccentric disciform scar 330, 348
Eccrine hidrocystoma 19
Echothiophate iodide 164
Ectasia 22 *see also* Keratoconus
Ectatic disorders **88**
Ectopia lentis et pupillae 10
Ectropion 125–127
    cicatricial 125, 126
    congenital 126
    involutional 125, 126
    mechanical 125
    neurogenic 125
    paralytic 125, 126
    severe 127
Edinger-Westphal nucleus 109
Edrophonium 213
Ehlers-Danlos syndrome 39
Elevated intraocular pressure 219
Embolic retinal artery occlusion 268
EMGT *see* Early manifest glaucoma trial (EMGT)

Emmetropic eye 44
Encephalitis 223
Endocyclophotocoagulation 210
Endogenous endophthalmitis 205
Endolaser retinopexy *352*
Endonasal dacryocystorhinostomy 203
Endophthalmitis 16, 52, 195, 242
    postoperative 361
       acute 51
       chronic 52
    vitrectomy study 364
Endoscopic dacryocystorhinostomy 198
Endothelial dystrophies 81
Endothelial failure 160
Endothelial function 91
Endothelial keratoplasty (EK) 90
Endothelial rejection 91
Entropion 128–130
    cicatricial 128, 129
    congenital 129
    involutional 128, 129
    spastic 128, 129
    surgical correction of 129
Epiblepharon 129
Epidemic keratoconjunctivitis (EKC) 73
Epidermal tumours 324
Epidermoid cyst 19
EPI-LASIK *see* Epithelial laser-assisted in situ keratomileusis (EPI-LASIK)
Epiphora 131–133, 201
    functional 132
    medical treatment 132
    surgical treatment 133
Epiretinal membrane 22, *357*, 358
Episclera 134, 135
    vessels 308
Episcleritis 15, 134–136, 307
    nodular *135*
    simple 134, *134*
Epistaxis, severe 42
Epithelial basement membrane dystrophy (EBMD) 79
Epithelial defect 92, *182*
Epithelial dystrophies 79
Epithelial laser-assisted in situ keratomileusis (EPI-LASIK) 265
ERD *see* Exudative retinal detachment (ERD)
Erythema 243
Erythrocyte sedimentation rate (ESR) 157, 268
Escherichia coli 183
Escitalopram 7
Esophoria 137
    decompensating 138
Esotropia 137–141
    causes of 137, **137**, 138
    constant 140
    cyclical 138
    infantile 137, 139

Index

minimal 138
surgery for 142
ESR *see* Erythrocyte sedimentation rate (ESR)
ETDRS *see* Early treatment diabetic retinopathy study (ETDRS)
Ethnicity 43
European Medicines Agency (EMA) 193
Evaporative dry eye 123
Examination under anaesthesia (EUA) 170
Excyclotorsional deviations, large 115
Exophoria 142
decompensating 142, 143, 145
Exotropia 142–145, *144*
secondary 142
Exposure keratitis 102
Extensive panretinal photocoagulation *119*
Extensive suprachoroidal haemorrhage 365
Extracapsular cataract extraction (ECCE) 48
Extraocular muscles 212
Exudative retinal detachment (ERD) 271
Eyelid trauma 146–148
Eyelid tumours
aetiology of 323
types of premalignant and malignant **324**

F

Facial dysesthesia 102
Facial nerve 101
Familial exudative vitreoretinopathy (FEVR) 205, 206, 348
Fat adherence syndrome 314
Fatigue 163
Fat-saturated sequences 178
Femtosecond laser 149, 264
Femtosecond laser-assisted
cataract surgery (FLACS) 149
phacoemulsification 149–151
FEVR *see* Familial exudative vitreoretinopathy (FEVR)
FFA *see* Fundus fluorescein angiography (FFA)
Fibroepithelial polyp 19
Fibromuscular dysplasia 39
FLACS *see* Femtosecond laser-assisted cataract surgery (FLACS)
Fleischer ring 84
Floppy eyelids, treatment of 127
Fluorometholone (FML) 136
Focimetry, pre-operative 48
Folate deficiency 239
Forced duction tests 313
Forme Fruste keratoconus 86
Foville's syndrome 98, 107 *see also* Medial inferior pontine syndrome
François central cloudy dystrophy 81
Frontalis muscle immobilised 36
FTMH *see* Full-thickness macular hole (FTMH)
Fuchs endothelial corneal dystrophy (FECD) 79, 81, 82, 90, 92

Fuchs heterochromic
cyclitis 14, 187, 306, 307
uveitis 159
Fuchs uveitis syndrome 159
Full-thickness macular hole (FTMH) 152–155, 358
Fundus 48
autofluorescence (FAF) 2, 60, *60*
Fundus fluorescein
angiogram (FFA) *3*, *4*, *277*, 288
Fungal endophthalmitis 195
Fungal infections 242
Fungal keratitis 76, *182*
Fusion maldevelopment nystagmus syndrome 223

G

Galactosaemia 56
Gass classification 152
Gaze palsy 178
GCA *see* Giant cell arteritis (GCA)
Ghost cell 307
glaucoma 306
Giant cell arteritis (GCA) 114, 156–158, 172, 173, 269
non-ocular complications of 158
Giant papillary conjunctivitis (GPC) 78
Giant retinal tear *351*
Glands of Zeis 326
Glaucoma 6, 16, 18, 46, 57, 58, 91, 158, 166, 169, 227, *232*, *249*, **306**
eye drop combination preparations **164**
hemifield test 250
inflammatory 159–161
medical management 162–164
necessitates treatment 58
phacolytic 46
phacomorphic 46
potential causes of secondary 220
primary childhood 169
primary open angle 165–168
secondary 42, 52
childhood 169
surgical management 160
with acquired condition 169
with non-acquired
ocular anomalies 169
systemic disease or syndrome 169
Glaucoma in children 169–171
Glaucoma surgery 170, 218
incisional 216
Glaucomatous optic neuropathy 7, 161
Glaucomatous visual field loss 252
Glaucomflecken 7, 43
Glial tumours 346, 348
Globe rupture 321
Goldmann applanation tonometry 226, 227
Goldman-type bowl perimeter 248
Gonioscopy 7, 159, 167, 170
Goniotomy 170 *see also* Trabeculotomy

GPC *see* Giant papillary conjunctivitis (GPC)
Gradenigo syndrome 107
Graft failure 92
    risk of 127, 130
Graft material depends 129
Graft rejection
    risk factors for 91
Granular corneal dystrophy 80, 81, *81*
Granular-lattice dystrophy 81
Granuloma 348
Granulomatosis with polyangiitis (GPA) 288
Granulomatous panarteritis 157
Graves' disease 316
Guillain-Barré syndrome 35

H
Haab's striae 169
Haemoglobin 283
Haemophilus 72
    influenza 181, 198, 242, 364
Haemorrhage
    subconjunctival 5, 72, 195
    submacular 365, *368*
    subretinal 330
    suprachoroidal 51, 368
Haemorrhagic chemosis *320*
Haptic vaulting 26
Harada-Ito procedure, modified 115
Head injury 98
Headache 172–175
Heidelberg retinal tomography (HRT) 160, 227
Hemiretinal vein occlusions (HRVO) 290
Hereditary endothelial dystrophy, congenital 82
Hereditary retinoblastoma *295*
Herpes simplex 229
    keratitis 160
    keratouveitis 159
    virus 159, 261
Herpes zoster virus 261
Herpetic disease 230
Heterochromia, congenital 342
Histiocytosis X 243
Hordeola 63, 64 *see also* Chalazion
    external 65
Horner's syndrome 10–13, 35–37, 98, 104, 110, 174
Horseshoe tears *351*, 253 *see also* U-tears
Hotz procedure 129
House-Brackmann score 102
HRVO *see* Hemiretinal vein occlusions (HRVO)
Human crystalline lens *44*
Humphrey visual field analyser 226, *249*
Hydrus *209, 209*
Hyperacusis 102
Hypercholesterolaemia 114
Hyperglycaemia 45, 116
Hyperhomocysteinaemia 290
Hyperlipidaemia 20, 118, 290

Hyperlipidaemic states 63
Hypermetropia 137, 263
Hypermetropic eye 44
Hyperosmotic agents 164
Hypertension 109, 118, 158
    malignant 246
Hyphaema 307
Hypocalcaemia 43
Hypochromia 159
Hypokalaemia 163
Hypoplastic abducens nucleus 138
Hypotony 195
Hypoxia 216
    acute 78
Hypoxic complications 76

I
Iatrogenic ectasia 88
Iatrogenic pressure 159
Ice test 213
ICRS *see* Intrastromal corneal ring segments (ICRS)
Idiopathic intracranial hypertenion (IIH) 245, 246
Idiopathic polypoidal choroidal vasculopathy (IPCV) 193
Idiopathic retinal vasculitis 196, 288
IIH *see* Idiopathic intracranial hypertension (IIH)
ILM *see* Internal limiting membrane (ILM)
Imipramine 6
Immunosuppression 106
In vivo confocal microscopy 33, 77
Incontinentia pigmenti **205**
Indocyanine green *343*
    angiogram *277, 279*
    angiography 3, 60
Infantile nystagmus syndrome (INS) 222, 223
Infarctions 111
Infection
    risk of 146
    sources of 242
Infectious endophthalmitis 155
Infectious keratitis 78, 181–184
Inferior oblique
    muscles 110
    weakening 314
Inferotemporal disc haemorrhage *165*
Infiltrative disease 37
Inflamed lacrimal sac 132
Inflammation, adequate control of 160
Inflammatory bowel disease 14
Inflammatory cells 159, 307
Inflammatory choroidal neovascular membranes 31
Inflammatory disease 37 *see also* Infiltrative disease
Inflammatory episodes 159
Inherited retinal disorders 272
    examples of 272
Inkblot' pattern *60*
Insulin-derived growth factor 298

Index

Intermediate uveitis 185–187, 288
  prognosis 187
Intermittent exotropia 142, 143
  management of 144
Internal carotid artery 109
  aneurysm 110
Internal hordeolum 64
Internal limiting membrane (ILM) 152, 358
International vitreomacular traction study (IVTS) 153, 358
Internuclear ophthalmoplegia 223
Intracameral tissue plasminogen activator 161
Intracapsular cataract extraction (ICCE) 48
Intracorneal ring segments 265
Intracranial haemorrhage, high risk of 41
Intracranial hypertension 98
Intracranial level 308
Intraocular gas tamponades, characteristics of **354**
Intraocular haemorrhage 365
  management of 365
Intraocular inflammation 132, 161, 195, 259
Intraocular lens (IOL) 57, 188, 190, 307, *362*
  malposition 53, 160
  material 188
  subluxed 160
  trans-scleral fixation of *363*
Intraocular pressure (IOP) 7, 47, 67, 92, 150, 159, 162, 166, 169, 208, 217, 219, 226, 305
  control of 218
  temporary raised 195
Intraocular tamponading agents **354**
Intraoperative optical coherence tomography imaging *150*
Intraretinal haemorrhages 40
Intraretinal microvascular abnormality (IRMA) 117
Intrastromal corneal ring segments (ICRS) 86
Intravitreal anti-vascular endothelial growth factor injections 61
Intravitreal injection therapies 193–197
Intravitreal procedures **195**
Intravitreal steroid 120
  therapies 196
Intravitreal tissue plasminogen activator injection 368
IOL *see* Intraocular lens (IOL)
Iopidine 13
IPCV *see* Idiopathic polypoidal choroidal vasculopathy (IPCV)
Ipsilateral eyelid 12
Iridectomy, primary peripheral 57
Iridex oculight 210
Iridocorneal endothelial (ICE) syndrome 10, 11, 305, 306
Iridoplasty 8, 9
  selective 308
Iridotomy 308
Iris 9, 149, 340, 341
  abscess 342
  atrophy 10
bombe 161
clip *363*
coloboma 11
constrictor pupillae of 109
crowding, peripheral 6
cyst 342
  differential diagnoses of **342**
  haemangioma 342, *342*
  hooks 10
  implants 10
  inflammation 10
  melanocytic
    lesions 342
    tumours of 340
  melanocytoma 342
  melanoma *341*, 342
  metastases 342
  naevus 342
  neovascularisation of 216
  prolapse 10, 51
  stromal cyst 342
  surface 159
  transillumination defects, mid-peripheral *256*
  trauma 10
  tumours of 216, 340
  vascular tumours of 340–342
IRMA *see* Intraretinal microvascular abnormality (IRMA)
Irvine-Gass syndrome 196
Ischaemia, anterior segment 157, 314
Ischaemic optic neuropathy 42, 156
  posterior 239
Ischaemic retinopathy 196
Ischaemic third nerve palsies 111
IVTS *see* International vitreomacular traction study (IVTS)

J

Juvenile idiopathic arthritis 14, 159, 161
Juvenile open-angle glaucoma (JOAG) 169

K

Keratectomy, superficial 80
Keratic precipitates (KPs) 14, 307
Keratitis 15
  marginal 76
Keratoacanthoma 17, 18
Keratoconic anterior corneal shape *85*
Keratoconus 22, 84, 94
  associations 84
  clinical signs of 86
  grading 85
Keratoepithelin 79
Keratoglobus 88
Keratometry 26
Keratopathy, risk of exposure 42
Keratoplasty, during 82

Keratoprosthesis 70
Khodadoust line *91*
Kissing lesion 17
Koeppe's nodules 15
KPs *see* Keratic precipitates (KPs)
Krachmer's spots 91
Krukenberg's spindle 16, 256, 257

L

Lacrimal duct scintigraphy 132
Lacrimal gland 122
    hypersecretion 131
    infiltrative disorders of 123
    lesions 201
Lacrimal infections 198–200
Lacrimal pump failure 125
Lacrimal sac
    excision of 198
    infection 198, 201 *see also* Dacryocystitis
Lacrimal scintigraphy *202*, 202
Lacrimal surgery 201–204
Lagophthalmos 126
LASEK *see* Laser-assisted subepithelial keratomileusis (LASEK)
Laser
    clinical application of 282
    delivery, incorrect 149
    iridotomy 8, 256, 258
    lenses 284
    photocoagulation 61, 353
    refractive surgery 263
    retinopexy 283
    tissue interactions 149
Laser-assisted stromal in situ keratomileusis (LASIK) 264
    surgery 89
Laser-assisted subepithelial keratomileusis (LASEK) 265
LASIK *see* Laser-assisted stromal in situ keratomileusis (LASIK)
Latanoprost (xalatan) 162
Lateral canthopexy 103
Lateral medullary syndrome 107
Lattice corneal dystrophy 80
Lattice degeneration 254
Leber congenital amaurosis 273
Leber's hereditary optic neuropathy (LHON) 239, *240*
Lens capsule opacification 205
    cataract surgery *206*
Leptomeningeal angioma 18, 20
Lester-Jones tube 133
Leucocoria 55, 205–207, *206*, 294, *294*
    causes of **205**
Leukaemia 107, 243
Levator function 36
Lid
    hygiene 32
    malpositions 131
    mass 36

retraction 111
traumas 146
Lid laxity 129
    horizontal 127
Lid margin 64, 125, 128
    disease 123
    eversion of 129
Limbal cell transplantation 70
Limbal hyperaemia 76
Limbal ischaemia 68
Limbal relaxing incisions 265
Limbic keratoconjunctivitis 77
Lincoff's rules 270
Lowe's syndrome 56
Lower lid 125, 130
    cicatricial ectropion *126,* 129
    ectropion 125
        involutional *127*
    entropion 128
        involutional 128, *130*
    orbicular muscle 129
    punctum, abnormal 131
    stages of repair of *147*
Lumbar puncture 111, 237
Lyme disease 14, 186, 240, 261
Lymphadenopathy 72
Lymphoid hyperplasia, benign 338
Lymphoid tumours 338
Lymphoma, secondary 179

M

Macula 234
    OCT of *120*
Macular corneal dystrophy (MCD) 81
Macular laser 283
Macular oedema 151, 158, 193
Macular photocoagulation 120
Macular retinal thickness analysis *234*
Maddox rods 114
Malyugin ring 10
Manual kinetic perimetry 248
Map-dot-fingerprint dsytrophy *80*
Marcus-Gunn jaw winking syndrome 35
Marcus-Gunn pupil 12
Marfan's syndrome 50
Margin-reflex distance 36
Masquerade syndrome 66
Mechanical ptosis 36
Medial inferior pontine syndrome 107
Medial orbital fracture 137
Medial rectus, recession of *313*
Medication intoxication 223
Medulloepithelioma **205**
Meesmann corneal dystrophy 79
Megalocornea *25*
Meibomian gland 33, 122, 326
    chalazion *64*
    dysfunction 32, 134

Index

Melanin 283
Melanocytic iris freckle *341*
Melanocytic lesions 337
Melanomas 329
Meningioma 110
Meningitis 223
   headache 172
Meretoja syndrome 80
Metabolic disorders 223
Metaherpetic ulcer 159
Metastases 340
   from cutaneous melanoma 348
Metastatic carcinoma 243
Metastatic potential, tumour size for 334
Microbial keratitis 75–77
Microbial orbital cellulitis 242
Microcornea 206
Microhyphaema 159
Microphthalmia 206 *see also* Microcornea
Microphthalmic eyes 57
Microtropia 137, 138
Mid-peripheral bone-spicule retinal pigmentation *273*
Migraine 172, 173, 174, 219
Millard-Gubler syndrome **107** *see* Ventral pontine syndrome
Minimally invasive glaucoma surgery (MIGS) 208–211
Mitochondrial optic neuropathy 239
Mittendorf's dot 56
Modern cataract surgery 50
Moebius syndrome 107
Mohs micrographic surgery 327
Moll glands 63
Molluscum contagiosum 19
Monoclonal antibody inhibits 119
Monovision 266
Motor nucleus supplies 109
Muir-Torre syndrome 336
Multifocal choroiditis 261
Multifocal intraocular lens 190, *266*
Multiple sclerosis 223, 235, 288
Muscle specific kinase 212
Myasthenia gravis 35–37, 108, 114, 138, 142, 212–215
Myasthenic crisis 214
Myasthenic muscles 213
Myasthenic signs 37
Mydriasis, congenital 10
Myelinated retinal nerve fibre layer 205
Myopathic ptosis 36
   congenital 36
Myopia 43, 219, 263
   high 53, 138
   pathological 193

N

Naevoid basal cell carcinoma syndrome 323
Naevus flammeus 18
NAION *see* Non-arteritic anterior ischaemic optic neuropathy (NAION)

Nasolacrimal duct
   obstruction (NLDO) 33, 131, 198
   system *131*
Nasolacrimal system 146
Necrotising scleritis *303*
Neisseria gonorrhoea 73, 181, 229
Neoplastic cells 307
Neovascular glaucoma (NVG) 196, 216–218, 305
Nephropathy 118
Nerve palsies
   congenital fourth 113
   congenital third 35
   incomplete third 111
   seventh 103
   third 35, 37, 110
Nerve stimulation
   repetitive 214
   tests 214
Neurofibroma 330
Neurogenic ptosis 35
Neuromuscular ptosis 35
Neuromyelitis optica spectrum disease 237
Neuro-ophthalmic problems 109
Neuro-ophthalmology 104
Night blindness, congenital stationary 274
Non-arteritic anterior ischaemic optic neuropathy (NAION) 239
Non-axial flash photography 205
Non-contact tonometer (NCT) 227
Non-giant cell arteritis 239
Nonglaucomatous optic neuropathy 220
Non-infectious systemic disease 261
Non-proliferative diabetic retinopathy (NDPR) 117
Non-Sjögren's syndrome dry eye 123
Nonsteroidal anti-inflammatory drugs 52, 111
Normal tension glaucoma (NTG) 166, 219–221
   prognosis 221
   risk factors for **219**
Norrie's disease 205, 206
NPDR *see* Non-proliferative diabetic retinopathy (NDPR)
NSC *see* National screening committee (NSC)
Nuclear cataract 44, 56
Nutritional deficit optic neuropathy 239
Nystagmus 222–225
   asymmetric dissociated 223
   classification 222
   downbeat 223
   infantile 222
   manifest latent 57
   rebound 223
   upbeat 223

O

Obstructive sleep apnoea 219
Occipital neuralgia 172
Occulomotor palsy, painful 41, 172

Index

Ocriplasmin 195
Ocular bruit 105
Ocular cicatricial pemphigoid (OCP) 128, 132
Ocular herpetic disease 159
Ocular hypertension 159, 226–228
    treatment study (OHTS) 166
Ocular ischaemic syndrome 157, 196, 216
Ocular lymphoma 216
Ocular malignancies, radiation of 216
Ocular myasthenia 212
Ocular surface 126, 128, 132
    burns **68**
    inflammation 32
    irritation 131
    squamous neoplasia (OSSN) 336
Ocular toxoplasmosis 195
Ocular trauma *319*, 319, 365
    score 320
Ocular tumours 179
Oculomasticatory myorhythmia 223
Oculomotor nerve 35, 109
    palsy 109, 143
    supplies 109
Oculomotor palsies, management of 111
Olivary nucleus, degeneration of 223
Olsen's formula 24
Ophthalmia neonatorum 229–231
Ophthalmic lasers 284
Optic disc 205, 246
    assessment 170
    haemorrhage 219
    neuroretinal rim pallor 220
    optical coherence tomography *165*
    pallor *273*
Optic disc imaging 232–235
Optic neuritis 172, 236–238, 348
    treatment trial (ONTT) 236
Optic neuropathy 178, 239–241 246
    compressive 240
    infectious 240
    infiltrative 240
    inflammatory 240
    post-radiation 240
    post-traumatic 241
    post-vaccination 241
Optical coherence tomography (OCT) 30, 176, 186, 206, 232, *233*, 237, 268, *277*, 279, 348, 373
    anterior segment 92, 308
Orbital apex syndrome 107
Orbital cellulitis 242–244
    anatomy 242
Orbital infection 178
Orbital metastases 179
Orbital proptosis 40
Orbital trauma 178
Orbital tumours 179
Ozurdex 31, 194

P

Pachymetry 91, 95
Panretinal photocoagulation (PRP) 118, 196, 216, 283, 284
Panuveitis 16, 259
Papillary conjunctivitis 125
    degree of 126
Papilloedema 235, 245–247, 348
    acute *245*
Paralytic ectropion 131
    causes of 125
Paraneoplastic optic neuropathy 241
Parotid gland 101
Pars plana vitrectomy (PPV) 152, *352*, 353, *353*, *355*, 361
Pavingstone degeneration 253, 254
PCV *see* Polypoidal choroidal vasculopathy (PCV)
PDR *see* Proliferative diabetic retinopathy (PDR)
Pellucid marginal degeneration (PMD) 88
Pendular nystagmus 223
Penetrating keratoplasty (PKP) 82, 87, 90, *90* 92
Perilimbal hyperaemia 122
Perimetry 248–252
Periodic alternating nystagmus 223
Peripheral vestibular nystagmus 223
Persistant hyperplastic primary vitreous 57
Persistent foetal vasculature (PFV) 205
Persistent pupillary membrane 10
Phacoemulsification *360*
Phakic (piggyback) IOL 191
    surgery 265
Pharmacologic vitreolysis 358
    with ocriplasmin 153
Photophobia 14, 32, 52, 72, 76, 84, 129, 173
Photopsia 30, 154
Photorefractive keratectomy 265
Phototherapeutic keratectomy (PTK) 82
Phthisis 52
Pigment dispersion syndrome 256, *256*
    prevalence of 256
Pigment epithelial detachment (PED) *2*, 5, 59
Pigmentary glaucoma 220, 256–258, 342 *see also* Uveitis
Pigmented chorioretinal scars *260*
Pigmented epithelium, tumours of 348
Pituitary tumours 110
Plateau iris syndrome 6
Platelet-derived growth factor 316
Plexiform neurofibroma 36
Pneumatic retinopexy 353, *353*
POHS *see* Presumed ocular histoplasmosis syndrome (POHS)
Polyarteritis nodosa (PAN) 288
Polymyalgia rheumatica (PMR) 156
Polypoidal choroidal vasculopathy (PCV) 279
Poor glycaemic control 116
Port-Wine stain 18

Posner-Schlossman syndrome 160, 307
Posterior capsular complications 50
Posterior capsular rupture, management of 50
Posterior capsule opacification (PCO) 53, 188
Posterior communicating artery (PCA) 11, 109, 111
Posterior polymorphous corneal dystrophy (PPCD) 79, 81
Posterior uveitis 259–262
    examination 260
Posterior vitreous detachment (PVD) 152, 153, 270, 352
Postrefractive corneal surgery 26
Presbyopia 263
    refractive surgery in 266
Preseptal cellulitis 242
Presumed ocular histoplasmosis syndrome (POHS) 195
Pre-trabecular meshwork level 305
Primary acquired melanosis 337, *337*
Primary angle closure glaucoma (PACG) 6, 7, 9
Primary congenital glaucoma (PCG) 169
Primary headache syndromes **174**
Primary open angle glaucoma (POAG) 165, *165*
Proliferative diabetic retinopathy (PDR) 118, 195, 196, *356*
Proliferative retinopathy 42
Proliferative sickle cell retinopathy 310, *355*
Proliferative sickle retinopathy (PSR) 309
Prophylactic retinopexy 254
Propranolol 174
Proptosis 105, *179,* 243
Prostaglandin analogues 160, 162
Proton-beam radiotherapy 333
Pseudoesotropia 137
Pseudoexfoliation syndrome 50
Pseudoexotropia 142
Pseudomacular hole *357*
Pseudopapilloedema 246
Pseudotumour cerebri 245
Pseudoxanthoma elasticum 39
Ptosis 10, 35, 36, 173
    chronic 36
    involutional 35
    partial 110
    simple 36
    surgery, type of 37
Punctal occlusion 201
Punctate epithelial erosions *123*
Punctate erosions 122
Punctate inner choroidopathy 261, *374*
Punctum ectropion 127
Purulent discharge, severe 72
Pyogenic granuloma 19, 64, *65*

R

Racemose haemangiomas 346
Radial keratotomy 265
Ranibizumab (lucentis) 4, 5, 119, 193, 194, 196
Recombinant tissue plasminogen activator 367

Red reflex, loss of 55
Refraction 170
    pre-operative 48
Refractive error 137, 263 see also Hypermetropia
    correction of 263
Refractive lens surgery 265
Refractive lenticule extraction 265
Refractive pentacam corneal tomography scan, four-map 95
Refractive surgery 122, 263–266, **264**
    clinical assessment for 263
    lasers in 264
Refractive surprise 53
    postoperative 26
Reis-Bücklers corneal dystrophy 80
Relative afferent pupillary defect (RAPD) 12, 220, 236, 239
Reticular degeneration 253, 254
Retina
    capillary haemangioma of 345
    congenital hamartoma of 347
    glial tumours of 348, 349
    opaque whitening of *287*
    tumours 345
    ultrasound of 280
    vascular tumours of 345
Retinal ablation 300
Retinal angiomatous proliferation (RAP) 1, 193
Retinal arterial occlusion 267–269
Retinal astrocytic hamartoma 205
Retinal breaks 350, *351*
    multiple *352*
Retinal degenerations
    inner 253
    peripheral 253–255, **254**
Retinal detachment 52, 53, 195, 205, 217, 270–271, 330, 350, *351*, 352
    pathogenesis of 351
    risk factors 53
    surgery for 352, 354
Retinal dysplasia 205
Retinal dystrophies 43, 272–276
Retinal haemorrhage *366*
Retinal imaging 277–281
Retinal inflammation 260 see also Retinitis
Retinal laser 282–285
    types of 282
Retinal lesions 283
    differential diagnosis of **348**
Retinal macroaneurysms 365
Retinal necrosis
    acute 288
        peripheral *287*
Retinal nerve fibre layer (RNFL) 160, 232, 233, *233*, 245
Retinal pigment
    absorption spectra of **283**
    epithelial cells 305
    epithelium (RPE) 119, 153, 348, 352, 358, 366

Index

Retinal surfaces, apposition of 51
Retinal tufts 254
Retinal vascular disease 119, 150
Retinal vasculitis 260, 286–289, 365
Retinal vein occlusion (RVO) 193, 195, 196, 290–293, 365
Retinal vein, cuffing of *287*
Retinal-choroidal interface 1
Retinitis 260
    and retinal vasculitis 261
Retinitis pigmentosa (RP) 43, 272
    arteriolar attenuation of *273*
Retinoblastoma (RB) 205, 216, 294–297, 342, 348
    genetics 295
Retinochoroidal biopsy 364
Retinopathy
    progression of 118
    risk factors for developing 116
Retinopathy of prematurity (ROP) 142, 196, 205, 298–301
Retinoschisis 205, 252–254
Retrolental fibrosis 205
Rhabdomyosarcoma 243
Rhegmatogenous retinal detachment 270, 350, *355*
    differential diagnoses of **352**
Rheumatoid arthritis 123
Rhinorrhoea 173
Rigid gas-permeable contact lenses 86
Roper-Hall classification **68**
Rosacea 17, 64
RPE *see* Retinal pigment epithelium (RPE)
Rubeotic glaucoma 119
RVO *see* Retinal vein occlusion (RVO)

S

Salmon-patch haemorrhages 310
Sarcoid 288
Sarcoidosis 14, 160, 216, 261, 288, 342
Scanning slit Scheimpflug principle 95
Scheie classification 8, **8**
Scheimpflug-based systems 85
Schirmer's test 102, 122
Schlemm canal outflow 208
Schnyder corneal dystrophy 81
Schnyder crystalline corneal dystrophy 81
Schwartz-Matsuo syndrome 307
Scleral buckling 353, *353*
Scleral perforation 314
Scleritis 15, 135, 136, 286, 302–304, 307
    posterior 330
Sclerochoroidal calcification 330
Scleroderma 132
Sclerotomy incision *369*
Sebaceous gland 63
    carcinoma 33, 323, 326 *see also* Nasolacrimal duct obstruction
    lesions 18

Seborrheic dermatitis 63
Seborrhoeic keratoses 17, *18*, 20
Seclusio pupillae 159, 161
Secondary open angle glaucoma 305–308
    prognosis 308
Sectoral iris atrophy 159 *see*-saw nystagmus 223
Selective transmission laser 168
Senile' retinoschisis 253
Sensory esotropia 137
Sensory exotropia 142, 143
Sentinel episcleral vessels *341*
Serous retinal detachment (SRD) 59
Sickle cell retinopathy 309–311, 348
Single fibre electromyography 214
Sinus histiocytosis 132
Sinusitis 242
Sinus-related headache 172
Sixth nerve palsy, investigations for 99
Sjögren's syndrome 122, 123 *see also* Ocular graft vs host disease
    primary 123
Sleep apnoea 59, 125
Small choroidal melanoma *331*
Small incision cataract surgery (SICS) 48
Small stellate keratitic precipitates 159
Snailtrack degeneration 254
Solid state laser 282
Space-occupying lesions (SOL) 246
Spaeth system of angle grading **8**
Spasmus nutans syndrome 223
Spectral domain optical coherence tomography (SD-OCT) 153, *153*, 291
Spheno-cavernous syndrome 107
Spherical aberration 190
Spine pathologies 46
Spontaneous retrobulbar pain 316
Squamous cell
    carcinoma (SCC) 323, 336
    papilloma 336, *336*
Squamous papilloma *18*, 19 *see also* Fibroepithelial polyp
Squint *294*
    convergent 137
Standard automated perimetry 248
Staphylococcus 58, 72, 198
    aureus 17, 72, 198, 229, 242, 364
    epidermidis 34, 52, 72, 75, 242
Stargardt disease 274
Static perimetry 248
Stereopsis 145
Stereotactic radiosurgery 41
Sterile peripheral corneal infiltrates 78
Steven-Johnson syndrome 128, 129, 163
Strabismus 46, 138, 144, 205
    amblyopia 55
    divergent 143
    esotropia 137

management of adult 145
type of 142
Strabismus surgery 139, 144, 312–315
   early 139
   indications 312
   postoperative care 314
   techniques 312
Strawberry naevus 17, 19
Sturge–Weber syndrome 18, 169, 307
Stye 64
Subarachnoid haemorrhage (SAH) 42, 246
Subcapsular cataract 45
Subepithelial corneal infiltrates 72
Subepithelial dystrophies 79
Submacular haemorrhage, treatment of *368*
Subretinal fluid 352
Sub-retinal heavy liquid *370*
Subretinal pigment epithelium (RPE) 59
Subtarsal foreign bodies 131
Superficial keratopathy, corneal ulceration 34
Superior limbic keratoconjunctivitis (SLK) 77
Superior oblique
   muscles 114
   surgery 314
   tendons 115
Suprachoroidal haemorrhage, acute *369*
Susac syndrome 288
Suture granuloma 314
Swedish interactive thresholding algorithm 248
Swelling of arcuate nerve fibre layer (SANFL) 155
Symblepharon formation 70
Sympathetic ophthalmia 216
Synechiae, posterior 10, 15, 161
Synkinetic ptosis 35
Synthetic materials 126
Syphilis 14, 288
   infection 91
Syringoma 19
Systemic antibiotics 33
Systemic chemotherapy 106, 132
Systemic disease 72, 288
   secondary to 43
Systemic hypertension 219
Systemic hypotension 219
Systemic immunosuppression 31
Systemic lupus erythematosus (SLE) 288
Systemic steroids 57
Systemic vasculitides 288

T

T sign *303*
Tarsal fracture 129
Tear
   film 33, 63, 122
   outflow 131

production, imbalance of 131
U-shaped 253, *351*
Temporal artery biopsy (TAB) 156
Tenonplasty 70
Thiel–Behnke corneal dystrophy 80
Thyroid
   disorders 316
   orbitopathy 137
Thyroid eye disease 108, 114, 138, 140, 178, 307, 316–318, *317*
   severity classification in **318**
Tolosa-Hunt syndrome 41, 107
Tonic pupil 11, 13
Toric lens
   calculation 26
Torsional nystagmus, pure 223
Toxocara 261
Toxocariasis 205
Toxoplasma 240, 261
Trabectome 209
Trabeculectomy 160
Trabeculitis 159, 307
Trabeculotomy 170
Trachoma 73, 128, 129
Tractional retinal detachment (TRD) 271, 354
Transient ischaemic attack (TIA) 268
Transpupillary thermotherapy 333
Traumatic mydriasis 10
Travoprost (travatan) 162
Triamcinolone 31, 194, 196
Trichiasis 128, 131
Trigeminal nerve 40
Trigeminal neuralgia 172
Trochlear nerve 113
Trochlear nerve palsy 113
Trochlear palsy
   congenital 113
T-sign 303
Tumours of choroid 329–335
   prognosis 333
Tumours of retina 345–349
   differential diagnosis 347
   pigment epithelium 345
Tumours of uvea 340–343
   pathogenesis 340
   prognosis 343

U

Ulcer, geographic 182
Ultrasound biomicroscopy (UBM) 256
Ultra-Widefield imaging 280
Upper lid 125, 127
   cicatricial entropion 128
   ectropion 125
   entropion 129

Urrets-Zavalia syndrome **10**, 11
Uveitic glaucoma 160
    management of 160
Uveitis 14, 30, 43, 131, 220, 307
    active 159
    herpetic 159
    idiopathic posterior 29
    non-infectious posterior 196
    phacoanaphylactic 46
    severe anterior 186
    trauma 46
Uveitis-glaucoma-hyphaema syndrome 307
Uveoscleral outflow, increasing 209

V

Valve of Hasner 132
Varicella zoster virus (VZV) 159
Vascular endothelial growth factor (VEGF) 4, 116, 290, 305
Vasoproliferative tumours 348
Vena cava syndrome, superior 307
Venous stasis retinopathy 42
Ventral Pontine syndrome 107
Viral conjunctivitis 63, 73
Viral keratitis 181
Viral retinitis 195, 288
Visual field 237, 248, 308
Visual impairment, causes of 116
Visual loss 157, 161, 267, 292
    irreversible 50
    pathogenesis of 366
    progressive 41
    unexplained 220
Visual rehabilitation 48
Visual-evoked potentials 237
Vitamin supplementation **4**
Vitelliform macular dystrophy, adult 275
Vitrectomy
    and drainage 367
    and macular peeling 358
    irradiation 43
    surgery *371*
Vitreolytic agents 195
Vitreomacular adhesion (VMA) 153, **153**, 358
    classification system of **358**
Vitreomacular interface disorders 350, 356
Vitreomacular traction (VMT) 153, 195, 356, *357*, 358

Vitreoretinal complications *370*
Vitreoretinal interface 24
    disorders *357*
Vitreoretinal lymphoma, primary 187
Vitreoretinal surgery 119, 350–361
Vitreous 48, 364
    detachment 187 *see also* Vitreous haemorrhage
    floaters 154, 195
    haemorrhage 42, 57, 116, 187, 195, 365
    loss 51
Vitritis 185
    anterior 52
VMA *see* Vitreomacular adhesion (VMA)
VMT *see* Vitreomacular traction (VMT)
Vogt-Koyanagi-Harada syndrome 160, 216, 260, 352

W

Wallenberg syndrome 107
Watery eye 125, 131, 132, 201 *see also* Epiphora
Weber's syndrome 109
Wegener's disease 303
Wernicke's encephalopathy 223
Whipple disease 223
White cataracts 45, 50 *see also* Intumescent cataract
White dot syndrome 29, 372–374
    multiple evanescent 261, *373*
White pupil 205
White without pressure (WWP) 253, 254
White-dot syndrome 261
Wide-field angiography 31

X

Xanthelasma 19
Xen gel stent 210
Xeroderma pigmentosum 336 *see also* Muir–Torre syndrome

Y

Yamane's technique *363*

Z

Zentmayer ring 257
Zonular dehiscence 50
Z-plasty procedure 126